Some of the things teens talk about in this book . . .

➤ "I hate it when people say, 'Oh, you're just acting that way because you're a teenager.' It's like they don't give us any respect for being a human being with feelings. They make you feel like your feelings aren't worth anything. You're just put in this category: Teenager."

➤ "My parents are worried because I don't go out yet. I mean, I go places with my friends, but I don't date or go to parties. And I don't have a boy that I like. They make me feel like there's something wrong with me, like I'm unpopular or something."

➤ "Three years ago in seventh-grade gym class, I spent a lot of time comparing myself to other guys. I felt like I was much smaller than everyone else. I started worrying if I was okay, if I had all the same things going on that everyone else did."

➤ "When I got to school the first day, everyone looked at me like I was from outer space or something. It was like, Who's that? Look at her hair. Look at what she's wearing. That's all anybody cares about around here: what you look like and what you wear. I feel like a total outcast. As soon as I got home I locked myself in my room and cried for about an hour. I was so lonely."

➤ "A lot of people don't want to admit their feelings, even to themselves, because they're afraid that their problems will scare their friends away. I usually think, well, if they knew I felt that way, they'd think I was weird."

➤ "I was in sixth grade, and a friend told me I should wear a bra. I had never thought of it before, never thought I was big enough, and she said, 'You should wear a bra.' Who is she to be telling me I need a bra? After that, I got all self-conscious."

➤ "I can't talk to my parents anymore. If I told them what me and my boyfriend do, they'd tell me I couldn't see him anymore. They think I'm so innocent."

➤ "We're at the age where we're having real sexual feelings, and if I want to act on them, my conflict is that I can't just be natural about it—whatever that means—because the feelings I have get so mixed up. It gets to the point where I don't know what I'm really feeling and wanting anymore. Sometimes I wonder if I'm just doing things that I think someone my age is 'supposed' to be doing."

➤ "When you first find out that you're gay, it's a real shocking experience for a lot of people. Like, I called myself sick. It was like I was mentally disturbed."

➤ "Sometimes you just get to the point where you say, I hate myself. How could I have done that? How stupid! Or you say, I'll never be able to do anything right."

➤ "The hardest thing is coming to grips with who you are, accepting the fact that you're not perfect—but then doing things anyway. Even if you are really good at something or a really fine person, you also know that there's so much you aren't good at. You always know the things you don't know and what you can't do. And however much you can fool the rest of the world, you always know how much bullshit a lot of it is."

Changing Bodies, Changing Lives

ALSO BY RUTH BELL

Talking with Your Teenager
(with Leni Wildflower)

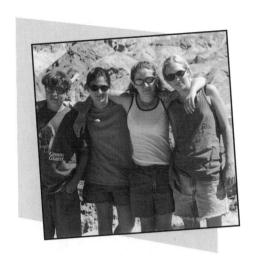

Changing Bodies, Changing Lives

EXPANDED THIRD EDITION

A Book for Teens on Sex and Relationships

Ruth Bell and other co-authors of
Our Bodies, Ourselves and *Ourselves and Our Children*,
together with members of the Teen Book Project

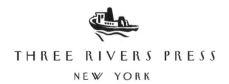

THREE RIVERS PRESS

NEW YORK

Clinic Discount

Changing Bodies, Changing Lives is available at a discount to clinics, groups, and organizations licensed by the state to operate entirely or in part as counseling services, health clinics, or mental health clinics offering health education and information to teenagers, for distribution to their members or clients. The discounted price is $6.90 per copy, plus $1.40 per copy to cover shipping. The following requirements must be met:

(1) A minimum of twelve (12) copies must be ordered (on a nonreturnable basis).
(2) A copy of the state or federal license (or other document filed with the state or federal government indicating as one of the organization's purposes the teenager education function as described above) must be included with the order.
(3) Payment must be by money order or cashier's check.
(4) Money orders and cashier's checks much be made out to Random House. When ordering, write to Random House, Inc. (Dept. CBCL, Westminster, MD 21157). Orders that do not fulfill the above requirements will be returned.

While we hope the information contained in *Changing Bodies, Changing Lives* will help you make healthy choices and give you useful tools and ideas, this book is not intended to replace professional health and medical care.

Published by Three Rivers Press, New York, New York.
Member of the Crown Publishing Group.

Random House, Inc. New York, Toronto, London, Sydney, Auckland
www.randomhouse.com

THREE RIVERS PRESS is a registered trademark and the Three Rivers Press colophon is a trademark of Random House, Inc.

Originally published in 1998 by Times Books.

Printed in the United States of America.

Book design by H. Roberts Design.

Library of Congress Cataloging-in-Publication Data

Bell, Ruth.
    Changing bodies, changing lives : a book for teens on sex and
relationships / by Ruth Bell and other co-authors of Our bodies,
ourselves and Ourselves and our children, together with
members of the Teen Book Project. — 3rd ed.
        Includes index.
        Summary: Candidly discusses teenage sexuality and the many
physical and emotional changes that occur during adolescence.
        1. Sex instruction for youth.   [1. Sex instruction for youth.]
    HQ35.B44   1998   613.9′ 07—dc21   97-29249

ISBN 0-8129-2990-X

10   9   8   7

"You must be the change you wish to see in the world."
—Mahatma Gandhi

With courage and commitment,
young people throughout the world
are working to make our planet a healthier
and more compassionate place to live.
This book is dedicated to them.

Acknowledgments

We have worked on this book and its subsequent editions over the course of twenty years. During that time scores of people have offered support and assistance in many ways. With thanks for their help, we mention their names below.

To those of you who participated in individual or group interviews, please accept our heartfelt appreciation. Your comments helped us shape the content of the book.

We would like to acknowledge Vicki Legion of the Community Health Workers Training Program of San Francisco State University. Convinced that a new edition was necessary, Vicki inspired us with her enthusiasm and persistence to make it happen.

Our deep gratitude goes to David Alexander, Elsa Burt, and Charlotte Mayerson, who gave not only support and encouragement, but also an enormous amount of time during the long rewriting phase of this project. Their expertise enriched our work.

The following individuals were always available to offer assistance whenever we called upon them.

Special thanks to:

Poppy Alexander

Polly Attwood

Shannon Del Rio

Cindy Irvine

Betsey McGee

Jane Pincus

Wendy Sanford

Tovah Walters-Gidseg

Special thanks also go to:

Charon Asetoyer, who interviewed teens for the chapter "Changing Things"

Boston Women's Health Book Collective, for support, encouragement, and research assistance

Sally Bowie, for her contribution to the original edition of this book and her support throughout

Patricia Florin, who helped with word processing and added her wisdom to the chapter "So You Think You Might Be Pregnant"

Wendy Schaetzel Lesko, Executive Director, Activism 2000 Project, whose work embodies the theme of the chapter "Changing Things." She has been both a resource and an inspiration

Judy Lipshutz, Bonnie Richardson, Laura Ewing, Tracy Smith, and Laurie Baum, who organized interview groups and helped formulate several chapters

Andrea McNichol, for help interviewing teens for the "Living with Violence" chapter

Bruce Reinstedt, who gathered anecdotes and offered important advice

Lauren Schaffer, for interviewing teenagers active in the arts

Carla Turner, who reported on her class's project for the chapter "Changing Things"

Enthusiastic thanks go to our team at Random House—Olga Seham, Elsa Burt, Nancy Inglis, John Rambow, and especially our executive editor, Elizabeth Rapoport—for their dedication and commitment to this book.

We are grateful to these clinics, centers, schools, and organizations for participating in our research:

Alameda Senior High School, Denver, Colorado

Alive Together Teen Theatre, Grants Pass, Oregon

Ashland Adolescent Center,
Ashland, Oregon

Beaver Country Day School,
Brookline, Massachusetts

Bikes Not Bombs, Roxbury,
Massachusetts

Boston Women's Health Book
Collective:
Women's Health Information
Center,
Somerville, Massachusetts

Boys and Girls Aid Society, Portland, Oregon

The Cambridge Friends School,
Cambridge, Massachusetts

Centers for Disease Control and
Prevention:
National AIDS Clearinghouse,
Atlanta, Georgia

Chicago Women's AIDS Project,
Chicago, Illinois

Children of the Night,
Los Angeles, California

Committee for Gay Youth, of the
Cambridge Women's Center,
Cambridge, Massachusetts

The Commonwealth School,
Boston, Massachusetts

Community Health Center,
Ashland, Oregon

Community Health and
Education Program,
Center for Population and
Family Health,
Columbia University, New York,
New York

Crater Cabaret, Medford, Oregon

Delta Women's Clinic,
New Orleans, Louisiana

The Door: A Center of
Alternatives,
New York, New York

Duct Tape Theatre,
Ashland, Oregon

Eastern Women's Center,
New York, New York

Feminist Women's Health Clinic,
Los Angeles, California

Free At Last: Community Recovery
and Rehabilitation Services,
East Palo Alto, California

Gay Community Services Center,
Los Angeles, California

The Gloucester Prevention
Network,
Gloucester, Massachusetts

Hamburger Home, Los Angeles,
California

HOY: Help Our Youth, Arcadia,
California

IMAGES: Theatre for Young
Hearts and Minds,
San Diego, California

Los Angeles Free Clinic,
Los Angeles, California

Lulu Belle Stewart Center,
Detroit, Michigan

Madison Park High School,
Roxbury, Massachusetts

Multnomah County
Library Services,
Portland, Oregon

Native American Women's Health
Education Resource Center,
Lake Andes, South Dakota

Oakwood School,
North Hollywood, California

Open Adoption and Family
Services, Inc.,
Portland, Oregon

Peace House, Ashland, Oregon

Planned Parenthood's Teen Theatre in Detroit, Detroit, Michigan

Planned Parenthood,
Des Moines, Iowa

Planned Parenthood,
Los Angeles, California

Planned Parenthood League
of Massachusetts,
Cambridge, Massachusetts

R.E.A.L. School, Windham, Maine

Rocky Mountain
Planned Parenthood,
Denver, Colorado

Routh Street Clinic, Dallas, Texas

Sex Information and Education
Council of the United States
(SIECUS), New York, New York

Spence-Chapin Services to
Families and Children,
New York, New York

Temple Isaiah, Los Angeles,
California

To Make The World A Better
Place (of The Door:
A Center of Alternatives),
New York, New York

University High School,
Los Angeles, California

Workers of Wonder Program of
the Columbia University
Liberty Partnership Program,
New York, New York

WorldLink, Berkeley, California

Yo!, Youth Outlook News Service,
San Francisco, California

Youth as Resources,
Washington, D.C.

Youth and Family Center,
Lawndale/Inglewood, California

YouthBuild, Somerville,
Massachusetts

Youth Communication/
New York Center, Inc.,
New York, New York

Youth Expression Theater,
Planned Parenthood League of
Massachusetts

Youth Radio, Berkeley, California

Many adults went out of their
way to assist in the creation of
this book. Their individual willingness to help and in many cases
their significant contribution of
time and energy to our project
was and always will be greatly
appreciated.

Gail Abarbanel

Ashana Abu-Jefferson

Stephanie Allen

Susan Allen

Myron Arnold

Susan Bell

Zachary Bell

Terry Beresford

Alan Berger

Pamela Berger

Denise Bergman

Denise Bisaillon

Richard Borofsky

Peg Bowden

Paula Bowen

Dennis Boyd

Cheryl Bradley, JD

Liza Brown

Mira Brown

Marcia Bullock

Scott Burnham

Jan Calvin

Elizabeth Canfield

Ginny Cassidy

Gwindale Cassity-Miller

Judy Chason

Stuart Chason

Mavis Cloutier

Jan Cobble

Bill Connet

Mary Cosey

Ruth Coulthard

Joni Craig

Andre Cunningham

Jerald Davitz, MD

Page Dickinson

Hannah Doress

Paula Doress-Worters

Carol Downer

Pam Dungan

Ben Eastman

Mary Linda Eccles

Jesse Epstein

Rob Evans

Ellen Fader

Lyndi Farmer, RN

Judy Favor

Aida Feria

Janice Fialka

Emily Fiore

Jane Fleisher

Michael Foley

Rabbi Robert Gan

Cindy Garboden

Ada Gearan

Dinah Gilburd

Michael Gilburd

Carol Gilligan

Sharon Gillin

Abby Gilmore

Fran Goldfarb

Julie Goudy

Louis Bowie Graves

Tony Greenberg, MD

Judith Greene

Priya Karim Haji

Katrina Hammond

Florence Hanson, RN

Daphne Hawkes

Nancy Miriam Hawley

Keith Hefner

Liz Hoskinson

Debra Hurt

Dei Iaroli

Selden Illick

Nels Israelson

Jake

Jan Janssen

Maggie Jensen

Anna Jimenez

Jana Johnson

Jean Johnson

Ron Johnson

Joyce Jones

June Kailes

Antra Kalnins

Susan Kandel

David Kantor

Meredith Kantor

Temma Kaplan

Jerrold Katz

Bobbi Kidder

Joyce King

Polly Kirkpatrick

Vera Kirkpatrick

Joette Krupa

Ricky Lacy

Judith Lennett

Margo Levin

Amy Levine

Shari Levine

David Lewis

Gene Leyden

Allen Loots

Peggy Lynch

Judith Anne McBride

Molly McBride

Ron McClain

Brooke McIntyre

Andrea Marks, MD

Nick Masi

Alice Michelson

Michael V. Miller

Kahrin Mishan

Sonya Mittelman, JD

Freida Mizrahi

Monica Mizrahi

Dane Morgan

Larry Morgan

Nancy Morgan

Judy Norsigian

Pat Nichols

Katie Olsen

Cindy Orrell

Mary Owen

Randy Paulsen

Mark Pecker, MD

David Pendleton

Ed Pincus

Aaron Rapoport

Lin Reicher

Sandra Ripberger

Eric E. Rofes

Michelle Rogers

Esther Rome

Joan Samuels

Matthew Sanford

Lisa Schaeffer

Mary Scofield

Irene Selva

Jim Shames, MD

Larry Shapiro

Matthew Small

Ann Smith

Anne Smith

Leslie Smith

Steve Smith

Kathy Sommerich, CSW

Judith Steinbergh

Cil Stengel

Nannette Stevens

Jane Stewart

Dorothy Stoneman

Sarah Swales

Lisa Tackley

Charlotte Taft

Robert Takahashi

Lois Tandy

Sherrie Tepper

Mary Ann Terrall

Liz Thompson

Richard Thompson

Virginia Valian

Merry Vediner

Alice Verhoeven

Tom Vinetz

Cyndee Wallace

Ellen Walsh

Esther Walter

Donald Wasson

Susan Watts

Barbara Waxman

Andrea Weiss

Michaele White

Leni Wildflower

Gayle Wilson

Sidra Winkelman

Lauren Wise

Janet Witkins

Lanita Witt, MD

Allen Worters

Francie Young

Linda Young

Donna Zaengle, CSW

Margie Zamudio

Irv Zola

For their assistance with photographs and/or graphics for the latest edition, we thank:

David Alexander

Poppy Alexander

Jenny Arden

Emily Bixler

Christopher Briscoe

Josh Crane

Aaron Cruz-Garcia

Jesse Epstein

Nels Israelson

Tina Lewis

Paula Maloof

Stephan Phelps Ransom

Daniele Robbiani

Leslie Stone

Tom Vinetz

Sandy Wasserman

Hundreds of teenagers have read our writing, offered their comments, shared their stories, discussed philosophy and point of view with us, and reminded us over and over again not to preach, lecture, or moralize. We hope they know how important their contributions have been. Indeed, their comments and stories remain the backbone of this book.

The teens listed below were particularly generous with their time and their ideas:

Tyler Abel

Clarice Albert

Poppy Alexander

Ronnie Allen

Tara Anderson

Elijah Apilada

Coya Artichoker

Jaime Ballard

Bernadette Barbaran

Desiree Bartak

Darlyne Baugh

Sarah Baum

Zack Bell

Ethan Berdanier

Katherine Bergmann

Paula Binkley

Sweet Black

Kyle Blount

Rena Blount

Nadine Borofsky

Angel Boyd

Lisa Bryant

Rachel Burnson

Leslie Ann Campbell

Ana Carreon

Linda Carter

Sarah Cedarface

Stacy Chanin

Aaron Chapman

Kate Chason

Liz Chason

Louisa Chavez

Angie Christianson

Kim Cook

Tina Costanza

Alicia Cox

Aaron Cruz-Garcia

Elias DeChristo

Cyndi Dionne

Leah Diskin

Daa Shanda Doakes

Irina Doty

Melinda Doty

Charles Douma

Hilary Eustace

Bob Fehlau

Kathy Finnerty

Desi Fischer

Roberto Fletes

Jose Gabilondo

Aaron Garcia

Emile Garcia

Melanie Garrison

Aaron Goldman

Antonio Gonzalez

Lance Goodrich

Jace Green

Almon Grimsted

Mona Hamedani

Joshua Hawley

Melissa Hovis

Lynn Hudson

Bryon Hunt

Ivan Hunter

Cathy Jacobs

Elton Jimenez

Chris Johnson

Ursula Joseph

Melody Judge

Rebecca Katz

Dana Michael King

Lori Kleban

Sara Kontoff

Shelly Krieb

Laurel Kronsky

Clarinda Lattoure

Lorien Leyden

Noah Lindsay

Jonah McBride

Noah McIntyre

Christine MacNeil

Joan Mankin

Kelly Mead

Heidi Meiser

Jaime Michaels

Heidi Milham

Mica Miro

Ahrin Mishan

Jessica Mizrahi

Chelsea Morgan

Chris Myers

Djuna Myers

Jackson Myers

Ati Nasiah

Lily Neuffer

Ellen Newman

Kyra Zola Norsigian

Guthrie Nutter

Sokly Ny

Brandon O'Connor

Andrew Pailas

William Perillat

Brian Peterson

Kathi Peterson

Courtney Philbrook

Kathy Phillips

Sami Pincus

Sol Prandini

Stefan Phelps Ransom

Braxton Reed

Dane Reinstedt

Ben Richards

Toni Rivero

Chaske Rockboy

Nora Romero

Erica Rosen

Erica Ryan

Rachel Saloma

Travis Sapp

Brigitte Serville

Uma Small

George Smith

Janell Smith

Emile Snyder

Eric Sudeth

Stuart Swerdloff

Nakia Thomas

Sean Thommen

Cory Thompson

Tom Vance

Lauren VanderLind

Kirsten Vannice

Sarah Visser

Tovah Walters-Gidseg

Justine Warner

Christy Wilton

Christine Wood

Frances Young

Rachel Zaslow

Julie Zimmerman

Nicole Zuck

Beverly

Erin

Ishiah

Nicole

Tiffany

Trina

The girls at Ashland Adolescent Center, Ashland, Oregon

The girls at Hamburger Home, Los Angeles, California

The teens at the Boys and Girls Aid Society of Portland, Oregon

The teens of Pax Panis, Peace House, Ashland, Oregon

The teens at *Teen Voices* magazine

The teens in W.O.W., Columbia University, New York, New York

NOTE: We think it only appropriate to mention that some of the people listed above were teenagers in 1978, when this book was first conceived. They may be parents now with preteens or teenagers of their own!

Illustration credits:

Unless otherwise credited, all drawings and diagrams were done by Leslie Stone of Leslie Stone Design, Santa Monica, California, and all cartoons were drawn by Paula Maloof, New York City.

Contents

Thanks to Leni Wildflower for her work on the original chapter,
"Sex Against Your Will."

Preface

Those of us who worked on *Changing Bodies, Changing Lives* joined together on this project because we think teenagers—and all of us—have a right to accurate and thorough information about health and sexuality. We believe that unwanted pregnancies, epidemics of sexually transmitted disease, and exploitative sexual relationships are dangerous and unnecessary. They can be prevented. We know that information is powerful; it gives us the opportunity to make healthy and responsible choices for ourselves. With that in mind, our main goal for *Changing Bodies, Changing Lives* is to give you the information you need to take good care of yourself as you go through the teenage years.

The inspiration for this book came from *Our Bodies, Ourselves,* a book on sexuality and health written by and for women. *Our Bodies, Ourselves* taught us that people feel better about themselves when they understand how and why their bodies work the way they do. Facts empower us when they are put in a context that lets us understand how the facts are relevant to our lives.

This completely revised, updated, and expanded edition of *Changing Bodies, Changing Lives* presents facts and information about important teenage issues in a personal context. Within each chapter you will hear from teens who are faced with the same changes and challenges you face. They talk to you about their lives, their needs, their problems, and their successes. For the most part, we've changed their names and sometimes even the cities from which they come to offer them more anonymity. But while the names have been changed, the stories are real. You will probably identify with some of the stories, and you may find that many are different from what you know and experience. In any case, we hope that by reading what other teenagers have to say you will learn to feel better about yourself and make choices that will keep you healthy and safe.

A NOTE TO PARENTS ABOUT THIS BOOK: Many parents have an underlying feeling that sex information will shock or disturb their children, or, even worse, that it will interest them too much. Some fear that by giving teenagers information about sex we encourage them to rush out and "do it."

That isn't what happens. Good sex education gives young people the tools to think before acting. It teaches them how to protect themselves; how to make good choices; how to evaluate whether a situation is dangerous to their well-being. Most significantly, it helps them to see the consequences of the actions they take. Good sex education teaches people how to be responsible and respectful.

Studies confirm that teens who are taught about body functions, safer sex protection, sexually transmitted disease, and good relationship behavior are LESS likely to get pregnant before they want to, LESS likely to catch a sexually transmitted disease, and LESS likely to engage in thoughtless, promiscuous, or exploitative sexual activity than teens who haven't received that education. Indeed, it's when we don't teach our young people about sex and relationships that they get into trouble physically and emotionally. We don't want that to happen.

ABOUT THE AUTHORS

Many people helped write this book. There were the hundreds of teenagers we interviewed; their contributions are the core of our writing. There were the parents and health educators and junior and senior high school teachers who talked to us about their experiences living and working with teens. There were the medical practitioners who read over the chapters and made sure our facts were accurate. We had teenage editors and commentators who met regularly with us to share ideas and philosophies, and who read and criticized our work in progress. Teenage poets and writers contributed poems and essays; teenage photographers and artists offered their photos and artwork. And finally, there were the authors of each chapter who, working independently and together, completed the actual research and writing. We would like to tell you something about who we are:

Ruth Bell, Project Coordinator. As a founding member of the Boston Women's Health Book Collective, a co-author of *Our Bodies, Ourselves, Ourselves and Our Children,* and *Talking With Your Teenager,* and a mother of a son in his twenties and a teenage daughter, I have long been convinced that teenagers need a book like *Our Bodies, Ourselves* that directs itself exclusively to them and addresses their real concerns. I hope *Changing Bodies, Changing Lives* does that without compromise, euphemism, or moral judgment. I would like preteens and teenagers to be able to turn to this book whenever they have a question or a problem and find within it the help they are looking for.

When young people are given the information they need to make good choices, when they can trust that the questions they ask will be honored and answered truthfully, they develop faith in themselves and respect for others. The goal of this book is to help in that process.

Breanna Farmer. I am a young woman who has struggled with an eating disorder for many years. I agreed to help write the chapter on eating disorders because I believe it is so important to educate others about this baffling disorder. I have researched this subject, and I have conducted interviews with others, but most of my words come from knowing the pain and confusion that you feel when struggling with an eating disorder. For me, the path to recovery is one of honesty, self-acceptance, and self-love. It is a path I tread respectfully every new day.

Bonnie Folick. For the past twenty-three years I have worked with children, teens, and families as a social worker and psychotherapist. I have reared three wonderful sons, now young men, and I believe that the healthy emotional development of our youth is the foundation of our society and our most important task. It was an honor and a joy to participate in the writing of the Emotional Health Care chapter. It is my hope that this book will continue to educate and empower teens in their journey toward self-fulfillment and healthy, responsible choices.

Joanne Gates. Helping to write this book and revise it has been a culmination of twenty years of my life. It crystallized my experiences as a mother and as a psychologist. I wanted to share in writing something that would really matter to teens and touch their lives the way *Our Bodies, Ourselves* touched mine. I wanted this to be a book that I could give to my own daughter and son to learn more about life, love, and relationships and about their bodies so they might meet the challenges of their sexuality in today's context of the threat of AIDS.

I have learned the most about teens by being a parent. My professional work with teens includes being a counselor in an abortion clinic, writing and teaching a course on teenage health and sexuality, making a film and a six-part cable TV program on teenage sexuality, and being a counselor in a New York City alternative high school. I have worked as a sex and family planning counselor in a multi-service center for adolescents, and I have worked with college students at a city university. At present I am also a psychotherapist in private practice.

Naomi Krupa. I am a graduate of Union College in Schenectady, New York, with a BA in history. My interest in eating disorders stems from my own personal struggle with one throughout most of my life. Two main reasons drew me to work on this chapter: First, I felt that writing my feelings down would help me deal with and understand the problems I have faced with my own weight. Second, I hoped that hearing about my constant battle with anorexia might possibly prevent it from happening to others and might comfort those who suffer from this affliction too. Having an eating disorder is frightening. You feel crazy and alone, but you don't have to. I hope this chapter gives people hope and lets them know that it's okay to ask for help.

Carolyn Myers. I am a teacher, writer, and theater director. Since 1987 I have worked primarily with teens. I started two teen theater companies that create and perform original plays about issues of concern to young people. I like to teach in alternative high school programs for "at risk" students. My wish is to help build a society where adolescence is recognized and supported as a time of great discovery of self, community, and the world.

I live in Ashland, Oregon, with my husband and two daughters, Uma and Mica.

Wendy Sanford. Working on *Changing Bodies, Changing Lives* has been one of the joys of my life. I am co-author of *The New Our Bodies, Ourselves* and have co-authored all the editions since 1970. I serve on the Board of the Boston Women's Health Book Collective. For nearly a decade, I served as Protestant chaplain at a commuter university in downtown Boston where I was pleased to be able to use this wonderful book as a resource for my students.

Steve Smith. I have been a certified alcohol and drug counselor for nine years and have learned a lot about the issue of substance abuse from the young people with whom I work. Having a chance to be part of this book has allowed me to share some of that cumulative experience with others. Too much of what I do is not science but a day-to-day challenge to help people who struggle under the weight of substance abuse and face its dangers.

I live in the great small town of Ashland, Oregon, with my wonderful wife and two beautiful children, Claire and Jesse, who keep me focused on what is really important for me.

Tim Wernette. During the writing of previous editions of this book I worked as a sexuality educator with Planned Parenthood and taught human sexuality classes at Pima Community College in Tucson. Currently I work at New Frontiers, Arizona's educational equity program, and at the University of Arizona, where I coordinate diversity education in the Human Resources department. I am also the director of the Gender Awareness Program at Pima Community College. I have been active in the profeminist men's movement and lead Sierra Club service, rafting, and international trips. During my adolescence I struggled with many of the issues that *Changing Bodies, Changing Lives* addresses. I hope this book can help make this challenging time of life easier and more joyful.

Introduction

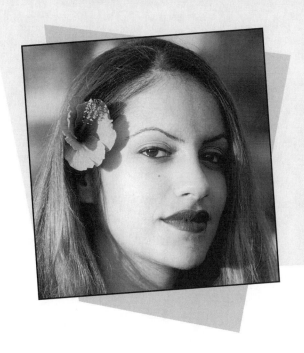

Change can take place so gradually that you don't notice it's happening until something pulls you out of the day-to-day flow of your life and makes you stand back. Maybe you haven't seen a friend for a long time, or you go back to an old neighborhood for a visit, and you suddenly see how different things are. When it comes to yourself, one day you look in the mirror and instead of merely adjusting your clothes or combing your hair, you actually see yourself. Barry, a thirteen-year-old from Texas, told us:

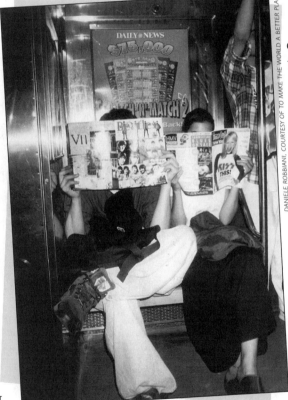

One day when I was about nine, I caught a look at myself in the hall mirror as I was going out to a baseball game and I saw this grown-up kid, chewing gum, wearing his baseball uniform, and I remember thinking, Hey, I'm a real kid now. In that second I remember feeling like I'd changed. I wasn't little anymore.

Just a few years later, you look and see that you're not even a kid any longer. You've moved out of childhood and into the teenage years.

Then changes start to happen so fast it's hard not to notice them. Hair grows in places it's never been before. Breasts develop; muscles form. Voices change. Important "firsts" take place: first kiss, first date, first job, first license, first bra, first ejaculation, first menstrual period, first love. Of course, these things don't happen for everyone precisely during the eight years from twelve to twenty, and there isn't any rule book to let you know when, where, or how to make the moves; you just know you're expected to come out the other end "grown up" and able to take care of yourself.

Everyone goes through these changes, but that doesn't make them any easier to handle. They involve a lot of experimenting and, usually, making a lot of mistakes. You test your abilities, make false starts, take risks, push yourself into new things, and often feel lonely and misunderstood. We all do, because that's what growth is all about.

In the middle of all this, many people say they sometimes feel pretty mixed up. They feel they're in a hurry to grow up, but at the same time feel uneasy about being pushed into doing it too quickly. Fourteen-year-old Raoul, who lives in New York, told us:

> A lot of weird things I do are just a matter of trying to prove to everybody, and I guess prove to myself, that I'm not a kid anymore. But sometimes I think to myself, Hey, wait a minute, I *am* a kid. Don't make me grow up too fast.

As your body gets bigger and develops sexually, people may treat you differently even before you start to feel very different inside yourself. They may expect you to act older or more grown-up in ways that don't feel comfortable to you yet. Or they may treat you like a child when you feel quite mature. All this can be confusing.

Also, as you get older you have more choices to make. When you were little, most new experiences were filtered through your parents or guardians. Now decisions come up daily, and you're the only one who can make them: Do you do what your friends want you to do? Do you take this class instead of that one? Do you ask so-and-so out? Do you have sex with your boyfriend or girlfriend? Do you take a drug or have a drink along with your friends? For the most part, the decisions you are faced with are hard ones, with serious consequences. It's no wonder several teenagers we met said they feel as if they're on a seesaw—sometimes soaring gracefully, sometimes coming down with a hard crash. Cassie, an eighth-grader from Ohio, put it this way:

> Everyone my age is trying to grow up really quick, and I can't stand it anymore. There are all these decisions to make—like about drugs and sex and trying to act older. Sometimes I get so sick of it I just want to get away from it and crawl back into my mom's lap.

Changing Bodies, Changing Lives is about the ups and downs of the teenage years. As in the previous editions, in this book teenagers talk about the changes, choices, and feelings in their lives right now. We've included a lot of information that many teens can't get very easily—information about sex, physical development, personal relationships, and emotions.

The teens we interviewed were from all across the United States. They were different ages, from eleven through their early twenties. They were from different backgrounds and ethnic groups. They had different ideas and different interests. But they were all coming face-to-face with the issues that affect teens: body development, sexuality, self-esteem, changing relationships with parents and friends, fears and frustrations, and the need to establish independence and look toward their future.

You'll hear stories and anecdotes from many of

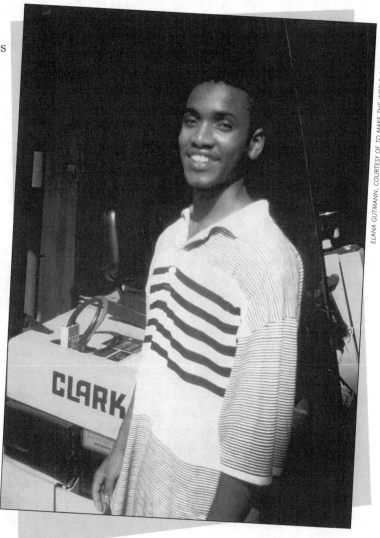

ELANA GUTMANN, COURTESY OF *TO MAKE THE WORLD A BETTER PLACE*

these teenagers in the following chapters, because we've learned that listening to real people talk about their lives is usually more helpful than pages of advice written by "experts." As you read you'll probably discover that some of the problems you're dealing with are other people's problems too, and that many of the questions you have are also being asked by other teenagers. The important thing to remember is that each of these stories comes from a real teenager somewhere, and probably speaks for many other teenagers throughout the country.

We've changed people's names and the cities they come from to protect their privacy. Many of the quotes are very personal, telling about deep feelings and intense frustrations. Some quotes are quite frank, describing sexual activity or other intimate details. We are glad that the teenagers we met were willing to share those things with us, because their openness allowed us to discuss important issues that are often left unsaid. We hope that hearing about other people's experiences won't make you feel pressured to do one thing or another just because some-

one else has done it. There's no "right" way or "right" age to have life experiences.

Along with the personal anecdotes are facts and practical information about body changes, health care, and sex. You may not be at all interested in sex right now, you may already be having sexual relationships, or you may be somewhere in between. In any case, you deserve clear and accurate information to help you take care of yourself now and in the future. We think people have a right to know about how their bodies work, a right to have their questions about sexuality answered, a right to choose when and if they want to become parents, and a right to keep themselves and others safe from sexually transmitted diseases.

Some of you may not want to read this book from cover to cover. Some parts of it will be relevant to your life now, and other parts you may not need for years. We hope that you and your parents will be able to use *Changing Bodies, Changing Lives* to open a dialogue with each other, and that groups of friends will use it as a basis for discussions about what's going on in their lives.

Changing 1 Bodies

IT HAPPENS TO EVERYONE

Sometime between the ages of nine and seventeen, your body will change dramatically. As Jenny, aged fourteen, said, "This year my body is going crazy! I look more like my older sister than myself!"

This time of change is called puberty (*pu*-ber-tee), and everyone goes through it, although each person grows and changes at his or her own pace. When it happens, your body may become fatter, skinnier, taller, more pimply, hairier, rounder, more big-breasted, more muscular, and more awkward. You may feel full of energy or lie around and sleep a lot. Your moods may shift uncontrollably, surprising you and those around you.

These changes occur when your body reaches a certain stage of growth and a part of your brain called the pituitary (pih-*too*-ih-ter-ee) gland signals your sex glands—your ovaries if you are a girl, your testicles if you are a boy—to start working. These glands in turn begin signaling other parts of your body, telling them to grow.

Hormones carry the signals. Hormones are chemical substances that travel in your bloodstream. Testosterone (tess-*tahs*-ter-own), the main hormone special to males, is made in the testicles. Estrogen (*ehs*-tro-jin) and progesterone (pro-*jess*-ter-own), the main hormones special to females, are made in the

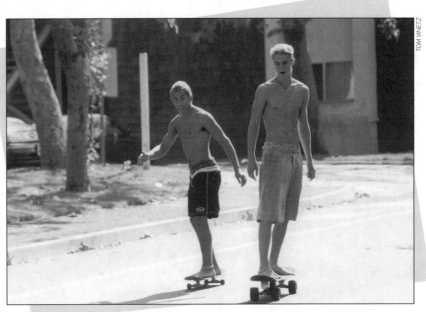

ovaries. These hormones cause most of the body changes of puberty—growth, facial hair, pubic hair, breast development, voice deepening, menstruation, and so on.

Almost all the physical changes of puberty have some connection with the ability to reproduce. While becoming a parent may be the last thing on your mind, once you go through puberty your body will be ready to create or bear children. That's why it's so important for you to get decent information now about the best ways to prevent unwanted pregnancy (see sections on Sexuality, page 89; Safer Sex, page 279)

"I Feel Like I'm the Only One Who . . ."

You can fill in the blank for yourself. Maybe you feel like you're the only one who hasn't gotten her period yet. Or the only one who wakes up in the morning with "come" (sperm and seminal fluid) all over his sheets; the only one who has a bad case of pimples at age eleven or the only one who has one breast bigger than the other or one testicle hanging lower. Maybe you think of yourself as the only boy who hasn't grown since fifth grade, or the only girl whose breasts haven't even started to develop.

If you don't know about how and why people's bodies change during puberty, you're likely to wonder if your changes are normal. In this chapter you'll hear from a lot of teenagers who have wondered about the same thing, and you'll see that wondering if you're normal is actually a very normal thing to do!

SEXUAL CHANGES

Many changes that happen during puberty are sexual. Your sexual organs are growing and your sexual feelings may become more intense. At a girls' discussion group in Denver, thirteen-year-old Roxanne said:

> I used to be such a goody-goody and always pay attention in class and follow all the rules, and now all I can think about is my boyfriend. Actually I have a lot of boyfriends now. I'm not Miss Perfect anymore.

Eleven-year-old Darlene told us:

> I get these weird sensations in my stomach all the time. My friend read to me from this book about sex, and I got this weird feeling down here, like my stomach was flipping over.

When all this is going on, it can be hard to pay attention to your schoolwork or carry on with life the way you used to. Luke, a fifteen-year-old boy from Boston, put it this way:

> I swear I woke up one day and everything changed. It was like somebody put up a big flashing neon-light sign in my head that said SEX. I am always turned on—I mean always—and all I have to do is sit across from an attractive woman in the subway and I get a hard-on.

You may read these quotes and think, But I'm not feeling sexy all the time, and I'm a teenager! Many times in this book people will talk about feelings you don't have right now. Or they will talk about doing things that you don't do, even though you may be the same age or older. Bodies change at different speeds. Sexual feelings are stronger or weaker at different times in our lives. Think of this book as having a conversation with lots of teenagers who are being honest about things people don't usually talk about. Some of them will sound like you and some won't. The main point is for you to understand better what's happening with *your* body and *your* feelings.

Does Sex Have to Be a Mystery?

Since so many teenage body changes are sexual and many adults are uncomfortable about sex, often teenagers aren't given much information about what's going on.

When your parents were your age, sexuality might have been a mystery to them too, something that wasn't discussed openly, perhaps something seen as "dirty" and shameful, so it's no wonder they have a hard time talking to you about sex. Even parents who want to talk to their kids in an open way generally feel awkward about it, probably as awkward as you feel listening to them talk about it. As Tina said,

> I'm lucky. My parents are very easy to talk to. But when it comes to sex, they fumble around and turn red. So I say, "It's okay, I already know that." So they say, "Well, just remember, you can ask us anything when the time comes. You can always come to us." Sure. That's great. But right now it's easier to get my information from my friends, who don't know a whole lot more than I do!

Society's negative attitudes about sex cause many of us to be more embarrassed, shy, and ignorant about it than we want or need to be. We feel stupid if there's a joke we don't get or someone tells us something about sex that we don't understand.

EMERGING

The shine,
The yellow,
The golden
is rising.
Can this be
the beginning?

My shining
My glow
My green
sight
so slowly
it opens
and buds into
a spotted flower.
I rise
my limbs
they open
and the dried skin peels
and reveals
the shining flesh
that will take over.

The step into
a wonderful vegetable
I hide,
and sleep,
and come out new
and blue,
I step back,
one step,
but a million steps
to all
in the wooden world . . .
My old world . . .
My wooden world
seems old
seems dark
seems gruesome.
And all who live there,
without stepping
into the light
into the glow
are still speaking
the wooden language
that I have left behind
long ago.

—LYN BIGELOW

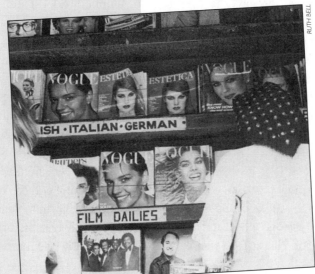

This happens to everyone, even people who seem to know everything. We can help one another feel less awkward by sharing information, talking honestly, not making fun of one another's differences. After all, if we don't learn about our own bodies, how can we ever expect to feel comfortable with ourselves? If we don't learn about the opposite sex, how can we be caring partners and friends?

We're talking about "sex education." And although most teens get some form of sex education at home or in school, it is often too technical to be interesting. Most of the time you don't get to ask the questions you really want to ask. Instead, much of our introduction to sex comes informally, from jokes we hear in locker rooms or on street corners or from gossip about who's doing what; it comes from what we read in books or see in movies and on TV and from what's available in pornographic magazines and pictures. Sex is portrayed as either superromantic or supersmutty, which usually ends up confusing us even more.

You may be fortunate and find some really helpful sources of information—an open-minded parent or teacher, an older brother or sister, a well-informed boyfriend or girlfriend who's comfortable talking about sex. But however we get our sex education, we usually take in only what we're ready to learn or need to know about, and sometimes we're just not ready or interested. That's okay. As long as you know how to find the information when you need it, you don't have to rush. That's the main reason we wanted to write this book. So you could have a resource to turn to when the time is right for you.

DO I LIKE MY BODY?

This is a heavy question for most of us. Thirteen-year-old Charlene said:

Sometimes when I'm all alone, I stand in front of the mirror and stare at myself. I stare at all the things I can't stand about myself, like my legs. They're so short and my thighs are so huge. There's this white bump on my neck that really bothers me. It's not a pimple. It doesn't hurt. It's just there and I don't know what it is, but I can't stand it. And the worst part is my chest. I'm so flat-chested I look like a boy.

Fifteen-year-old Pablo said:

I can't stand what I look like right now! Sometimes I just want to put a bag over my head to hide my face. It's all broken out with zits and oily places. I can wash it ten times a day and it's still the same.

What one person wants may be just what another person hates:

Sally: I wish I had bigger breasts.

Tai: Believe me, you don't want to be big. Once you got there, you'd want to get back down. I wish I could give you some of mine.

Some adolescent conditions are genuinely distressing and embarrassing. Teens who have a bad case of acne, for example, or those whose sweat glands come on strong at first are likely to want some real relief from these problems. There are special dietary measures and vitamin supplements that can be prescribed

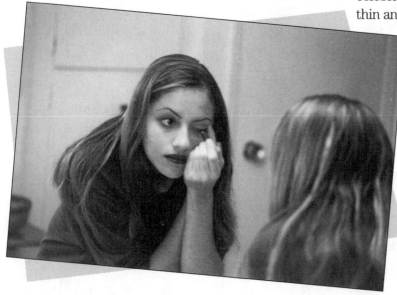

by a physician or a nutritionist. There are also acne preparations you can use and special deodorants to buy for body odor. These conditions will go away with time, but while you are suffering with them that's not much consolation.

For the most part, we spend a lot of time and effort during these years trying to look different from the way we are. We diet to lose weight or gain weight. We work out, lift weights, dye our hair, wear makeup, shave, don't shave, get our hair permed or straightened, buy trendy clothes. We have ourselves pierced and tattooed. We try cosmetic surgery, sun-lamps, tanning clinics. We buy mouthwash, hair spray, hair coloring, bleaches and hair-removal products for body hair. Just think how much energy and money, at any one moment all over this country, are going into changing people's looks.

Who says we're not great just the way we are? Those companies that put unbelievable amounts of money each year into advertising their "body-beautifying" products do a terrific job of making us dislike our bodies and ourselves, because if we liked ourselves we might not rush out to buy their products. And we believe them when they tell us we need this lipstick or that hair dye, especially during adolescence, when we're feeling the most unsure of ourselves anyway.

That's not to say that looking good isn't important to us. Most people want to look good. But unfortunately, we are being fed a line that says there is only one way to look good. During adolescence in particular we look for role models, and what do we see? We see supermodels! We see movie stars and celebrities. People who earn their livelihood by being thin and beautiful and perfectly toned. They work at it, sweat over it for hours every day, diet relentlessly, have cosmetic surgery, but we grow up believing that they look beautiful naturally and that unless we do too, we're less than we should be. So girls starve themselves to be thin. Boys work out furiously to build muscles and look buff.

Pay attention to the effect constant advertising and media pressure have on you and your friends. For a laugh and an eye-opener, the next time you watch TV look critically at the ads. Try to figure out what they're trying to sell you before they say it.

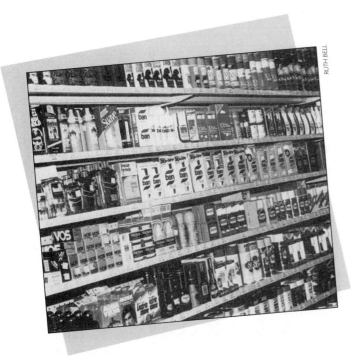

Read magazine advertisements for the hidden message; see if they try to convince you that you need their product to be more beautiful or sexy or manly.

Probably no one can talk us out of disliking some parts of our bodies, but it may help to look at some of the reasons why we worry:

FEELING JUDGED BY THE OTHER SEX: Boys and girls check each other out a lot, and they often judge each other harshly. Ellen complained:

> There's this kid who has a crush on me and drives me crazy wanting to sit with me at lunch and stuff. He's built like a Raggedy Ann doll—real weak and floppy.

Dan, a high school junior, said this about hairy legs on girls:

> What grosses me out is the bristly part. When you think of a girl, somehow her sensuality is involved in softness, so that hard bristliness is a turnoff.

With judgments like those, is it any wonder boys spend hours lifting weights or girls feel they have to shave their legs every day?

FEELING JUDGED BY YOUR FRIENDS: Chances are that the friends you hang out with have a certain

idea of what looks good—and you'll feel pressured to look that way. Fourteen-year-old Sandy recalls:

> If you want to be popular the expectation is that you should wear eye makeup and get tit implants and wear tight, skimpy clothes. I know so many girls who are starving themselves because they think they're too fat. It makes me feel fat just looking at them.

COMPARING YOURSELF WITH OTHERS: Our society emphasizes competition between people, companies, countries, so it's not surprising that we feel competitive. Annie, who turned out to be a fashion model, suffered from her height:

> All through junior high school, I was taller than *everybody*. It was embarrassing for me. I had a really tiny friend, and I used to envy her.

Ben, fourteen, has the opposite problem:

> I hate the way I look. I'm shorter than everybody in my class. I look like I'm ten years old. Even the girls are taller than me.

The competition may be most painful in your own family, as Anita remembers:

> When I was twelve or thirteen, my mother told me about periods, but she said, "I don't think you'll be getting yours for a while yet." Then when my sister was only eleven, she told *her* about it. She said, "You girls should be expecting periods any time now." So it became really important to me that my sister didn't get hers before me.

FEELING JUDGED BY YOUR PARENTS: Parents may get hung up on wanting you to look a certain way. Often they say, "It's for your own good." Sometimes they're right, and sometimes they have other motives they're not aware of—they may feel that how you look is a reflection on them, or they may be haunted by memories from their own adolescence. This is what Jeff told us:

> My dad is always bugging me to go on a diet. I think it's because he was fat and unpopular as a

kid. I'm heavy, but not *that* heavy. But when he looks at me with that look in his eyes, I feel like I weigh three hundred pounds.

Molly's mother has a picture in her head of how her daughter should look:

Every morning my mom says, "Don't you think you ought to put your hair up? It looks so nice up." Can't she get it that if I liked the way my hair looks up I would put it up? I mean, I brush my hair. It's clean. What does she want? She makes me feel like she doesn't like the way I look, and that makes me feel bad.

It helps a lot when our parents let us know they think we're fine just the way we are. Josh, eighteen, said:

When I was in seventh grade and complaining about how skinny and small I was, my dad said, "Napoleon was only five foot three. So just remember, greatness has nothing to do with what you look like. It has to do with who you are and how you feel about yourself."

Your Body Is Okay

The next time you catch yourself saying, "I hate my legs [or breasts, chest, face, hair, body, height, weight]," stop for a minute and ask yourself: *Who* says they're not good enough? Do you really agree? Look at yourself in the mirror and pick out the things you *do* like. Compliment yourself. Compliment your friends, help them like themselves better. Marge Piercy, a poet, writes: "Live as though you liked yourself, and it may happen."

Your body is okay. In fact, as one boy reading this section remarked, "Your body isn't just okay! It's great! And it does some amazing things!"

"I Feel Like I'm in the Wrong Body"

For some teens the dissatisfaction with their body is not about whether or not they like the way their body looks; it is deeper than that. These teens feel they are in the wrong body altogether. You've proba-

bly heard about big people saying they feel like a small person inside, or small people saying they feel big. Well, some girls feel like a boy inside and some boys feel like a girl inside. It's usually during adolescence, when people's bodies begin changing and maturing, that these teens experience their differences most acutely.

This condition is called cross-gender identification. If you would like to read more about it, see page 134. Also look in the Resource section on page 150 for a good book on the subject.

BOYS' BODIES

NOTE TO GIRL READERS: When we talk to the reader of this section as "you," we mean a boy. When we asked a group of girls who they thought would read the different parts of this book, however, they said, "Girls will read the parts about boys, and boys will read about girls!" So we figure a lot of girls will be reading

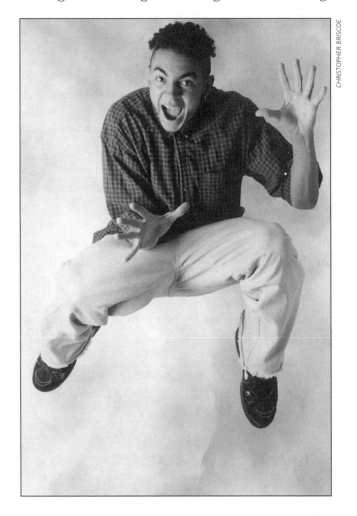

CHRISTOPHER BRISCOE

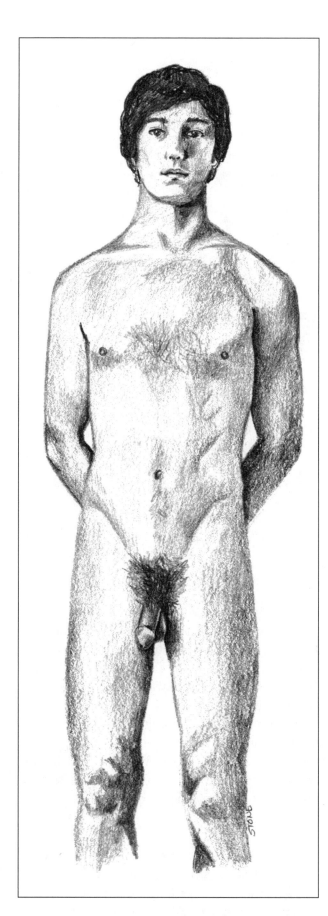

this section. This is great, because girls have been ignorant about boys' bodies for too long. Just don't be surprised when we talk about "your" penis!

In a few short years a boy experiences these things:

➤ Your penis and testicles get bigger.

➤ You grow pretty close to what will be your full height.

➤ Your voice gets deeper.

➤ Your skin becomes oilier; you may get pimples on your face, neck, chest, and back.

➤ Your testicles start to make semen and millions of sperm.

➤ Pubic hair grows around your testicles, your anus, and the base of your penis.

➤ Your body hair gets thicker, you grow hair under your arms, and whiskers start to grow on your face.

➤ You start to ejaculate ("come") when you have an orgasm—either in dreams when you are asleep (called wet dreams), or when you are masturbating or having sexual activity with someone else.

➤ You may start having more frequent and stronger sexual feelings.

➤ Your sweat glands begin working and you sweat more.

➤ Your muscles and strength increase.

Not all of you will go through every one of these changes. But most of them will happen at some point during the teenage years.

How you feel about what's happening to your body depends on what you know about body changes; what your idea of "manly," "good-looking," and "handsome" is and how you accept the ways you *don't* match that image; whether your family and friends pressure you to grow up fast, to have a deep voice, a developed penis, and a "he-man" body.

Joe thinks competition in body development is worse among boys than girls:

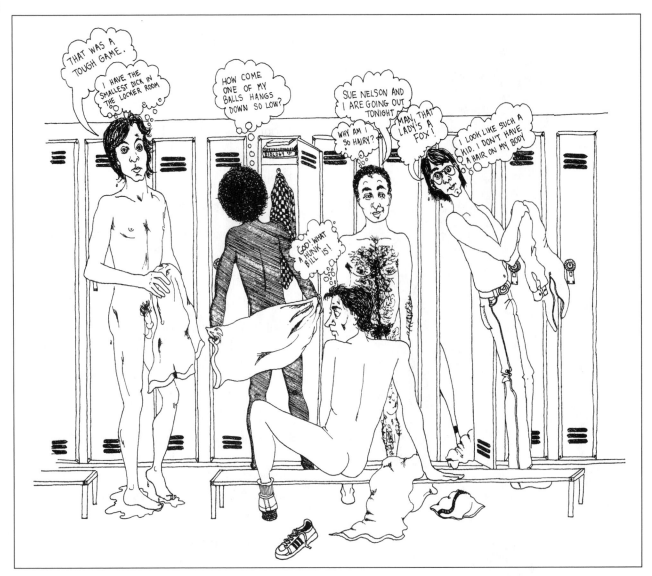

Guys notice it more than girls. Especially in the locker room. Because somehow for the guy it's so much more important. He's supposed to be the virile one. He feels more inadequate if he's not as developed as his friends.

How society treats you is another big factor. Once you start growing and looking like a man, people may react to you differently. Other boys may start expecting you to be tough; they may pick fights with you. You may get accused of doing things you didn't do, just because many people have an attitude about teenage boys. You may be treated as though all you have on your mind is being macho and having sex.

When girls' bodies change, they may be harassed or get a lot of comments on the street that are sexually suggestive. Boys may get some of that too. It can make you feel very uncomfortable, even frightened.

Something else that will influence how you feel about yourself is how educated your friends are about boys' bodies and the changes boys go through. Can you talk honestly with your friends about yourself and your feelings?

There's a myth that girls are more self-conscious than boys, and that boys breeze through their teenage years never worrying what they look like or how fast they are developing. Of course this isn't true. Steven, a seventeen-year-old from Los Angeles, speaks for many boys:

Well, for me it was weird because I didn't even start growing until last year. Everybody thought there was something wrong with me because I still looked like a ten-year-old up until I was fifteen or sixteen. That has been really a bad experience for me, because everybody was changing around me and I was standing still. I was changing in my head but not my body. My parents were even going to take me to the doctor to see if I was deformed or something like that, but they didn't, and finally last year I started to grow. My voice started changing and everything, so I guess I'm normal after all, but I think it's going to be a while before I stop feeling like I'm different from everybody else.

Proper Terms and Slang

The words for sexual organs have a lot of power. While "penis" and "testicles" (so-called proper terms) are quite sober and unemotional, they are not often used. The words that are used most frequently can be silly or personal or full of attitude. We asked a bunch of teenagers what they called the parts of a male's anatomy and here is the list they came up with:

penis		*testicles*
cock	schmuck	balls
prick	schlong	nuts
dick	pecker	jewels
stick	thing	rocks
rod	dink	cubes
gun	dinkus	nugies
wee-wee	privacy	eggs
wang	banana	
wiener	putz	
pisser	dork	
peter	meat	
hot dog	dong	

Slang is tricky, because we use these words in many different ways: to express fondness and pride (then they are funny, friendly, loving, playful); to put down or humiliate someone or to hurt someone (then they are hostile and ugly).

Try this exercise: Say each of these words in different tones of voice, and notice how they change according to your intention. The same word can be an endearment or an insult. Some people use slang without realizing how it sounds.

Body Parts: What Your Genitals Look Like on the Outside and Inside and How They Work

PENIS: Your penis has three functions. You urinate from it. It gives you sexual pleasure when it's touched, rubbed, or stimulated, as it's the most sexually sensitive part of your body. It is also the passageway through which semen, containing sperm, leaves your body.

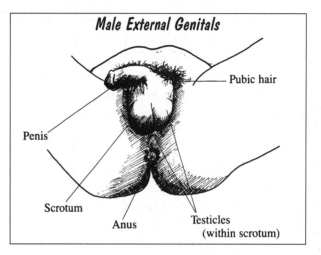

Male External Genitals

Pubic hair

Penis

Scrotum

Anus

Testicles (within scrotum)

Next time you are naked, take a careful look at your penis. It has two parts. The *glans* is the rounded head or tip and is the most sensitive to touch. The *shaft* is the long part of the penis—the part that gets hard during an erection. Inside the

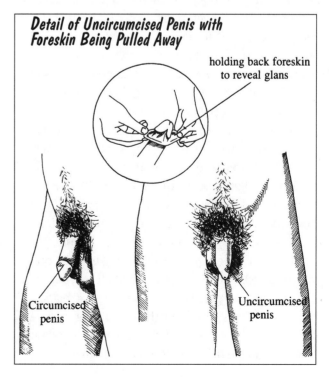

Detail of Uncircumcised Penis with Foreskin Being Pulled Away

holding back foreskin to reveal glans

Circumcised penis

Uncircumcised penis

shaft is spongy erectile tissue that fills with blood when you become sexually excited. (See page 17 for more on erections.)

If you have been circumcised (see diagram on page 15), your glans will be visible. If you have not been circumcised, there will be skin covering the glans. This is called the *foreskin*. Circumcision is an operation performed on some boys soon after they are born in which the foreskin is removed. It may be done for religious reasons. It may be done for health reasons too, so that a thick, whitish substance called *smegma*, which appears around the glans, will not collect under the foreskin and cause infection. In modern times, because of the convenience of baths and showers, this is not a problem as long as you keep your penis clean.

TESTICLES: Your two *testicles* are glands that hang in a skin sack called the *scrotum*. One testicle may hang lower than the other. This is normal. Your testicles are where sperm are produced. The scrotum's function is to keep your testicles at just the right temperature for sperm production.

Sperm are extremely tiny living cells. When one of them unites with a woman's egg, conception takes place (see page 38). Since sperm are made at a few degrees *lower* than your body's temperature, your testicles hang from your body so that air can get in around them and keep them cooler than the rest of you. When the weather is very hot, after you take a hot shower, or if you have a fever, your scrotum relaxes completely so that your testicles hang as far away from your body as possible. In cold weather, the scrotum brings your testicles closer to your body for more warmth. Also, when you are frightened, your scrotum tightens up to keep your testicles close to your body for maximum protection.

Inside your testicles, the *vas deferens* tubes carry sperm from the testicles to the *seminal vesicles,* where sperm are stored. The seminal vesicles and the *prostate gland* make semen, the fluid that carries sperm out of your body during ejaculation (see page 18). Semen travels through the *urethra,* a tube inside your penis that connects to the bladder. Urine also leaves your body through the urethra. A valve closes the urethra off from the bladder when you ejaculate so urine and semen can't mix.

As every boy knows from painful experience, your penis and testicles hurt when they are hit. This is why a lot of athletes wear protective cups around that area when they are playing sports.

Changes: Your Penis and Testicles Grow

During puberty your penis and testicles start to grow bigger, usually when you are between the ages of eleven and fifteen, but sometimes earlier or later. Because puberty starts at a different time for each individual, some boys' penises are much bigger than others' even though the boys are the same age. Comparisons frequently happen, and many boys wonder if their penis is normal. Roger said:

Three years ago in seventh-grade gym class, I spent a lot of time comparing myself to other guys. I felt like I was much smaller than everyone else. I started worrying if I was okay, if I had all the same things going on that everyone else did.

Sometimes there is teasing and outright cruelty, as Greg reported:

Gym teachers in our junior high are always using sex jokes to keep everybody in line. One teacher in particular used to try to influence the guys by making jokes about them in the locker room. He was real hard on us. Like in the shower he'd go

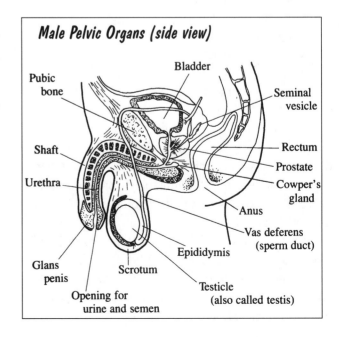

Male Pelvic Organs (side view)

Pubic bone · Bladder · Seminal vesicle · Shaft · Rectum · Prostate · Urethra · Cowper's gland · Anus · Vas deferens (sperm duct) · Glans penis · Epididymis · Scrotum · Testicle (also called testis) · Opening for urine and semen

around saying, "Hey, look at that big cock over there," or to someone else he'd say, "Look at that guy, he couldn't even fill up a keyhole." I always did everything I could to avoid the shower line when that teacher was around. I mean, that was really humiliating.

This gym teacher is not just being cruel, he is sexually harassing his students. (For more about sexual harassment, see page 221.) It is illegal for teachers, or anyone else, to make sexual remarks to keep people in line or to establish control or discipline.

The fact is that the size of your penis has *nothing* to do with how manly you are, how many erections you can have, how good your orgasms will feel, or with your ability to satisfy a partner. Two of the young men who helped us with this book said they try to ignore the hype and put-downs around penis size.

George: I read a book on sex that said small penises could get very big when they were hard and cocks that started out big when they were soft might not grow so much when they were hard, so I didn't really ever worry about the size of my cock. I figured it would work when it had to, and that was pretty much all I cared about. [The book that George read was right, by the way.]

David: When my cock is soft it shrinks up so much you can hardly see it, and I used to look at these guys who had cocks halfway down their thighs and I'd wonder, Hey, what's my problem? But when I get excited, mine looks like everybody else's, so I've got no complaints.

Erections

HOW AN ERECTION HAPPENS AND WHAT IT LOOKS LIKE: During an erection (a "boner," or "hard-on"), your penis gets longer, harder, and wider. It stands erect, away from your body. When you are sexually aroused, a nerve center at the base of your spinal cord sends messages that cause some of your blood to rush into the blood vessels and spongy tissue in your penis. The muscles inside the base of your penis tighten so that this extra blood can't easily drain out.

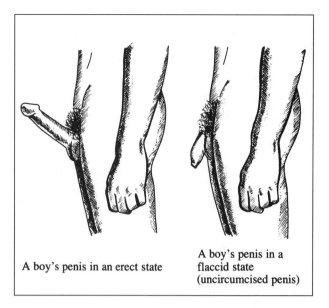

A boy's penis in an erect state

A boy's penis in a flaccid state (uncircumcised penis)

An erect penis looks very different from a soft one. A seventeen-year-old girl told us:

I've seen my brother naked, but I'd never seen an erect penis until the other night. When my boyfriend pulled his out of his pants, I nearly croaked. "My God, where have you been hiding that thing?" No way it could have been in his pocket all that time!

When a penis is fully erect, it almost seems as though there were something rigid inside it, like a bone. People even call an erection a "rod" or a "boner." But in fact there's no bone inside, only blood and tissue.

WHEN AND WHY YOU HAVE ERECTIONS: You have been getting erections all your life, ever since you were a baby. Lots of boys and men wake up in the morning with erections. Sometimes having to urinate will give you an erection. The friction of your pants on your penis when you are exercising can make your penis hard. One nine-year-old boy said, "Whenever I get excited about anything, my penis gets hard." Even sounds can do it, as Tony remembered:

Whenever I hear a vacuum cleaner, I start getting hard. That must be because I used to love those days when I'd stay home from school, sick, and I'd be up in my room while my mother was vacuuming downstairs. That's a real good memory.

Mostly, erections come with sexual arousal. Stroking and touching your penis and testicles in a sexual way, or having them stroked by someone else, leads to an erection. Thinking sexy thoughts, reading sexy books, or daydreaming about someone can cause it too. Jerry, who's twelve, was surprised at first:

> When my penis first started getting hard, like at a movie during a love scene, I remember thinking, Hey, what's this? Why is this happening?

When you get an erection suddenly without planning on it and when your penis hasn't been touched, it's called a "spontaneous erection." Teenage boys have these a lot because of the high or fluctuating level of the hormone testosterone in their bodies. Here's what a few boys said about spontaneous erections:

> Jim (sixteen): It's really embarrassing to have an erection just when you have to go out onto the field in a gym class when there are girls on the field too. That's happened to me a lot.

> Tom (seventeen): I get a hard-on in drama class almost every time I have to go up on stage. I can never tell if they are laughing at my performance or at my bulging cock.

Some boys worry about the number of erections they have. They may think they have too many, or compare themselves with friends and think they have too few. Jason said:

> I thought I had a real problem because I would get hard-ons about fifteen or twenty times a day, for no reason at all. I'd be sitting at my desk, and maybe my mind would be wandering and all of a sudden, ZAP! there it would be. I used to put a book down in my lap and read it from there. When I asked my friend how many times he would get hard during the day, he said not so much, so I was sure there was something wrong with me.

There is in fact *nothing* wrong with Jason. There is no such thing as too many erections. When you are older and past puberty, if you don't ever get *any* erections, you probably should discuss your condition with a doctor.

A spontaneous erection goes away by itself after a while if you don't touch or rub your penis to add to the stimulation. An erection caused by touching can end in one of two ways. If the touching or rubbing keeps up long enough—if you are masturbating (see page 96) or someone is fondling you—you will probably have an orgasm. After an orgasm, your penis will lose its erection and become soft again quite quickly. Or if the touching, friction, or rubbing stops without your having an orgasm, the extra blood will slowly drain out of your penis and it will get soft again. This may take a little longer. You may feel sexually frustrated and your testicles may ache slightly, but they will return to normal on their own after a short time. In slang, the condition is called "blue balls." It is not harmful.

Making Semen and Ejaculating (Coming)

About a year after your penis and testicles start to grow, and just about when your pubic hair begins to come in, your testicles start to make semen.

How do you know that semen is now being made? This boy describes it:

> The first time that I really came and this whitish stuff came out of my cock, I thought, Wow, this is really great, this feels great!

When fluid spurts out of your penis like that, it's called ejaculation (ee-ja-cue-*lay*-shun). Maybe you know it by another word, like coming, creaming, climaxing, juicing, milking, letting go, shooting off.

The milky whitish fluid that shoots out of your penis is called semen or ejaculate or "come." It has millions of sperm in it, as well as other fluids that help carry the sperm along. Contractions of the muscles in your penis push the semen out at the peak of your sexual excitement. This is called an orgasm. Orgasm usually feels very good.

Usually a man ejaculates when he has an orgasm, though it is possible to ejaculate without one. (It is also possible to have orgasms without ejaculating.) Some people think that because guys ejaculate when they have orgasms, women do too. They don't.

Starting to ejaculate is, for a boy, like a girl's having her period for the first time. It's a major sign that your body is growing up. Colin said:

I heard everyone talking about coming and jacking off, and at fifteen I hadn't experienced it

yet. It was real mysterious to me. I would try and try, masturbating every night, and even though that felt good it didn't bring results. Finally one night, bang. It happened.

A boy's first ejaculation often happens while he is masturbating or sleeping. Mike, who is thirteen, told us:

Ejaculation, Sperm, and Conception (You Can Conceive a Child Now)

Once you begin making sperm and semen, you are able to conceive a child. Sperm are made inside each testicle, in tightly coiled tubes located in 250 little compartments. These tubes grow during the early stages of puberty, which is why your testicles get bigger then. If you unwound all the tubes and put them end to end, they would stretch the length of several football fields!

Once made, sperm move into a special compartment attached to each testicle called the epididymis (eh-pih-*dih*-dih-mis). Here they take six weeks to mature. Sperm that don't ripen or are less mature die in the epididymis and disintegrate. Only the healthiest sperm are ejaculated.

When the sperm mature and are ready to fertilize an egg, they go from the epididymis into a tube called the vas deferens, one for each testicle. These are the tubes that are cut and sealed if a man has the sterilization operation for permanent birth control called a vasectomy.

From the vas deferens, sperm move to the seminal vesicles and are stored in two compartments until you ejaculate.

Your ejaculate contains both sperm and fluids made by the seminal vesicles and the prostate gland. This seminal fluid carries the sperm and protects it from the very slight acidity in a woman's vagina which could be harmful to sperm without that protection.

Sperm comes out through your urethra. When you are sexually aroused, a valve closes off the bladder entry so no urine can come out. That's why it takes a while to urinate just after you've been sexually excited.

The Responsibility of Being Sexually Active: When a man and a woman have sexual intercourse, his ejaculation sends about *400 million sperm* into her vagina. The sperm swim rapidly up through her cervix and uterus into her fallopian (fel-*low*-pee-yan) tubes. One of her ovaries releases an egg each month in a process called ovulation (ah-vue-*lay*-shun). If a woman ovulates around the time she has intercourse, her egg

The Inside of a Testicle

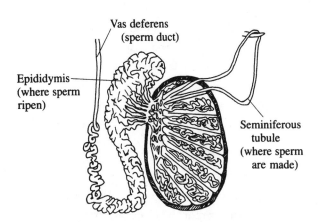

Vas deferens (sperm duct)

Epididymis (where sperm ripen)

Seminiferous tubule (where sperm are made)

may meet a sperm in the tube and the two will join to start a pregnancy. Since sperm can stay alive in the fallopian tubes for up to six days, there are about eight days each month when it is possible for sperm and egg to unite to start a pregnancy. It's hard to determine just when those eight days occur each month, and miscalculations often lead to unplanned pregnancies. (See pages 37–38 for more on ovulation.)

There are usually some live sperm in the drops of fluid that come from your erect penis even *before* you ejaculate. These drops of pre-ejaculate can cause pregnancy too. They can also contain germs from sexually transmitted diseases if you have one.

If you have sex with a girl and you don't want to start a pregnancy, you must use birth control (see page 279). *It's very important.* Becoming a parent before you are old enough to feel mentally, emotionally, and financially ready is a burden on you, on your partner, and on a child.

In addition, if you start having intimate sexual encounters, you must use safer-sex methods to protect yourself and your partner from sexually transmitted diseases such as HIV/AIDS and other dangerous infections. (See chapters 9 and 10 for more information.)

Puberty is a time to celebrate and enjoy; it is also a time to be cautious, thoughtful, and responsible.

I have fantasies just about every night before I go to sleep. I lie there with all these sexy things going on in my head, and of course my hand always seems to make it down to my cock. This one time I got real hard and my balls started itching, like, and then there was this liquid shooting out of my cock. It felt amazing. So I went to sleep with a big smile that night.

If it happens during sleep it is sometimes called a "wet dream." Dennis said:

I was about thirteen. I felt like I had this total sexual experience in my dream and I woke up and thought, Wow, did this really happen or not? It blew my mind it felt so real. After a second I realized my pajamas were wet. I sort of knew what it had to be, but still I was a little surprised.

Andrew said:

I think a first wet dream is a powerful moment. It marks becoming a man. It happened to me in the bathtub the other night, and it felt amazing.

The formal term for wet dream is "nocturnal emission." It is your body's way of relieving your testicles when a lot of sperm have built up in them. If you have orgasms once in a while when you're awake, you may not have many nocturnal emissions.

Some boys wonder if they will run out of semen if they come frequently. If you ejaculate several times in a row, there won't be as many sperm in the later ejaculations, but there will be some. You will not run out of sperm or semen.

Pubic Hair, Body Hair, and Whiskers

The hormone testosterone causes boys to grow pubic hair around their genitals. Over the course of a year or two, it grows over the pubic bone and covers the genital area, including the anus. The function of pubic hair may be to help keep people's genitals warm and protected.

Most kids know that adults have pubic hair, so they expect it. Dan, an eleven-year-old, said:

I keep looking for it, keep expecting to find one any day. A couple of my friends are already growing pubic hair, and I can see fuzz around my balls, but so far, only fuzz.

Pubic hair starts with just a few hairs. Gradually, more hair grows, and it gets coarser and curlier. For a while, it covers a limited area, and then it fills out in a kind of upside-down triangle at the base of your abdomen all around your genitals. Usually it is dark. People with naturally light or red hair may have pubic hair of the same color as the hair on their head, or it may be darker. Some people have a lot and others not much at all.

Your first pubic hair may begin to grow without your noticing. Or it may be a shock. Three boys in a discussion group in Providence found they had feelings in common:

Juan: Pubic hair scared the shit out of me. I saw all these little bumps and I didn't know what they were. I thought maybe I had VD but I hadn't even had sex.

Eric: I thought I was growing pimples.

Juan: I told my father right away, because I was so scared.

Richard: I didn't say anything to anyone. I just waited. And then I noticed hair was growing out.

As with most of the changes in puberty, the kids who get pubic hair early are usually teased, and the ones who get it late are teased too.

You may also grow new, thicker body hair. To get an idea of how much hair you will have, look at the men in your family. If they have lots of hair, then you probably will too. How you feel about body hair is basically up to you. Some people are turned on by thick body hair, and some people prefer bodies with hardly any hair. It's personal, and a matter of individual taste. Having a lot of body hair doesn't mean you are more "masculine" than someone else.

The hair on your face usually starts to grow between the ages of fourteen and eighteen. A sixteen-year-old said:

I had to shave a lot earlier than most of my friends. I was already shaving every day by the time I was fifteen, and even though I felt macho about it, it really was a pain in the neck. My dad's the same way—he has to shave twice a day to look good.

Shaving can be another real symbol of growing up. One man remembered:

I was late in getting a beard; it was a big deal if I had to shave once every couple of weeks in high school. I looked up to this friend who had a full growth of face hair when he was a junior. I couldn't have grown a beard if somebody paid me a million dollars.

Usually, facial hair first starts coming in as sideburns and a mustache. A seventeen-year-old said:

When I was fourteen, I went around for about two weeks with this dirty smudge on my upper lip. I kept trying to wash it off, but it wouldn't wash. Then I really looked at it and saw it was a mustache. So I shaved!

Voice Change

One of the cartoon stereotypes of a teenage boy is a guy who's talking along in a deep, impressive voice and all of a sudden his voice cracks and he starts squeaking. Voice change, brought on by testosterone, happens somewhere around fourteen or fifteen years. The deepening of your voice isn't necessarily any big drama. Tony said:

All of a sudden I realized my voice was low. On the telephone people started thinking I was my father, not my mother.

For George, it was more noticeable, but brief:

Last year it happened over two weeks. My throat was really killing me. I was feeling this scratchy thing every night when I called my friend. My voice would start cracking, and he'd say, "What's the matter, you got a cold?" and I'd say "What?"

because I didn't notice it. Then when I listened to myself talk, I heard my voice get heavier. In two weeks it was stronger, more mannish. It didn't bother me that much.

Some boys have a harder time. Dave reports:

I know a kid whose voice has been changing for a year. It cracks all the time and kids tease him.

Ian said:

You feel self-conscious, especially talking to a girl. I hear my brother talking on the phone with his girlfriend, and he seems to be controlling his voice. He doesn't let himself sound angry or real happy or surprised. Your voice usually goes high when you get emotional or angry. So you try not to get too emotional. That way your voice will keep steady and low.

Your Breasts

Boys have breasts too, but since their breasts are not designed to provide milk for babies, their breasts don't develop in the same way girls' breasts develop.

Most boys have some temporary breast growth during the early stages of puberty. It is called gynecomastia (guy-ne-co-*mas*-tee-a). Both breasts may get larger, or sometimes one breast gets bigger than the other. Most of the growth will disappear within a year, but some boys find it embarrassing. It happens to nearly all boys to some degree. Sometimes this condition appears in the form of a lump, which can make you worry that something is wrong. You may want to see a health practitioner about it for reassurance. In most instances, the lump will go away by itself.

Sometimes during puberty boys' breasts will feel painful or sensitive. Eddie said:

When I was in eighth grade, my nipples felt so sore that it hurt to wear any shirt at all.

If this condition persists, discuss it with a health practitioner to see if she or he can recommend a treatment for the soreness.

Taking Care of Your Genitals

To take care of your penis and testicles, wash them with soap and warm water every day if you can. Clear away any smegma (page 16) that collects around the glans, especially if you are uncircumcised. Also, get in the habit of checking your testicles once in a while, maybe once a month when lying down, to feel for any changes or lumps, just as a girl checks her breasts for lumps.

Most of us know what our bodies look like, but we also want to be conscious of the ways our bodies feel as they change and develop. That way we can be the experts on our own bodies and know when everything's normal and also when something needs medical attention.

Some of the signals that should send you to a clinic or doctor are:

➤ An open sore or persisting sore spot around your penis.

➤ A burning feeling when you urinate.

➤ An undescended testicle.

➤ Discharge (pus or whitish fluid) coming from the end of your penis.

➤ A pain in your testicles that doesn't go away.

➤ A lump that wasn't there before.

Many of these things are more likely to happen once you are sexually active, because they may indicate a sexually transmitted disease. Check your genitals for sores or rashes. Sores, rashes, painless bumps, or a burning sensation during urination can indicate an infection. Have yourself checked by a health practitioner, and do not have any sexual activity until the health worker says you are not contagious. **Using a condom during sexual activity is the easiest and most effective way to help protect yourself from disease.**

You'll want to find a doctor you feel comfortable with. Many pediatricians are now trained in health care for teenagers (adolescent medicine). Ask your parents to help you find a good doctor. If you need medical attention but don't feel you can tell your parents, find a clinic in your area that works with teenagers. Ask a friend to go with you. To learn what to expect from a good medical exam, check pages 246–52.

DISCHARGE FROM YOUR PENIS: This is a common problem, which may have a number of causes. Always have yourself checked by a health practitioner, because a discharge might be a sign of gonorrhea if you are at all sexually active, or chlamydia or some other infection in the urethra. Most of these diseases require antibiotic treatment.

If you stop yourself regularly from ejaculating during masturbation or sex play, you may develop a condition known as retrograde ejaculation. That means that the semen has gone back down the urethra into the glands and is building up there. That buildup can cause pain and a discharge from the penis. The best way to avoid retrograde ejaculation is to let yourself come at least occasionally when masturbating or during other sexual activity. Just because you feel the need to come doesn't mean you *have* to come inside a partner. There are many safe ways to enjoy ejaculation without having intercourse. If you do choose to have sexual activity with a partner, be sure to use protection to keep yourselves safe from disease and pregnancy. (See the Sexuality chapter, beginning on page 89.)

Your body may also eliminate excess sperm buildup naturally in a wet dream.

PAIN IN THE GENITAL AREA: Pain in the groin or genital area can be caused by many things. It might be a swollen lymph gland or a hernia or an infection. If it lasts more than a day or two, you should have it checked by a doctor. Sometimes when you stay sexually aroused for an extra long time without ejaculating, you'll feel a painful discomfort around your testicles, which can be relieved by masturbating. Or else it will go away by itself after a while. It is no cause for alarm, and certainly no reason to feel you have to talk someone into having sex with you.

UNDESCENDED TESTICLES: Ordinarily a boy's testicles descend shortly before or just after his birth. Sometimes, especially in the case of premature babies, the testicles do not descend for several months. When they have not descended by themselves, the condition can be corrected by surgery or hormone treatment.

A partially descended testicle can become twisted and cause you a great deal of pain. An operation is called for to untwist the cord that supplies blood to the testicle. If you have pain in your testicles that hasn't been caused by an immediate injury, or if you've been hit in the testicles and the pain lasts for a very long time, see a health practitioner.

CANCER: Teenagers very rarely get cancer. When they do, the best chance of cure is early discovery of the disease. So it is crucial to have your symptoms checked out by a medical person as soon as you suspect something may be wrong. Symptoms to have checked are a lump that doesn't go away; sores that aren't healing; blood in your bowel movement; and irregular bleeding from a mole.

Skin cancer has become much more common, because of the partial depletion of the protective ozone layer in the atmosphere. Teenagers who enjoy being outdoors and sunbathing should wear sunscreen to protect themselves from ultraviolet rays. Have suspicious moles or spots checked by a doctor.

ATHLETIC ITCH (JOCK ITCH, OR JOCK ROT): If you have itching and a damp feeling in your genital area, you may have jock itch. The skin will be sore and red around your testicles and on the inside of your thighs, and it will usually itch a lot. There may even be tiny blisters.

Jock itch is a fungus condition. It can be caused by wearing clothes that are too tight or that are made of fabrics that don't let the air circulate. Rubbing cornstarch, which you can find in any supermarket, lightly on the area will often be enough to cure it, but you may need to use an antifungal powder or cream that can be purchased without prescription at a drugstore. If the condition doesn't go away, you may want to see a health practitioner, especially to make sure nothing more serious is involved. Keep the area clean and dry. Wash your

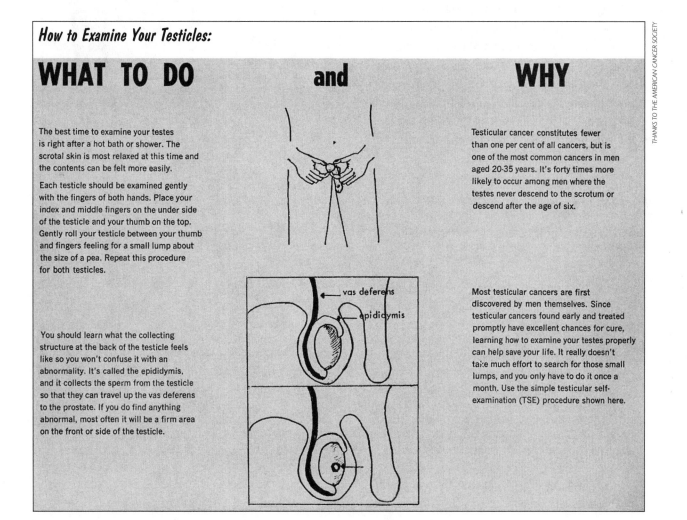

How to Examine Your Testicles:

WHAT TO DO and WHY

The best time to examine your testes is right after a hot bath or shower. The scrotal skin is most relaxed at this time and the contents can be felt more easily.

Each testicle should be examined gently with the fingers of both hands. Place your index and middle fingers on the under side of the testicle and your thumb on the top. Gently roll your testicle between your thumb and fingers feeling for a small lump about the size of a pea. Repeat this procedure for both testicles.

You should learn what the collecting structure at the back of the testicle feels like so you won't confuse it with an abnormality. It's called the epididymis, and it collects the sperm from the testicle so that they can travel up the vas deferens to the prostate. If you do find anything abnormal, most often it will be a firm area on the front or side of the testicle.

vas deferens
epididymis

Testicular cancer constitutes fewer than one per cent of all cancers, but is one of the most common cancers in men aged 20-35 years. It's forty times more likely to occur among men where the testes never descend to the scrotum or descend after the age of six.

Most testicular cancers are first discovered by men themselves. Since testicular cancers found early and treated promptly have excellent chances for cure, learning how to examine your testes properly can help save your life. It really doesn't take much effort to search for those small lumps, and you only have to do it once a month. Use the simple testicular self-examination (TSE) procedure shown here.

pants, underwear, and jock strap frequently, and don't wear tight clothes that rub or irritate your genital area.

GIRLS' BODIES

NOTE TO BOY READERS OF THIS SECTION: Many boys look at girls' bodies—a lot—because they are curious and fascinated, because it's a pleasure, and because they are trained to look by a culture that "sells" women's bodies along with products. Girls, too, look at girls' bodies almost as much as they look at boys' bodies.

There's a big difference between *looking at* and *knowing about.* A group of teenage boys helping us with this book were "experienced" lookers: they always knew whether a girl was wearing a bra or not; they had opinions about hairy legs and body shape. Yet they still had many questions about girls' feelings and about what goes on inside their bodies. Boys helping us with this book asked: Do you care how big your breasts are? Does getting your period hurt? Do you like it when boys make comments about how good you look? As the girls in the group answered these questions, you could actually see the boys moving from looking at the girls to really understanding their feelings. There's a lot we can learn from one another, and the more we talk to one another, the better friends we can be.

Girls' Changes

Somewhere between the ages of nine and eighteen, a girl will experience these changes:

➤ Your breasts will grow, a little or a lot, depending on the body shape you inherited from your family.

➤ The hair on your legs will grow thicker and maybe darker, and hair will grow under your arms.

➤ Pubic hair will grow around your vulva (the whole genital area, where your legs come together).

➤ You will get taller, growing to what will probably be your full height.

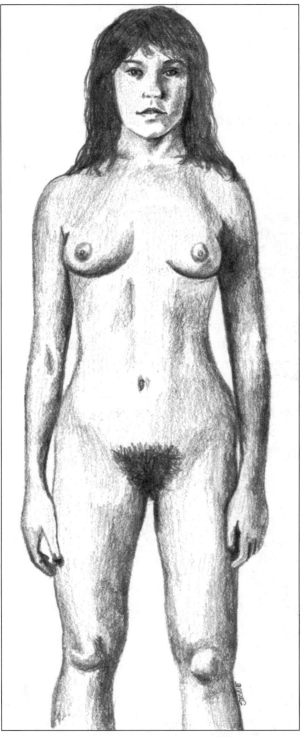

➤ Your hips will get bigger, and your body weight may shift.

➤ Inside, your uterus and vagina will grow. Eggs in your ovaries will start to mature each month. You will be able to get pregnant.

➤ Your period will come, though it may not come regularly for a few months.

➤ Your skin may become oilier, and you may get pimples on your face, neck, chest, and back.

➤ Your romantic and sexual feelings may become more insistent.

➤ Your sweat glands begin working and you sweat more.

All these changes are caused by hormones, which become strong and active in a teenager's body somewhere between the ages of eight or nine and sixteen or seventeen.

Your Feelings About the Changes

How you feel about these changes will depend, as it does for boys, on how much you know about the way bodies grow, on what your idea of "beautiful" or "attractive" is, and whether you accept the ways you *don't* match that image. Your feelings will also probably be influenced by how your family and friends react toward your growing up. Are they supportive? Hostile? Competitive? Too interested?

On the streets men who notice your growing breasts and hips may call out, hoot, ogle you, and make suggestive remarks. While it's possible they think they are complimenting you, many girls find those kinds of remarks annoying, if not downright hostile and frightening. Because of this, many girls say they feel a level of fear and tension whenever they are in unfamiliar surroundings, afraid of potential verbal and even physical attack. (See pages 221–43 for more on harassment and sexual abuse.)

Cathy (sixteen): How about guys whistling at you and bugging you on the street? I hate that. And it's pretty scary, too, people whistling at you when you're walking home late at night.

Denise (twelve): Since I've gotten more physically mature I get a lot of stares when I go out. Sometimes it feels nice or funny when I'm with my friends, especially when it's someone nice. But when it's some weirdo or when some older man says something like "Ooooooooh," then it's scary and I want to say, I'm only twelve, leave me alone.

When you apply for an after-school job, the boss may make sexual remarks. A neighbor who used to treat you like a kid may begin teasing you suggestively. Some adults may come on to you in ways that are demeaning or downright frightening. This is not okay. When someone makes a sexual remark to them, girls sometimes wonder if they "asked for it," if it's their fault. No, it is not. The fault may lie with our society's attitude, which encourages males to treat females as sex objects, not as equals. Jenny, a seventeen-year-old from Washington, remembers:

During the seventh and eighth grade I always wore a coat to school. It didn't matter what the weather was. I was embarrassed about my body, because the guys at our school would always go around grabbing parts—you know, sexual parts—and I hated that.

Most of women's clothing is made to be provocative. And some boys feel they have the right to make lewd comments when they think a girl is dressed in a sexy way. It is not their right. In fact, it is called sexual harassment, and under certain circumstances it is considered a criminal act (see page 221). Boys and men have to be educated that it is *not* all right for them to make remarks about your body, just as they wouldn't want you making statements about the size of their penis or the sexiness of their anatomy. Let people know that you don't appreciate their stares and their harassing comments.

You certainly have a right to grow into your woman's body, to feel good and look good and wear whatever you feel comfortable wearing without being teased or harassed. Talk with other girls about these situations if they come up. You can give one another much-needed support. Talk to the boys you know about these situations too. Many boys are unaware that their actions are hurtful or frightening, and most of them appreciate having honest discussions with girls about sexual feelings and other teenage concerns.

Slang and Girls

There are many names for girls' body parts. The proper terms—vagina, vulva, clitoris, hymen, and breasts—are used much less frequently than slang words. Here is a list arrived at by some of the teens who helped us with this chapter:

vagina	*vulva*	*clitoris*
cunt	snatch	clit
box	twat	button
hole	pussy	joy button
honeypot	meat	panic button
	poontang	clint
	beaver	pearl tongue
	muff	

hymen	*breasts*
cherry	tits
maidenhead	knockers
	bonkers
	melons
	boobs
	caldoons
	mammies
	tetons
	honkers
	jugs
	pair
	knobs
	hooters

In the section on boys' slang (page 15), we discussed how tricky slang can be, because the same words can be used in different ways. Try saying each one of these words in a loving tone, then in a hostile tone, and notice how they differ in impact.

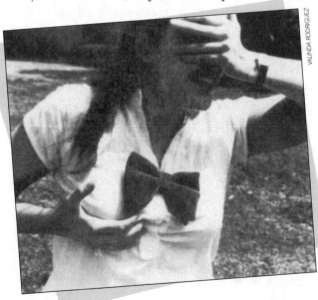

Even so, some of these words for parts of women's bodies have been used as insults for so long that it's almost impossible to avoid frightening a girl or hurting her just by saying them. There's really no way to make someone feel loved if you call her vulva "meat." If the word "cunt" (or "prick") is spat out in anger against someone you hate, it's hard to use those words again with affection. Think about how often our vocabulary for sex is used hatefully or—especially against women—to degrade other people.

Changes: Your Breasts Develop

Your breasts develop because of the increased production of estrogen, one of the female hormones in your body, at puberty. Estrogen causes the growth of mammary glands inside your breasts (enabling you to produce milk), as well as increasing the amount of fat tissue surrounding them.

The changes in your breasts come in stages. The areola (ah-ree-*oh*-la), the area around your nipple, is usually the first part to change. It gets thicker and darker. Depending on the amount of color in your skin, it can range from a light pinkish color to a very dark brown. Some hairs may grow around it.

When your breasts are cold (while you are taking a cold shower, for example), when you feel sexually excited, or when your breasts are touched or stroked, your areola may get bumpy-looking and your nipples may stand out more than usual. Otherwise, the areola can be quite smooth.

During the next stage, before your breasts really start to form, your nipples will probably get larger, and they will become more prominent. A fourteen-year-old girl said:

One day I realized that my nipples had started growing and one was really pretty big. I thought, this is weird, everybody else has breasts and I'm going to have big nipples. I didn't really get breasts for another year, until I was about twelve.

Another girl said:

A boy came up to me at school the other day and said, "Ginny, you're totally flat!" I wanted to say,

Well, you haven't seen my nipples, they're enormous! Instead I said, "Give me time, just give me time."

A sophomore from New Jersey told us:

My little sister says she feels embarrassed to wear tight shirts because her nipples are showing, but my mom says she's too young for a bra. I remember when I felt the same way—glad that I was starting to develop but embarrassed about people noticing, especially at school.

Some people have nipples that stand out a lot and other people's nipples hardly stand out at all. Some nipples sink into the areola. These are called inverted nipples (see page 30).

Starting to develop is exciting. It's a sign of growing up and in many families a special time to acknowledge:

Billie Jean (thirteen): My mom and I are really close, and when I first started getting breasts she took me out to celebrate. It was around my tenth birthday, and it made me feel very grown-up.

Pauline (fifteen): I have three sisters who are older than me, so I was real charged up when I started popping out in front because that made me feel I was joining their club. In fact, when I got big enough, my oldest sister took me downtown to get my first bra.

BREASTS: WHEN? Some girls begin to develop breasts at eight or nine, others not for years after that. Several girls said it was hard being the first among their friends to develop:

Janet: I started maturing physically when I was very young. And I never wanted to. When I was about nine I already started having breasts, and I hated it. I was still a tomboy, and I used to do anything to hide my chest, like wear baggy shirts and overalls all the time. Now that I'm older I realize that I just didn't feel ready to grow up then. My body was leading the way and my feelings about changing were about a mile behind.

Judy: When my breasts first started growing I used to wear really supertight shirts—my little sister's T-shirts. I'm serious—to flatten me. Then I'd wear another shirt over that because I was really self-conscious. I was only in third grade, and every other girl in the class was flat as a board.

Sometimes breasts grow slowly:

I must have been about ten or eleven when I first started getting breasts—well, not exactly breasts but swellings on my chest. I was so proud I went around showing everybody who was interested—you know, everyone in my family and some close family friends. But now I'm fourteen, and my breasts are still pretty small. My mother says just wait, but it's hard to wait when you don't know what you're waiting for.

For some girls, the change can be more dramatic:

And my breasts, wow! Those just started going nuts. They were popping out. My sister used to call me "squished strawberries" and "busted egg yolk." Now she calls me the names I used to call her—basketball woman, grapefruit. I'm almost up to her. Another year of this kind of growing, I'll be up there.

The changes may not be even. For example, one breast often starts to develop before the other one, or seems to grow at a faster rate:

When I first started growing I was totally lopsided. My left side was a size-A cup and my right side was absolutely flat. It seemed to me that it was like that for a long time. I remember thinking, Uh-oh, I'm going to look very strange if this keeps up.

Usually breasts eventually grow to be about the same size, but many women have one breast larger than the other. Ellen is twenty-two:

One of my boobs is bigger than the other one. It's not noticeable with clothes on, but when I'm naked I can really see the difference. It seems like my whole left side is bigger than my right side, all the way up from my foot to my hand to my boob.

Some girls don't begin developing until much later than their friends, and some remain small-breasted throughout their lives. But the size of a girl's breasts does not indicate how sensitive to touch her breasts will be or how much milk she'll produce once she has a baby. Annie is the mother of two. She said:

> I didn't even start getting breasts until the tenth grade. It was okay with me, because I was on the basketball team and the soccer team and I liked not having that extra weight bouncing around on my chest. I used to wear an athletic bra, but I didn't really need it. By the time I was twenty-three, when my first baby came, I went from an A cup to a C. I had so much milk, I could have bottled it.

BREASTS: HOW BIG? The size and shape of your breasts depend mostly on the amount of fatty tissue they have: if there is a lot of fat in your breasts, they will be large; if there is little fat, they will be small. The major factor is heredity—that is, the body shape you have inherited from your mother or from women in your father's family. Weight has less to do with it. We've all seen thin women with large breasts and heavy women with small ones.

One group of teenagers working on this book talked about all the ways people try to develop their breasts. Candace said:

> I don't think it's fair that when you go on a diet your boobs get smaller, but when you gain weight you usually gain it everywhere but your boobs!

Exercises make your pectoral muscles (the muscles under your breasts) bigger. That doesn't really affect the amount of fat in your breasts, but since most of the girls in the room had tried the exercises, they demonstrated a few. Kate chanted, "I must, I must, I must improve my bust!" One of the boys asked, "Is it true that if you put butter on your tits they get bigger?" Charlene had heard this too:

> Last year I went to my girlfriend's house and her younger sister was in the bathroom rubbing butter and onions on her boobs, because someone told her that makes them grow. It hasn't worked yet, but you never know!

The Mammary Glands

From the time of puberty onward, your mammary glands are ready to change elements of your blood into milk if you should get pregnant and give birth.

A mammary gland is made up of areas that make milk, called alveoli (al-vee-oh-lie), and passageways, ducts through which the milk travels to the nipple. You can see a few small openings in your nipple: these are the ends of the ducts. Sometimes a little bit of discharge (some liquid) will come out of these (see page 29).

Internal View of the Female Breast

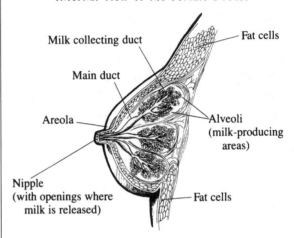

Milk collecting duct
Fat cells
Main duct
Areola
Alveoli (milk-producing areas)
Nipple (with openings where milk is released)
Fat cells

While a woman is pregnant, her mammary glands get bigger as hormones make them ready to produce milk. Hormones released during the birth process trigger the production of milk a couple of days after the baby comes. When a mother holds her newborn to her breast, the baby instinctively sucks on the nipple. This sucking pulls the milk through the ducts and into the baby's mouth. Since the baby's sucking causes milk to be made within a few hours, there will be more milk for as long as the mother wants to keep nursing, no matter how big or small her breasts are. If she doesn't want to breast-feed her baby, the first milk will dry up and no more will be made until another birth.

Some women with extremely large breasts wish theirs were smaller. If you are overweight, losing weight may help. Once you are fully grown (past adolescence), there is an operation available that removes some breast tissue and reduces the size of your breasts. As with any other surgical procedure, it involves risk and discomfort, and it can cost several thousand dollars. But some women feel it's worth it if having very large breasts has caused them physical and/or emotional suffering.

BREASTS: WHAT THEY LOOK LIKE: Breasts come in many shapes and sizes. It would be great if we could all accept who we are and what we look like; if we didn't tease each other about who's big-breasted and who's small-breasted; if "girlie" magazines and advertisers didn't produce endless images of what they consider to be "perfect" female bodies. It would be even better if boys didn't grow up learning to judge a girl by her breasts or judge their friends by their girlfriends' breasts.

As women have started to see how much they have suffered over having the "wrong"-shaped breasts, they have come to realize that what was "wrong" was not their shape, but society's attitudes. So whether your breasts are big or small, pointed or rounded, we hope this section will help you hold your own against all those voices that say they should look different. It's all part of the same problem: being judged not for who we are but for how we look.

TAKING CARE OF YOUR BREASTS: Whether or not to wear a bra has become an issue for a lot of girls. If you have small breasts or very firm ones, you may not need a bra. If your breasts are large, they probably need some support, especially during sports or dancing or any other vigorous activity. Your breasts may feel much better with the support that comes from wearing a bra. Often, however, your decision about whether or not to wear a bra will be based more on what your friends do than on what your body needs. Shannon said:

> I was in sixth grade, and a friend told me I should wear a bra. I had never thought of it before, never thought I was big enough, and she said, "You need a bra." Who is she to be telling me I need a bra? After that, I got all self-conscious.

Mary's friends had the opposite opinion:

> I had a few friends who thought it was sick to wear one. So if I ever wore one I'd wear a lot of sweaters over it. By that time I wouldn't even need to wear one.

Ellie added:

> I know girls whose mothers bought them bras and said they should start wearing them. But I don't think you should start wearing a bra until you want to yourself.

MONTHLY SWELLING: Many girls and women have swelling and tenderness in their breasts just before their period arrives. Your tissues tend to hold liquid before menstruation; this often makes your breasts feel heavier than usual. Wearing a well-fitting bra may be more comfortable during this time of the month. Also, since eating salt can cause tissues to hold water, cutting down on salty foods may help.

GETTING HIT IN THE BREASTS: Your breasts are sensitive. If you bump them or if they are hit, it can be painful. Your body is able to handle bruising and minor accidents, so unless your breasts are badly bruised you probably don't have cause for concern.

Some girls worry about having their breasts handled roughly during sex play. Sucking and rubbing won't cause them damage, but if it hurts or makes you feel uncomfortable, ask your partner to stop.

HAIR: Lots of women have hair on or around their breasts. Sometimes it's just one or two strands; sometimes it's quite a bit more. The hormones in the birth control pill may, in some people, cause hair to grow around their breasts. If this hair bothers you, check with a medical person.

SECRETIONS: You may sometimes notice a discharge coming from your nipples. This is normal and occurs naturally as your body's way of keeping the nipple ducts open. The discharge may look like very thin milk, or it may be clear or light-green, grayish or light-yellow. Women who take birth control pills may have this discharge. It can come during sexual arousal and at certain times in your menstrual cycle. Be sure to keep your nipples clean by washing with warm water and soap so the discharge won't dry and accumulate. If the discharge has pus or blood in it, or if it is brownish in color, see a doctor; it might be a sign of infection.

INFECTIONS: If you have an infection in or near your breasts, you will probably feel soreness and heat and see swelling or redness. Have it checked by a doctor; antibiotic or other treatment may be necessary. Sometimes nursing mothers get infections if one of their milk ducts gets plugged up and doesn't drain properly. Keep your nipples clean by washing them at least once a day.

INVERTED NIPPLES: Some nipples turn in instead of sticking out. In some cases, as your breasts continue to grow, the nipples will be pushed out. If not, don't worry. It won't stop you from enjoying sex, nor will it stop you from breast-feeding your baby if you have one. There are now special nipple shields made especially to help women with inverted nipples breast-feed. Lots of women have inverted nipples, so it's nothing to feel strange about. The only problem you might have is that if your breasts discharge any fluid, the secretions might get caught in the folds around the inverted nipples and dry there, possibly creating a chance for infection to develop. Be especially sure to keep your nipples clean to avoid this. *If your nipple has been sticking out and suddenly becomes inverted, you should see a doctor right away.* It might be the sign of a tumor.

LUMPS: Breasts can be very lumpy. Some girls and women find changes in breast tissue throughout their monthly menstrual cycle. *If a lump stays in one place for several weeks, see a doctor.* Most lumps will be benign (noncancerous). If a lump hurts—if it is tender or sore—it may mean you have an infection.

Teenagers of both sexes may get a kind of lump called an adolescent nodule, a sore swollen spot right under the nipple. The nodule will disappear by itself, but it can be scary if you don't know that. Teens very seldom have breast cancer. Occasionally, though, a lump can indicate cancer. So if you feel a lump, have it checked by a doctor.

If there is a history of breast cancer in your family, be vigilant about checking your breasts each month, but even if breast cancer does not run in your family, it's important to get into the habit of checking your breasts regularly for lumps. Cancer that is detected early is more easily treated and cured than cancer that is ignored.

If you or someone you love does have a malignant or cancerous lump, be sure to learn about alternative forms of treatment.* Doctors often disagree about treatment, so remember: always get a second opinion. You'll want to choose the doctor whose approach seems most sensible to you.

EXAMINING YOUR BREASTS IS IMPORTANT: Learn how to do a breast self-exam each month. (See the diagram below.) Many women don't examine their breasts, because they haven't learned how. Others are too busy, too embarrassed, or too afraid they

---

Breast Self-Exam

Undress from the waist up and stand in front of a mirror. Look at your breasts, first with your hands at your sides; then with hands raised above your head; then with hands pushing firmly on your hips or with your palms pressed together. Look for differences in shape, not size. Look for a flattening or bulging in one but not the other, for puckering of the skin, for discharge from a nipple when it is gently squeezed, for a reddening or scaly crust on a nipple, for one nipple harder than the other.

Then lie down on a bed or couch, or in a bathtub. Or stand in the shower. Hands glide more easily over wet skin. As you examine each breast, raise the arm on that side above your head. Or bend your arm and put your hand under your head, your elbow lying flat. If you are lying down, putting a small pillow or large folded towel under your shoulder will help flatten out your breast tissue so it's easier to examine. Use your right hand to examine the left breast, your left hand for the right breast. With your fingers flat, move them gently over every part of each breast. Move your fingers in small circles or with a slight back-and-forth motion, being sure to examine the whole breast. Pay special attention to the area between nipple and armpit, for most tumors are located there. Check for any lump, hard knot, or thickening.

Breast self-exams should be done frequently at first (every few days), so that you can learn about the different ways your breasts feel during the course of a month. Later, examine them once a month at the same time each month. A few days after menstruation is a good time, as they will be less full then.

If you feel a definite lump or thickness that doesn't go away after a week or so, see a doctor.

---

* See Boston Women's Health Book Collective, *The New Our Bodies, Ourselves* (New York: Simon & Schuster).

How to examine your breasts

1

In the shower:

Examine your breasts during batch or shower, hands glide easily over wet skin. Fingers flat, move gently over every part of each breast. Use right hand to examine left breast, left hand for right breast. Check for any lump, hard knot or thickening.

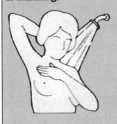

2

Before a mirror:

Inspect your breasts with arms at your sides. Next, raise your arms high overhead. Look for any changes in contour of each breast, a swelling, dimpling of skin or changes in the nipple.

Then, rest palms on hips and press down firmly to flex your chest muscles. Left and right breast will not exactly match—few women's breasts do.

Regular inspection shows what is normal for you and will give you confidence in your examination.

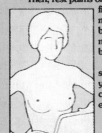

3

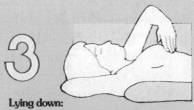

Lying down:

To examine your right breast, put a pillow or folded towel under your right shoulder. Place right hand behind your head—this distributres breast tissue more evenly on the chest. With left hand, fingers flat, press gently in small circular motions around an imaginary clock face. Begin at outermost top of your right breast for 12 o'clock, then move to 1 o'clock, and so on around the circle back to 12. A ridge of firm tissue in the lower curve of each breast is normal. Then move in an inch, toward the nipple, keep circling to examine every part of your breast, including nipple. This requires at least three more circles. Now slowly repeat procedure on your left breast with a pillow under your left shoulder and left hand behind head. Notice how your breast structure feels.

Finally, squeeze the nipple of each breast gently between thumb and index finger. Any discharge, clear or bloody, should be reported to your doctor immediately.

might find something wrong. *Take the time to do it.* You'll learn about the normal (for you) changes in your breast tissue. With practice, you'll feel comfortable touching your breasts. Rarely will you find something wrong. Remember, though, a breast self-exam can save your life if you do find a malignant lump early enough.

Pubic Hair and Body Hair

Pubic hair grows around your genitals—over your pubic bone and around your vulva, vagina, and anus. When it starts growing, it covers only a small area. Then it fills out in a kind of triangle or diamond shape over your pubic area. You may have just a little, or it may extend up to your navel and down the inside of your thighs.

Your first pubic hairs sometimes begin to grow without your noticing, but many people remember it as a big moment. Ann, an eleven-year-old, said:

Me and my friends go swimming at the college every week. In the shower there aren't any doors, so we kind of check each other out. A couple of weeks ago one of my friends showed me these hairs that were starting to grow down there, and I thought, Oh my God, I don't have any yet. Then I examined myself closer and I had three hairs there too. Three little dark hairs.

Also during puberty, the hair on your body—in your armpits, on your legs, maybe on your forearms or upper lip and chin—gets longer, thicker, and sometimes darker. Some women have very little body hair, and others have a lot. It can grow on their face, on their chest, on their neck, and on their back.

Boys usually welcome their thicker hair as a sign

of manhood. For girls, it's different. In our society, girls get the message that smooth, hairless skin is supposed to be beautiful and body hair is supposed to be ugly. Did you ever see a magazine model with lush curly hair on her legs and tantalizing tufts under her arms? New body hair may be a sign of growing up, but for most girls *shaving* is the true sign of womanhood. Many girls are eager to start shaving:

Vicky: When I was fourteen and not even much hair had grown yet, I had a contest with my friend to see whether my mother's electric shaver or her razor could get a closer shave under our arms. I forget which won, but, boy, do I remember how sore and raw my armpits were.

Cindy: When I started getting hair under my arms it was in the spring. People were starting to wear bathing suits, and I had these hairy underarms. I wanted to shave, but I was afraid to because my mother never talked to me about it. So finally I said, "Ma, is it okay if I shave?" She said, "Oh, yes. I just thought you were liberated." Because I always talk about women's rights and stuff, she thought that meant I wouldn't want to shave my underarms.

Many girls shave so as not to look different from everyone else. Three girls in Boston discuss shaving:

Eileen: I shave in the winter when it's time for gymnastics, because you don't want to be the only one on the team with hairy legs.

Iris: Yeah, you're under a lot of pressure to shave your legs.

Liz: There's a difference between what you want and what you think other people want. I don't think hairy legs are that bad. It doesn't bother me on me, and it doesn't bother me on other girls. But still I shave it at times.

Many girls who have dark hair on their arms or thighs, or on their faces, wish they didn't have it and dream of ways of getting rid of it. They tweeze it out or remove it with wax. They use chemical bleaches and hair removers sold commercially; they go to the expense of electrolysis or laser hair removal—methods for permanent hair removal. Sometimes they feel fine about having hair but are pressured to use one of these methods by parents or older women in their families. The idea "No hair is beautiful" goes deep. It's up to each of us to decide how we want to look, and how much body hair we are comfortable with. It's good to remember that body hair doesn't cause health problems, but the ways we try to remove body hair do sometimes cause infections, allergies, and irritations.

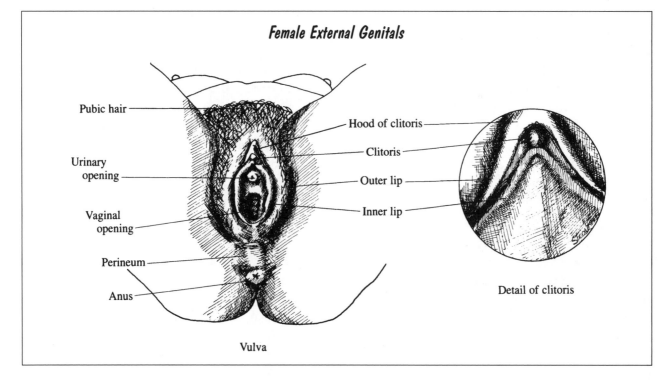

Female External Genitals

Pubic hair

Urinary opening

Vaginal opening

Perineum

Anus

Hood of clitoris

Clitoris

Outer lip

Inner lip

Detail of clitoris

Vulva

Your Genitals and Reproductive Organs

Your genitals are easy to see: Take a hand mirror and squat over it or hold it between your legs as you sit on the edge of a chair or toilet. Be sure you have plenty of light. Make sure you have enough time, too, and enough privacy so you can feel relaxed.

You may be surprised to read, "Take a mirror and flashlight and look at your genitals," or "If you reach your finger up inside your vagina you can touch your cervix." You may be shocked that we'd suggest such a thing. Doreen said:

> I know a lot of girls who think they're dirty down there and are taught not to touch themselves.

Becky, a sixteen-year-old helping with this book, said:

> I absolutely can't stand to think about doing that. It gives me the shivers. Even when I have to wash myself, I can barely do it.

Becky had been taught that it was wrong, dirty, and shameful to touch herself. When she was a child, her parents punished her when they found her masturbating (see page 96). She learned that "nice" girls don't have anything to do with that part of their bodies.

The funny thing is that Becky didn't mind when her boyfriend touched her down there or even when he looked. Her genitals were only off limits to herself. The other girls in the discussion group tried to help her feel more comfortable with the idea of touching herself. They explained that the more she knew about her body, the better care she'd be able to take of herself. As Doreen said to her:

> I figure it's a part of my body, just like any other part, except it's not right out there like your boobs are. Anyway, I sure as hell don't want someone else playing with it if I don't know what it is myself.

Lots of girls start out feeling like Becky. One of the best lessons to come out of the new consciousness many women have is that we owe it to ourselves to know our bodies. We have a right and a responsibility to be aware of how our bodies look and feel. That way we know when everything's normal, and we also know when something needs medical attention.

YOUR GENITALS: WHAT YOU CAN SEE ON THE OUTSIDE:

Starting from the front, you'll first see a soft, fatty mound called the *mons*. It's sometimes called the mound of Venus or mons veneris: Venus was the goddess of love. The mons is the pad of fatty layers that covers your pubic bone. If you press it, you can feel the bone right above where your legs join. Pressing it may feel good in a sexy kind of way. If you have pubic hair already, this mound will be covered with hair.

Next you'll see the *labia majora*, the outer lips, two pads or flaps of skin covering the entrance to the inner organs. Unless you spread your legs apart, these lips fall together, protecting the rest of your genitals as they were meant to do.

If you gently separate these lips, you'll see the *labia minora*, or inner lips, another set of folds of skin with no hair on them. These give more protection. They may hang below the major lips. They are sexually sensitive.

As you carefully spread open the inner lips, you see that where they come together at the front they form a hood over a small, sensitive pea-shaped bump, which is the top of the *clitoris* (*klit*-or-iss). The clitoris is densely packed with nerves, extremely sensitive to touch, and the center of sexual sensation for a woman. This sixteen-year-old said:

> It's not hard to find your clit. Just put your hand down there and feel around. When you get to the place that feels great and turns you on, that's your clit.

Your clitoris, like a penis, has a *glans*, or head, which is the most sensitive part, and a *shaft* under the skin, which is the main part of the clitoris. Glans and shaft contain the same spongy tissue that makes a penis erect. When you are sexually turned on, extra blood rushes into the spongy areas (erectile tissue) and causes your clitoris to get a little bigger. The whole area around it swells too, and becomes sensitive to touch. Rubbing the area around the clitoris can feel very good and may make you have an orgasm—a climax of sexual excitement. Your clitoris is so sensitive that rubbing or touching the glans directly may hurt.

Your clitoris is special; its only purpose is sexual arousal. In some cultures girl children are required to undergo an operation to remove the clitoris, which leaves them unable to experience the deep sexual pleasure this organ brings. Many women in our own culture have sex without knowing about the role the clitoris plays in their sexual pleasure. Their partners often share this ignorance. We recommend that you read Chapter 3, beginning on page 89, for more information about the role of the clitoris.

Next in line from your clitoris, also inside the inner lips, you'll find a small dot or slit which is the opening of your *urethra.* You urinate through this little round opening. The urethra is about 1½ inches long; it is the tube that carries urine from your bladder, where the urine is stored.

Your *vaginal opening* is next. It is larger than the urethral opening. It leads into your vagina. Menstrual blood, vaginal discharges, and, if you give birth, babies come out through the vaginal opening.

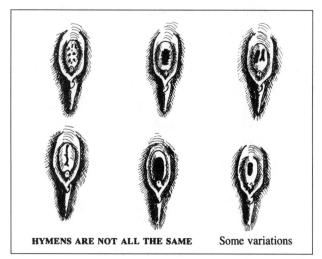

HYMENS ARE NOT ALL THE SAME   Some variations

Look around the opening. You might see your *hymen* (*hi*-man), a membrane (a special kind of tissue) that covers the vaginal opening partway. It almost never blocks the opening all the way, since there must be a way for menstrual blood to leave your body once your period begins. The hymen gives your body extra protection. It becomes stretched if you are very active or if you have had intercourse or if you use tampons to soak up your menstrual flow.

You can stretch your hymen open by yourself. Wash your hands and put one or two fingers into the vaginal opening. Move them slightly from side to side. You can use a tampon instead of your fingers. Do this every day until it stretches. Be gentle, and take your time. Even after stretching your hymen, you may see little folds of hymen tissue around the vaginal opening.

Over the centuries a big deal has been made of the hymen. For many people, it is the symbol of a young woman's "purity," the sign that she is still a "virgin"—that she hasn't had sexual intercourse with a male. The sexy parts of lots of books have dramatic scenes where the hymen (the "cherry" or "maidenhead") is torn during first intercourse, with lots of blood and anguish and passion. These accounts are wildly exaggerated! (See the section on virginity, page 120.) Having a hymen or not is no sign of virginity. Some girls are born with no hymen at all; some have a naturally large hymen opening; some stretch their hymen open during the normal play of childhood, including masturbation.

Now put a finger into your *vagina,* which is the passageway leading to your uterus. A moment ago, the vaginal walls were touching each other, but now they are spreading around your fingers. The walls seem to hug them. Feel the soft folds of skin. The stretchy walls allow the vagina to change shape, to accommodate whatever is inside. This may be a tampon or fingers; it could be a penis; it could be a baby being born.

Maggie was surprised to find these walls touching each other:

I always pictured my vagina as open, like a box or something, a hole I carried around between my legs. It's nice to realize I'm not so wide open.

Now move your finger. Notice whether it slides around easily. Sometimes the walls of the vagina are almost dry, sometimes they feel moist. The walls of your vagina give off a liquid, called *mucus,* most of the time. Mucus is your vagina's natural way of cleaning itself—which means that you don't have to douche (a special bath for the vagina). The mucus is slightly acid, keeps many infections from starting, and tastes salty. You may find signs of this mucus discharge on your underpants at times, which is normal. If it is very thick or foul-smelling, however, it may be a sign of a vaginal infection (page 273).

The degree of moistness depends on your age, on where you are in your monthly cycle, or on whether you are sexually excited. Do you notice that when you are turned on sexually, even by a picture or a fantasy, the lips of your vagina get wet? The vagina's natural mucus increases when you are sexually excited (see page 123).

Push gently against the vaginal walls. Try it all the way around. The outer third of the vagina, closest to the entrance, is very sensitive because it contains many nerve endings. This sensitivity is important in lovemaking.

If you squeeze the muscles around the entrance of your vagina and then relax them, you'll feel the *pelvic floor muscles.* These muscles hold your pelvic organs—your uterus, bladder, and ovaries—in place. When these muscles are weak, you may have trouble holding urine or having orgasms. The pelvic floor muscles, like mucus and nerve endings, play a role in lovemaking.

To locate these muscles, spread your legs apart while urinating and try to start and stop the flow of urine. Exercise these muscles by contracting (squeezing) for a second and then releasing completely. Repeat ten times in a row (which takes about twenty seconds). You can do these exercises anytime—while you are sitting, talking, walking, reading.

You may realize when you feel inside with your finger or when you look at the diagram that your vagina doesn't go straight up into your body. It goes back at an angle toward the small of your back. This is a good thing to know when you are trying to put in tampons for the first time. Your vagina ends after a few inches. Nothing that goes into your vagina can get lost in the rest of your body.

If you reach your middle finger as far up as you can, you should get to a smooth lump that feels like the tip of a nose—or larger, if you've had a baby. This is your *cervix,* the lower part of your uterus, or womb. (If you have trouble reaching it, bring your knees and chest closer together.) Marie said:

I had always thought my womb was so far up in there that I could never touch any part of it. The

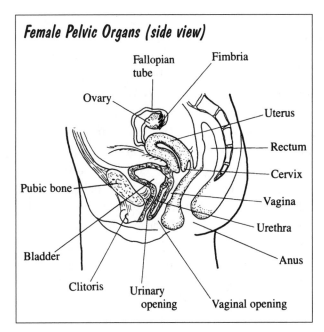

Female Pelvic Organs (side view)

Fallopian tube · Fimbria · Ovary · Uterus · Rectum · Cervix · Vagina · Urethra · Anus · Pubic bone · Bladder · Clitoris · Urinary opening · Vaginal opening

first time I touched my cervix, you could have knocked me over with a feather. Amazing!

You may not always feel your cervix in exactly the same place every day, because your uterus moves slightly during your monthly cycle. Some days you can barely reach it. It also shifts when you are sexually excited.

In the center of your cervix, you should be able to feel a small dimple, called the *os.* About as wide as a straw, it is the opening to your uterus. Blood comes out through your os when you have your period. Believe it or not, when a pregnant woman goes into labor, the os opens up wide enough to let a baby through. Most of the time it is very tiny. No tampon or finger can go through it. No penis can, either. But germs can, so to avoid infections make sure that *everything* you put into your vagina is clean. And if you have intercourse, make sure you are protected against sexually transmitted disease (see page 253). Of course, sperm can go through the os too, so use birth control if you don't want to get pregnant.

An instrument called a speculum can hold the walls of the vagina apart during medical examinations. It opens your vagina, giving a clear view of your cervix, which looks like a small pink doughnut. A doctor or practitioner uses a speculum during a gynecological exam (see page 251), but you can use one too, with a flashlight and mirror. Women's clinics often sell inexpensive clear-plastic speculums for girls and women who want to examine their vaginal walls and cervix.

Your *anus* is the third opening you will come to in your examination. It is where your bowel movements leave your body. It leads from the rectum, where solid wastes are stored. In fact, since only a thin wall of skin separates the vagina from the rectum on the inside, if you have your finger in your vagina you can sometimes feel the feces in your rectum right through the wall. They will feel like a lump in the bottom or back side of the vaginal wall. By the time your pubic hair is fully grown, you will also have hair around your anus.

Your bowel movements have germs in them that can cause infection if they reach your vagina and urethra. After urinating or defecating it is important to wipe yourself from front to back so that the bacteria from the anus do not get into the vagina. Also, in sex play be careful: if a penis or finger has been on or in the anus, don't put it in your vagina without cleaning it first with soap and water.

FURTHER INSIDE: YOUR INTERNAL REPRODUCTIVE ORGANS: Except for your cervix (the lower part of your uterus), internal organs are too far up inside your body for you to see or feel them.

Your *uterus* (*you*-ter-russ) or womb (woom) is an organ about the size of your fist and the shape of an upside-down pear. It has thick walls of strong, stretchy muscles.

Two tubes, called the *fallopian* (fel-*low*-pee-yan) *tubes,* lead out from the top of your uterus, one on each side. They are about 4 inches long, and narrow, about the width of a fine needle. The outer end of each tube has fingerlike fringy ends (*fimbriae*—*fim*-bree-ay) that wrap around your ovary but do not touch it.

You have two *ovaries* (*oh*-vah-rees), one on each side. An ovary is the size and shape of an unshelled almond. Your ovaries make the important female hormones estrogen and progesterone. These hormones are chemicals that travel through your bloodstream when triggered by certain glands and organic processes. They cause most of the changes of puberty.

Both ovaries contain eggs. These eggs, stored in little pockets called *follicles,* are in a girl's ovaries from the day she is born. When you reach puberty, one egg matures each month and leaves the ovary.

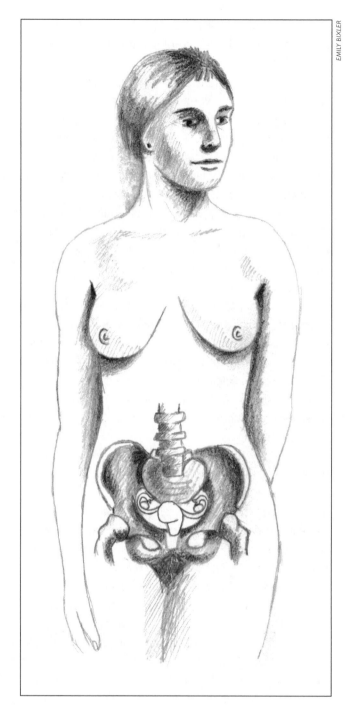

EMILY BIXLER

The fimbriae guide the egg into the fallopian tube. If the egg meets a sperm and becomes fertilized, you get pregnant. If the egg goes unfertilized, you have a period.

Menstruation, or Getting Your Period

Menstruation (men-stroo-*ay*-shun) is part of the process of creation. It connects women to the cycle of life and death and regeneration. In many cultures, it is a time for celebration.

Unless they are pregnant, nursing a baby, very underweight, ill, or have some problem with their reproductive system, all women menstruate for many years of their lives. Yet, in our own society, many girls and boys know very little about menstruation—in fact, many think of it in a negative way. For each young woman, the first time she menstruates is a rite of passage; it means she is joining all womanhood in a monthly cycle of cleansing and renewal. Menstruation is the way a female's body flushes out the old uterine lining and begins to prepare a new lining, making the uterus ready to accept a pregnancy, should one occur. This happens every month.

A woman usually begins her period between the ages of nine and eighteen. The time of the first period is called *menarche* (meh-*nar*-key), and once they begin their period, women usually continue to menstruate for the next thirty to forty-five years. Some women's periods occur at a set interval every month and almost never vary from that schedule— for example, every twenty-eight days or every thirty days. Most women are not this regular, however. Their periods come about every twenty-one to forty days and last from one or two days to a week.

Though there are negative words (like "the curse") for a menstrual period, getting your period is a normal, healthy, important process. Without the female's menstruation or the male's ejaculation, there would be no new human life. Women menstruate when their bodies are able to get pregnant and nourish a developing fetus. They continue to menstruate until their bodies stop producing ripe eggs, sometime between the ages of forty and fifty-five. This is called *menopause* (*men*-oh-pause).

YOUR MENSTRUAL CYCLE: Medical people count your menstrual cycle from the first day your period comes. This is called Day 1. They talk in terms of a twenty-eight-day cycle, just for simplicity. We will, too, to help you understand what goes on. Very few women, in fact, have a twenty-eight-day cycle.

Look at the cycle at Day 5—that is, five days after your period begins. At this point, the pituitary gland near your brain sends a signal to several of the thousands of eggs in your ovaries. Some eggs begin to ripen, but usually only one egg will mature completely. Meanwhile, the ovary sends out the hormone estrogen, which signals your uterine lining to become thicker with blood and tissue.

About Day 14, the ripened egg breaks out of its follicle and rises to the surface of your ovary. This is called *ovulation* (ah-vue-*lay*-shun). You may feel a

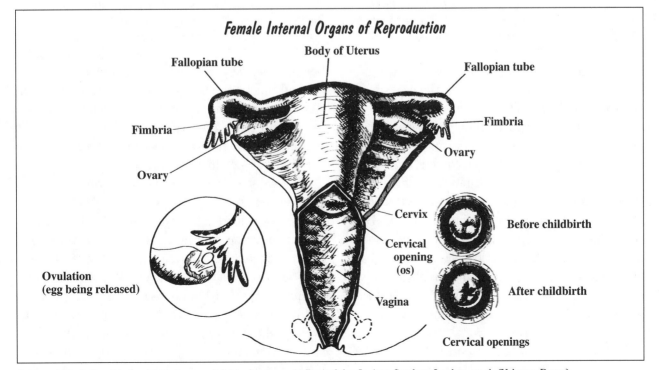

Female Internal Organs of Reproduction

Fallopian tube
Body of Uterus
Fallopian tube
Fimbria
Fimbria
Ovary
Ovary
Cervix
Before childbirth
Cervical opening (os)
Ovulation (egg being released)
After childbirth
Vagina
Cervical openings

* A great book for girls (and boys), ages eight to fourteen, is *Period*, by Jo Ann Gardner-Loulan, et al. (Volcano Press).

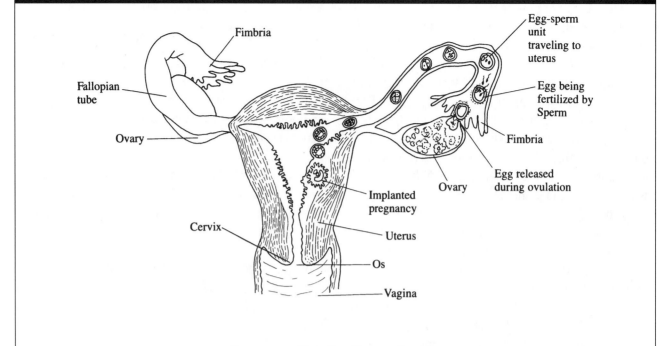

Labels on diagram: Fimbria · Fallopian tube · Ovary · Cervix · Egg-sperm unit traveling to uterus · Egg being fertilized by Sperm · Fimbria · Egg released during ovulation · Ovary · Implanted pregnancy · Uterus · Os · Vagina

Conception: How You Become Pregnant

If you have had sexual intercourse with a man and used no birth control, if your birth control method hasn't worked, or if some semen from a man's penis has gotten close to the lips of your vagina and sperm have swum in, then the sperm will swim up the vagina through the cervical os into the uterus and then into the fallopian tube. The egg just released by the ovary may be penetrated by sperm. This is called *fertilization* or *conception*. Fertilization most often takes place in the fallopian tube. From there the fertilized egg takes about six days to move through the tube to the uterus, where it attaches itself to the inner uterine *wall*, or *lining*, and grows for about nine months.

While you are *pregnant*, hormonal signals sent to the uterine lining keep it thick and nourishing for the developing fetus. Because the lining is in use, you don't get your period. Not getting your period is one of the signs of pregnancy (see pages 49 and 313).

cramp or twinge in your lower abdomen or back when you ovulate. After it is released, the egg is guided into the fallopian tube. Meanwhile, the ruptured follicle produces the hormone progesterone, which causes the uterine lining to continue its buildup. If the egg has *not* been fertilized (if it has not accepted sperm), after two or three days it breaks apart and disintegrates. At that point, the estrogen and progesterone signals to your uterus weaken. By Day 24, they have stopped. The uterine lining starts to break up. By Day 28, it has loosened so much that bits of it start to break off and come out of your cervix and vagina, and menstruation begins. This is Day 1 again. Five days later the cycle starts all over again. We call this the *menstrual cycle*.

As you can see, ovulation occurs before menstruation. That is why it is possible to get pregnant before your first period ever comes. Some girls get a kind of "practice" period a few times before ovulation starts, as their body adjusts to the new level of hormones, but other girls ovulate first. If they are having unprotected intercourse, they can get pregnant even before they begin menstruating.

What comes out of your vagina during your period looks like blood and is usually called blood, because the blood in it makes it red, but it's really a mixture of tissue, mucus, and blood. So when a clump of it comes out all at once we may call it a clot, but it is not a blood clot. You do lose *some* blood during your period, but not as much as it may seem.

You may have *cramps* when the muscles of your uterus tighten up to push the menstrual fluid out, and when the muscles of your cervix open the os a little bit to let it out. Some girls experience very heavy cramping with menstruation; some girls experience little or none (see the box on page 44, Helping Yourself Feel Better).

WHEN WILL YOUR FIRST PERIOD COME? You have no definite way of knowing when you will menstruate for the first time. Usually, you start about two years after your breasts begin to develop and one year after your pubic hair begins to grow. When *you* begin will depend on your health and on when the women in your mother's or father's family began their periods. There's no particular time when you "should" start. Menstruation comes according to your body's own time.

Two girls talk about waiting for their first period:

Lisa (eleven): I'm glad I haven't gotten my period yet. I'm still a kid. No way do I want to worry about that every month.

Toni (sixteen): I wish I would get it already. Just about everyone I know has it, and I feel like a freak not having it yet. Like friends come up to me and say, "Oh, do you have a Tampax I could borrow?" and then they'll say, "Oh, sorry, I forgot you don't have it yet."

When your period comes for the first time, it can be a big event. Sally, a twelve-year-old from Buffalo, described her first time:

The whole weekend I had this terrible stomachache, but I just thought it was a stomachache. Then on Saturday night while I was in the bathroom, I saw this brownish stuff in my pants and I thought, No, it couldn't be . . . because it was brown and I thought a period was red. So I didn't put a sanitary napkin on or anything. Then in the morning I had this big mess in my pajamas and that's when I knew for sure. I was really excited. I was sort of waiting for it to come, because I have an older sister who got her period around her twelfth birthday.

As Sally described, sometimes the menstrual fluid is not bright red, but brownish or dark reddish-brown. This is normal and has to do with the

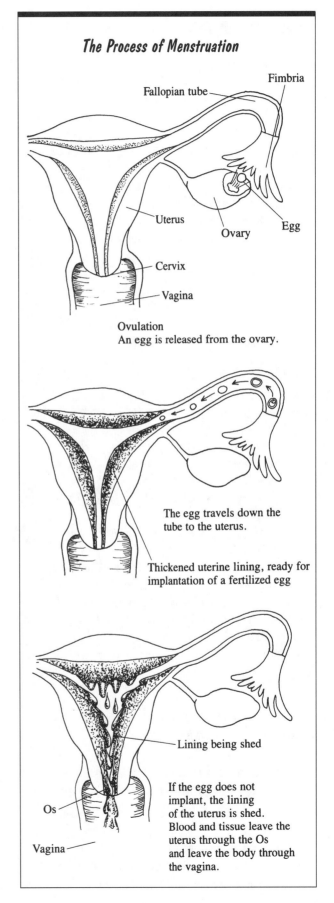

The Process of Menstruation

Fimbria
Fallopian tube
Uterus
Ovary
Egg
Cervix
Vagina

Ovulation
An egg is released from the ovary.

The egg travels down the tube to the uterus.

Thickened uterine lining, ready for implantation of a fertilized egg

Lining being shed

Os

Vagina

If the egg does not implant, the lining of the uterus is shed. Blood and tissue leave the uterus through the Os and leave the body through the vagina.

I AM WOMAN

As time goes by,
the memories remain, the laughter, the joys,
even the great depth of pain.

Remembering when you started to walk,
remembering when you fell—that first fall
      was great.
Knowing someone was there.
I wonder what it would have been like
if no one was there,
      that first step may have been the last.
The first day of school and you couldn't
      reach the water fountain,
      tried to get up to your chair—it was too
      tall.
When you had to go to the bathroom and
      couldn't undo your clothes.

As time goes by
the memories remain,
that first pain and discomfort of being a
      woman
not knowing who to tell—or what to do.
Your body flows of red rivers and your
      mind races in time,
remembering your mother walking in your
      room saying,
"You're a young lady now, and ladies don't
      run around
with a lot of little boys playing boyish
      games.
You should sit properly and dress neatly."
Never did she tell me that it was okay that
      I am
      Woman.

                                   —ANNETTE BARNES

makeup of the discharge and the way it changes color when exposed to air over time.

NOT FEELING READY: Some girls are not ready for their period to begin. Either they haven't been told it will come, or they don't feel grown-up enough:

Crystal: I didn't know what was happening. I had these cramps and a headache, so I went to the bathroom, but it wasn't like I had the flu or anything. I didn't know what I had. When I got up from the toilet I noticed this blood in there, and then I saw some blood on my thigh, so I started to scream. I thought I was bleeding to death. Nobody told me about periods; nobody told me about anything. I was in the fifth grade and I still thought babies grew in your stomach and came out your belly button. I can't believe how scared I was.

Holly: When I got my period it wasn't okay with me, and I cried and cried, because I never thought I'd ever actually get my period. I was eleven and I remember crying and thinking, Oh, now I'm a woman and I'm too young to be a woman. I was such a kid. I was so upset I didn't want to tell my mom at first. I had this crazy idea that she was going to be mad at me for getting it, but when she saw how upset I was, she asked me what was wrong. I finally told her. She turned out to be wonderful about it and really made me feel better.

BEING READY: Being ready for your period makes a big difference. It helps if someone—a parent, aunt, sister, friend, teacher—has told you ahead of time what to expect. Most schools try to teach girls (unfortunately, rarely the boys!) something about menstruation, but often those classes start after half the girls already have their periods. A good idea might be to get together with a few friends and talk about it. Or encourage your school to start a good discussion group for both sexes, so that more of you will understand what is happening and be prepared for it.

Darlene is luckier than some girls. At twelve, she said:

I'm ready for it when it comes. I sent away for that Kotex kit—you know, where they send you this book about it and some pads and stuff. And my mom showed me how to wear a pad, so when it comes I'll be prepared.

There are a lot of mothers like Darlene's, who give their daughters the help they need in getting ready for their period. If your mother hasn't been much help, remember that *her* mother may not have told her anything. She may have no practice in talk-

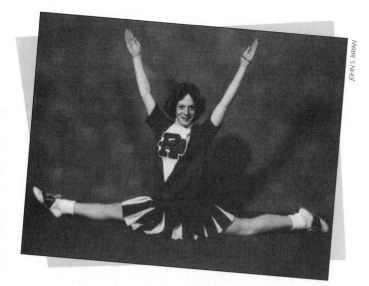

JOHN S. BRYAN

ing about these things. Maybe reading this chapter with you would give her a chance to talk with you in a way she'd really like to. But even if you can't learn what you need to know from your mother, you do have a right to information. Perhaps a teacher or school counselor or another relative will be able to help.

Many cultures have strong traditions surrounding menstruation, but our western culture doesn't. It is reassuring when a girl grows up in a society that has a ritual for celebrating the arrival of menses. Short of those rites, many families find ways to start their own menstruation rituals. Some parents take their daughters out for a special dinner or they prepare a family feast in her honor. Some girls go out for a special day just with their mothers or another important adult woman in their life. Some girls light a candle to signify the onset of a new stage in their development.

YOUR FEELINGS ABOUT BEGINNING TO MENSTRUATE:
Girls have a lot of feelings about menstruating. Some are proud, like Karen and Ginny:

> I got my period early, when I was in fourth grade, and all my friends were jealous. They wanted to get theirs too.

> I told everybody when I got my period. Everybody! I celebrated and went out and bought myself a present.

Menstruation makes a big change in your life. What's happening to your body is new. It's natural to feel strange at first, full of mixed emotions.

Some, as we have seen, are embarrassed about being the first one of their friends to get their period, embarrassed to be so young, shy to tell their parents and their friends:

> *Alice:* My friends sort of teased me when I got my period—like something was wrong with me for developing faster than them. I think I was a little ashamed of myself for getting it. No one told me it was something to be proud of.

> *Charlotte:* When my best friend moved away, we swore to each other that we would tell the other one when one of us got our period. Well, she got it and she didn't tell me, and I had a funny feeling about that. She sort of got shyer. It was like she was ashamed she got it.

> *Ruthanne:* I didn't want to tell my mother when I got it, because I thought she would be mad at me for knowing what it was. I thought she was going to think I was dirty for having it so young.

We believe that girls feel embarrassment and shame not because menstruation is shameful but because our society has a negative attitude toward menstruation. Many people in our culture are uncomfortable about bodies, and women's bodies in particular. Too many girls and women suffer needlessly because of these attitudes.

ATTITUDES TOWARD MENSTRUATION: Throughout history in many societies women have been sent to special houses on the days they menstruate. Some cultures consider menstruation such a powerful event they have special rules about what menstruating women can and cannot do. In many societies, men are not supposed to have sexual relations with menstruating women. If you were a girl growing up in a society that had definite rituals associated with menstruation, you would know what you could and could not do and you would not be alone. Everyone menstruating at the same time you were would be with you. Your menses would not be secret and private; it would be part of the natural order of things and public knowledge. You wouldn't feel ashamed to be having your period.

Menstruation was and is revered as a sacred activity in some cultures. Women who menstruate are honored as a symbol of the earth's regeneration process, which allows that each month the cycle will begin anew, like the moon's cycle. Menstruation is seen as a sign of hope. There are special festivals to honor a girl at the onset of menstruation.

Imagine what it would be like to grow up in a society that honored you just for becoming a woman, in a society in which bodily functions were considered normal and positive aspects of life.

Menstrual blood *is* a special kind of blood. It doesn't come from sickness or injury. It is related to a woman's ability to give birth, and that ability was and still is a power that only women have. Thousands of years ago, before much was known about the physiology of periods and childbirth, some men might have been jealous of that power or afraid of it, and some of the negative attitudes we in this society have learned about menstruation may come in part from that fear or jealousy. Here are some untrue statements about menstruation you may have heard: "Menstruating women shouldn't water plants." "Menstruating women shouldn't exercise." "You shouldn't have sexual relations during your period." You may have been told that you shouldn't take a bath or wash your hair or feed your dog or cook or go swimming when you have your period. These false beliefs restrict women and make them think they are helpless and less "normal" than men.

Today women in our society are questioning attitudes like these. You and your friends can too. If you ever find yourself or a friend feeling ashamed or bad about having her period, remember that it's a healthy event, an event to celebrate. While you are having your period you may not feel like doing certain things, and you can honor that, but you don't *have* to restrict your activities if you don't want to. You and your friends can learn about women through the ages who have menstruated, borne children, made history, healed one another, been strong.

SOME DIFFICULT MOMENTS: Our attitudes about menstruation won't change overnight, and even if they did, people would still get embarrassed at times, for hundreds of reasons. Many girls, and older women too, talked to us about their fear of getting

caught without a pad or tampon, or of getting blood on their clothes. Nancy remembers:

> This didn't happen to me, it happened to my friend Paula, but I've always prayed it wouldn't happen to me! She went to the movies with a bunch of kids. She sat on her legs for some of the movie. Her period came right in the middle and she didn't know it. When the lights came on there was blood all over her white knee socks. She was so mortified!

Your period won't necessarily start when you're at home. Some months, it comes when you're in school, on a date, or at work, when you're not expecting it. Because we were raised to think about menstruation as something to keep private and secret, when our periods become "public" we may find it difficult to accept. Debby, a thirteen-year-old from Denver, said:

> My mom and I were out shopping and I got my period right then and we didn't have anything with us, so we had to go to the drugstore to get some pads. Just as we were going up to the counter I saw a boy I knew from school. I almost died. He didn't see me, but my heart started beating like mad and I turned bright red. As soon as the lady at the counter put my stuff in a bag I felt so much better, but then as we were walking out, we ran into him and I could hardly even say "Hello" to him, I was so nervous, thinking, Oh my God, what am I going to do if this bag rips!

A fifteen-year-old from Los Angeles said:

> That was the most embarrassing thing I've ever done in my whole life, buying my first box of tampons. I'll never forget. I was in the store and I kept waiting until the guy at the register went into the back. I waited and waited until there was a lady there, and then I bought something else that I absolutely did not need just so I could hide the box of Tampax behind it. I really needed a big box, but I only bought a small one so I wouldn't be so conspicuous.

Belinda's story is one of the most dramatic:

> My mother always told me, when you have your period you take off the used pad and wrap it up in toilet paper and throw it in the wastebasket right away. Well, I was at my girlfriend's house and I was in the bathroom and I had my period, so I took off the old pad and put it up on the top of the toilet while I was putting the new one on because I couldn't find the wastebasket. For some reason, I totally forgot about the old pad sitting up there on the toilet and I walked out of the bathroom and left it there. Her brother went into the bathroom a few minutes later and found it. I wanted to die. He was older and he knew about girls getting their periods—plus he had three sisters, so that had probably happened to him before anyway—so he was pretty understanding. He made a little joke about it and made me laugh, but still I was dying inside. I made some excuse and went home real soon after that and I went into my room and started crying. My girlfriend was really nice about it the next day in school, and she didn't tell anybody, but I waited a long time before I went over to her house again.

Those kinds of experiences are common. When Belinda was telling her story, one of the other girls in the room said, "Oh my God, the same thing happened to me, but it was my cousin who saw it and he teased me about it for weeks."

Lots of girls are teased by boys about having their period. Most boys can't be blamed—probably no one has told them what is going on, and they are nervous. If someone takes the time to talk to boys about menstruation, they are usually interested in a serious way.

PREDICTING YOUR MENSTRUAL CYCLE: Some women have regular menstrual cycles; others have irregular cycles. Many teenagers have unpredictable cycles, at least in the beginning. In a discussion group, Carrie said, "My sister went for almost a year with only one period. When I first got mine, six months passed without another one." Mark commented, "It must be scary if you sleep with a guy because you never know if you are pregnant or not."

He's right: if you have very irregular periods and you have sexual intercourse without using protection, you may not be able to tell if you are pregnant for several months. Sometimes just worrying about being pregnant can make your period come late.

Being irregular can be puzzling and frustrating. You may be regular for a while, then skip a month, or be late because of events and pressures in your life. You may lose or gain a lot of weight, go on a trip, get sick, or worry a lot about something, and all these can affect your period. It's amazing how connected our minds and bodies are. At some point your menstrual cycle will probably settle into its own pattern. As you grow older that may change again.

There are ways of knowing when your period is due:

1. Find out the average length of your cycle. You have your own rhythm. Even if your periods seem to come in no regular pattern, try keeping track of them on a calendar for six months. Each month mark an X on Day 1, the day your period starts. After six months, count the number of days from Day 1 of one cycle to Day 1 of the next. Add the number of days in all the cycles together and divide by six (the number of months) to find out your average cycle length. If the length of your cycle varies greatly from month to month, the calendar method won't be helpful for predicting, but it is always useful to have a record of when your last period came.

2. You may notice some body signs. For instance, when you ovulate you may get a pain or cramp in your back or abdomen. Two weeks after ovulation, your period should start. Often your breasts feel bigger, heavier, and lumpier after ovulation and before menstruation. Familiarize yourself with how your breasts feel. If they change, mark it down and notice when your period comes.

You may get headaches or backaches just before your period. You may not sleep well. Your face may break out in pimples, or you may feel depressed, moody, or cranky. Some or all of these signs can mean that your period is about to begin.

3. Another way of figuring out your cycle may seem complicated at first but in fact is pretty accurate. It's called the mucus method. At the time of ovulation, your vaginal mucus is runny and wet.

Closer to your period it gets thicker and dryer. You can learn to tell the difference simply by how wet or dry the lips of your vagina feel, or by putting your finger into your vagina to test the mucus closer to your cervix. About fourteen days after the day of runniest mucus, you'll get your period. (This method is used by some women as a form of birth control. See page 309.)

KNOWING ABOUT SIDE EFFECTS: Menstruation brings a number of side effects. Some women experience none of them; others experience just a few. Some of these side effects are headaches, backaches, skin problems, mood changes, depression, cramps, nausea, and water retention (when the liquids you drink tend to stay in your body and you feel puffy and heavy). Many women find that as they grow older some of the painful symptoms become less severe or go away.

You may not even notice that your period is coming and not feel any different at all. You may feel heavy or more tired than usual before your period but be fine once the flow starts. Gini, at sixteen, is a swimmer and a lacrosse player:

My period is no problem, and it never really was. When I first got it, I got it when I woke up one morning, and even now, four years later, it still usually comes in the morning, so I almost always know I have it before I go to school. I also had no trouble learning how to use tampons—I used them right from the beginning. And I hardly ever get cramps. I mean, I feel so lucky about that. Some of my friends really get pretty bad cramps, they even have to miss classes sometimes, but for me my period doesn't affect my life at all.

For other people, it's not so easy. Ruthanne is sixteen too, and has the opposite experience from Gini:

Helping Yourself Feel Better

If you have painful periods and/or depressing premenstrual moods, here are some things that women have discovered help to make them feel better. You and your friends may also discover some of your own remedies. Since each woman's body is unique, some of the remedies will work for you and some won't. Pay attention to how the remedy you choose affects you.

1. Watch your own body signs so you can begin to notice when your period is due. Then you'll be able to plan your schedule around whichever days are hardest for you. You'll be able to take steps like watching your diet or getting exercise or getting enough sleep when you know you'll need it. (See the section "Predicting Your Menstrual Cycle," page 43.)

2. Watch what you eat. If you know when your period is due, cut down on salty foods before and during. Salt makes your body retain water. Water retention can add to your feeling of heaviness and swelling during your period, as well as to tension and depression beforehand. Salt—in chips, pretzels, nuts, spicy foods, soy sauce—can make you more uncomfortable than you need to be. For about ten days before your period, also cut down on sugar, white flour, and caffeine. This list covers a whole lot of what you eat and you may not be able to cut down on them all at once. But try to avoid cola drinks, chocolate, coffee, soft drinks, junk foods, and most cakes, pies, and breads.

Alcohol, too—especially wine and beer—may increase cramping and headaches. Drink natural fruit juices. Some herbal teas—raspberry-leaf tea, for instance—are soothing and may help relieve cramps.

If you have very painful periods, you might ask a nutritionist to recommend a special diet with vitamin and mineral supplements. Experiment to see what works well for you. Eat well-balanced meals. You might find that when you change your diet you'll feel better in general.

3. Some women find that taking several dolomite calcium tablets and vitamin C supplements each day for a week before their period helps to relieve tension and depression. You can buy these tablets in a drugstore or health-food store.

4. If you have heavy menstrual flows, iron supplements are recommended to help you avoid anemia. Blackstrap molasses contains B vitamins, which help you absorb iron, and calcium, which reduces cramping.

5. If your cramps are severe, you may feel better if you lie down and relax your whole body. That's easier said than done, because when you are in pain your body almost automatically tenses up. Tenseness often comes from a fear that there's something wrong because you're hurting so much. Tell yourself there's nothing wrong. Remind yourself that your body is just working to let out the old uterine lining. Many women have learned to keep themselves from tensing up by breathing deeply and slowly, and by keeping their bodies as relaxed as possible.

Childbirth breathing techniques are very helpful. Lie on

I hate my period. I almost always get really bad cramps, and for about a week before it comes I am the biggest bitch and I cry at the drop of a hat. I hate it. I never know when it's coming, and even now, after I've had it for three years, it's so irregular that sometimes I skip a whole month. I know a lot of people who don't have any problems with their period at all, but for me it's the biggest problem of my life.

Connie is a senior from Los Angeles who is on the drill team and exercises all the time. She said:

You know, I thought that I was going to die the first few times I got my period, the cramps were so bad. Even now, even with all the exercise I get, I still have at least a day with such bad cramps that I can't even go to school. The only thing that helps is if I stay in bed with a heating pad. And I bleed so much I always have to bring another pair of pants with me to change into. I go through everything, even when I wear a tampon and a napkin both.

Some people, like Connie, suffer from bad cramps and heavy bleeding. Usually the worst cramps last only a day or two, but for these girls, these are days each month when their lives are disrupted.

For other women, the week or few days before their period arrives is the most difficult time. They feel tense and depressed. They are even more likely to fall or hurt themselves accidentally. Molly keeps being surprised:

This month it happened again! I was feeling real depressed. I had this terrible fight with my best friend, and I thought we'd never talk to each other again. When I woke up the next morning, I wanted to crawl back down under the covers and not go

---

your side or sit up with your back supported by pillows. Get as comfortable as you can. Then take a full breath in and blow it all out. Repeat that deep breath. Then begin breathing deeply so that you can see your stomach rise with each breath in and fall as you breathe out. Make sure you blow out all the air very slowly. Keep up that deep stomach breathing for as long as you feel cramps.

You may notice that your cramps come in waves. Their strength rises and falls. Try breathing with the waves.

6. Gently massaging your stomach or your back may help. In childbirth this gentle rubbing is called effleurage. It is very relaxing. Someone else can do it for you, or you can do it for yourself while you are breathing deeply.

A back rub or whole-body massage will often relieve cramps caused by tension. Apply pressure on your tail-bone (coccyx) by hitting or pounding it with your fists or pressing into it with your knuckles or fingers. Work only as hard as is comfortable. You can do this yourself or ask someone else to do it. You can find other kinds of menstrual and general massages in books on yoga, shiatsu, polarity therapy, etc.

7. A hot-water bottle or a heating pad on your stomach or back may help. Also a warm washcloth on your forehead may make you feel better. Some people prefer a cold washcloth. That's up to you.

8. Sometimes curling up in a knee-to-chest position with a hot-water bottle or heating pad on your back helps. Try to keep yourself relaxed, though.

9. For some women, having an orgasm or being sexually aroused helps to ease the pain and tension and also helps to start the flow of your period.

10. Many women find that aspirin brings fast and complete relief from cramping. Unless you are allergic to aspirin—which is rare—small doses should not cause any serious side effects.

11. Exercising throughout the month and getting enough sleep in the week before your period can relieve your symptoms and will make you feel better in general.

12. Some doctors prescribe the birth control pill to help ease the side effects of menstruation. The birth control pill causes you to stop ovulating, which means your hormone balance of estrogen and progesterone will be more steady. Consequently, some women feel less tension and pain during their periods when they are taking the birth control pill. Also, women on the pill tend to have shorter periods.

We do not recommend the birth control pill for young teenage women, and many doctors don't, either. Since it takes your body about a year, and sometimes more than a year, to get used to the cycle of ovulation and menstruation, it doesn't seem like a good idea to tamper with that process—at least not until it is firmly established. Also, introducing human-made hormones into your system has its own dangers. (See pages 301–305 for a complete discussion of the birth control pill.)

to school or see anyone. Then that afternoon I got my period. You'd think I'd remember when I'm feeling bad that my period's due soon. When it comes it doesn't change my situation, but it changes how I'm looking at it. I'd save myself some grief by remembering.

For Molly, keeping a calendar would help (see page 43).

Some people say they appreciate the changes in their moods. "Usually, I try to act happy a lot even when things are troubling me," said one woman in her thirties. "So when I get real moody and vulnerable for a few days before my period, it gives me a chance to know the darker part of my feelings."

A number of people feel better than usual around the time of their period, especially when they are feeling good about themselves that month. There are many different ways you can feel.

WHY SIDE EFFECTS? We don't know as much as we'd like about the side effects of menstruation and why some women seem to suffer more than others. People may try to tell you that your menstrual side effects are "all in your head." Those girls who get bad cramps know the pain is not just in their head! But what causes cramps and premenstrual tension?

While most people agree that there *are* real physical causes, they don't agree on *what* causes menstrual side effects. Three theories have been suggested:

1. Muscle contractions in your uterus and cervix may cause pain and cramping. Your uterus contracts to push out the old lining. It clenches like a fist, especially when there are "clots" to expel. At the same time, your cervix pulls itself open a tiny bit to let the blood and tissue out.

2. The low level of estrogen and progesterone in your body just before your period causes many of the side effects, including depression.

3. An excess of hormone-like substances called *prostaglandins* may cause your uterus to tighten with more sustained force than the normally pain-free rhythmic contractions of the uterus. This tightening may block oxygen from reaching the uterine and intestinal muscles, and it is the lack of oxygen

that creates the pain. (There are some antiprostaglandin drugs, which help some women. Check with your local health facility.)

TAKING CARE OF YOURSELF DURING MENSTRUATION: If you suffer from cramps or weight gain or depression because of your period, you can do certain things to make yourself feel better. Women have been passing these hints along and making up new ones for generations. In the box beginning on page 44, you'll find a list of ideas, some old as the centuries and some new.

Lorie, a twenty-five-year-old woman from Massachusetts, described how she learned to take care of herself:

When I first got my period, I was twelve and a half, and for the next three or four years I had very painful periods. I used to get so tense when I felt the cramps that I'd just curl up in a tight ball or run around the room or just cry because I couldn't stand it and I didn't know what else to do. My mother and I found some things that seemed to work to make me feel better. Like first of all, when I learned to stop fighting the cramps and just go with them, just relax and breathe with them, I found they were really not constant pain, but just kind of short waves of pain. When the wave would come, my mother or I would rub my stomach and I'd try to relax. I liked using a hot-water bottle or a heating pad—the heat always made me feel more comfortable. And my mother—she really was pretty terrific—would make me some tea, and I'd sip that hot tea, and something about that ritual made me feel so much better. Even now when I'm feeling tense or sick, I like to crawl into bed and have a cup of hot tea. It makes me feel taken care of.

WHAT TO USE FOR THE FLOW: Women in different cultures have used many different methods to soak up the menstrual flow. Since earliest times, women have made tampons and pads using natural materials like sponges, grasses, or bits of cloth. Your great-great-grandmother may have used rags, which she washed out in cold water each night, because while cold water washes blood stains away, hot water sets them.

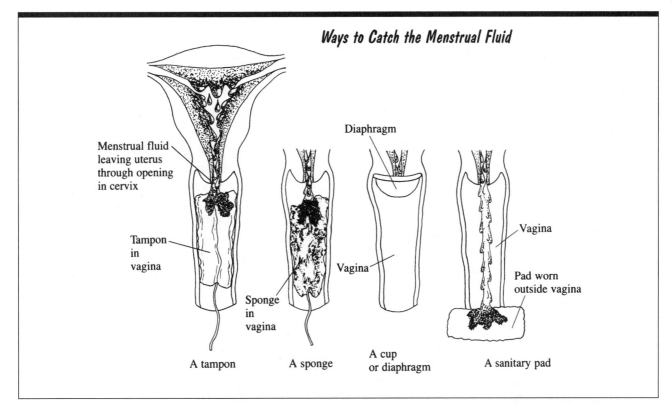

Ways to Catch the Menstrual Fluid

Menstrual fluid leaving uterus through opening in cervix

Tampon in vagina

Sponge in vagina

Diaphragm

Vagina

Vagina

Pad worn outside vagina

A tampon   A sponge   A cup or diaphragm   A sanitary pad

A woman today in the United States has a choice among commercial sanitary pads and tampons, natural sponges, and cups. You might end up trying all of them before you find the one you like using best.

Sanitary Pads. Most girls start out using *sanitary pads.* These are rectangular pads of cotton, usually with a plastic lining either between the cotton layers or on the outside. They have a sticky strip that sticks to your underpants. You wear one in your underpants until it is nearly soaked with menstrual flow, then change it for a fresh one. Pads come in different sizes and thicknesses, and a few different shapes.

NELS ISRAELSON

Sanitary pads come in different sizes and thicknesses.

When the menstrual fluid hits the air outside your body, it dries and can develop a stale odor, so you'll probably want to change your pad several times a day and wash the area daily with water and mild soap. Do not use pads with deodorant or perfume, as these chemicals can irritate your vagina.

Pads may seem bulky and strange at first. Alice said:

> When I tried on a maxi pad for the first time, I felt like a cowboy—like I was walking bowlegged. I was so self-conscious all day long. I was sure that everybody could tell by the way I walked that I was wearing one.

Actually, no one can tell you have one on—it just feels that way.

Some girls feel embarrassed at first when they buy pads or when they carry around a purse just for their extra pads. A sixth-grader from San Francisco devised a very imaginative way to handle her embarrassment:

> What do you do when you have to change your pad at school? That really worried me when I first

got my period, because I always felt kind of obvious carrying my backpack to the bathroom on the days when I had my period. Also, it was creepy for me to have to buy pads in the machine in the girls' room, so I always wear knee socks under my pants when I have my period. I stick an extra pad in each sock and then I always have them with me when I go to the bathroom and have to change. It works fine. But I can't wait until my mom lets me use Tampax.

Tampons. A *tampon* is made of soft cotton pressed together into a hard, compact cylinder. It fits into your vagina, where it expands as it soaks up the menstrual fluid. You push a tampon in with your fingers or with the applicator that comes with some brands. It has a string that hangs from it outside your vagina; to take it out, you pull the string.

The material in a tampon holds lots of fluid, so you may not have to change it as often as you would change a pad. On the other hand, if you are flowing heavily, you may have to change the tampon often and use a pad or minipad too, for extra protection.

Since the tampon sits inside your vagina, it can't be seen. And since no air gets at it, it doesn't have any odor. You can swim more comfortably with a tampon than with a pad.

Each package of tampons comes with directions explaining how to insert them. But even with written directions, it's sometimes hard to figure out the first few times you try. Lots of girls have spent hot, sweaty hours in the bathroom trying to get their first few tampons in. The best thing is to have a friend or mother or sister show you how to put it in. Remember, your vagina angles back; it doesn't go straight up. Allison, eighteen, told us:

I was away at boarding school when I got my period for the first time, and my friends all came into the bathroom with me to teach me how to put in a tampon. One girl gave me this hand mirror to use so I could see my vagina better. So I was like wandering around in the bathroom holding this mirror up to my vagina trying to stick this tampon in at just the right angle. It's a good thing nobody had a camera!

Lisa, who's now thirty-five, said:

We were raised Catholic and didn't know anything. One of my big sisters conned me into putting the tampon up my urethra. *Ouch!*

Some girls worry that the tampon will get lost, but except for the tiny hole in the cervix leading up to your uterus, your vagina doesn't open into the rest of your body. There is *no way* you can push the tampon up too far or lose it in there. You *can* forget to pull them out, though. So if you use tampons when you menstruate, remember to check for one each time you urinate.

Pull on the string to remove the tampon, and when you remove it, wrap it up with tissue or toilet paper or newspaper and throw it away in a wastebasket. That goes for pads too. Do *not* throw them in the toilet. Pads will definitely clog plumbing, and tampons often do too.

Sonya, aged thirteen, told us:

My mom told me I couldn't use tampons. She said I was too young. I think that's stupid. What's age got to do with it?

Sonya's mother might think she's too young because she is associating tampon use with sex. Many girls have been taught not to put anything inside their vagina, and of course that means a penis most of all. Tampons are not going to affect your virginity because the term "virginity" applies to whether or not a person has had sexual intercourse. As we explained on page 34, many girls are born with no hymen at all, and many others have a large opening in their hymen. Actually, using a tampon may stretch a tight hymen, but this is not harmful.

There is another reason to be careful about using tampons, however, and that is a disease called toxic shock syndrome.

TOXIC SHOCK SYNDROME: Toxic shock syndrome (TSS)* seems to strike a small number of menstruating women under thirty years of age, about one in

---

* Thanks to the Boston Women's Health Book Collective, especially to our late dear friend and colleague Esther Rome (1945–1995), for the information on toxic shock syndrome and tampon use.

10,000. Some young women have died from it. Not much is known about how or why the disease affects certain women and not others, but researchers have linked the disease in many cases to the use of tampons. The higher the absorbency of the tampon, the higher the risk of TSS. The disease also seems to be associated with how long the tampon is worn.

CHANGE YOUR TAMPON REGULARLY,
AND DON'T USE TAMPONS DURING
THE NIGHT WHILE YOU SLEEP.

TSS may be linked to the acid-base balance in a particular woman's vagina. This balance can be affected by a variety of factors, including what form of birth control a woman uses. (See *The New Our Bodies, Ourselves* for more information.)

You can reduce your risk of getting TSS by not using tampons during menstruation. But many women enjoy the comfort and convenience of tampons so much, they have continued to use them despite the TSS scare. Here are some hints for using tampons that will lower your risk of getting the disease:

1. Use a tampon with the lowest absorbency you can. Absorbency is the amount of liquid or blood a tampon will hold. A used tampon should slide out easily when you pull on the string. It is too absorbent if it sticks to the inside of your vagina. Use the smaller tampons and change them frequently.

2. Do not use perfumed or "deodorant" tampons. These tampons have chemicals in them that may irritate your vagina and cause soreness. You don't need deodorants in your vagina at any time, since the vagina has its own natural cleansing process. Menstrual odor can be avoided by regularly changing your pad or tampon and bathing every day. Some girls have been told not to bathe or shower when they have their period. That is poor advice. Keeping clean is especially good for you during menstruation.

3. Find out the ingredients of the tampon. On the box, it tells what the tampon is made of. Plain non-chlorine bleached cotton is the first best choice; plain rayon is the second. Avoid "superabsorbent" materials.

4. Plastic applicators can pinch. If you use them, be sure the tampon is completely inside the applicator, so the flap edges are not exposed. The flap edges can pinch, causing tears in the vagina lining, which may lead to infection.

Symptoms of Toxic Shock Syndrome

➤ Fever, especially over 102 F

➤ Nausea and vomiting

➤ Diarrhea

➤ Dizziness or feeling faint

➤ A painless, red sunburnlike rash

If you get any of these symptoms during your period and you are using a tampon, REMOVE IT IMMEDIATELY AND GET MEDICAL ATTENTION RIGHT AWAY. TSS can be life-threatening. Tell the doctor you think you might have toxic shock syndrome, so he or she knows what to look for.

SOME PROBLEMS RELATED TO UNUSUAL MENSTRUAL SYMPTOMS

Pregnancy. If you have been having sexual intercourse or petting heavily, with a boy ejaculating in or near your vagina, and you miss a period, the first thing to consider is pregnancy. Go to the local health facility and have a pregnancy test. (See pages 316–317 for more information on pregnancy testing, including home tests.)

Ectopic Pregnancy. If a fertilized egg doesn't implant in your uterus but gets stuck in your fallopian tube and starts growing there, you have a tubal, or ectopic, pregnancy. When the fetus grows too big, the tube usually bursts. You will probably miss your period as you would with a normal pregnancy, and before the tube bursts you will feel very severe sharp pains in your abdomen, chest, and/or shoulder. Go to a doctor immediately; a burst tube brings internal bleeding and other serious symptoms that can lead to death.

Ectopic pregnancies are not common, but if you have had an infection in your fallopian tubes because of pelvic inflammatory disease (see below), your chances of having an ectopic pregnancy are greater.

During the healing process after an infection, scar tissue can form, creating pockets and obstacles in the tube, which sometimes block the sperm–egg unit from reaching the uterus.

Endometriosis (en-doh-mee-tree-o-sis).

When the tissue that usually grows in the lining of the uterus begins to grow in other places, such as your vagina, urinary tract, or bowel, you have endometriosis. Its symptoms are very painful periods that may last a long time and be quite heavy. Your period may also come more frequently than usual— for example, every twenty-four days or less.

Some Problem Signs

Many of the premenstrual and menstrual symptoms we've discussed happen to most of us at one time or another. When we lose or gain a lot of weight, when we travel or get sick or worry a lot, our period might be affected. Sometimes it just doesn't come at all, or sometimes it comes early or late. There may be times when we have a very heavy flow and other times when our flow is really light. Our mind and our body work together, so whenever we experience problems or changes, we might also experience irregular menstrual symptoms.

Sometimes, however, our body is signaling us that something is not working right. In that case it is important to have a medical checkup to find out what's going on. Some signs that mean a checkup is in order are:

➢ a very heavy menstrual flow that lasts more than four or five days
➢ severe menstrual cramping or pain that lasts more than three days each month
➢ a sudden irregularity in your cycle that isn't due to sickness, travel, or weight gain or loss if suddenly your period doesn't come one month and there's no reasonable explanation
➢ bleeding in the middle of your cycle or at any time other than during your period
➢ severe cramps at times other than when your period is due

These five symptoms are warning signs that something might be interfering with the normal functioning of your body, and they mean you should see a doctor.

Endometriosis is more common among twenty-, thirty-, and forty-year-olds than it is among teenagers. Treatment for this disorder varies. If your doctor advises surgery to remove the extra tissue, you may want to check the diagnosis with another physician. (Check *The New Our Bodies, Ourselves* for more on this subject.)

Pelvic Inflammatory Disease (PID).

"PID" is a general name for different infections in the pelvic area, the area around your uterus and vagina. Symptoms of PID are extreme cramping during periods, irregular bleeding, cramps even when you're not having your period, general pelvic pain, and sometimes chills and fever. Gonorrhea and chlamydia are major causes of PID, but other infections cause it as well. Sometimes PID is a problematic side effect if you use an IUD for birth control. Treatment for PID is a heavy course of antibiotics, lots of rest, and no sexual intercourse for at least two weeks after you begin treatment. PID can cause scar tissue to form in your fallopian tubes, which may result in ectopic pregnancy or infertility (inability to get pregnant). If you have severe, long-lasting abdominal pain and have been sexually active, go to a physician at once.

Fibroids and Cysts.

"Tumor" is the medical word that means growth or swelling. Fibroid tumors are noncancerous growths in the uterus. Growths can also develop in the ovaries. Cystic growths are generally filled with fluid, and most will go away on their own without surgery. Any type of uterine or ovarian tumor can affect your period, either by blocking the flow or causing extra bleeding during menstruation or at other times during the month. Tumors that occur in teenagers are almost always benign (not caused by cancer). Nonetheless, they should be checked by a doctor.

Since in most cases fibroids stay rather small, they don't always cause problems, and some women live with them for years. They usually disappear during menopause. If they get large enough to create pain or heavy or irregular bleeding, they can almost always be removed by surgery without removing your uterus. Ovarian cysts may also be removed if they become big enough to cause problems. If the doctor suggests taking out the ovary too, get a second opinion before proceeding.

Cancer. Teenagers get cancer very rarely. The best chance of cure is early discovery of the disease. So it is crucial to have your symptoms checked out by a medical person as soon as you suspect something may be wrong. Symptoms to have checked are vaginal bleeding not during your period, a breast lump that doesn't go away, sores that aren't healing, blood in your bowel movement, and irregular bleeding from a mole.

Skin cancer has become much more common, because of the depletion of the protective ozone layer in the atmosphere. Teenagers who enjoy being outdoors and sunbathing should wear sunscreen to protect themselves from ultraviolet rays. Have suspicious moles or spots checked by a doctor.

BUTTERFLY

I am shrouded, here, in my cocoon,
I go through the motions of life, and
            enjoy it,
as best I can.
I am growing.
Slowly.
I am blossoming into adulthood.
Growing my wings.
Everything seems so confusing now.
My brain is crowded.
Is this a crash course in life and liv-
            ing?
All the chaos shall bust.
Soon.
Too soon, perhaps.
My cocoon will burst.
I will be left open.
Alone.
Vulnerable.
A butterfly at last.

—JANIE LEIVE

Changing 2 Relationships

It's not just how we look that changes during the teenage years. How we see also changes. It's as if we're wearing a pair of "life" glasses, and as we go through each new stage of growth we replace the lenses. What used to look really big suddenly appears a lot smaller. What used to seem like the whole picture now becomes only a part. New interests and ideas come into view. Parents and family slip out of the foreground, as our focus shifts to school and friendships and the future. This chapter is about those changes.

PARENTS

NOTE: While we refer to "parents" in this section, we know that many teens live with only one parent, with their grandparents, or with some other relative. Still others live with foster parents or in group homes with "house parents." In this chapter, when we say "parents," we are referring to the essential adults in your life, the one or ones with whom you share the ups and downs and ins and outs of daily living.

Parents are the key people in our lives when we are younger. During adolescence, that relationship undergoes a significant shift. As you read the following pages, try to keep this in mind: You and your parents are saying goodbye to one sort of relationship with each other—a relationship based for the most part on your dependence on them—and you're trying to find a new way of being together, a relationship based on your growing independence. If there is a lot of stress between you now, it's probably directly related to that change.

Although you may still be living at home, it's likely that things are different now. You probably have more responsibilities, like caring for younger siblings,

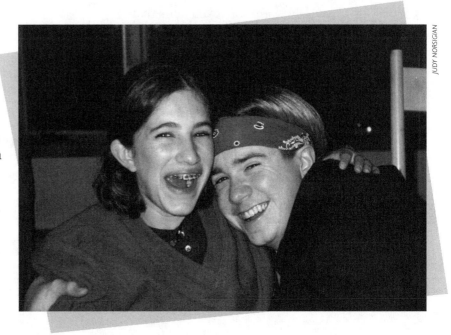

helping out with meal preparations, running errands, washing and putting away your clothes, making sure your homework is done, and maybe earning money to help with your own and/or the family's expenses. Along with these responsibilities comes a certain amount of new freedom. You probably spend more hours away from home. Your bedtime may no longer be regulated by a parent. You are able to get from one place to another on your own, and you don't always have someone keeping tabs on you. Alexandra, a seventh-grader from Seattle, described what becoming a teenager has meant to her:

> You start doing more stuff. You're out of the house more, meeting more people, getting more friends. You can get around by yourself now, so you want to be out more. You don't want to always be with your family.

Twelve-year-old Duncan explained:

> Even though even I think I'm too young to be doing some of the things I'm doing, it just happens. You're out there and it's happening and before you know it you're doing it too. My parents just wouldn't understand. They'd never let me do half the stuff I do.

Your growing independence means your parents have to relinquish some of the control they once had over your activities and acquaintances. As a result you may find that they worry about you more than ever now. John has a sixteen-year-old son and a thirteen-year-old daughter. This is how he put it:

> This is a dangerous world, what with all the drugs and drunk drivers and violent crime and kids disappearing and you name it. I know my kids are pretty responsible, but can I trust all their friends? Are they going to end up in some situation that they can't get out of? Are they going to get in over their heads? You can never be sure, so I worry and I set curfews and make rules about where they can go and who they can go with. Not because I want to be a tough dad, but because I want them to be safe.

As John explains, parents can't help still wanting to have some control over what you're doing and with whom you're doing it, if only to make sure you stay healthy and safe. You, on the other hand, may feel as Joanna does:

> I'm old enough to make good decisions; I'm careful and responsible. I don't want to die or get in bad trouble or flunk out of school. Why can't my parents just trust that I'm the one who cares most about me? I'm not stupid.

The struggle between parents and kids that takes place in most U.S. households during adolescence stems from the difference between what John is saying and what Joanna is saying. "Trust me," teens demand. And most parents reply, "We do trust you, but you still need guidance." As a result, there are times when you feel completely misunderstood and unappreciated by each other, times when anger erupts and feelings get trampled. Julia, fourteen, said,

> I just hate my mom sometimes. She doesn't understand anything about what I'm going through, and most of the time it seems like she doesn't even care. She treats me like I'm a child.

Elizabeth, a seventh-grader from Des Moines, described the confusion she feels:

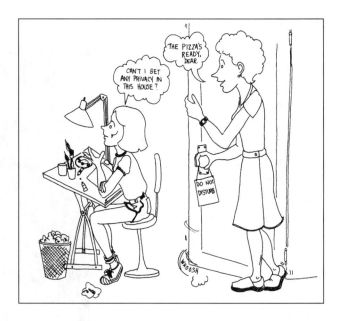

One minute my mother treats me like I'm old enough to do this or this—like help her out at home by doing the marketing or making dinner or babysitting my little brother. And she's always telling me, "You're thirteen years old now, you should know better than that!" But then the next minute, when there's something I really want to do, like there's a party that everyone's going to, she'll say, "You're too young to do that."

Timothy, fourteen, is from New Orleans:

Physically I matured much faster than my friends—and emotionally I feel older too, and that causes a lot of problems between me and my parents. They're always saying to me, "Stop going out with people so much older than you. Why don't you hang around some kids your own age?" They still see me and treat me as if I were a child, and I resent that because it's not who I am.

As a teenager you are old and young simultaneously—old enough to be able to take care of yourself in more and more situations, but young enough to be still living at home. Many teens feel eager to free themselves from home and parental rules, but Steve, a sixteen-year-old from Denver, feels ambivalent about it:

Some of my friends say that once you're eighteen you're *free* and you can do anything you want. You're out from under your parents' control. But for me . . . I'm going to get out in that world and I'm going to say, "Uh-oh, now what do I do?"

Here's how Lara, fourteen, put it:

We're not children anymore so we know there's something out there, but we're not adults, so we don't know what it is. And that's what I'm scared about!

Independence doesn't happen overnight. It takes time. Like Steve and Lara, you may not feel completely ready to go "out in that world." If you feel anxious when you think about leaving home, you're not alone. Most teens worry about how they'll be

able to take care of themselves, how they'll earn money, how they'll survive. At the same time, part of you may be ready to find out. Jenny, an eighth-grader from Louisiana, complained:

Parents are always telling you what to do, but we have to do things our own way. We have to make our own mistakes.

Sixteen-year-old Jonah said:

When I'm home I'm still my parents' kid. When I'm out in the world, I'm a person, and I like the way it feels.

You are older, and you have a right to expect that you will be treated with more trust than when you were a small child, but while you are living at home, most parents insist that you abide by their rules. Todd, a seventeen-year-old from Rhode Island, said:

I'm independent, and I like to come and go as I please, but it's hard because you've got to listen to what your parents say, and even though they're pretty lenient—like they tell me I can come home around one or two in the morning sometimes—I still have to be home when they say. And I always have to let them know where I'm going. They have certain rules for the younger kids, like no TV during dinner, and homework before phone calls, and when I'm there I have to go by the rules too, whether I think they're right or not. They tell me I have to set a good example for my sisters and brothers. So mostly I stay away as much as I can.

Betsey is fourteen. She lives in Miami:

When I got into eighth grade, I started going out to parties with my friends, and that's when my parents started setting curfews for me. I felt that was really unfair, because I was always the one who had to come home first. My parents are European, and they have strict rules. They just couldn't understand that it would be okay for me to stay out past midnight. That was really embarrassing for me.

You may think your parents are holding on too tightly when they set strict limits for you and question every move you make. From your perspective, they may not seem willing to accept that you're old enough to take care of yourself and make reasonable decisions for yourself. Jane, an eighth-grader from Boston, said:

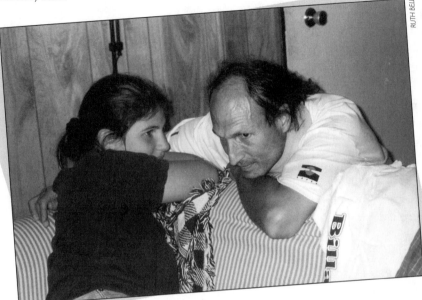

I told my mom about this party that was either going to be at this boy's house or a teenage nightclub in the city. I asked her if she'd let me go if it was at the club, and she said no, because she knew that club had a pretty bad reputation with drugs and make-out rooms and stuff like that. Well, I had sort of heard those things too, so I wasn't too interested in going there anyway, but I told her that if I knew that it was a safe place to go, I would want to go, because now I feel like I'm old enough to have good judgment about things like that.

Jane's situation might have turned into an angry battle had she insisted on going to the party even against her mother's wishes. In many families a scene like that would lead to harsh words, punishment, and resentment. If you and your parents can keep the lines of communication open, however, if you are both willing to compromise a little, it's possible to figure out ways to redesign the rules to meet both your need for independence and your parents' sense of concern. This is what happened to Dorene, a high school sophomore from Chicago:

My mother told me I couldn't go with a guy in a car until I was in my senior year of high school. I argued with her about that, but in a nice way. We ended up compromising, and she said I could ride with someone as long as she knew who the person was. So now whenever I go out on a date, my mother invites the guy in and sits and talks to him for a while. At first it embarrassed me, but then I started liking it, because it calmed a couple of those guys down and we ended up having a nice time together instead of just being wild.

Your growing independence and desire to spend more time on your own has another side to it as well. Stephanie, a ninth-grader from New York, told us about her situation:

Last year I started doing more things on my own. It was exciting—I started meeting people, going to parties, sleeping over at friends' houses, but my mother felt that I wasn't spending enough time with her anymore. She's divorced and I guess she feels lonely, but she makes me feel guilty.

Fifteen-year-old Joseph said he has the same problem:

With me, every time I'm with my friends my mother tells me, "You're never home. You don't care about your family anymore." And it's sort of true,

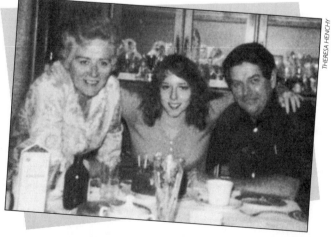

because these days I don't really enjoy doing that much stuff with them. I have other things I want to do.

Many parents find themselves feeling neglected or rejected when all of a sudden their kids, who were always there before, can barely be counted on to show up for dinner. They may complain about being completely left out of your life when they don't even know what classes you're taking in school or who your friends are. If you've had a close relationship previously, it's a big change for your parents. They miss you. Barbara, a mother of two high school students, put it this way:

Suddenly, in the last six months, I look at my kids and they're like strangers living in my house. I don't know them at all. I don't even know what they like to eat anymore. All of a sudden one's not eating dairy. The other's only eating protein. Just last year we could say, "Oh, let's all do this or go here together," and we'd do it and have a wonderful time. But now everyone's into his or her own thing, and no one's ever home anymore. There's been a real breaking away this year, and it's sad. It's sad for us as parents, anyway.

Parents who have been very involved in their children's lives do have to find a way to let go during these years, and that's not easy. Remember, when you think your parents are being controlling and intrusive, it's not because they really want to ruin your life, as it may seem. More likely it's because they aren't ready to say goodbye to your childhood. Most parents have invested so much time and energy into taking care of you, that they find it a challenge all of a sudden to stand back and watch you make your own mistakes. If you are able to respect each other's needs enough to compromise and keep communication open between you, it will be easier on both of you. If you can arrange for some special time together, like a "family night" once a month or a weekly family dinner, that can make the transition easier still.

In some households, the problem is not one of too much parental control; it's the opposite. There are many teens who wish their parents would spend

more time with them. They wish their folks *would* set some limits and watch out for them. Brandy is thirteen:

My mom's always going out and leaving us alone. She wants me to cook dinner for my little brothers and put them to bed. I'm old enough now where she doesn't feel like she needs to be here. But I'm scared staying alone. I want her to come home before I go to bed. But most of the time she doesn't.

Fourteen-year-old Julian agreed,

My parents are never home. They're either off on a trip or away at work or something. Like, I get home from school and there's a note on the table about what I can make myself for supper and not to expect them. They don't show up at my games or band concerts. I mean, am I an orphan or what?

Noreen, sixteen, said once she got old enough to find her way around town alone, her parents basically stopped being parents:

My dad does drugs. My mom too. Once I got to be eleven or twelve, they kicked me out of the house every weekend so they could party. I don't know what they expected me to do, but after a while I felt like I couldn't just sponge off friends. A couple of nights I slept out on the street. But then my

He told me I was pretty
  My mother told me I smell like some
  chemical.
He told me that we will run away together
  My mother told me I better clean up
  my room.
He told me, "You are my ultimate friend."
  My mother told me, "Get off the phone."
Then he suddenly disappeared
  And that's when my mother, smelling
  of warm milk, told me that I was
  beautiful.
                                    —*ANONYMOUS*

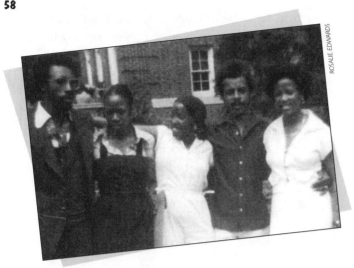

ROSALIE EDWARDS

friend Heidi's mom said, Why don't you just bring your things over here and you can stay with us as long as you want to. It was so great there. They actually had family dinners where everybody sat down at the table and talked about their day and things like that. And her parents would help me with my homework. But they had to move last year, so I'm living at home again. It's not too bad now, because I'm older. I can take care of myself better.

It takes years to become fully independent, and it also takes support. All teenagers deserve to have responsible, committed adults in their lives who can help them achieve independence in their own time and at their own pace. If you are not getting that kind of help and support at home, like Noreen, you may be able to find it at the home of a friend or with relatives. Take a look at Chapter 4, beginning on page 178, for some suggestions.

Your Style

Lots of people, no matter what their age, use their appearance to make a state-

ment. Whether they spend hours in front of the mirror studying and adjusting how they look, whether they dye their hair green or shave it off altogether, whether they dress only in black, go barefoot to their brother's wedding, shower three times a day, or wear spotless $150 tennis shoes, their appearance says something about who they are.

During these years of change, you begin shaping a style that will be yours in the future, and in doing so you may try out many different roles, costumes, accents, hairdos, and attitudes before you settle on the you *you* like best. This can be another source of conflict. You and your parents may end up in all-too-frequent battles over how you look. Allen, a fifteen-year-old from Denver, said:

> My parents are always on my case that my hair's too long. Every time I walk into the house, my mom tells me I need a haircut. And if we go anywhere, they're always complaining about how I look—my pants are too big, my hands aren't clean, I have zits. I swear they spend every minute telling me what's wrong with me. So I just say, "Sure, Mom—right, Mom," and go up to my room and close the door.

Susan, who's now eighteen, had a particularly hard time with her mother's idea of how she should look:

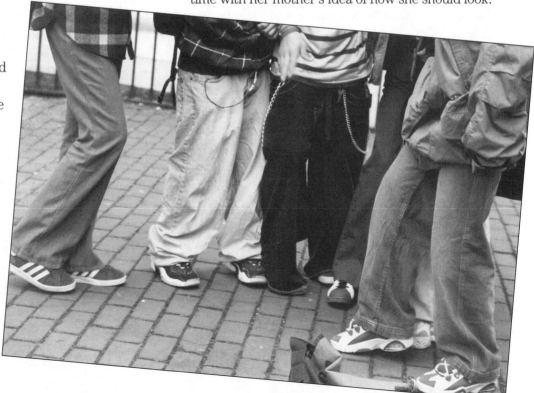

JESSE EPSTEIN

When I started junior high, my mom always wanted me to wear these special little outfits to school functions. I couldn't believe it. Everyone is wearing jeans, and I'm supposed to wear mix-and-match outfits. Give me a break!

The conflict comes when *your* idea of who you are and how you want to look is different from your parents' idea of who their child is and how he or she *should* look. Here's what Cheryl-Ann, a fourteen-year-old from Connecticut, said:

I want to grow my nails long, but my mom makes me cut them. She makes me cut them even though I say, "It's not fair. They're *my* nails." It's like her

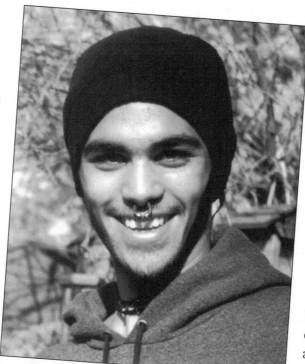

saying to me, "I'm going to cut your hair whether you like it or not." It's my hair and I should be able to wear it any way I want to. And they're my nails. I want long nails so my hands will look good. I wish she would let me grow them, but if I go against her she punishes me.

Daniel, twelve, said:

I dress different now that I'm in middle school. I used to not care about my clothes—I'd wear whatever my mom bought for me. But now I really care about what I'm wearing. I really take time to think about it. So it bugs me when my mom yells at me for wearing jeans with holes or big shirts. It's a big deal to her if my clothes aren't clean. She thinks my teachers will think she's a bad mother or something.

Some teens we met say they have to resort to subterfuge. Anthony told us about his girlfriend:

My girlfriend's parents are, you might say, old-fashioned. They won't let her wear tight shirts or

makeup or short skirts or anything like that. So sometimes she'll wear whatever she needs to to pass inspection, and then she'll have all this other stuff in her purse and she'll make me drive her to the nearest gas station and she'll change into what she wants to wear.

And sometimes parents resort to devious measures to get their way too. Jonah said:

My jeans disappeared. Vanished without a trace. So I asked my mom where they were and she said she tossed them because they had too many holes. She cut them up to use for rags. My favorite pair of pants.

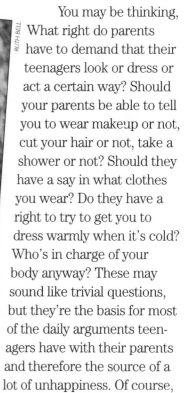

You may be thinking, What right do parents have to demand that their teenagers look or dress or act a certain way? Should your parents be able to tell you to wear makeup or not, cut your hair or not, take a shower or not? Should they have a say in what clothes you wear? Do they have a right to try to get you to dress warmly when it's cold? Who's in charge of your body anyway? These may sound like trivial questions, but they're the basis for most of the daily arguments teen-agers have with their parents and therefore the source of a lot of unhappiness. Of course, there is no one answer to these questions. If what you are doing or wearing is unhealthy for you or may affect your future or represents values that your parents consider completely antithetical to their own, they will undoubtedly feel they have a right to try to influence you. The younger you are, the more say they are likely to want to have. They'll push and you'll resist. Or you'll push and they'll resist. Ideally, a compromise will evolve that works for you both. Fourteen-year-old Sarah said:

I don't wear hats, but my mother thinks I'm going to catch pneumonia if I don't wear one, especially when I go out at night. We're always fighting about it, so finally I said, "Look, Mom, I hate wearing hats, but I'll take one and keep it in my pocket. Then if I get really cold I can put it on." It worked. She was okay with that, and last week when it was pouring I even wore it.

Fifteen-year-old Olivia said:

I'm not at all an appearance-obsessed person, but for some unknown reason I wanted to get my nose pierced. I wanted to do it for a long time, but my parents wouldn't let me. Since you are required to have a parent sign the form, I waited. Last year my parents told me it was my decision—they didn't condone it and they wouldn't pay for it, but they said they'd sign the form. And for me it became a statement to myself of independence in a way, since it was a big decision I was able to make for myself. It kind of stands for the fact that I'm no longer just my parents' child—I'm also my own human being. I definitely feel like a separate human being from my parents, with separate values and a separate identity. Of course, I also think it looks good!

Parental Expectations

Another area of potential conflict is directly related to your parents' expectations: Are you turning out the way they think you should be turning out? If and when you choose to become a parent yourself, you'll discover it's almost impossible not to have some expectations. Parents want their kids to be healthy and happy, and the list goes on from there. They want the best for their kids, but what parents don't realize is that sometimes their idea of "the best" is not what's right for their child. A sixteen-year-old from Chicago said:

I find that I fit a lot of gay stereotypes—how I dress, how I walk, how I talk. My style is gay and I like it. But my parents and grandparents, who are still under the impression that I'm heterosexual, think that I should fit in with how straight sons should act. Straight sons should want to ogle girls and stare at *Playboy*. Straight sons should be interested in cheerleaders at school. I almost want to scream at them, *"HELL-O!! I'm GAY!!"* because I'm taken aback when they think I'm straight. I don't act the part well, nor do I want to.

Some parents express their expectations in the form of worry. Their seemingly constant anxiety about your size, your shape, your grades, your social life, your athletic ability, your popularity makes it seem as if they want you to be perfect. Lewis, a sixteen-year-old from Los Angeles, said his parents are making him upset:

My dad and my brother are both over six feet tall and I'm only five-five at sixteen. They keep telling me, "Oh, don't worry, there's still plenty of time for you to grow," but the more they talk about it, the more it feels like they couldn't stand it if I didn't

LEMON

They try to tell me I'm not what I think.
They dye me and feed me full of their
things.
Conform me.
   I am myself.
   I am fresh and sunny.
   Me.
They take me and reap me. Stamp me.
Sun Kissed.
They use my juice. Squeeze my life out
   of me.
They take my scent to clean dishes and
   make hands softer.
They use my seeds to grow more.
They throw away my skin, my shell.
   Nothing left.
   I want to peel my skin off and
   show you the sun!
Well damn you. Yes you
I want you to see me.
You don't know me.
Don't say I'm fake.
I'm not unreal.
I am me!

   —AMY C. ROSEN

grow. I'm getting pretty disgusted with the whole thing. I mean, I am who I am, and if I take after my mother's family, maybe I won't grow much more. They make me feel like there's something wrong with being short.

Patty, who just turned fifteen, has to deal with her parents' concern over her "popularity":

My parents are worried because I don't go out yet. I mean, I go places with my friends, but I don't date or go to parties. And I don't have a boy that I like. They make me feel like there's something wrong with me, like I'm unpopular or something.

A thirteen-year-old from New England said his mother has the same concern:

Every time I get off the phone, my mom wants to know if I was talking to a girl. Or if a girl calls, my mom says, "Peter, it's a girrrrrrl for you. Anything serious?" She makes me feel like I'm not normal if I'm not always wanting to go out with girls.

Whitney, sixteen, is an excellent student, but she feels her parents put way too much pressure on her. She told us:

I got an 88 on a math test, and my dad's all, "What happened? Why didn't you get 100?" I mean, give me a break! Do I have to be perfect?

Some teenagers with severe physical disabilities told us how important it is to them to feel accepted for who they are, especially by their parents. Lois, a sixteen-year-old from New York, was born with a spine problem. She said:

My mother and I have such a hard time communicating. She's not affectionate with me at all—I guess because I'm disabled. She makes me feel like there's really something wrong with me. I keep saying to her, "Don't put me down. I'm just like everyone else. I have the same feelings as everyone else. The only difference is I have to walk with leg braces."

And fifteen-year-old Paul, who's spent most of his life in a wheelchair, told us:

My mom just can't deal with my handicap because she blames herself for it. But I don't think she should. I don't blame anybody for it. It was something that happened. I just want her to be able to accept me as a person. I mean, I do have limitations and I can't do certain things, but disabled people always try to find a way to get around those things. I would rather that she treat me the same way she treats my brother than to keep treating me like there's something wrong with me.

All the teens quoted above are saying they want their parents to love them and feel good about them no matter how they look or act, how they do in school, whether they're popular, or physically able. They are looking for acceptance just for being who

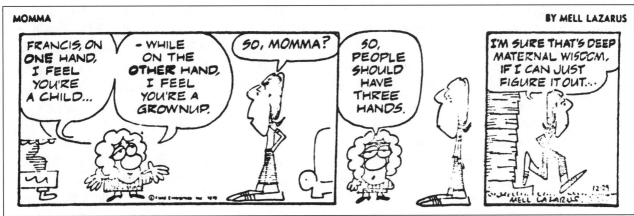

they are. Parents need to remember how it was for them when they were teenagers. Perhaps they had to conform in order to be accepted by their own parents. If so, maybe they can remember how much they hated being held to someone else's standards of how they "should" be. You can help your parents ease up on you by talking to them calmly and without anger about how much it hurts when they expect you to achieve their idea of perfection without taking into account the reality of who you are and what's important to you.

In many ways, you are a beginner, facing certain adult problems and situations for the first time. You need as much understanding, guidance, encouragement, and love as you can get. Here's Carl's story. He is a seventeen-year-old from Los Angeles:

> The few times I tried telling my parents what was going on in my life, it was disastrous. They just couldn't understand, and they would yell at me and punish me without even the tiniest bit of understanding. So finally I ran away from home, and my best friend's family took me in and I lived with them for about six months. His parents became my second parents, and to this day they still are. Because they weren't my real parents, I could tell them stuff, because they didn't get threatened by it. They didn't have a lot of negative feelings around it like, "Oh, we're failures. Our son's doing this, this, and this." They didn't expect me to be perfect the way my real parents did. Plus they showed me a lot of love, and I really needed that.

This is your time to find out who you are. When all you hear is criticism, it can be difficult to hold on to a positive sense of self. None of us is perfect, but in order to be as good as we can be, we need to feel accepted and appreciated. When your parents make you feel like you're a bad person or put you down for not meeting their expectations, you have to dig inside to find the parts you appreciate and respect about yourself. Teens who aren't getting much support from the adults around them have to try to develop their own internal support system. Look for more on this in the Emotional Health Care chapter, beginning on page 153.

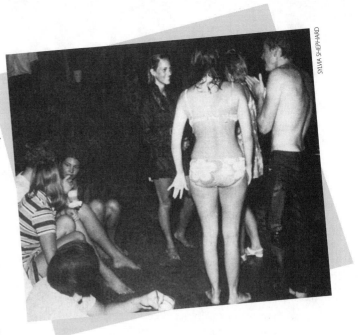

Parents and Your Sexuality

A father of two teenage daughters said:

> I watch my daughters grow and I think, "This is beautiful." It's exciting to see children turn into adults. That's when I see it objectively. But when I look at them and see *my little girls*, when I say to myself, "Those are my children and they're becoming adults and they're going to have to deal with that outside world without me along to protect them," that's when I get emotional. They're beautiful and they're sexy. My daughters are sexy young women, and I worry for them. This world is rough, and they could get hurt, and I know there's nothing I can do about it except teach them good values and hope they make good choices.

Almost all parents have mixed feelings about their children's sexuality. In our society, sex is considered part of the "adult" world, and as your body becomes sexually mature, you step closer and closer to the border of their world—whether you want to or not and whether your parents are ready to let you or not. Just seeing you now forces them to think of you in a new way. Joanne, a mother of four, said:

> With my first son, it affected me very strongly. I think when he became really physically grown it made me feel strange to think that he would be going out with girls and sleeping with girls someday. With my daughters, it didn't affect me so much, maybe because I'm a woman.

A father of a thirteen-year-old daughter said:

> I can't help pulling away from Jenny now. She's getting so womanly, so sexy. I don't want to say that I'm aroused by my daughter, but sometimes I look at her and she looks so beautiful and sexy that it takes my breath away.

As this father says, during adolescence, when your body starts looking more like that of an adult, parents may feel uncomfortable hugging you or touching you the way they used to when you were smaller. It's another sign of parent-adolescent separation when around this time even families who used to walk around naked in front of one another start covering up. You may feel more shy about hugging and kissing your parents now too. Some preteens and teens try to avoid the issue by hiding their development altogether. They wear layers and layers of oversized clothes, try never to undress in front of anyone, avoid swimming, and basically go "underground" for a few years. Some of this behavior is a sign of simple self-consciousness.

When teens completely shut themselves off from their friends or family, however, when they overeat to the point where the extra fat on their bodies covers up any sexual development, or when they stop eating and lose so much weight that normal growth functions, such as menstrual periods in girls, cease, and normal adolescent body changes disappear, their behavior needs attention. If you or someone you know is becoming extremely introverted or developing strange eating habits, it's a good idea to seek out help. Check out the Emotional Health Care chapter, beginning on page 153, for advice on how to find competent adult helpers with whom to discuss these issues. (Also, see the chapter on Eating Disorders, beginning on page 185.)

Once your parents begin to notice that you are looking older, it may trigger their concerns about your sexual activity. Fourteen-year-old Brenda, an eighth-grader from Massachusetts, told us that her parents became very suspicious when they found out she had a boyfriend:

> The most important thing to me is that I know my parents love me and respect me. But they just can't accept the fact that I'm growing up and I have a boyfriend. Now, I never or rarely ever lie to my parents, but when they asked me if I ever made out with my boyfriend, I said no. I felt I had to say no, because if I told the truth, they'd say, "No more Brian. No more seeing him, no more phone calls, no more parties." I'd like it so much more if they were just a little more realistic. Like if they said, "Just don't have intercourse, but you can make out. We know that's normal." I mean, I don't want them to get mad at me for kissing Brian for more than two seconds. If they could only understand that I have my limits, that they can trust me.

Parents have concerns about sex for many reasons. No responsible parent wants his or her child to experience an unplanned, unwanted pregnancy or the dangerous health consequences of a sexually transmitted disease (STD). In this era of HIV/AIDS (see page 256), parents worry that casual sexual experiences can be potentially life-threatening. Good sex education is more important than ever now, and the best sex education is the result of an open dialogue between parents and children. When your own parents teach you the facts of sexuality, explain to you about safer-sex methods, and answer your questions honestly, they help you develop healthy, responsible attitudes toward sex and sexuality. You and your parents may want to take a look at the information starting on page 89 to begin a dialogue about sex.

Sexual relationships have emotional as well as physical consequences, and parents don't want you getting hurt before you have enough self-confidence or emotional maturity to handle it. Corinne, a fifteen-year-old from Duluth, told us about her mom's feelings on the subject:

> My mom will say, "Well, I don't expect you to be a virgin till you get married," since she knows I don't expect to get married until I'm in my late twenties. But she also says, "I do expect you to wait until you feel that you can handle it, until you feel responsible, until you're on your own and taking care of yourself." She doesn't think I could handle it until I'm out of high school, and she's probably right.

Corinne and her mother have talked about sex openly. She thinks that's helped her to have a more responsible attitude about what she wants for herself. Sixteen-year-old Tom said the same about his parents:

If I was going with someone for a long time and we were getting into some heavy sex, I'd want to talk to my folks about that. They're very understanding. After all, they went through the same thing. They wouldn't try to tell me what to do. But they also wouldn't say, "Hey, man, go ahead and do what you want." They would probably tell me to think about the consequences. They trust me.

If you know that your parents are willing to listen to your ideas and questions, it will be easier for you to discuss sex with them than it is for many of the teens we interviewed who were of the opinion that their parents could not accept their growing sexuality. In fact, they just assumed their parents didn't want them to think about sex until after they were married. Fifteen-year-old Mariellen tried to talk with her mother, but the results were not good:

My mother says I shouldn't be interested in sex because I'm handicapped and will probably never get married. That drives me crazy. I say, "Well how do you know? You don't know me. You're not inside me. You don't know what I feel."

In Portland, Maine, sixteen-year-old Patrick said:

My father's so strict, if I look at him funny he knocks me under the table. That's how he was raised; that's the way he treats me. So if he doesn't ask, I don't tell.

And Bobbi-Jo, a sixteen-year-old from Memphis said,

My father never talked to me at all about sex. Never one word. But one night we were out to dinner and my boyfriend was with us. As we were walking into the restaurant, I put my arm around my boyfriend and my dad gave me the dirtiest, angriest look and said to me sort of under his breath, "You don't do that!" I was really shocked by how angry he looked. I felt like saying to him, "Well, if you think that's bad, you should see what we do when you're not around." But I didn't say anything.

Teens whose parents feel comfortable answering questions and concerns about sexuality generally have higher self-esteem and more self-confidence when faced with challenging sexual situations. They've been given the opportunity to establish their own limits and to feel okay about enforcing them.

Teens whose parents get angry or very closed off when sexuality comes up, sometimes feel the need to rebel, as Rachel did:

When I told my mother we played Spin the Bottle at my sixth-grade graduation party, she was so angry she told me I could never go to another party until I was in high school. I was totally shocked at her reaction, but for the three years of junior high I never went to a party. Then when I got to high school, I was wild. I got into all sorts of trouble. I think I was taking revenge on her.

In some families parents are more open and lenient with their sons than they are with their daughters, as David, a sixteen-year-old from Kansas, told us:

There's definitely a double standard at my house. My fifteen-year-old sister will talk about bringing her boyfriend home and it will be a tense subject, and my parents let her know that it's really not okay with them. But with me, my dad's always joking around asking me how things are going with my girlfriend and stuff like that. Whenever I go out on a date, he says, "Well, I'll see you in the morning." Like whatever I do or whenever I come home is okay with him.

If you are female, you may find that your parents are concerned about your "reputation." They want to protect you from being labeled "loose" or "cheap." Unfortunately, those kind of labels are still around, and girls seem to bear the burden of them much more than boys do. (See page 105 for more on the double standard.)

Perhaps your parents, for religious or health reasons, put a high value on your remaining abstinent (having no sex) until you are married. There are a lot of good reasons to abstain from intercourse until you are older. Many teens we met have decided to wait until they are married or engaged before introducing sex into their relationships. For more on this topic, see pages 107 and 121.

While a teenager's developing sexuality usually creates at least some tension at home, in a number of families the tension comes not from your parents wanting to limit you, but from *you* wanting to limit them. Your relatives, family friends, and/or neighbors may be taking more notice of your sexuality than you feel is appropriate. Adults or older teens may be acting sexual with you in ways that scare you, disgust you, hurt you, or make you just plain uncomfortable. Their attention may include touching or hugging or kissing or fondling or even sexual assault. They may try to make you think that what they are doing is perfectly normal and okay, but trust your own feelings. It is not normal and okay; it is sexual abuse. If after you tell them to stop they continue to mistreat you, *find someone to talk to about it.* Even if they tell you not to tell or threaten to hurt you if you tell, find a friend or a relative or a teacher or a religious leader who will listen to you and help you decide what to do. No one has the right to sexually abuse another person. See page 227 for a more complete discussion of sexual abuse.

Seeing Your Parents as People

As you get older, you may find yourself criticizing your parents for the way they act, the way they dress, the way they look, the values they have. This is a normal part of the separation process, but it can be extremely hard on your parents. Paul's mom said:

> I can't do anything right. I'm too fat. I'm not cool. Why can't I be more like Jonah's mom, always smiling, always looking beautiful? I'm telling you, for someone who's tried as hard as I have to be a good mother, it really makes me feel bad. I know he's just telling me to back off, but does he have to be so mean about it?

Your parents are people: ordinary people with faults and weaknesses and insecurities and desires and problems just like everyone else. That may sound like the most obvious statement in the world, but during adolescence, you may begin to realize for the first time that your parents are separate from you and different from the way you might wish them to be. Many children learn this about their parents early on—especially children who've been mistreated or neglected. But if you've grown up thinking of your folks as shining examples of perfection or the ultimate authorities on most important topics, seeing them as regular people for the first time may be a surprise and a disappointment. Fourteen-year-old Arlo said,

> My mother came to this meeting at my new school and she was so loud and obnoxious I pretended I didn't know her.

Bernard, a fifteen-year-old from Chicago, said:

> My parents are always picking on each other, always arguing. It seems so stupid. I don't see how they can stand it.

As a little child you may have accepted the fights between your parents or their funny habits or their unusual style of doing things as just the way life was. As a teenager you have more exposure to the world around you, and when you meet other people who do things differently, you have a chance to compare your life with theirs. This gives you a broader picture from which to develop your own values and standards. It's another part of the separation process. Sixteen-year-old Maurice has a particular concern. He feels his parents aren't making an all-out effort to support the values they say they believe in:

> I like going to church every week, and I get so mad at my parents for not going. They're such hypocrites. They're always talking about people who don't have religion, but then they only go to church on the big holidays or when it's convenient. My dad has his golf game on Sunday morning, and nothing can interfere with that.

Whether it's religion, politics, sexuality, honesty, or simple human kindness, if your parents don't practice what they preach, you may think, like Maurice, that they're acting like hypocrites, and you may feel like telling them they're setting a bad example.

Or maybe you think your parents have the *wrong* values altogether. Once you begin to form your own opinions about important subjects, you may find yourself fighting with your parents over whose ideas are "correct." Violent arguments occur in families over some very complicated issues, like whether homosexuality is okay, whether interracial or interreligious dating is acceptable, whether homeless people should be helped by the government, whether capital punishment is right or not, whether there is more than one "true" religion. Matthew had this experience:

> My best friend came out to me last summer, and it kind of freaked me out a little, because, I mean, he was my best friend. We were together a lot. How could I not know that about him? Well anyway, after I got over the initial shock, I wanted to be there for him, support his telling other people and everything. But when my parents found out that he was gay, they totally went berserk and said, "He's not welcome in our house." It's been like hell here ever since.

Fifteen-year-old Barry told us:

> I'm having a really hard time with my parents. I had to get away from them, because we keep having these fights about whether I should be allowed to visit my mother's parents. My folks don't talk to them, and they want to keep us kids from seeing them because I think my parents want to punish them for something that happened before I was even born. Well, I think that stinks. I think it's really childish and selfish on my parents' part to do that, and now I feel like I'm old enough to do something about it. That's why I decided to come here this summer to be with my grandparents even though my parents were dead set against it. I worked during the year to save the money for this trip.

Sixteen-year-old Rosie, from New Jersey, was really disappointed by her mother:

> I got this great job at the market, and they wanted to put me on a career path, which meant they would send me to a five-week training class where I could earn twice as much as minimum wage. I thought my mom was going to be so proud of me, but she wasn't. She freaked, because it takes ten hours a week and she didn't think I should drop the ten hours I was working to take the class. She said we need the money, but I know it's really her. *She* needs the money for her Bingo.

Maturity doesn't come automatically; it takes work. As we become adults, our goal is to try to become more and more conscious of the commitment and responsibility we have to the people around us, especially the people we love. Unfortunately, for some adults that goal is hard to achieve. Eighteen-year-old Phil knows his father is one of those people who can't seem to get it together:

> When my dad gets drunk, he gets out of hand. He's beating up on us or pushing my mom around, and I can't stand it. I caught him punching my little brother out a couple of weeks ago, and I jumped him and started punching him. I had to move out after that until he settled down.

Gayle is now seventeen. She grew up in a small Eastern city with a mom who had a drug problem and a dad who never lived with her or supported her or her mother. Last year, her mom moved them both to be near relatives, in the hopes of kicking her drug habit. Here's what Gayle told us:

> I never could adjust to the new school. I never went to class and was always getting into trouble. I was used to my old school and my old friends, so after a couple of months I left. I saved enough money and hopped a bus back and stayed with one of my girlfriends. Her folks were really nice about it and let me stay for a month. Then we got word that my mom had died. She overdosed and died at the hospital. I didn't know where to go. My dad called and said, "You can come and live with me by my

rules if you want to." But I said, "I don't even know you. Will you come here and visit me?" Basically he just screamed at me, "I made you an offer. Take it or leave it," and he hung up the phone. So Alison's mom and dad said that I could stay with them until I got my life together. And I'm still here.

If your parents have chronic abuse problems with drugs or alcohol or a violent temper, you've probably learned by now that you can't depend on them. Like Gayle, you may have family friends or relatives who will help you. But if you find yourself alone and feeling uncertain about your future, there is help available for you. Talk to a counselor at school or a favorite teacher to begin with. Check the Resource section of the Emotional Health Care chapter, beginning on page 181, for more suggestions.

Parents Go Through Changes Too

Adults go through changes over the years just the way you do, and one of the stages many adults experience somewhere between the ages of thirty-five and fifty-five is called a "midlife crisis." It's a time when people look at themselves and their lives and say, "I'd better start doing some of the things I've always wanted to do before it's too late."

For a number of parents, watching their children become young adults increases that longing. They see your strong young body, and suddenly their wrinkles look wrinklier, their sags look saggier, and they feel it's time to do something drastic. We met seventeen-year-old Gordon in Wisconsin. He said:

Everything was going along like usual and then all of a sudden my dad started doing crazy things— like staying out real late, not telling my mom where he was, showing up late for work or not showing up at all. My parents were arguing a lot and he would get real defensive, so it just kept building up and up. I could see it, but I didn't want to say anything. I knew something was going on. I was expecting something. And pretty soon my dad came to me and said, "Well, you know me and your mom are having problems and I think I'm going to have to leave." And we both started crying. It was a heavy scene. My little sister, who's

only eight, didn't really know what was going on. I didn't want to cry, I was trying not to cry, but I couldn't help it.

Ellie, a thirty-nine-year-old mother of three, put it this way:

I'm ready for a giant change, because a little change just won't do it for me. My kids are getting ready to leave home soon, and I want to sell the house and do something crazy, like go around the world for a year, or move back into the city and get a job or go back to school. I'm not willing to wait till I get cancer or until somebody dies, or until Peter and I get a divorce to make a change. At least now we can still enjoy ourselves.

When you are going through your own ups and downs, it's hard to watch your surroundings disintegrate. It's easier to leave home and go off to college or get a job, if you know "home" will still be around when you want to come back for a visit. This is *your* time to change, so it may feel quite upsetting to hear your parents express their own need to get away and change their lives. Their actions undoubtedly will have an effect on your life too. Wendy, from San Francisco, said:

My mom's just starting her career now. She's going to become a legal assistant and she's going back to school and all, but she's saying, "All these years you kids have been able to do what you've wanted, and I've always been there putting you first. Well, now I'm coming first for a while. Now I need you to watch the little ones while I go back to school. Now I need you to take care of the house." And I say, "Gee, Mom, that's great for you, but where am I supposed to come from now? I mean, what about the job I wanted to get and the money I wanted to save for college?" She really came on strong and I could understand, but I thought, This isn't fair. This isn't like my mom.

Wendy said she feels selfish when she thinks, No, Mom, I don't want you to give up being a mom yet. Wait until I have my life in order. But she can't help feeling that way.

Mario is eighteen. His father was just diagnosed with cancer:

> When you've been planning your whole life around going to college, it's not easy to let go of that dream. But I'm going to have to. It's hopeless. My dad's going to have to stop work and I'm the oldest. I never wanted to be flipping burgers for a living, but what else am I going to do? My family needs me.

When Mario confided his dilemma to his counselors at school, they arranged for him to meet with the college financial aid officer and an adviser. These people put together a schedule and a financial aid package that allows Mario to work part-time and go to school part-time.

If your family is in transition, if your parents are getting separated or divorced, if one or both of them lose their job or change careers or decide the family has to move, if someone in your family gets very sick or dies, you may think that no one will understand or accept the way you feel. You may worry that others will judge or criticize your family's problems, so you may try to keep your feelings to yourself. But one thing to remember is that whatever is happening in your family has probably happened in many other families too. You're not alone. Again, what we have been saying over and over applies here too: find someone to help you. Talk to someone at school or church, or discuss your mixed feelings with a close relative. Don't give up your dreams. Find a way to make them work.

The "Double Life"

Of the hundreds of teenagers we interviewed for this book, nearly all of them said they had things going on in their lives that they just couldn't or wouldn't tell their parents about. Things like sex, drugs, smoking, and drinking were the most commonly mentioned, but people also talked about staying out late, picking up strangers, skipping school, fighting, going around with friends their parents didn't like, and going to places their parents wouldn't approve of. Anything you are doing that you don't tell your parents about comes under this category. Rebecca just turned thirteen:

> I can't talk to them anymore. If I told them what me and my boyfriend do, they'd tell me I couldn't see him anymore. I know my parents. My mom says to me, "You're too young to have a boyfriend." She treats me like I'm so young. She thinks I'm so innocent.

Teenagers don't tell their parents about some of the things they do, because they know their parents wouldn't approve; they know their parents would say, Think of the consequences. Lou, a sophomore from Arizona, put it this way:

> I'm doing things that my mom wouldn't want me to be doing. I know that. But I'm levelheaded; I can say no when I want to. The thing is, sometimes I want to smoke pot or stay out to see the sun rise, or do other things that would worry her, and I don't think she'd understand that I know what I'm doing. I think she'd get mad, so I don't tell her.

Part of the reason you feel you can't be open with your parents may have to do with their idea of who you are. Here's what fifteen-year-old Suzanne said:

> My parents think I'm so much more innocent than I am. That makes me feel bad, like they'd be disappointed in me if they knew the things I do. Even I think I shouldn't be doing some of the things I'm doing, but I can't help it. You're with your friends and things just happen.

Cassie, an eighth-grader from San Francisco, said:

> In seventh grade I started getting drunk, going out with friends to parties and stuff. I stopped talking to my parents except for little bullshit things. I would tell them I was sleeping at a girlfriend's house, and they wouldn't ask what we were going to do. In a way I feel good doing things they don't know I'm doing, because it makes me feel important. I have a separate life from them, and I don't think they're on to it at all. Like I'm sure they feel, Oh, my daughter wouldn't do anything like that. They wouldn't believe half of what I'm doing, and they want reassurance that I'm not doing that stuff, so I can't tell them the truth even if I wanted to.

Many teens wish they could share more of their life with their parents. You, too, may wish that your parents would be willing to listen to your stories objectively, without feeling the need to give you advice or punish you. Tyler is sixteen. He speaks for many teens when he says:

If I could let my parents know what's going on with me, that would help so much. If I could let them know and not get judged by them, that would be such a relief. If only they could understand that parties and staying out late and pot—and sex— are part of growing up for me.

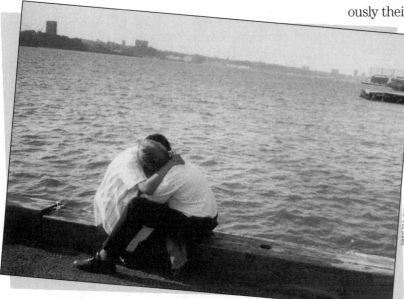

Seventeen-year-old Karen felt her parents' idea of how she ought to behave while living under their supervision was an impossible standard for her to uphold. She decided to find a way to support herself so she could live on her own:

My parents didn't let me do anything. They always had to know exactly where I was going and exactly who'd be there and exactly what time I'd be home, or they wouldn't let me go anywhere. And they never let me go on a single date, only on double dates, so we had to pretend we were doubling just to please them. We had to go through this whole thing of getting two other people to act like they were going with us, when they really weren't. I felt like I was too old for my parents to still be treating me like a baby. I wanted

to talk to them and be friends with them, but they just couldn't handle that. I love my parents, but I just couldn't talk to them because they have a thing: what they think is right goes and that's it. They wouldn't let me express my feelings about anything, so I just closed them out of my life.

Being the parent of a teenager is almost as challenging as being a teenager. Your parents see your life through their own experience. They remember what they were like as teens, or they remember stories of other teens they knew who pushed the boundaries and found themselves in dangerous situations as a result. Since most parents take quite seriously their responsibility to raise you and keep you safe, they want you to be cautious and they want you to survive these years intact, both physically and emotionally. In direct contrast, it's part of the teenage experience to want to do things without being too cautious, and sometimes you will end up getting yourself into spots you'd rather have avoided. It's at those times especially that you may really want your parents to be there for you. Sometimes it takes a crisis to bridge the gap. Eighteen-year-old Meagan was in a group we interviewed in Iowa. She said:

I finally broke down and told my mom that I needed an abortion, and she just about got hysterical. She started shouting, "My baby, my baby," like I was a three-year-old. But when she calmed down, we had the first good talk we've ever had. And after the abortion, she helped me decide what kind of birth control to use and she was much more open with me about her life.

You may be surprised to find that if you talk to them, your parents will be more willing to come through than you think. In fact, since you're getting older, they may want to talk to you, too, about things that are upsetting them in their lives, things they've been keeping secret from you. It won't necessarily be easy for you to hear their concerns or for them to hear yours; it may take a lot of strength and self-

MY OLD MAN

My father,
Boy can he drive you crazy!
He sits down after dinner
With his head buried in the world's
gossip which he calls a newspaper.
Dad I gotta talk to you.
Silence
Ya see dad I've got this problem.
Silence
Dad I'm PREGNANT!!
Did you say something, honey?
No dad, go back to sleep.
—ANDREA MINTZ

control just to listen to each other. But the alternative, which is cutting yourself off from your parents altogether, is painful for everyone. Gretchen, a senior in high school from Milwaukee, told us she's really glad she finally opened up to her mother:

> I never was very close to my parents, but when my first boyfriend broke up with me last year, I was really depressed, and he kept saying I should talk to my mom. So I did. And she made me feel a lot better. Now I talk with her about a lot of things—anything, really. I still can't talk to my dad. I know I can't, because my mom tells him everything and he never responds to me, so I know he doesn't want to talk about that stuff. It's okay, though. We love each other. But my mom and I are really close now. I feel like she's a friend, not just my mother.

FRIENDS

Our friendships take on new meaning during the teen years. Friends help us build the bridge away from dependence on family toward a more independent life on our own. They accept us in ways our parents may not, and they understand what we're going through, because they're going through the same things themselves.

Groups

Many teens say that being part of a crowd of friends makes life more fun. They agree that going to a movie or a party, going shopping, participating in sports or academic contests, joining clubs, doing community service, or just hanging out can all be more enjoyable when you do them with friends. Jennifer is an eighth-grader from Tennessee. She told us why it's important to her to have a group of close friends:

> You know sometimes you feel scared to do stuff, but because everybody's doing it, you do it too. Like dancing. For me dancing was really hard to do. I always felt like everybody's eyes were right on me, so I was too embarrassed. But at the dance the other night one of my friends pulled me out on the floor to dance with her and everyone was helping everybody else learn the steps, so I didn't feel too self-conscious. It was great. I had a lot of fun.

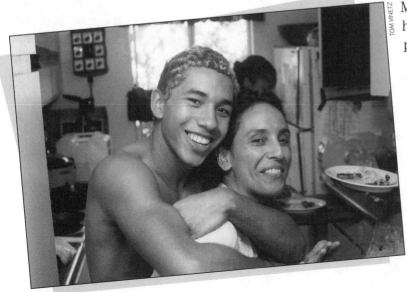

TOM WINETZ

Mark, a fourteen-year-old from Idaho, said his friends keep him from feeling completely alone at school:

> You would not exactly call me an athlete. You know how every guy is supposed to love sports? Well, I'm the exception to that rule. I am totally unable to play any sport that involves a ball. I can't catch. I can't throw. I can't hit. I'm too small to tackle. I can't kick. And you better believe I take plenty of shit for it, too, from the so-called jocks. They always say, "Oh no. Does Mark have to be on our team? Not

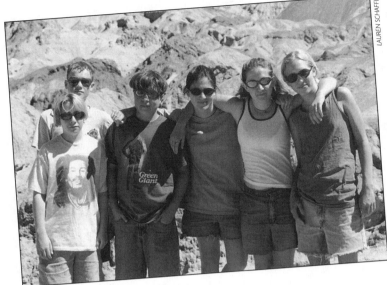

alternative or whatever. There's lots of different groups, but once you start hanging out with one group, you pretty much get labeled, which kind of sucks, since I think, if anything, you find your group because of who you are, not because they influenced you to be like them. It's like you seek out people who you like, and you go hang out with them.

Even if *you* know that the people you hang out with are all different from one another, with their own individual personalities and priorities, people on the outside of your group may see you all as a unit. Whether you like it or not, you may be labeled. Gina said she hates that.

him!" Lucky for me I've got my friends. We're into other things, like we have a band, and we're writing a movie. Otherwise I'd probably kill myself.

Vicki, a tenth-grader from New York City, told us:

Some people I know like to say that groups are the pits. They say they want to be an individual. But I mean, what fun is it to be an individual if you don't have a group of friends too? What are you going to do? Be an individual with yourself? Sit at home and say, "Oh, I'm an individual." Sure.

Vicki's question brings up an issue we heard discussed by a number of teens: Can you be an individual and still be part of a group? Can you maintain your separateness at the same time you're hanging out with the same bunch of friends and doing the same things they are? Maria admitted that it *is* pretty easy to lose sight of people's individuality when you see them with one group all the time:

Like it's really easy to go, He's a jock, or he's a punk, or she's

I'm labeled as one of the rah-rah girls. I'm just put in this box, and people think they know me. So when I overhear somebody saying something about the rah-rahs, as if we're not people, I go up to them and say, "Is it really me you're talking about? Or are you just making a big generalization?" Then they always say, "Oh, we didn't mean you." But they don't get that they're being so stupid to label people just because they go out for something like sports or cheerleading or student government. Everybody's not the same who does those things. It's like saying that everybody who likes to swim is the same.

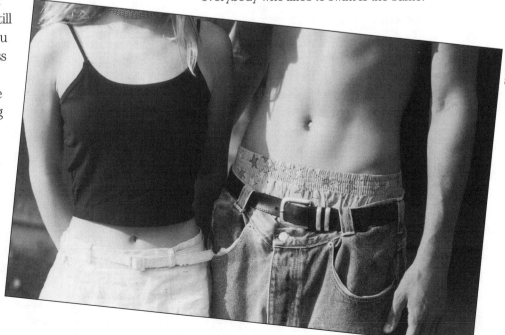

Many of us are concerned about fitting in, and during the teen years that usually becomes a top priority. How do you act, what do you do to be considered "cool," or at least not different or weird? Tyrone, a fifteen-year-old we interviewed in Chicago, said:

> In my school there's the "in" group and the "out" group, which is everyone else. And whatever the "in" group does, that's the thing to do. They can go out and stand in the middle of the street and get run over by trucks, and sure enough, the next day everyone will be standing out in the middle of the street getting run over by trucks. You know what I mean? It's pretty bad.

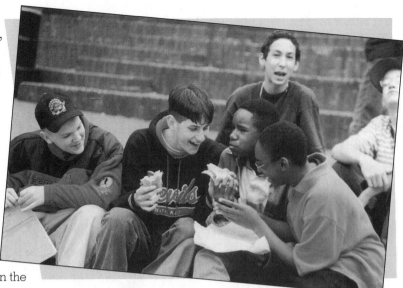

Tyrone was laughing when he told us about the pressure to be like the "in" group, but it's a concern that affects all of us, no matter what our age. There's a difference between doing and saying and being what we want because that's who we are and that's what we believe, and doing things or saying things or acting a certain way because that's how we think people want us to be. How much of our true selves do we have to give up to be part of a group? It's especially confusing during adolescence, when we're only just becoming aware of who our "true selves" are. Conrad, thirteen, said:

> For me, I'm exploring who I am—trying to find out who I am, because I'm not really sure anymore. Because up till about seventh grade, I was just a kid. I was me and I never really thought about it. But now I've thought about it a lot more and I'm starting to have to make decisions about who I want to be and who I want to hang out with. There's pressure that goes along with it too. You have to think about how you dress and how you act. If you do something dorky, it gets around. It's bad for you.

And Janie, a seventh-grader from Ohio, said:

> I know it sounds crazy, but I think clothes really do make a big difference in how people perceive you. I know in sixth grade it made a big difference

in who my friends were, because I would wear sweatpants to school, and all the popular kids were like totally driven crazy by that. It was like I was offending them by dressing that way. And I thought, I'm not going to let that bother me. I'm not going to care about what other people think. But this year I *am* more concerned about what other people think of me and how they look at me. I do care more about my clothes now.

Bill, a seventeen-year-old from New England, told us:

> In junior high especially, it was like everyone had to be cool and fashionable and taking the right drugs and going to the right parties to be in the popular crowds. I never really fit in and I felt terrible most of the time. Since I've been in high school, though, it's been different. I'm finding some friends who accept me for who I am now. I don't feel I have to dress a certain way or act a certain way to have friends. Now I'm sort of glad that I didn't really fit in in junior high, because I know I don't want to be that way anyway. When you're so caught up with fitting in, you lose a lot of chances to find out who you are.

Schuyler, a fourteen-year-old from Oregon, felt the same way:

> You know, I always had friends and things but I always felt different from them. I just never really fit in. They would always want to do the same things over and over—like hang out downtown

and try to pick up boys and act cool or sit around and watch dumb shows on TV—I just never really wanted to do that stuff. But you know, you want to have friends, so you go along. But now I've got these friends who are like me. We like the same music. We do homework together. We talk about the books we've read. We talk about the future. Finally, I feel like I'm not a freak.

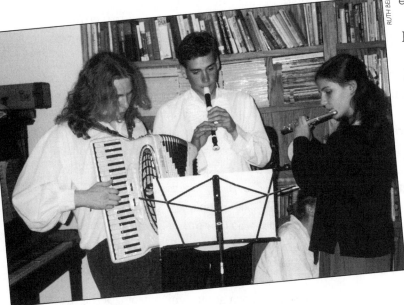

RUTH BELL

Adolescence is a time when people tend to feel extremely exposed, as if they're always under surveillance. Since it takes a lot of courage to stand out from the crowd and express a different opinion or cultivate an interest that everyone else thinks is a little strange, that means, for many teens, keeping parts of themselves hidden. Austin, a high school sophomore from Delaware, said it this way:

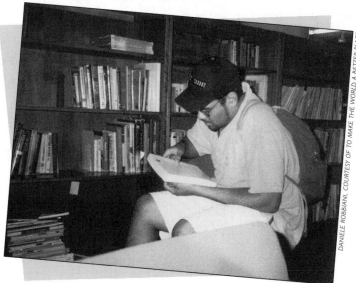

DANIELE ROBBIANI, COURTESY OF TO MAKE THE WORLD A BETTER PLACE

I hate school because I have to stifle a lot of myself and I can't say a lot of the things I feel because I'd just be made an outcast. Like in English class, if you're into reading poetry or something or if you have an opinion on it that's different from the rest of the class, you can very rarely express it without them all jumping on your back. You have to do and say what everybody else is doing and saying.

Fourteen-year-old Dana said:

I don't know what's wrong with me. I must have some genetic imbalance or something, but I do not feel the need to dye my hair like the other ten thousand kids I know who do.

There's the issue of wanting to "fit in" and doing what you have to do to conform, but there's another side to it too. While some people who feel unsure of themselves withdraw, others go to the opposite extreme, like Janine, an eighteen-year-old from Cleveland:

I've been thinking of all the times I've been rejecting of people. Like even in grammar school I'd walk down the hall and go, "Oh, there's so and so, she's weird." Or "Eeeuuu, stay away from Ricky, he's a creep." It was so cruel, but that really happened, and I used to do it. Other people I know did it all the time too, and sometimes I'd think to myself, That's so mean. I don't want to be like that. But like if *you're* doing the rejecting, then you're not the one being rejected. You know, you don't feel good about yourself being mean, but at the same time, you're so worried about being accepted yourself that you don't stop to think about that for others.

Derrick described it this way:

I really think there is a basic tribalism that most people need. It can turn kind of ugly, though, when one group of people thinks they're better than everyone else. Or people put each other down for being different.

Fifteen-year-old Pedro said:

> It all turns into a big Dr. Seuss book. Thinking
> about this reminds me of the Sneeches and the
> Star Bellies and how the Star Bellies think that
> they're better than the Sneeches, so they say
> we're going to have some parties and you can't
> come. And so the Star Bellies are always having
> fun and the Sneeches are always trying to be
> included. It's just like that in school. Except in the
> book everything turns out all right.

Lots of social clubs, sororities, fraternities, country
clubs, and other exclusive organizations are based on
the same idea: people in this group have fun and
know what's cool. What's implied is that if you're not
in this group, you must not be so cool or have as
much fun.

A similar concept comes through in any organized association that says, "We're the best. We
know the right way." The implication is that anyone
who feels differently must not know the "right" way.
People who insist their ideas are the *only* right ideas
may actually be worried somewhere deep inside that
they're nothing if they're not the "best." And while
they may derive a certain kind of comfort from feeling they're better than other people, they have, by

definition, a rather limited perspective. Generally,
that's the kind of thinking that creates prejudice and
stereotyping, not tolerance or understanding.

A few teens we met said it was different at their
schools. Jenna, a fourteen-year-old from New England, goes to a small school where, she said, people
try to be accepting of one another. She didn't feel
there was much competition there at all to be in an
"in" crowd, because everyone was friends with
everyone else and there really was no "in" crowd.
Zack, a fifteen-year-old from Colorado, had a similar
experience. He said:

> Last year I started going to this school where it's
> really incredible. It's like a family. You get to know
> everybody, even the teachers. Of course you don't
> have to like everybody, but it's not like you feel like
> you have to stick with just one group of friends to
> be popular. Everybody's accepted as an
> individual. It's like people appreciate each other
> for just being who they are.

Zack and Jenna and many other teens we met
say it makes school life a lot more enjoyable when
there's less concern about which group is the most
"popular" and more appreciation of each person as
an individual.

Going Along with the Crowd

Being part of a group of friends can give you self-
confidence and help you do things you might not try
on your own, but being part of some crowds can
work against you. Fourteen-year-old Lionel, from
Newark, gave us an example:

> Friends can push you into doing stuff you know
> you shouldn't be doing. You try and say no
> and they'll probably end up beating you up or
> something. My friends tell me to do something and
> I do it. They're a lot older than me. Like they tell
> me we're going to play basketball, so they come
> by and pick me up and we end up going to the
> liquor store. And I say, "Hey, man, what's in the
> bag?" and they say, "Gin. Now shut up and take
> a drink."

JULIE JUNG

That's a no-win situation. Lionel said he didn't want to drink, but he felt he had to or else it wouldn't have been cool, since he was younger than most of the other guys. He liked playing basketball with them. They were good, and he was glad they accepted him on their team, but he felt a lot of pressure to do the things they did.

Fourteen-year-old Matt told us how he got involved with a friend who was really mixed up:

There was this guy at our school, Jimmy. One day he came up to me and I was really surprised, because Jimmy had never said anything to me before. So he was like, "Hey, Matt, you want to have some fun?" and I was like, "Uhh, sure Jimmy." "You want to go upstairs and spit on people?" And so we did. And then almost every day he would come up to me with more weird shit to do. It could get really perverted, and I don't know why I was doing it, except Jimmy wanted me to do it with him. So I did. Like one day Jimmy caught this puppy and told me to throw it in the creek, so I did. Jimmy said he would stand by and keep a lookout, but I guess he didn't see this woman coming. She started yelling at me to get the puppy out, so I did. I had to jump in the stream, and I got all wet too. Then she gave me this really weird look like she couldn't believe that a person would do such a thing as throw a poor, defenseless little puppy in a creek. I couldn't believe it myself. I don't know if that puppy would have drowned if I hadn't jumped in after it. That kind of opened my eyes. After that I didn't hang out with him anymore.

When Matt listened to the tape of his interview he was struck with how many times he said, "So I did." It bothered him that he would just go along with someone else's ideas without giving it any thought of his own. He said, "It's like I was a zombie, just waiting for someone to give me directions."

Sometimes the pressure is less direct. In Boston, Ben, also fourteen, told us about his experience:

I'm part of the crowd who are considered the "cool" kids at school, and it always gets into who's the coolest in the crowd. Like who's done the most or who knows the most stuff. There's this competition around who's going to lead the group—who everybody else will follow. Sometimes the so-called leaders do a drug and don't let me or some of the others do it, because that makes them more experienced than us, and we sort of end up feeling less mature than them. It makes doing that stuff very appealing, because you start thinking, Oh yeah, that looks like fun. I want to do it too. It's not that anyone's telling you to do it. In fact, they may be telling you not to do it, but since they're doing it, and since they make it seem so great, you naturally want to do it too.

Most of the teens we met say they do what they do because they want to, not because other people are doing it. But even so, everyone agreed there are times when they personally know they shouldn't be doing something, or maybe they feel that they're not quite ready to do something, and they end up doing it anyway because their friends are. Inside, they're unsure or they're worried about getting caught or having their parents find out or hurting themselves, but they go along. MaryLee is eighteen; she told us this story:

I went to this coffee shop with my friends and this guy comes over to our booth and you could tell he was high by the way he was sort of buzzing and talking and he came and sat with us and he's all, "You guys want to buy some crack?" And I said no. So he said, "You wanna give me a ride home?" And he had like this huge knife on him, and I was so scared because he was definitely loaded and you don't know what they're going to do. He was scary. But my friend's super nice, so she said we'd give him a ride. Him and his friend. And I went along. Lucky for us they didn't kill us.

The choice to go along with your friends does, at times, get in the way of what you know is right. When other people are doing something that is dangerous or destructive or humiliating or illegal or just plain not what you want to be doing, you're faced with the decision Do I do it too, or do I say no?

These kinds of tough decisions appear all the time throughout a person's life. Situations come up that test your values—whether to cheat on an exam, drive without a license, shoplift, fight with someone who provokes you, try a drug, have sex with someone you hardly know, or for that matter, with someone you know very well. No parent is standing over you at those times telling you what to do. It's up to you alone. And if you do take a stand that is different from other people's, you risk having to put up with their teasing or their anger or their rejection. It takes courage and self-confidence to stand apart from the crowd. In the long run, the question is whether you want to be responsible for making your own choices in life based on what you believe is right, or whether you're willing to let others make your choices for you.

If your crowd values the opinions of its individual members, that makes it easier to express yourself honestly, to be "who you are." In Connecticut, fourteen-year-old Aaron said:

> If the kids in my group are smoking marijuana, they say, "You want to try it?" If you say no, they say, "Fine." That's all there is to it. No one forces you. And no one puts you down.

If you're in a crowd of friends who take care of one another, that helps too. LaShawna, a seventeen-year-old from Detroit, said her crowd is like that:

> Usually the kind of drinking or smoking that goes on with us is just social. People just sitting around and smoking a little weed or having a little wine. But if you see your friends getting wasted or messing up, if you're a good friend you'll say something to them. Like if somebody's totally bombed and they want to drive home, you tell them, "Oh no. I'll drive tonight." We watch out for each other.

Some people we met are in the opposite kind of crowd, in which people are admired for doing things that are dangerous, things that can hurt them or get them into trouble. Seventeen-year-old Annie told us about her experience when she first entered high school:

> Big, bad, and bitchin' was the thing in my school—at least with my crowd. If you cut school and got away with it, that meant you were all right. You had a scam

on those teachers. If you could still pass, you had an in. Everyone thought that was great. You'd be stoned in class and sit back and make a fool of yourself and everybody would laugh and you'd be considered fun. Like you'd be entertaining everyone. And if you didn't get caught you were cool, you were okay. The thing was—just don't get caught.

Fifteen-year-old Josie was in a similar kind of crowd. She said she couldn't count on her friends for anything but trouble:

> When I was twelve, I started hanging out with this crowd at school, and they really had an influence on me. I always looked up to this one guy who was like the leader of the crowd. He was a couple of years older than me, and he'd be the one who'd think up the stuff to do, and we'd all do it. Like ripping off a store or smashing car windows or setting fires. He'd supply the drugs and we'd supply the action.

Josie was arrested and put in a county home for girls. That's where we met her while we were interviewing for this book. She said:

> When you don't feel too sure of yourself and somebody says, "Hey, you're cool," well then, you appreciate that so much, it makes you feel so good, you just want to be with them. You want people to notice you. I think everybody does, probably. If the kid who was class president or somebody who got straight A's wanted to be friends with me, I'd probably have ended up getting straight A's too.

Most people we met say they want to feel accepted, especially if they aren't getting much support or acceptance at home, or if they're going through a tough time—like parents splitting up, or moving to a new place, or changing schools, or if someone in the family or a friend has an accident or gets really sick or dies. At times like these, people feel particularly vulnerable, and it really hurts more than ever not to have friends who like you and appreciate you. Josie wrote this poem and gave it to us to put in the book:

Loneliness is a terrible thing.
It rules in some way every human being.
"Help" is what some people cry—
Can you just sneer and pass them by?

Feeling Alone

As we were interviewing teenagers around the country, we found out just how common it is for teens to feel "out of it" because they don't think they're like the other teenagers they know. Monica put it this way:

> It seems like everyone else has the script. Everyone else knows what's happening and I look around and say *Duh*.

The funny thing is that no one has the script because there *is* no script. Some people just forge ahead anyway and hope for the best, and others have a tendency to stay on the sidelines and watch. Brian, a ninth-grader from Cleveland, said he stays back because he doesn't think he would measure up if he put himself out there:

> I'm not a tough guy, and I don't like to fight. But in my school it seems like people get respected for their physical strength—I mean boys, that is. Everyone goes around bragging about how many kids they've beat up and how strong they are and how much they work out. I'm not big and I have a lot of fears that keep me from doing the things that those kids do. Like, I'm even afraid of roller coasters, and I don't like deep water so I don't really know how to swim. And I always worry that someone will dare me to do something that I'm scared to death of, or that someone will start fighting me and I'll lose. Of course I'll lose. I've never fought before in my life. And then everyone will see how chicken I am and they won't respect me anymore. That's one of my biggest worries— not being respected by the other kids.

Brian is an excellent student and a fine musician, but still he has those deep feelings of insecurity. Adolescence is a time when many people think they *should*

be feeling more confident than they do. They're down on themselves for not being tough enough or popular enough or smart enough or attractive enough or talented enough. Nobody we met told us exactly what "enough" would be; they just know they aren't it. They look around and see other people who seem to have it all together, who seem to be attractive and fun to be with and full of self-confidence, and that makes them worry all the more that they're the only one in the world who's afraid to try out for a team, or too shy to say something in a crowd, or too timid to ask someone out on a date. If you're like most people, you probably have some of your own private issues that cause your stomach muscles to tighten up and your heart to beat faster.

The truth is, *we all feel that way.* There isn't anyone, no matter how mature, who doesn't feel scared and out of it at times. Some people know how to cover up their insecurities with a pretty good per-formance. But once you start seeing through the per-formance, you find that underneath, everyone—at least everyone we've ever met—has the same desire to be liked and respected that you have, and every-

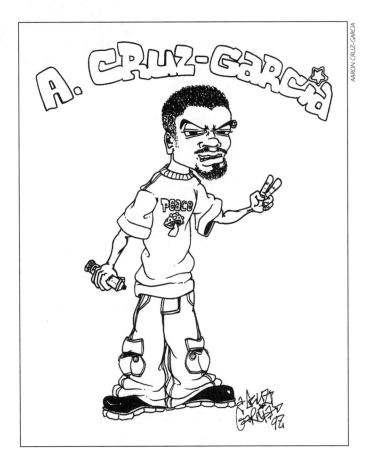

one has the same worry that they may not be able to "measure up" in one way or another. That's one of the secrets most people carry with them throughout their lives. If you talk with your friends about it, you'll probably find they feel the same way. Nan, a seventeen-year-old first-year college student who helped us write this chapter, told us she thinks that's the biggest problem she's facing right now:

> The hardest thing is coming to grips with who you are, accepting the fact that you're not perfect—but then doing things anyway. Even if you are really good at something or a really fine person, you also know that there's so much you aren't. You always know all the things you don't know and what you can't do. And however much you can fool the rest of the world, you always know how much bullshit a lot of it is.

When you're feeling particularly critical of yourself, it's important to remember the things you do know and the things you can do.

People change as they get older. They develop different interests and start becoming serious about specific parts of their life, like sports, or academics, or the arts. Even if you grew up with the same kids you know now, because of this shift in priorities, friendships have a tendency to go through changes when people get to adolescence. Sometimes that can be very painful—for example, when you and your best friend start to drift apart and go different ways. Thirteen-year-old Myla put it this way:

> Maddy and I were friends since first grade. We really loved each other. She was probably the person I felt closest to in the whole world. But then this year she started hanging out with the

"popular" kids, and I kind of think they're creeps and I didn't want to hang out with them. So we don't talk to each other as much anymore, and I guess it's like there's kind of a hole in me now. I kind of haven't really adjusted yet.

Moving to a new neighborhood and a new school disrupts your life and your friendships too. You have to establish yourself in a brand-new scene, which can be difficult. Fourteen-year-old Tina moved from a small town in New York to Los Angeles. Without her old friends around to appreciate her, she felt lost and out of step. She said:

DANIELE ROBBIANI, COURTESY OF TO MAKE THE WORLD A BETTER PLACE

> When I got to school the first day, everyone looked at me like I was from outer space or something. It was like, Who's that? Look at her hair. Look at what she's wearing. That's all anybody cares about around here: what you look like and what you wear. I felt like a total outcast. As soon as I got home, I locked myself in my room and cried for about an hour. I was so lonely.

Stuart, a fourteen-year-old from Iowa, told us a similar story:

> I moved to Des Moines in the middle of the year last year, and everybody in my new school was going around in their own little groups. It's hard to get into a group of people. I would sort of hang around, but no one would really notice me or pay attention to me. I started making a couple of friends this year, but last year was really tough.

For Daniel, a junior from a town outside Detroit, it isn't anything in particular. He just hasn't found anyone with whom he feels a close connection:

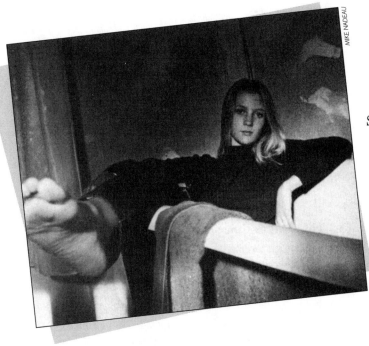

MIKE NADEAU

There are a lot of people in my school, of course, and they're okay, but I get to homeroom and I sit there and do my work and I walk to my next class and I sit there. I might say hi to whoever's the person sitting next to me, but I go through the day pretty much by myself. I know most of the people, but no one's really more than an acquaintance.

We met a number of teens who, like Daniel, feel unattached. Sometimes it's because they like keeping to themselves. Sometimes it's because they feel different from the people around them, maybe older and more mature or simply interested in different things. This is how fifteen-year-old Brett put it:

When you're aware about stuff and you can take a mature attitude about things, it can sort of be a hindrance because you can talk to some people, sure, but I know so many kids that I can't share that with. And I don't want to say, "I'm more mature than you," because that sucks. But it seems that some kids are so superficial. It feels like they don't care about anything important.

Polly, sixteen, told us:

I have some so-called friends, people I hang out with at school, and we can have fun together. But I

don't feel close to them. Like, when I have a problem I can't go to them because they just don't understand. They talk behind people's backs. You can't trust them. I'm looking forward to college. At least I'll meet some new people.

Stephanie, a ninth-grader from Texas, said:

I spent just about my whole seventh-grade year wishing I could be in the popular crowd. I would watch the kids in that crowd and sit near them at lunch and I'd pray that one of them would call me and ask me to go somewhere with them on the weekends. Well, in the eighth grade I did become friends with them. I went to their parties and I dated the guys in the crowd, but I never really felt like I fit in. I found out I wasn't really into drugs, and I didn't feel comfortable at make-out parties. So this year I stopped hanging around them. I guess you'd say I'm not exactly in any group now.

A LONE WOLF

A lone wolf with no companion
The sun shining reflecting off the snow
makes his fur seem glossy, thick, soft
 and warm.
And his eyes show wisdom and wild-
 ness,
but kindness, loneliness and sadness.
Isn't he something like me.
He is strong, cunning, skillful
But merciful and gentle.
He faces the elements
that would make him mighty
For he has no companion, no mate,
and no leader. He lives
but barely. But it is his wisdom
his kindness, his loneliness, his sad-
 ness,
his mercy and his gentleness that make
 me
feel pity and love for him. I say again,
isn't he something like me.
 —CHRIS KING

Some teenagers who didn't have a particular group of close friends said it was okay. They fill their lives with personal activities and interests. One fifteen-year-old girl we met in Rhode Island is writing a novel. She spends much of her time writing her ideas and feelings into her book. A senior named Bob who lives in Seattle is preparing himself for Olympic swimming competition, which means hours of practice every day. Gwen is a cellist with the youth symphony in her city. She, too, spends hours each day practicing, because her goal is to be a concert performer. Alex spends time corresponding with people on the Internet.

Without a goal or special interests or a job, however, you can get to feel pretty lonely if you spend long hours by yourself watching TV or doing nothing. Chris, a seventeen-year-old who works at a park in St. Louis, told us:

> I know a kid who doesn't have anybody at all. His mother's dead and his father's off somewhere, and he's staying with his great-aunt, who doesn't understand him, so he doesn't really have anybody. I met him at the park because he was hanging around all alone. So I asked him to come play on the football team I was coaching. I think he was hoping someone would ask him. After that, whenever he was having a problem he'd come a little early and we'd spend some time sitting around talking about what was on his mind. He just loved to come to that park when I was there. We got to be real good friends.

School isn't the only source of friends. There are teen groups at your church or temple, sports teams at the parks, or the Boys' or Girls' Clubs or YMCAs in your area. Local organizations that are doing important community work are always looking for volunteers. Chris said:

> If you really don't have anybody, it's best to try to go out and do a little bit. Like get into a sport and join a team, or go to a dance class or some after-school club or something. Get interested in something. You don't have to be good at it—just have some fun and be with other people. Or go volunteer someplace where they need help. Then you can find a friend.

Best Friends

Whether they hang out with a group or not, many teenagers find that they are drawn to one particular person, someone with whom they can be themselves. Here's what Sam, a thirteen-year-old from Idaho, told us about having a best friend:

> A best friend to me is someone you can have fun with and you can also be serious with about personal things—about girls, or what you're going to do with your life or whatever. My best friend, Jeff, and I can talk about things. His parents are divorced too, and he understands when I feel bummed out about the fights between my mom and dad. A best friend is someone who's not going to make fun of you just because you do something stupid or put you down if you make a mistake. If you're afraid of something or someone, they'll give you confidence.

Conrad and Josh, both eighth-graders, have been best friends for about a year. Josh said:

> Conrad's somebody I can be myself with. Like when I just don't feel like having to think about what somebody's going to think about me, when I want to do whatever I want to do, I can still be with him. Like the other night we were hanging out watching a movie and we decided to dye our hair. Right then. We went out and got all the stuff and just did it. It was fun.

Best friends appreciate you for who you are. When you need someone to listen to you, they're

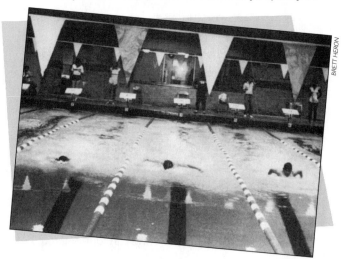

BRETT HERON

there for you. When you want to do something fun, they're there to enjoy it with you. And when you're going through a hard time, they can reassure you. Marlianne, a senior from Chicago, told us about her best friend Julie:

Julie was on the swimming team with me, and she was scared to compete because she thought she wouldn't beat the other person. I was trying to tell her, "Come on, you can do it." But she always thought she wasn't good enough. And that was the way she felt about everything, not just swimming. Since I was her best friend, I really talked to her. I kept telling her, "You can do it. You're great. Do it for our team." I kept boosting her confidence, and you know, after a while she did it. We all cheered for her and she was terrific.

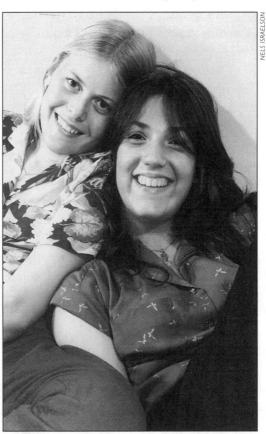

NELS ISRAELSON

Most friendships just evolve naturally over time. Seeing someone all the time, working or playing or going to school with them, gives you a chance to get close. Sometimes a person you were best friends with in elementary school is still your best friend in middle and high school. Ben said:

I have this one friend who I've known for nine years and I can really talk to him. He knows what I'm going through, and I know what he's going through. We're always together.

It's especially reassuring to have a friend who'll listen to you when you're feeling down about something. In fact, that's one of the best things friends can do for one another, just be there. Sarah, a sixteen-year-old from Des Moines, told us this story:

My closest friend got so mad at her parents that

she said, "Well, I'm going to swallow this whole bottle of pills." I was with her, and I just started crying because I hadn't ever heard anybody say anything like that before, and I was scared. I tried to talk her out of it by saying, "No, don't do anything like that. It can't be that bad." I said, "You can talk to me about it." So she did, and it turned out that she didn't really want to do it. She was just so mad. I told her to talk to me about how she was mad, and she said her parents just have too tight a hold on her. She feels like she can't move.

Being able to share intense feelings without being afraid that your friend will think you're weird is what friendship is all about. It's also important to find out that you can get mad at each other and still remain friends, for in most close relationships disagreements crop up every now and then. When this happens, it's healthy to be able to tell each other what's making you angry and then to make up.

Best friends may experience physical closeness as well as an emotional closeness. They often spend hours together each day, sleeping over at each other's homes, taking showers together, touching and wrestling and laughing and whispering together. They can do all that without feeling sexually aroused, as Jennifer, a high school sophomore from New Jersey, said:

Me and my best friend Erica always go around with our arms around each other or holding hands. And one time some guy yelled out from a car, "Hey, lesbos." It made us mad for a minute, but it really didn't bother us, because I mean if people are going to call you names just because you're holding hands with your best friend, well then forget them.

If the intimacy of a very close friendship does begin to create sexual tension, however, friends may not always feel comfortable with the results. Here's what happened to Laura, a seventeen-year-old from Pennsylvania:

My best friend and I—well, we were like sisters, and you know, I wondered about how much I loved her. Her boyfriend was jealous because we were so close. Sometimes we'd fool around and dance with each other, and once we got drunk together and we got a little too drunk and we started slow-dancing together. And I thought, This is weird, you know? But then I thought, Oh, what the heck. So we kept dancing and we kept putting on slow dances and we kept dancing. And then we both fell down and started kissing. We kissed for a long time, maybe a half hour or so, and then we stopped, and for the next few days we were real formal with each other. When we finally talked about it, she said, "I wish we hadn't done it, because you probably think I'm a lesbian now." And I said, "Oh, that's funny. I was afraid you were going to feel that way about me." So we laughed and everything and hugged each other.

Of course girls often hug and kiss each other without feeling that there's anything strange about it, but Laura said she and her friend felt funny about their experience because it wasn't just friendly kissing, it was definitely sexual and they both sensed it. The important thing for Laura was that instead of keeping her feelings about what happened to herself, she found the courage to share them with her friend. Talking about what was uncomfortable about the experience helped to clear the air between them.

The boys we interviewed

wondered if there isn't more of a taboo against physical closeness for males. Jason said:

It's like we finish a game and we're in the locker room getting dressed and it's like Ian and I are hugging each other or slapping each other's butts, and there's always that sense of Don't take this too far. What will the other guys think?

It's not unusual for close friends to be very physical, and even sexual, with each other without it signaling anything in particular about their sexual preference, except that they enjoy being intimate with people they love. Unfortunately, in our society, boys aren't usually given the same kind of freedom to kiss and hug each other that girls are, even though boys can, of course, have the same intense and affectionate feelings that girls have toward their friends. In many other cultures, male friends openly hug and kiss and touch each other, and it is expected that they do so.

Sexual feelings can be powerful and confusing. You may want to read the next section on changing sexuality, which has helpful information as well as thoughts and stories from many teenagers.

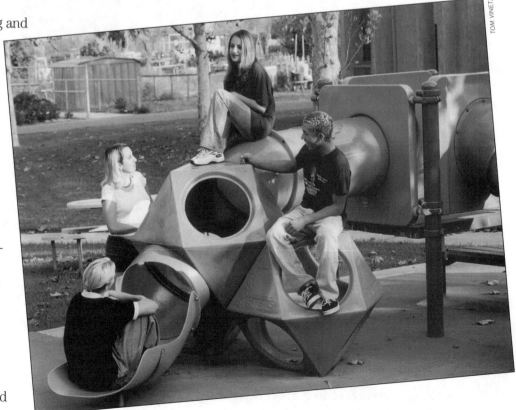

TOM VINETZ

Some people form their closest friendships with people of the opposite sex. They can confide in each other, go out with each other, and have fun together, without getting romantic. In Washington, D.C., sixteen-year-old Franklin said:

Sandy's just about my closest friend. I talk to her about everything, especially things I wouldn't talk to the guys about, like if I'm having problems with my girlfriend or something. We tried going out together in the ninth grade, but it lasted exactly one week. We're just not compatible that way, I guess, but it's great to have her for a friend.

Mary Elizabeth, a senior from Delaware, described what she especially likes about her relationship with Will:

I have girlfriends who are fun and stuff, but I just don't feel like I can trust them. There's so much competition between the girls I know. You never know who's going to turn around and spread a rumor about you. Will is really my best friend. We really love each other, but just not romantically. You know what I mean? It's comfortable. It's really comfortable—no games, no expectations.

We heard from many teens that they enjoy having a nonromantic, opposite-sex friendship because it's "neutral." You have the benefit of advice and caring from someone very different from you, but you don't have the tension or jealousy or possessiveness that often accompanies a romantic relationship.

Just because two people like each other in a romantic way, though, doesn't mean they can't really enjoy a friendship together too. In fact, several teenagers we met said that their boyfriend or their girlfriend *is* their best friend. And most of the married couples we know who are happy in their marriages say it's the friendship and trust between them that makes their marriage so satisfying.

Pairing Up

In this section we'll be talking mostly about male-female relationships, since most people in our society have heterosexual dates and heterosexual lifestyles. Of course, much of what happens when people begin to date is the same whether it's a heterosexual relationship or a homosexual relationship. For a more thorough discussion of homosexuality, read the chapter beginning on page 89.

No matter what part of the country we were in, teenagers agreed that they like going out in a group of friends rather than dating. Pairing up may happen at some point in the evening, but at least there is a bunch of people around to have fun with whether it happens or not. Brianna, a fourteen-year-old from the Northwest, said:

It's like we get together every weekend at somebody's house. We don't even call it a party, but it sort of is. Maybe five or six people, sometimes maybe even ten people or more, and we listen to music and watch movies and eat.

When pairing up does occur in these groups of friends, group support may be the catalyst. Fifteen-year-old Forrest told us that among his friends, everyone knows when two people like each other, and the group kind of fixes them up:

Let's say Matt says to me, Isn't Rosie cute. Then I say to Rosie, What do you think of Matt? And she says, I think he's cute. Then another friend Lauren says to Matt, I think Rosie likes you. And pretty soon Matt and Rosie are going out.

WOULD YOU?

If wisdom came in bottles
And kindness came in pounds
Would you talk to me?

If where to laugh and when to cry
And even how to live and die
Was found by looking under "I,"
Would you think about me?

If feelings came in vitamins
And I ate twice the daily dosage
Would you care about me?
—DAVID HASS

Of course, pairing up can and does also happen for a lot of teens without the input of others. Boys or girls call each other up or see each other at school and arrange to go out together. Victor, a tall, quiet boy we interviewed at a high school in New York, complained:

I'm already in the tenth grade and I've never even gone out with a girl, and that bugs me. I'm shy to an extent, but I think I could overcome it if I knew there were some girls who liked me. Then I could probably ask them out or something, but I haven't been able to be friends enough with a girl to give her a reason to like me.

A lot of boys feel that it's up to them to make the first move. Here's what Max, a fourteen-year-old from Philadelphia, said about that:

I think boys have it really hard. Once you get to be a teenager, suddenly everybody expects you to start calling up girls and going out with them. But hey, I think it takes a lot of courage to call a girl up and ask her out. You know, you always worry that she'll say no, and then you feel like shit. It's not so easy for me to just pick up the phone and act cool. I get nervous.

On the opposite side, if you're a girl and you've been taught that you're supposed to wait for a boy to ask you out, you may sit around getting just as nervous. Sixteen-year-old Leeann said:

Sitting around waiting for the phone to ring is a big part of my life—you know, wondering if the guy you like is going to call and ask you out. Like I'll sit there and say to myself, Well, the phone's going to ring by the time I count to twenty-five. Then if it doesn't ring, I count to a new number. It makes me so nervous I can't concentrate on anything else, and I'm always yelling at everybody to get off the phone if they're using it.

How do you meet someone? How do you ask someone for a date? A group of tenth-graders we met in Los Angeles were talking about exactly that. Allison, fourteen, said:

I think it's great when someone comes up to me, when they're wanting to meet me. It makes me feel good. But it depends on what kind of energy they give me. If they're nice and act like they just want to get to know me, I like it. But if they just want sex or something, I can tell that too, and I usually leave as soon as I can.

Peter explained his concern:

It's not always so easy to meet someone, though. Like, what if you see this girl going to class every day and you want to meet her, so you go up to the class and wait for her to come. Like, you plan to be there at the right time so she'll have to pass you on her way and you set the whole thing up. That's really tough for me, because I get more of a fear of her turning me down when I stand around and wait. My stomach goes crazy.

Allison said:

I know the feeling. When you planned something and you know you have to do this or this to make it happen. That's why I like it when my friends go out together as just friends, because then it's just friends. Then if you start liking each other, it kind of flows. It just happens.

In dating relationships, some people get stuck in the mover role—always making the first move, doing the asking, arranging the plans—and other people get stuck in the waiting-around-to-be-asked role. Sally, a senior from Boston, explained that she does what she thinks is right for her, and she doesn't like sitting around waiting to be asked.

I always approach guys when I want to. And I've met very few guys who are afraid of that or who shy away from that. It always blows me away when I run into a guy who says, "I can't go out with you because you asked me, I didn't ask you." I wouldn't really want to go out with someone who was so uncomfortable with himself that he'd feel that way.

There are plenty of guys around the country who

would appreciate Sally's willingness to make the first move. In Wisconsin, seventeen-year-old Alex said:

> I think it's great when a girl calls up a guy to ask him out. A lot of guys are shy, like I was shy for a long time. It was hell for me to ask a girl out. And a lot of the girls I know are much less shy than I am, so it makes me feel terrific when one of them asks me out.

Evie said that in her school in Seattle, people say they want things to be different, although she's found that's not necessarily so:

> A lot of guys I know *don't* like it when a girl comes on to them. So that makes me hesitate to ask a guy out, because I'm afraid that he'll be totally shocked by it and lose respect for me.

Evie's worried that if she asks a boy out he might say no. That's the same worry Max talked about. Whenever you put yourself out there, especially if you're going against tradition, it's a risk. But this is true for everything—relationships, jobs, school elections, applying for college. It hurts to be rejected. Yet as LeRoy, one of the teens we met in Detroit, said, if you don't try, you don't have any chance at all:

> All they can do is say no. And then you have to say to yourself, "Well, nice try LeRoy. You gave it a shot."

Falling in Love

When two people fall in love, each feels attracted to and appreciates the other. There's a joyfulness between them, and they have fun being together. As their love develops, the level of their trust and commitment and contentment with each other deepens too.

Many people fall in love during their teenage years. Sometimes it turns into a long-lasting relationship. More often it's an intense emotional experience that lasts a while and then changes. This kind of short-term relationship can be very exciting. Thirteen-year-old Dolores told us:

> I went to a party with my boyfriend, and at the party I was slow-dancing with another boy and I fell in love with him. I didn't want to hurt my boyfriend's feelings, but I really wanted to be with the other boy. When he touched me, I got shivers all over my body. While we were dancing, I felt like we were floating on a cloud.

If you've ever felt the way Dolores did, you know how passionate that kind of love can be. Some people find they can't eat or sleep or concentrate on anything other than the person they care about. Just being near them can bring intense pleasure. When you're apart, you fantasize and daydream about them and make up romantic love scenes in your head. Fourteen-year-old James described it this way:

> I'm reading a book or watching TV, and all of a sudden it's me and Wendy in the story, off alone somewhere kissing and touching and staring into each other's eyes.

Brandon, a sixteen-year-old from Ohio, told us about the girl he likes:

> I really have a pretty bad crush on my friend's sister. She's a little older than me, and I already know she won't go out with me, because I asked her and she said no. She was real nice about it, but it was still no. The trouble is, I can't stop thinking about her, thinking that we could really get it on together if she'd just give me a chance. But you know, you can like somebody all you want. If they don't like you, there's nothing you can do about it.

When one person is more involved in the infatuation than the other, it hurts. You want it so much, yet you know that it probably won't ever happen.

It can be even more painful when you are still in love with someone who's no longer in love with you. This happens to almost everyone at one time or another during their lives, and it is always excruciating. Several of the teens we interviewed for this book were going through deep depressions over breaking up with their boyfriend or girlfriend. They described feeling hopeless, saying that nothing else mattered to them. Seventeen-year-old Glenda told us:

> I just feel like my life is over, like there's never going to be anything to smile about again.

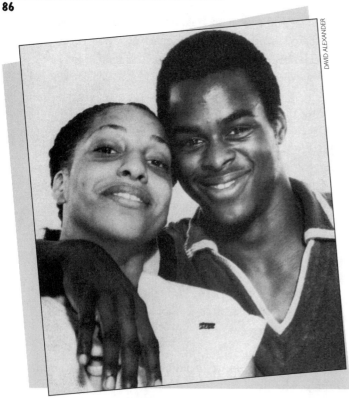

DAVID ALEXANDER

And David, a fourteen-year-old from Kentucky, said:

It hurts really bad. I see her with her new boyfriend and I want to run away and cry. We were going to get married. We were going to spend our lives together. I loved her so much.

Although time really does have a way of healing the wounds caused by a broken romance, while you are experiencing the grief you may feel, as Glenda and David did, that you'll never be happy again. People will say things like, "Don't worry. There are plenty more fish in the sea," and it's true. You will find love again. But right now, the pain you feel is real. Usually talking over your grief with a close friend or your parents, if you feel close to them, will help a lot. Some teens we met let themselves cry in their mother's arms or with a friend or even into their pillow, and they say that makes them feel better. Keeping busy helps a lot, and spending time with good friends can definitely raise your spirits. You may find some good ideas in the Emotional Health Care chapter, which begins on page 153.

One question many people ask is "How can I be sure I'm in love?" It's an important question that doesn't have a definite answer. Emotions can't be weighed or measured, so everyone has a different definition of what it is to be in love. Seventeen-year-old Rebecca said:

I've been going with Donnie since the ninth grade, and we've changed a lot together. That's why I know he's right for me. We're really compatible. We hardly fight at all. We really respect each other, so if something's wrong, we can work it out between us. That's not how it always was, so we've come a long way. In fact, I don't think I've seen a better relationship in people my age. But still, sometimes I think, I wonder what it would be like to be with somebody else. I see some guy and I think, Oh, look at him. I wonder what it would be like to be with him? When I think that, it scares me, because I worry about whether that means I don't really love Donnie.

Rebecca's relationship sounds very solid. She and her boyfriend respect and care about each other. They are able to work through their differences, and they enjoy being together. Yet she feels doubt.

During the romantic and absorbing early stages of love, you may not have any doubts at all. Everything may seem perfect. Then, when questions start coming up—and they *always* do—you may try to push them aside and get back to the way things were. Without this questioning stage, however, growth in a relationship is hard to achieve, especially when two people are still teenagers. Since it's impossible to know what life as adults will be like, it takes a great leap of faith to say, I'm certain that this is the person with whom I want to spend the rest of my life.

Several teens we met told us that they didn't want to be disloyal to their boyfriend or girlfriend but they wanted to see what it was like to go out with someone else. That often means breaking up a steady relationship. Nelson is seventeen. He's a senior in high school in Los Angeles:

I think it would be hard to break up, especially after three years. I wouldn't know where to begin if Debbee and I decided to stop going steady. I'd just be out in the cold, saying to myself, What do I do now?

Lots of people stay in relationships because they're reluctant to break up. It's so comforting to know that you'll always have a date for the weekend and that someone cares about you and is choosing to spend time with you. But fear of being alone, or of going out with a new person, or of hurting the other person's feelings, or of being rejected is not a healthy basis for maintaining a relationship. Also, fear of being physically hurt by the other person if you break up is definitely cause for seeking help from a counselor or trusted adviser. If your boyfriend or girlfriend acts in a way that threatens you or makes you afraid, please let someone know and find a way to leave the relationship. See page 211 for more on this subject.

Of course, just because you feel some doubts about your relationship doesn't mean you *have* to break up or go out with other people. But it does mean that you and your boyfriend or girlfriend have to find a way to discuss and work through your doubts and fears as they arise.

Sometimes people allow the comfort of a steady relationship to lead them into marriage before they really feel ready. Elizabeth, a second-year college student from Colorado, is very concerned about that. She said:

> I've been thinking about it so much lately, and I'm beginning to realize that I'm just not ready to make a commitment like that. There's no way I could settle down right now. My boyfriend is much more ready to settle down. He's older then me, and he's done more already, so he feels more prepared, I think.
>
> But it's really hard for me when I'm around these friends of mine who really think they love each other enough to get married. It's a lot of pressure on me, because it makes me feel like I want to be in love like that too and settle down. It

seems so romantic. They seem so sure that their lover is the person they want to be with for always and always. I just don't know that yet. I don't think I feel that way. Sometimes I wish I did, but I just don't. I've got too many things I want to do first.

You may hear people say, "Forget it. Love can conquer all." And love can seem so wonderful, so romantic, that some people do allow themselves to be swept into marriage without asking important questions. Marriage is a partnership. Before you decide to get married, it's a good idea to look closely at the partnership you have and ask yourself if it is one you can live with. Do you respect each other's values, religious principles, goals? Do you enjoy similar interests? Can you laugh together? Can you talk with each other about difficult subjects? Do you have complementary ideas about family and children? Making a long-term commitment to another person is a very serious matter. Take the time you need to examine your questions and explore your doubts. If you and your partner can be open with each other during this process, your relationship will benefit.

Of course, it's very difficult to know at age eighteen or nineteen what you will want for yourself at age twenty-five or thirty, much less at forty or fifty. You'll change a lot over the years. Lawrence, a seventeen-year-old senior from Ohio, put his feelings this way:

> I'm looking forward to going away to college next year even though me and my girlfriend think we want to get married someday. I'm ready to meet some new people and have some new experiences, and she says she is too. Not to take away from what we have, just to find out more. I can't imagine getting married before I find out as much as I can about myself.

Changing 3 Sexuality

Many people think you aren't sexual until you actually start having sexual activity with another person. Watch any naked baby and you'll see this isn't true. Babies explore their bodies all the time; they love to be held and stroked; and they often play with their genitals, when they can find them. From the beginning, we are all sexual.

Being sexual can mean having sexy thoughts or feelings, loving to be touched and hugged, enjoying the way other people's bodies look, touching your own body in places that feel particularly good, making up romantic or sexy stories in your head, feeling very attracted to another person, kissing and caressing someone you like. All these things are part of your sexuality.

Sexual Feelings

The physical changes of puberty often bring strong sexual feelings. You may find yourself thinking more about sex, getting sexually aroused more easily, and even, at times, feeling totally preoccupied with sex. Some teens say they feel as if their whole body is on fire with sexual energy and excitement. Thirteen-year-old Dominic said:

> Every time I catch sight of my neighbor, I get a hard-on. She is completely gorgeous. I am totally in love with her.

Of course, many teens get busy or excited about sports or school or music or a job or something else in their lives and don't think about sex very much. Sex may just not be on your mind right now. That doesn't mean you aren't sexual. It just means that right now you are putting your energy into other things.

Because how we feel about sex is so individual, this section makes no assumptions. You may have been taught that sex before

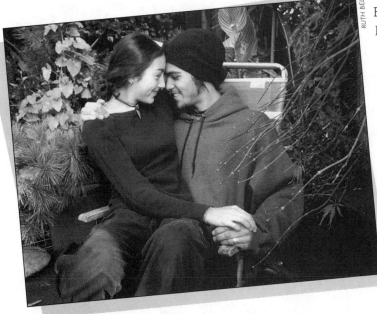

RUTH BELL

marriage is wrong. You may have been taught that sex before marriage is natural. You may be amazed that some fourteen-year-olds are having intercourse, or amazed that some eighteen-year-olds aren't interested. You may be attracted to people of the opposite sex or people of your same sex or both. You may have friends who say you're immature if you don't have sex, and you may have friends who say that people who "do it" are taking too much of a risk. You may be excited about reading this chapter on sex, or you may feel a little shocked and even worried that it will make you feel that you "ought" to be doing something that you don't feel ready to do.

The teenagers who contributed to this book all had different feelings about sex too. Some things they say will feel familiar to you; some things may feel unfamiliar. It's all okay. What's important is to go at your own pace and not let anyone pressure you into doing what you don't want to or feel ready to do.

We hope you will be very careful about sex. Sexually transmitted disease (STD) has become epidemic among teenagers, and some STDs—like HIV/AIDS, venereal warts, and herpes—currently have no cure. More and more teenagers are saying no to sex for that reason. Many have told us that they don't think it's worth risking their health or their future plans by having sex too soon or too casually. We hope that whenever and however you choose to act on your sexuality, you will treat yourself and your partner with thoughtfulness and respect, and that you will *always* try to protect yourselves from unwanted pregnancy and sexually transmitted disease (see Chapters 11 and 9).

A group of high school students in Boston wanted us to be careful that this book didn't pressure teens to act on their sexuality. Here is what they said:

> In your book you should say some things about not having sex early. Say it's okay to have sexual feelings, to get horny or excited, and *not* to go out and do it. . . . If you don't have sex with somebody, you don't have to worry about getting pregnant! . . . You don't have to worry about what you're supposed to do, or if you're doing the right thing to please your partner. . . . If you have a partner and you build into it instead of rushing into

At any point in the following section, we may be talking about something you don't believe is right or something you haven't done or experienced. Maybe you will someday. Maybe you won't. Don't feel you have to experience everything now. The beauty of sex and lovemaking is that we are always learning more about it, even as adults, so there's plenty of time. Allison, a seventeen-year-old girl from the West Coast, emphasized that point. She said:

> I have at least fifty, maybe even sixty more years of being sexual, and I'm sure I don't have to worry about doing everything this minute.

Whatever you decide, we encourage you to be respectful of yourself and others. This means

➤ Not letting yourself be rushed into anything.

➤ Not rushing anyone else into anything.

➤ Not feeling you have to prove how cool or mature you are by the amount of sexual experience you have.

➤ Never having sex with anyone you don't know very well.

➤ Learning from your mistakes.

➤ Not letting drugs or alcohol make your decisions about sex for you.

➤ Taking responsibility for your actions, which means using protection to avoid unwanted pregnancies and STDs.

it, what you do feels a lot nicer. If you rush into it, you feel like a piece of shit afterwards. . . . If you waited, you wouldn't have to worry, Did I do this right? Did I do that right? Was I being used? Should it have happened? . . . If you're worried about it at all, then it isn't time to do it. . . . The slower the better.

Aaron, a seventeen-year-old senior, put it this way: "If you're in doubt, *wait!*" The problem is that sexual feelings can be so intense and confusing, it's often difficult to be perfectly "sure" and "decided" about what you want to do. It could happen that only after trying something do you realize that you wish you hadn't. If this happens, you can stop and not do it again until you are ready. Just because you've done something once doesn't mean you're going to want to or have to do it again. People make mistakes in sex. Some mistakes are just part of growing up. In fact, a lot of what we learn about sex comes from making mistakes.

Some mistakes in sex are irreversible, however, as fifteen-year-old Johanna discovered when she found out she was pregnant:

I told Noah I wasn't using birth control, but he said, "Oh, don't worry, I know what to do." How could I have let him talk me into doing it? I was so stupid, but he kept saying, "Don't you love me?"

Lots of voices live inside our heads telling us "Do this" or "Don't do this." Your parents, friends, school, government, and religious leaders all have something to say about sex, and their views shape how you think. But when the moment comes, *you* are the one who has to decide what to do and what not to do; if you are

in a relationship, ideally, you will decide together. We hope this chapter will provide the information you need to make decisions that are right for you.

GETTING TO KNOW YOURSELF AS A SEXUAL PERSON

Learning About Sex

Much of what we learn about sex isn't told to us directly. We learn by watching and listening to what goes on around us. Karen, a fifteen-year-old from California, said:

I remember taking showers with my brothers all the time, so I always knew how boys looked naked. Then when I got in about the sixth grade and I started knowing about sex, and we had those sex ed movies, I'd think to myself, Oh yeah, that's like my brothers.

Lots of children go beyond Karen and do "research" on their own. Polly is from New York:

There was this one girl in my grammar school class—her name was Nancy—that me and my girlfriends used to play doctor with, and she was always the patient. We would make her take her pants off and we'd pretend to stick her with things, like giving her a needle, you know, and we'd go up to this room we have in our attic where we knew we could be private. Even now I can remember it being sort of thrilling to me that she would take her pants off.

Like Polly, you may have played games that let you do some early exploring of bodies and sexual feelings. Eighteen-year-old Jeff remembers:

I was always experimenting with sex, ever since I was really little. Like even at nursery school, it made no difference to me whether it was with a boy or a girl, we'd roll around together and feel each other and get naked together. It was no big thing, just fun. And of course it felt good. My

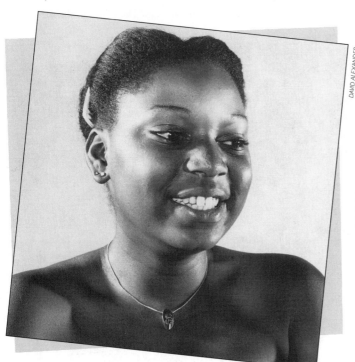

DAVID ALEXANDER

mother wasn't too crazy about it, though. She kept asking me why didn't I go out and play or ride my bike or something. She let me know she didn't think it was too cool to be doing what I was doing.

Indirectly, Jeff's mom was teaching Jeff something about sex. Maybe because of her reaction, a question entered his head: "Is what I'm doing okay?" Colleen's mother was more direct:

My mother came into my room and found me masturbating one day when I was ten, and she couldn't handle it at all. "Don't do that. It's wrong. You'll hurt yourself." I was terrified, and for years whenever I masturbated I felt this shame.

Colleen's mother had probably been taught that masturbation was wrong, and she was worried that Colleen was doing something that might hurt her. It's also possible that she just wasn't ready to think of her daughter as a sexual being. (For more information about masturbation, see page 96.)

Parents teach us about sex by their attitudes. Do they answer our questions about sex? Are they visibly embarrassed whenever the subject comes up? We learn from how they act with each other and how they feel about their own sexuality. Are they openly affectionate in front of their children? Are they very private about any display of sexual feeling? If your parents talk freely and in a relaxed way about their feelings for each other, that might make you more relaxed with sex. Or perhaps you find it embarrassing and think you're not ready to act like that. If they are very private, you may feel private about your sexuality too. Or you may have the opposite reaction and decide to be more open about your feelings.

We also learn by how our parents handle nudity. If nakedness is not allowed in your house, you may grow up feeling your body is something to hide. If bathroom doors are always shut and locked, you may learn that body functions are to be kept private. If people in your family walk around naked or carry on conversations in the bathroom or take baths together, you may grow up feeling that naked bodies are okay.

None of this is to say that one way is right and the other way is wrong, only that we all bring different attitudes to our sexual relationships based on what we are used to and grew up with, and it's good to remember that not everyone thinks the same way you do.

People also learn about sex (as we mentioned in the Changing Bodies chapter) through books, movies, magazines, TV, jokes, advertising, locker room conversations, and friends. These sources often provide inaccurate information, and they can make sex seem like one big exploitation, where people just use each other to feel good or show off. If you only had movies and TV teaching you about sex, you would probably think that everyone feels sexy all the time and that people come on to one another all the time, but this is a very different message from the one you might be getting at home or in a sex-ed class at school. So it's confusing. How do you know what's right for you? How can you sort through all the attitudes and messages to find the one that speaks to your heart?

It may not be until you first start having a boyfriend or a girlfriend that you learn how *you* really feel about sex. Whenever that time comes, the more you know about your own sexuality and the facts of how your body works, the better able you will be to make good decisions, which is the goal.

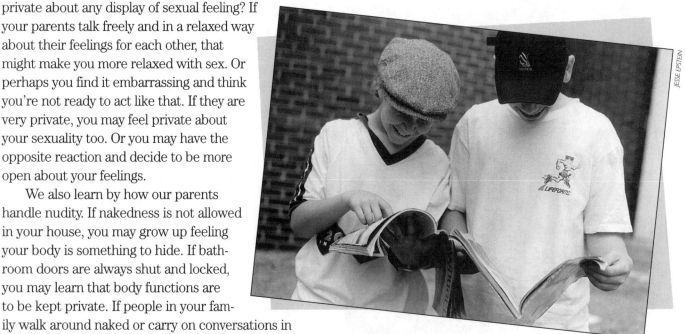

JESSE EPSTEIN

FEELING BAD ABOUT SEX: Along with the pleasure and joy our sexuality can bring, many of us find we feel bad or guilty about what we are doing.

Feeling private about sex is different. Many people feel private—or shy sometimes—about sexual activity, no matter how old they are. There is a natural mystery surrounding sex between two people, and no amount of sex education will ever take that away.

Sometimes, however, we feel guilty as well as private about sex. Lots of teens we met talk about feeling "dirty" or "sleazy" because of some sexual experience they've had. In many instances, it was because they ended up doing something before they felt ready to do it. That's what happened to Trish, a sixteen-year-old from Missouri:

> I felt dirty, I really felt dirty. I felt that I had deceived my mother in a way too, because she had always told me, "Wait till you're sure, wait till you're sure." And I wasn't sure. I just did it because everyone else was doing it. And it didn't feel good, and I didn't like it, and I thought it sucked all around.

Fifteen-year-old Amory said he feels guilty about masturbating. "I always wonder, Am I the only pervert, or is everyone doing this?" And Cedric, a seventeen-year-old from Providence, Rhode Island, said, "When I had my first wet dream, I was really excited about it, but I felt guilty at being so excited." Several girls spoke of feeling some shame when they started their periods. Other teens said they felt guilty about the sexual images that were often on their minds.

Our culture is mixed-up about sex, so it's no wonder we are too. On the one hand, signs of sex are everywhere, from advertising to porno movies to MTV to fashion. On the other hand, our families, social groups, and religious institutions often have strict rules discouraging or forbidding many aspects of our sexuality. Things like masturbation, oral sex, homosexuality, and sex outside of marriage are forbidden by some religions that teach that sex is only for procreating children and that any other kind of sexual enjoyment is sinful.

Our sexuality is part of being human. When we are made to feel guilty about sex, we may carry that guilt with us throughout our lives. Young men may have problems controlling themselves in sexual situations; young women may have a hard time enjoying lovemaking. It's not easy to let yourself go and feel all the pleasure if some part of you is saying, "I shouldn't be doing this." A couple may have trouble talking openly with each other about sex because they feel they "shouldn't" be having sex at all. Many teenagers say that they "forget" to use safe-sex protection because of that. They don't want to plan ahead and bring protection, because that means admitting to themselves that they are having sex. Feeling guilty, then, makes them risk pregnancy and sexually transmitted disease.

Some of you, as young children and teens, may have had a parent or sibling or relative or someone else force you or manipulate you to perform sexual acts with him or her. This is called sexual abuse, and it happens to millions of people. Because of having been sexually abused, many teens have feelings of anger and fear and guilt associated with sex that interfere with their ability to be able to enjoy their sexuality or feel comfortable in sexual relationships. You will hear from teens who have experienced sexual abuse and are finding ways to heal from the emotional pain of their experiences in the section on Sexual Abuse, beginning on page 227. In the Resource section on page 241, you will find books and organizations to which you can turn for support and information.

There's a lot to consider when you're deciding whether or not to have a sexual relationship, and feeling bad about your sexuality only makes it harder to be clear. We hope you will care for yourself enough to take your time and get to know your true feelings. We hope you will take care of your friends enough to respect their decisions to do the same.

Sex on Your Mind: Sexual Fantasies

Fantasies are a safe way to explore your sexual feelings. They are thoughts—they are under your control. You don't have to act on them unless you want to.

Thoughts can't hurt people; only actions can. Jerome, who's fifteen, put it this way:

My fantasies are all about things I'd never really do in real life—in fact, that's almost the definition of a fantasy for me: something I'd never really do. Then I feel free to do it in my mind without feeling guilty. Usually, the things in my imagination would be real embarrassing to me, really humiliating if I was ever in one of those situations. Like lying around naked in the lunch yard and having everyone standing over me, pointing at me, laughing at me. Or thinking about pulling someone's clothes off and being rough with them. I know I'd never do that, but just fantasizing about it makes it exciting.

Jerome understands that fantasizing about something doesn't mean he wants to do it or that he will do it. He's just enjoying some of the less-explored territory of his mind.

Here are three other fantasies people told us. Like Jerome's, they are about imaginary situations that are very erotic (sexually exciting) to the person having them:

I dream about diving naked into a swimming pool full of red Jell-O. I swim around and swim around, and it's thick and cool, and I bury my face in it.

I dream about being covered in whipped cream and some stranger comes and licks it all off.

Whenever I'm on the subway, I have this fantasy that all the women are naked. They have their shoes on and their purses and packages and everything, but no clothes on.

Thirteen-year-old Kathleen's fantasies are more about a real-life situation. They make the limits of her life more tolerable:

I think about my boyfriend all the time. Like especially when I'm watching TV or reading something romantic and they're kissing, then I think, Oh, God, I wish he were here. We barely ever get a chance to kiss, because school is just about the only place we see each other. My mom thinks I'm too young to have a boyfriend, so she doesn't let him come over. I mean we've tried to see each other, but it never works out. So mostly I just spend my time dreaming about him and what it would be like to be alone with him somewhere— just the two of us.

When Kathleen finally gets to be with her boyfriend, maybe things will be as terrific as she has imagined. This was true for Dan, who's sixteen:

Sometimes you fantasize about somebody you really like and then you find out that they really like you too. That happened to me with this girl I used to go out with. I used to daydream about how wonderful it would be to be with her and then we really did get together and it *was* wonderful.

For Oliver, however, the fantasies were better than the reality:

VALINDA RODRIGUEZ

When I was in junior high I found that my fantasies were a lot more pleasurable than the reality. In my imagination, I could make things work perfectly and be with just who I wanted to be with, but the reality of it at the time wasn't anywhere near as great. I was really awkward with girls and had trouble getting it on with them—but in my fantasy I was really smooth.

While your sexual feelings are blossoming, you may get a fierce crush on someone it's completely impossible to be with. It may be a teacher or camp counselor, a rock star, the older sister or brother of a friend, or the youth director at your church or temple. Crushes like these are normal, and if you don't suffer too much over not being able to have the person you yearn for, they don't do any harm. In fact, they give you a chance to explore your romantic feelings without acting on them.

A fantasy may be about someone of your own sex (a "homosexual" fantasy). This may mean that you are trying out feelings and possibilities that you will never choose to act on. It may mean that you find people of your own sex attractive, which is pretty healthy since it probably means you like yourself. It could also mean that you would like to have a sexual relationship with someone of your own sex—anything from kissing and hugging to making love. (See pages 130–150 for information on homosexual relationships.) Many people have homosexual relationships at some point. For some it is a brief experience; for others it is a way of life.

Having same-sex fantasies, however, doesn't predict one way or the other whether you will have a homosexual relationship in the future. Eric, a seventeen-year-old from Iowa, told us:

> I have a dream sometimes that I'm lying on the beach and these two big muscley guys come over to me and tell me what a great body I have. They stick around talking for a while and then we take our suits off and go swimming. I wake up excited and feeling sexy.

Sometimes people have fantasies of being hurt—being whipped, tied up, beaten—or of doing those things to someone else. We may dream or fantasize that sex is being forced on us. These fantasies can be repulsive or scary even though they are sexually exciting. Do I really want that? the person asks in a panic. The answer is usually no, but people do worry that fantasizing something means you really want it. Gloria speaks for the fears of many girls:

> I have these fantasies about being raped. Like when I'm walking home from school, I imagine that I'm pulled into a car and this man with dark hair and blue eyes pulls off my clothes and forces me to have sex with him. Right there in the car. It scares me to think about that, because it makes me wonder if I really want to be raped.

Real rape is very, very different from fantasy rape. Rape is when someone uses sex as a tool of violence against another person (see page 233). Yet many women who have been raped actually wonder if they were responsible, because they have occasionally had fantasies of sex being forced on them. *They are not responsible at all.* Rape fantasies often reflect a person's anxieties about the violence they know exists.

For many people, rape fantasies are a way of letting you imagine yourself having sex. Since the confusing messages in our society make many teenagers feel guilty about having sexual desires, sometimes the easiest way to picture having sex with someone is to imagine that it is being forced on you. Several teens told us that is how it is for them:

> *John (seventeen):* A lot of guys I know have this same fantasy about being with a couple of really huge women who are whipping them and forcing them to get undressed and have sex with them. In my fantasy, it's always in a sleazy motel room and there are two women who hold me down and take turns with me.

> *Susan (nineteen):* I have this very exciting daydream about a woman and a man coming into my house and making me have sex with both of them before I can leave.

> *Gary (fifteen):* I fantasize about older women. I like the idea of being seduced by an older woman, someone who knows what she wants, so you don't have to be put in that decision-making position. I get really turned on thinking about an aggressive woman who'll just lead me through the steps.

These fantasies all have the same theme. Thinking about being forced into sex or being seduced lets you enjoy the turned-on feeling of being sexually desired without having to imagine yourself being the one to start it. In real life, however, being the "victim" in a coercive sexual relationship does not lead to healthy self-esteem. The section on sexual abuse, beginning on page 227, discusses this issue in greater detail. Remember, fantasies are often your mind's way of dealing with real-life fears, so while your fantasies can't hurt you or anyone else, acting on those fantasies can be very dangerous and destructive.

Occasionally, a person will find herself or himself spending nearly all day and night in fantasies, which may come to seem more real than reality. Or your fantasies might be so strong and so vivid that you begin to fear you might actually act them out. This is especially scary if they are fantasies of violence, of hurting someone or of letting yourself be hurt. In cases like these, it is a good idea to talk about your fantasies and fears with someone you trust—a parent or other relative, a teacher, or a counselor. See the Emotional Health Care chapter, beginning on page 153, for suggestions.

Masturbation

Masturbation is something most people do at one time or another during their lives. Some slang phrases people use for masturbation are beating off, whipping it, hand job, jerking off, jacking off. You may have your own private name for it. Usually masturbation means touching, rubbing, or squeezing your penis or clitoris to give yourself sexual pleasure. Sexual thoughts and fantasies may fill your mind at the same time. If you keep it up long enough, you may have an orgasm—rhythmic waves of muscle contractions in your genitals and internal reproductive organs that feel very good. Masturbation is something you do with yourself, a way of giving pleasure to yourself, of loving and being tender to yourself. It also helps you to get to know your body's sexual responses.

Many teenagers told us that masturbating lets them enjoy their sexuality when they aren't in a relationship with someone or if they don't want their relationship to be sexual. It can also be a part of your relationship with yourself even when you have a sexual partner, and it can be part of your relationship with that partner too.

Not everyone masturbates, of course. Lots of people have never done it and don't want to do it. You may read this section to see what other people do and decide it's not for you at this point in your life. Cecile, sixteen, said, "I wouldn't masturbate, but if someone else does, that's their decision."

Most babies and little children masturbate. They touch themselves all over, exploring this part and that, finding the places that feel especially good. Greg, who's seventeen, said, "I've always masturbated, at least for as long as I can remember." Beth, who's sixteen, remembered:

When I was little I used to rub against things, like the corner of my mattress or this one stuffed animal I had which had a perfect nose for rubbing against my crotch. So I would go around rubbing this animal against me all the time. I don't think I really had an orgasm. It was more like after a while I would just get tired and stop.

Many children stop this kind of body play when they get to be a few years old, often because a grown-up pulls their hand away and tells them that touching themselves "there" is bad. Some religions forbid masturbation, so children growing up with those religious traditions learn early on that masturbation is not okay. Other children learn to have a good time masturbating privately. Sam, who's eleven, told us:

I like sleeping with my hand down there; I guess it just helps me feel relaxed. Sometimes I don't even know I'm doing it, but I'll wake up and that's where my hand will be.

A lot of people rediscover masturbation when they get to be teenagers and find their stronger sexual feelings need an outlet. A fourteen-year-old boy from Washington State told us:

Around the time when I was just starting junior high school I was changing a lot and feeling really sexy and all this tension started building up, and for me masturbating was a way of releasing it. It still is.

Emily also discovered masturbation when she was that age:

You know, I never even knew that you could masturbate. I mean I probably did it when I was a baby, but I don't remember. One day I overheard a conversation some kids were having at school, and one guy asked a girl if girls could masturbate, and she said, "Of course." And she was telling him how great it felt and everything, so that night when I was in bed I started feeling around down there, and I started getting these sexy sensations and I got really aroused. Right on that bone was the part I was pressing, I guess sort of rubbing. It felt amazing. I kept rubbing until these spasms and this incredible feeling started happening, and I couldn't rub after that because it was too tender, so I just lay there feeling good.

PRIVACY: Most people we talked to agreed that they like to masturbate in private, when they are alone with their own thoughts and feelings. Some mentioned masturbating with a friend or with a person they are having a sexual relationship with. But even then, they wanted privacy from others. Here's how Josh put it:

> It's a pretty vulnerable position to be in—caught with your hand on your cock, lost in your fantasies, working away at it. I don't think I'd want my mother or my sister walking in on that!

Getting privacy can be hard, though, especially for kids and teens, and especially in big families or if you share a bedroom. Darrell, sixteen, told us this story:

> One time I walked into my room to talk to my little brother, and he was whipping it and I scared the shit out of him. You know, he started yelling at me to get the hell out. He really was embarrassed—I mean, really embarrassed. Probably he felt like he was doing something he shouldn't have been doing. I couldn't help laughing, but then I told him it was cool. I told him, "Hey man, I do it too you know." But he acted like he was getting busted for robbery or something.

Almost everyone gets upset if his or her privacy is interrupted in the middle of a sexual experience. Even if we don't think what we are doing is wrong in any way, we may feel exposed, embarrassed, or even ashamed, because there is a natural privateness about sex. Johnny, a fifteen-year-old from Boston, said:

Even if you know it's normal and all that, you still lock the door! You don't go around advertising that you're doing it. There are all those jokes like, "What are you doing after school today?" "Oh I'm going home to beat off." You know, Ha-ha-ha-ha. That kind of thing. But even if everybody does it and everybody knows everybody does it, you still pretend you don't.

HOW DO PEOPLE MASTURBATE? Masturbation means using your hand to stimulate yourself sexually. Touching yourself is one of the most natural ways to explore your sexuality, to find out what excites you, what places are the most sensitive. There are lots of ways to masturbate, because it's a very personal thing.

Girls usually rub or press around or near their clitoris, since that is the most sexually sensitive part of their body and can be stimulated with the slightest touch or pressure (see page 33 for information about the clitoris). Many also enjoy touching their breasts or other places on their body. Some girls put their fingers into their vagina when they masturbate. Some masturbate using a spray of water from the shower or faucet; some rub against the sheets or pillow or some other soft object. Other girls don't use their hands or an object at all but squeeze the muscles in and around their vagina and anus. For some girls, fantasies are enough. One fifteen-year-old from Los Angeles had this experience:

> One time I was on this bus and I was sitting right over the wheel where it was vibrating a whole lot. I was fantasizing about this guy that I had just met in the street and I was getting more and more into it. I was wearing a skirt, so my thighs were touching and rubbing together, and with the vibrations and everything I was so aroused that I had an orgasm right there on the bus. In the middle of everything.

Boys usually masturbate by rubbing and stroking or pressing their penis and testicles. Some boys don't touch their penis with their hand at all but use sheets or a pillow or something else to rub around their genital area. Others tighten and release the muscles around their anus and pubic area. Still others bring themselves to orgasm by fantasy alone. Lots of boys combine fantasy and penis massage, as Brian, a fourteen-year-old from the East Coast, describes:

When I'm beating off I can get so much into a fantasy that it's almost like I'm really in it. There's this one very sexy girl that I always picture. I always watch her at school with her boyfriend. But when I'm masturbating, she's with me, you know what I mean? And it's a real shock when I come out of it, after I come and I open my eyes and see my own room in my own apartment. What a letdown! But it sure is great while I'm into it.

HOW MUCH DO PEOPLE MASTURBATE? Some people don't masturbate at all. Others do it once in a while. And some do it a lot. Bob, fifteen, was talking about this in a discussion group in Pennsylvania:

Sometimes when I masturbate a whole lot I begin to feel like I must be a sex-starved maniac or something. You know you always hear that if you masturbate too much you'll end up crazy. I don't really believe that, but a lot of the time I feel like I should stop myself from whipping it too much.

Bob doesn't have to worry. Masturbating doesn't hurt you, and you can't really do it "too much" unless excessive rubbing creates soreness, or unless you find yourself spending so much time alone that you're neglecting your schoolwork, your social life, your family, and your other activities. Doing any one thing to the total exclusion of everything else is not especially healthy for you.

IS MASTURBATION BAD/DANGEROUS/PERVERTED?
People are more accepting of masturbation these days. Movies even show people masturbating. But as we have already said, some religions denounce masturbation as sinful, and many adults grew up believing that masturbation was wrong and actually harmful to the body. Max ran into this theory head-on:

My grandparents gave me this book about bad little kids who masturbate. One of the bad little kids went blind, and another one had his thumbs

cut off. Can you believe that? There was no doubt about the message in that book: *Don't masturbate.* It was lucky for me that my parents were cool and didn't do that number on me.

If your parents or grandparents have punished you for masturbating or told you it would hurt you, it's probably because that's what they were told. Some doctors a couple of generations ago thought it was harmful. We know now that it isn't. Adults may disapprove of children masturbating because it is sexual. The thought that their children are doing something so sexual makes some parents uneasy.

You may hear from your friends that masturbation is bad for you. Ed told us this:

When I was about thirteen, I masturbated a couple of times but then I heard from the other guys I hang out with that it would sap your strength and that it leads to becoming a pervert. So I sort of gave it up.

Ed's friends were wrong. Masturbation does not sap your strength and it doesn't lead to your becoming a pervert. There's nothing that says you have to masturbate, however, so if you don't want to or don't feel comfortable doing it, don't.

Boys seem to talk about masturbation more than girls do, and although they usually talk about it in a joking way, listening to what they say might make you feel that there's something wrong with it. Not to mention the crudeness of some of the names people give to masturbation: slamming the ham, pounding the pud, jerking off. None of those terms express the tenderness that you might actually feel when you're enjoying being alone with yourself and getting into your fantasies.

Caddie, fifteen, describes her changing feelings about masturbation:

When I was really little, my best friend and I would sleep over at each other's house and we'd masturbate together in the same room. We even had our own name for it. We certainly didn't think there was anything wrong with what we were doing. It was just something we did that felt good. But in about fourth grade I found out more about sex, and I realized that masturbating was *sexual*. Then, as far as I was concerned, it was definitely not okay to do it anymore—especially not with somebody else in the same room. After that, I used to feel guilty when I was doing it, like it was kind of humiliating, and I tried to stop myself. Then last year when I heard from some of my friends that they do it too, I felt better about it.

Other cultures in the world teach people that sex is a natural part of life. They give their children a sense that feeling and being sexual is okay and perfectly normal. Fortunately, Caddie was able to hear from her friends that she wasn't the only one masturbating, and that it wasn't something she had to feel guilty about or worry about. She learned an important lesson too: Talking with people can help.

MASTURBATION AND LOVEMAKING: If and when you decide to make love with someone else, you may find that having masturbated helps you enjoy lovemaking more. It can help you discover what parts of your body are sensitive and what feels especially good. By communicating that to your partner, you can help him or her learn how to make sex more pleasurable for you.

Some people believe that once you are in a sexual relationship with someone else, you shouldn't masturbate anymore. They think masturbation isn't as good as making out or fooling around or having intercourse with another person. That's not the way it is: Masturbation isn't better or worse, it's different, as fifteen-year-old Angie described:

You know, you can have a boyfriend and everything, even lots of boyfriends, but when you're home in bed at night and you feel sexy right at that minute, what's wrong with doing it yourself? Sometimes people think you only masturbate because you don't have anybody to go out with and so you have to get off by yourself. But I don't see it that way at all. One thing doesn't have anything to do with the other.

Actually, many couples, even married couples, experience sexual closeness and give each other sexual pleasure through what we call mutual masturba-tion, in which partners use their hands to bring each other to orgasm. Sometimes people masturbate each other because they don't want to or can't have sexual intercourse; sometimes they do it as an added way to give each other pleasure.

Sexual Response

Our bodies are alive to sexual feelings. A scene in a movie, a sexy thought, the prospect of being with someone we're attracted to all bring physical responses. If the excitement keeps up, our whole body goes through a series of responses to the stimulation we feel.

We will describe this process, sometimes called the sexual response cycle, so you can recognize what is happening in your body when you are sexually aroused. This is what the cycle is like: A buildup of excitement, a climax of excitement (called orgasm, or coming), then a time when your body returns to a normal relaxed state.

People don't always go through the whole cycle, and for each person, each time may be a little different: sometimes the feelings will keep building and building, sometimes they won't; sometimes you'll have an orgasm, sometimes your body will return to normal without orgasm. There is no particular pattern your body and feelings "should" follow every time you get sexually aroused. Your body is individual, and your sexual responses are yours alone.

THE PHASES OF SEXUAL RESPONSE

Getting Excited: During the first phase of sexual excitement a boy's penis gets hard and a girl's vagina gets wet. This happens because extra blood from nearby blood vessels flows into the special spongy tissue inside the penis or vagina in a process called "vasocongestion." It is the same process in both girls' and boys' bodies.* In boys the spongy tissue in the penis swells up, making the penis longer, harder, wider, and erect (see page 17 for more details about this process). In girls the spongy tissue swells

---

* It's fascinating to realize that this same swelling process happens inside both boys' and girls' bodies. It's not surprising, since our sexual organs start out identical inside the mother's womb and don't become male or female until a few weeks after the fertilized egg attaches to the uterus and starts to grow.

up inside the walls of the vagina, making them secrete a liquid that lubricates the area. A girl's clitoris also swells a bit and gets erect. In fact, her whole pelvic area has a full, aroused feeling.

Stimulation: During this part of the excitement phase, your breathing and heartbeat speed up and your blood pressure rises a little. A girl's vagina gets slightly larger and longer inside, and her breasts may swell slightly. People can stay in this phase for a very long time, moving in and out of it as the stimulation varies.

After a while, if the stimulation keeps up—if your penis or clitoris keeps getting stroked or your fantasies intensify—you will move into another phase in which you reach a high level of body tension and sexual arousal. Your muscles tighten, especially around your pelvic area and buttocks. A boy's testicles pull in closer to his body, and a girl's clitoris pulls in under the hood of skin attached to her inner vaginal lips. In this position, her clitoris can be stimulated by friction from the hood if a finger or a penis or the pressure of her partner's pubic bone is rubbing against it.

If you stop suddenly once you get this excited, your pelvic area may feel congested (swollen, full) for a while until your body gets back to its regular, unstimulated state. This is what boys sometimes refer to as "blue balls," and girls may experience as an uncomfortable fullness or achiness in their lower torso. It isn't going to harm you physically in any way, but it might feel unpleasant.

Orgasm: Orgasm (slang names: coming, getting off, climaxing) is the second phase of the sexual response cycle. At the peak of sexual excitement and muscle tension, there is a sudden series of muscle contractions all along the penis or all through the vagina, clitoris, and pelvic area. It lasts about ten seconds, but it may feel a lot longer to you while you're going through it. An orgasm releases the body tension that has built up through sexual stimulation. It usually feels really good and really intense.

A boy nearly always ejaculates during orgasm— that is, semen spurts out of his penis. A girl doesn't ejaculate. Other than that, the experience of

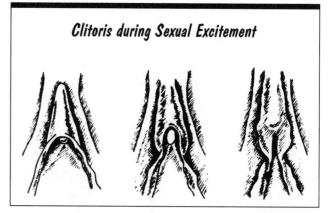

Clitoris during Sexual Excitement

orgasm is quite similar for both. Here's how Richie describes it:

> As I feel the orgasm coming I forget about everything else and get lost in this feeling that starts in the tip of my penis and spreads all over my body. It's like my body begins swimming all by itself, like there's something in me reaching out, welcoming the pleasure. As it becomes really intense, my body begins shaking with excitement. The sensations take me over, and just at the peak of it, I can feel this pulsing at the base of my penis and I feel the sperm shooting out of me like I'm sending it off, far away. It's amazing.

Dorie described her feelings during orgasm this way:

> How does it feel to have an orgasm? Well, for me it's like this buildup of excitement—you know, everything starts feeling better and better and with me, my fantasies get really vivid. Then as I get closer and closer to coming, it's like all my muscles tighten up down there, and I feel tingly all over. All my concentration is on my clit, because that's the place that is responding to every movement. I kind of cheer myself on in my head, Come on, come on, you're getting closer. Then I get to the point where I know it's going to happen, and my whole body relaxes, and with that I feel this flood of sensation—I don't know how to describe it—it's like these waves of pleasure that just take me over. When you're having an orgasm, you're just focused on that. Total involvement in that. Nothing else exists. It's the most wonderful feeling of just being alive in your body without your

head getting in the way telling you things. For me it's very peaceful.

Of course, each individual will experience orgasm in his or her own way, but most people say that it is a relaxing, deeply pleasurable occurrence.

Returning to Normal: After orgasm, your muscles relax, the swelling in your penis or vagina goes down, your breathing and pulse return to normal. This phase may take half an hour or more. For many people it is a peaceful, quiet, tender time, either alone or with someone else. Jasmine said:

> I like the time right after we make love, when we're just lying there together. Maybe we'll talk about really intimate things about ourselves. Maybe we'll just be happy to be together. I actually enjoy that even more than I enjoy intercourse.

After orgasm, most boys have a period of time during which they won't be able to get an erection again. That time can be as short as five minutes, or it can last several hours. Some girls feel sexier after they reach orgasm and want to continue the stimulation. Other girls have a period of time after orgasm during which they enjoy resting and letting their body settle down. Like so many things in sex, each individual will have his or her own experience. There's no one right way.

Having an orgasm can be a powerful experience. It can show you a wonderful, pleasurable side of your own nature. You don't have to be having sexual intercourse to be able to share that kind of mutual joy and closeness with someone you love. Many couples bring each other to orgasm by other means of lovemaking, like mutual masturbation or oral sex, or through sexual practices that they discover together. Since intercourse doesn't always provide the proper stimulation for girls, other techniques of sexual stimulation may actually make lovemaking more pleasurable for girls, and they definitely make it less risky.

IF YOU DON'T HAVE ORGASMS AND WANT TO: People can have an orgasm when they masturbate, through fantasies, in dreams, in sex play or lovemaking with another person. Some people don't have orgasms often or at all, others have orgasms when they masturbate but not with someone else around, some have orgasms with other forms of sex play but not with intercourse, and still other people seem to have orgasms easily and frequently. There's been a lot written and said about orgasms, and many teenagers (especially girls) complained to us of feeling that they "ought" to have them. Having an orgasm can become a *goal* that pressures people and makes them feel bad if they don't achieve it. That can definitely take the pleasure out of lovemaking.

Susan, who's fifteen, said something we heard from a lot of teenage girls:

> I hear all the time about orgasms and how great they are. But I don't think I've ever had one.

Julie, seventeen, didn't know what an orgasm was:

> I knew that there was this thing called a climax, because you read about it in books. It would say, "And they came to a climax." But I never knew that it was *someone's* climax. I didn't think women had orgasms at all. Then one time, making love, my boyfriend said, "Did you come?" and I said, "I don't know," because I didn't know what he was talking about.

Many of the teenaged girls we talked with hadn't experienced orgasm. They worried, "Will I ever be able to come?" "Is my body built wrong?" "Am I too screwed up about sex?" "Why do guys come so easily and I don't?"

It is not surprising that girls and women have orgasms less easily than boys and men do. First there's anatomy. A boy can't miss his penis. He touches it several times a day to urinate. Most boys discover masturbation, and it is pretty easy for them to figure out how to do it by just touching and rubbing and squeezing. But a girl's clitoris, and certainly her vagina, are more hidden. Also, if she was taught as a child never to touch her genitals, she may not have explored down there to find out what feels good and what doesn't.

Then there is sex education, or lack of it. If you aren't taught about your clitoris and what it does, you may not realize that sexual pleasure for a woman comes mainly from clitoral stimulation. Some women experience that stimulation through intercourse, when the penis rubs their clitoris from the inside. But for many women, internal stimulation isn't enough. They need direct, external clitoral stimulation to experience orgasm. If you don't know about that, it may be difficult to achieve orgasm.

Finally, girls in general are brought up to be less accepting and proud of their sexuality than boys are. This is part of the "double standard" we discuss on page 105. A teenage boy who is interested in exploring his sexuality may find that his sexual adventures are tolerated or even encouraged by his family and friends. But a girl is usually told she must be the one to say no. She rarely hears about her own sex drive, and she may not feel comfortable letting herself go sexually, since she's been taught that it's her responsibility to keep sex play under control. Furthermore, she knows that she'll be the one to get pregnant if they are not prepared with protection.

Many girls are taught that Prince Charming will come along someday to teach them about sex and love and to give them pleasure. They may feel they aren't supposed to explore sexual pleasure for themselves. This makes some girls shy about masturbating and even shyer about letting their partner know what pleases them. That puts a lot of pressure on their sexual partner to "perform" for both of them. In fact, many women find that the more willing they are to take the initiative themselves by touching their clitoris or moving their body in a way that stimulates their clitoris, the more likely they are to experience orgasm during sex play or lovemaking.

Feeling we "have to" have orgasms does nothing but add to the confusions and pressures many of us feel about sex. Furthermore, worrying about it generally makes people more tense and less able to relax and enjoy themselves. For most girls and women, having orgasms is simply a matter of time and practice. It may take you months or years of getting used to being sexual, but sooner or later, if you want to have an orgasm, you probably will.

IN LOVE

We laugh
not because it is funny,
but because it is funny
to feel so happy.

We rant and rave,
not because it is dreadful,
but because it is dreadful
to hurt so badly.

And when we love, at love,
our bodies communicating
in their own clandestine,
coded way . . .
We sigh—
not because we are frightened
but because it is frightening
to become each other
for one moment,
and still,
in the instant's shrieking sharpness,
to remain obliquely outside.

Forever together . . .
and yet,
together
alone.
and then,

We kiss,
not because it is loving,
but because it is loving
that makes us want to.
                    —MICHAEL SCOTT

EXPLORING SEX WITH SOMEONE ELSE

Loving someone and wanting to be closer, having a friendship that suddenly opens up to sexual feelings, feeling sexually excited by someone, getting just plain curious about sex—all these are reasons why people start exploring sex with each other. For you, "exploring sex" might mean kissing, hugging, and touching someone you're attracted to. It might mean staring at each other a lot and talking to each other privately. It might mean touching each other's bodies, or taking your clothes off with each other. It may include touching each other's genitals and/or having orgasms together. All of these are ways of having sex together and all can be ways to make love. At some point your lovemaking may include oral sex or sexual intercourse. *This chapter makes no assumptions about what you are doing or will do sexually.*

Bringing sex into a relationship between two people nearly always changes how they feel about each other and themselves. You may find your body aching to touch or kiss the person you care about. You may not be sure how or when or whether to attempt it. Deciding about sex isn't easy. In this chapter you'll hear how a lot of different teenagers deal with the sexual decisions they face.

Pleasure and fun and closeness are the best parts of being sexual together, but a sexual relationship can also bring unhappiness: for example, if someone's feelings are hurt when the relationship doesn't last, if someone you trusted goes around telling people what you did together, if it's not as great as you expected it to be, if you worry that you can't "perform" right or don't "know how" to do something, if you get a girl pregnant or get pregnant, if you catch a sexually transmitted disease, if the person you are crazy about doesn't care as much for you.

We hope this chapter and the information in this book will give you some of the knowledge and understanding you need to decrease those painful experiences and increase the positive ones.

When Does It Start?

Exploring sex with someone else starts early for some of us and a lot later for others. When *you* start will depend on how strong your sexual feelings are, what your standards are about sex, who your friends happen to be, and whether you are close to someone who also wants to explore sex.

A number of teenagers we interviewed experimented with sex when they were still in grade school. Usually it was not so much a matter of "being in love" with someone as of playing around with a friend and finding out about sex as a consequence. Marta told us:

In the fourth grade, me and this boy in the next grade used to meet in the garage in our apartment building where there were these storage rooms, and we'd spend hours down there making out and fooling around.

Sixteen-year-old Joe said:

My dad's *Playboy* magazine got me familiar with looking, and this girl in my fifth-grade class got me familiar with everything else. We used to sit around and talk about sex and stuff, and then we'd be playing around with each other, like making out and exploring each other.

Often this kind of sexual exploring is with a friend of your own sex. Lisa remembered:

I had my first sexual experience when I was seven years old. It was with my best friend. We were constantly together—we went to school together, we played together, everything. Then one day we started fooling around and touching each other all over. For about a year, we'd sleep over at each other's houses and do this.

For Connie, playing around sexually with boys at an early age was more of an adventure than a sexual experience:

When I was eleven, me and my best girlfriend were with some boys who were fourteen—we looked about thirteen ourselves. That night we were making out, and the guy I was with was feeling my breasts. I wasn't getting off on the feeling of it myself as much as I was thinking, Wow, look what I'm doing; wow, I'm making out; wow, he's feeling me up; wow, I can't wait to tell Jill about this! For me at that point, most of the excitement was in the fact that I was doing what I was doing.

Many people are older before they begin exploring sex with another person.

Jesse: On Monday morning when I was in middle school everyone would gather in the parking lot to discuss who did what with who over the weekend. I didn't have a boyfriend, and I was always wishing that I did so I could be part of the talk.

Molly: In the seventh grade I used to think it was gross to see a boy and a girl making out at a party. It was just about the same as going all the way in my mind. But this year we all make out at our parties, and everybody I know has boyfriends. I have two.

Paul: At thirteen I was into everything wild. I was in a gang, and we were bad, we got in a lot of trouble. Our gang was so tight, nobody else counted, not even our families. So girls were far from my mind then. Now, at fifteen, I'm a lot different. I'm not hanging out with the gang anymore, I have a girl and she's real important to me. We're into each other real deep. And a lot of the other dudes feel the same way too. They all have girls now.

Other teens don't get into a sexual relationship of any kind until they are much older—at the end of high school, in college, or out working. John said:

I'm pretty quiet and I changed schools a lot because my family was always moving, so I never really got into any crowd or got to know anyone real well. So I didn't have a girlfriend until this year. I'm seventeen and I met this girl who's a little older than me. I met her where I work at the market, so we see each other just about every day. She really has helped me get over some of my shyness. She takes the lead a lot, because she's had other boyfriends. We really like each other a lot.

Flo, who's a senior in high school, remembered:

I was in the eleventh grade the first time I really made out with someone. Before that it was just some kissing games at parties when I was much younger. I was so much slower than a lot of my friends.

NOT YET: For many of the teens who spoke with us, having a sexual relationship isn't an important part of their lives now. Sports, dance, photography,

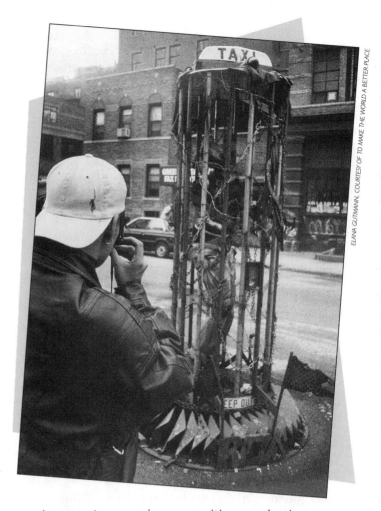

art, computers, music, cars, writing, academics, work that is very hard or very absorbing—all of these activities fill the lives of thousands of teenagers throughout the country (and throughout the world) to the extent that there is little room for anything else. Donna, who is fifteen, explained:

Right now my whole life is skating. I skate about seven hours a day, and that's all I think about and all I want to do.

Teens who have definite goals for themselves often put off having sexual relationships until they have achieved what they are going for, or until they are older and have more desire to find a partner in life. Tina, a sixteen-year-old from Detroit, said:

I have other things going for me right now. I'm just not into sex. I was into it when I was younger, but now I'm more involved in my schoolwork and my photography. I have a lot of plans for myself, and this is no time for me to be messing around with boys.

George, fourteen, has no special reason—he simply doesn't feel interested in having a sexual relationship right now:

> Every time I see my grandfather he wants to know if I have a girlfriend. It's like he wants to ask me, "How's your sex life?" but he doesn't come right out and say that. Well, I don't have a girlfriend now, and I don't think I'm going to have a girlfriend for a while yet. I'm just not into that. Not now, anyway.

THE DOUBLE STANDARD: Whether you are into having a sexual relationship or not may be influenced by societal and family values. Traditional values about sex—your own family's values, perhaps—can pressure you, if you're a boy, into feeling that you should be having sex, or make you feel the opposite if you're a girl. Many people have ideas about what's okay for boys to do and what's okay for girls to do. If you don't fit the stereotype, you may find yourself the butt of jokes or the subject of gossip. Kenny, a fourteen-year-old ninth-grader from Pennsylvania, said:

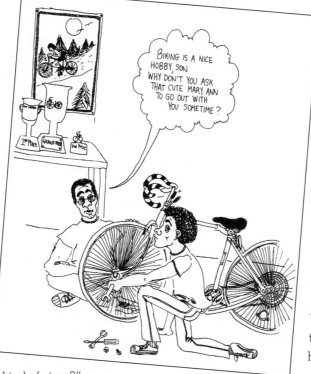

> Where I used to live, the guys had to go out and get laid. That was the attitude. All right, you're fourteen or fifteen, so go out and get laid. There was a real pressure on you, like they'd say, "Whatsa matta, you some kind of sissy?" or "Whatsa matta, you don't like girls?" If you weren't acting like a sex maniac, everybody thought there was something wrong with you. But it was the opposite for the girls. They heard, "Stay pure. Save yourself. Don't be cheap."

This is called a double standard because separate and opposite standards are set for boys and for girls. Boys are told they're supposed to "get as much as they can." Girls learn that it's up to them to keep boys from going "too far." Whether or not we agree, those old-fashioned ideas create a false sense of what's "normal," and since most people want to be considered "normal," we may feel pressure to conform.

We heard stories about the double standard all over the country. Here's how Henry, a fifteen-year-old from Texas, put it:

> In our school, if you don't go around bragging about how far you got and what you did with the girl you were out with, well, then they start calling you fag or queer or something like that. I think it's totally stupid. I think most guys lie about how far they go and what they do just to keep their image up.

Henry said there's a lot of pressure on the boys in his neighborhood to "get laid," and so for many boys, sex becomes a kind of contest: Who can get the most? On the other hand, in Detroit, sixteen-year-old Diana said:

> You know how it's okay for a guy to go around telling everybody about how horny he is and bragging about how he's going to get some this weekend? Well if a girl ever said those things, everybody would call her a slut.

We're supposed to get the idea that there are "nice" girls who know how to control themselves and "bad" girls who are loose and let boys get their way. Just think about the wording of that: "let boys get their way." The assumption is that boys are all out for only one thing, and if a girl wants to have sex, she's only doing it to accommodate the boy. We know from our interviews that many teenage boys aren't interested in having sex at this point in their lives, and many girls are very sexual, enjoying the feelings they get from sexual closeness. Leah, a sixteen-year-old from New York, told us that she's perfectly "nice" by most people's standards. She gets good grades and she's on the student council. She's planning to attend a top-ranked college when she graduates. But she said:

> I really shocked this boy I went out with because I had intercourse with him so soon. He kept expecting me to stop him, but I didn't. He told me afterwards that he never expected me to be *that* *way*. I guess he had this image that nice girls don't do that.

Leah said she felt that the boy would have been a lot happier if she had stopped him, because he didn't really want to have sex with her in the first place. He just thought that she'd think he was strange if he didn't try anything.

The problem with the double standard is exactly what Leah was describing: It doesn't allow people to act according to their own feelings. Many boys are pushed into having sex before they really want to, because they think that's how they are expected to behave. And many girls cover up or try to ignore their sexual feelings, because they worry about getting a bad reputation.

A lot of teens told us that they themselves buy into the stereotypes. Girls expect boys to want sex all the time—and think there's something wrong with boys who don't. Boys push for more but expect "nice" girls to stop them. Neither attitude allows teens any leeway.

Penny, an eleventh-grader from New York, learned how wrong her ideas were during an interesting experiment at her school:

> In our health class, the guys and the girls had to switch roles for a day. We were supposed to try to imagine what it's like to be the other one and act that way. The guy I switched with said he thought it would be so much easier to be a girl, because you wouldn't have to worry about knowing what to do or have to be smooth and cool and all that crap. He said the pressure is always on the guy to perform.

> I just couldn't believe he was saying those things, because I always thought how much easier it would be to be a guy. You wouldn't have to worry about how you looked or how you acted. You could do whatever you felt like doing without worrying about your reputation. But he said, Of course guys worry about their reputation, but it's the opposite kind of reputation. He said they have to put on this big act about how experienced they are. He told me it's really hard for him to take off his clothes in front of a girl, because he gets embarrassed. He worries about whether the girl will think he's attractive and everything. He worries that he won't do the right thing or say the right thing.

> That really helped me see how guys and girls have a lot of the same hang-ups. If only we would talk more about it with each other, that would take a lot of the pressure off. But everybody assumes the other person has it all together, so everybody's afraid to open their mouth.

You owe it to yourself to listen to what *your* body and *your* emotions and *your* values are telling you. If everyone around you is pressuring you to have sex or pressuring you not to have sex, you may feel uncertain about what's right for you. But remember: One of the nicest things about your sexuality is that it's *yours,* and it will be there for the rest of your life, to be enjoyed when you are ready to enjoy it. You don't have to rush into anything.

A NOTE ABOUT SEX AND MAKING LOVE: It's easy to forget that there is a distinction between sex and making love, because in our society the two terms are often used interchangeably. We don't want to do that in this book. There *is* a difference. Sex is uncoerced* mental and/or physical behavior that involves stimulation of the genitals and other parts of the body for individual or mutual pleasure. Making love is about mutual respect, tenderness, fun, and the desire to share physical pleasure with and give physical pleasure to someone about whom you care deeply. People can have all sorts of sexual activity, including sexual intercourse, without making love, and people

* Uncoerced means not forced. Sex that is forced on someone else is rape.

can make wonderful love without having sexual intercourse. If you've ever seen two lovers holding hands as they stroll down the street, you know what we mean.

ABSTINENCE: When we refer to abstinence in this chapter we mean choosing not to have sex. In our interviews, we met teenagers from across the country who have consciously chosen to avoid having a sexual relationship for now, even with a person they love. Seventeen-year-old Aaron told us:

> I'm in the STARS program at my school: Students Today Aren't Ready for Sex. We go to talk to sixth-graders, because there's a lot of feeling that if they're not having sex with their boyfriend or girlfriend, they're going to lose them. They don't understand that you don't just have sex to keep your boyfriend or girlfriend. We talk to them about the good reasons to have sex and the good reasons not to have sex. Most of the time, the kids see that there aren't a whole lot of good reasons to have sex, and there are a lot of good reasons not to. Like HIV/AIDS. Like unwanted pregnancy. Like being a teen parent and what that does to your life.

We discuss sexual abstinence throughout this chapter, because we believe many teens would prefer not having to deal with the problems a sexual relationship can cause. Abstinence is the only 100 percent sure way to avoid pregnancy and to keep yourself from catching a sexually transmitted disease. It gives you the opportunity to appreciate someone as a friend and companion, without introducing sex into the relationship. It sets your relationship off on the solid footing of mutual respect. Then if you do decide to have sex at a later point, you will really know each other and will be able to make important decisions together as a couple. (Check the Protecting Yourself chapter, which begins on page 279, for more on abstinence as a method of safer sex.)

BEING READY FOR A RELATIONSHIP: What if you feel as though you're ready to have a close, loving, maybe even sexual relationship with someone, but you aren't in love with anyone? What if you want to

be more active socially and sexually than you are, but there's no one with whom you want to share your desires? These can be especially confusing questions if they get mixed up with worrying that you aren't popular. Some people are waiting until they feel ready to have a lasting relationship, and they feel okay about waiting. Other people jump into relationships they don't really want, because they don't want to be alone. Some people feel frustrated, because they are ready to love someone but they haven't yet found that someone. They may wonder whether they'll ever meet anyone they like who likes them back.

If you worry that you'll never have a close relationship, you're not alone. Judging from the talks we've had with teens, lots and lots of people worry about that exact thing. Even people who talk about having sex a lot may be feeling worried underneath. Most of us want a good, close, caring relationship. We want to love someone special and to be loved by that person. It may take a while, but if you keep yourself open to it, it will happen and you will be glad you waited.

When and How Far: Making Decisions about Sex

Whether it's a first kiss, a French kiss, touching his penis, fondling her breasts, having intercourse, or lying around together making out, deciding what you want to do sexually with a certain person isn't always easy. At its best, the choice comes out of a close relationship, out of your values, and out of an understanding of the risks and responsibilities of sexual activity. Ideally, it is something you talk about and decide together, as a way of expressing your love and respect for each other.

But deciding about sex isn't always so clear or so mutual. Sometimes it's done in a split second—at a party, in a car, on the beach with others around, at home with parents about to walk in the door any minute. You're excited and the other person is excited and your bodies are reaching out for each other. Thoughts may rush through your head: Is this the right thing to do? If I don't do it now, will I get another chance? What will he/she think of me? What will I think of myself tomorrow? Will I be glad or sorry? Do I really love this person? Sometimes you consciously make a decision, sometimes you stop because your gut tells you to, sometimes you're caught in the moment and go ahead without thinking.

"Being sure" is something the teenagers working on this book talked about a lot. Sexual feelings are often so intense and confusing that it's hard to be sure. Manuel, sixteen, said, "I sometimes wonder whether I'll be glad the next day." Rita, seventeen, put it this way:

> We're at the age where we're having real sexual feelings, and if I want to act on them, my conflict is that I can't just be natural about it—whatever that means—because the feelings I have get so mixed up. It gets to the point where I don't know what I'm really feeling and wanting anymore. Sometimes I wonder if I'm just doing things that I think someone my age is "supposed" to be doing.

How "sure" do you want to be when you try something new? What can you learn about or think about in advance so that you can trust your split-second decisions to work out right? Reading books like this and talking with your parents and your friends may help you do some thinking ahead of time and help you figure out what your values, desires, and limits are. But we all learn by experimenting, and part of experimenting is making mistakes. Some mistakes may bruise your ego or make you unhappy or even fill you with shame, but in time they can be overcome. As Beverly, a fourteen-year-old from Detroit, said:

> Once you make a mistake and it really hurts you, you know you're not going to do it again. You've got to learn from your mistakes. You've got to learn how what you do affects other people around you too.

Some mistakes, however—like catching an incurable sexually transmitted disease or getting pregnant or getting your partner pregnant—are very serious. When this book was first printed, in 1981, before most people knew about HIV or AIDS, many teenagers felt it was okay to experiment with casual

sex—to have lots of different sexual partners and experiences. They told us they often had sex with people they barely even knew. They liked the excitement they felt being sexual, and it didn't matter to them who their partner was, so they made lots of mistakes and often ended up with more than just bruised egos. But those teens rarely felt they were going to die because of the mistakes they made. Now things are different.

Because of the explosion in sexually transmitted disease, especially the rapid increase in teenagers catching HIV, herpes, and HPV (see page 269), we want to be very clear about saying that CASUAL SEX IS DANGEROUS TO YOUR HEALTH. We urge you *never* to have sex with strangers. We urge you not to have sex with many different partners. *Every time* you have sex with someone, you are being exposed to all the germs he or she may have caught from all his or her previous partners. The more partners you have, the higher your chances of catching an STD (sexually transmitted disease). The more partners your partner has had, the higher his or her chances of passing an STD on to you. Jerome told us his story:

> My brother got AIDS from going to bed with a girl who got it from her old boyfriend, who used IV drugs. She didn't even know she had it until after she started being with Tony. She died last year, and he's going to die too.

Why are we telling you this? We're not trying to scare you away from sex forever. Sex is a wonderful part of being human, and our sexual experiences can be some of the most pleasurable of our lives. But we do want you to take care of yourself and learn how to be careful about sex. AIDS is killing thousands and thousands of men, women, and children every year, and the number of teenagers exposed to HIV is rising dramatically. At the time this edition went to press, there was no cure for AIDS and no preventive vaccine to keep you from getting it, although people are working on developing one.

People can have HIV for ten years or more without showing many symptoms. Very often, there is no visible way of knowing that a person is infected, so like Jerome's brother, you might be having sex with someone who has HIV and doesn't even know he or

Pressures and Influences: The "Voices" We Hear

Picture yourself in a situation where you are trying to decide what to do sexually. Put yourself inside your head at that moment, and imagine the "conversation" going on in there. There are probably many "voices" in this conversation, each with an opinion about what you *should* do. These are the pressures and influences on you as you decide whether to get involved with someone sexually and how far to go.

Voice One: Parents. If your parents or other adults who play a parental role in your life have talked to you about sex, their voice may be saying, "You're too young to be in the backseat of a car with a girl (or a boy)!" or "Enjoy yourself, but just don't go too far!" or "Boys won't respect a girl who's easy to get." or "Be careful!" or "If I ever catch you making out with that kid again, I'll . . ." You may feel you want to tune their voice out completely. Or you may realize that basically they care very much about you and want you to take care of yourself. In that case, their voice can help you make decisions you will be glad about. Whatever your parents' voices say inside your head, their voice will probably be powerful, because parents are so important in our lives.

Voice Two: Friends. Your friends' voices may be among the most influential. Inside a boy's head, the friends' voices may be saying, "Go ahead! Get as far as you can!" or "What are you, some kind of wimp that she hasn't let you inside her bra yet?" or "They always say no, but they don't mean it!"

In a girl's head, the friends' voices may encourage her to go ahead or warn her to stop, depending on what's expected in her particular crowd. So when a girl is about to make out with a boy, she may be hearing, "Watch out, you'll get a bad reputation." "You don't want to be called a slut, do you?" Or if all her friends are experimenting with sex, their voices may say, "You're so immature. You haven't even had sex yet," or "Being a real woman means at least doing X, or Y, or Z," or "Sex is great. Everyone's doing it." Both sets of voices can be oppressive, making it hard to know what *you* think is the right thing to do for yourself.

Voice Three: The Media. From TV, movies, magazines, and music, you have a lot of sexy images in your head that may influence your decision. The glamorous love life of movie stars and popular singers and sports figures makes us feel we're pitiful if we don't have at least one gorgeous admirer hanging all over us. Ads just reinforce the fact that we need

to buy this or do that to enhance our attractiveness and become sexually appealing. The media voice says, "If your love life isn't dazzling and exciting, then you must be unattractive." This voice makes a lot of us rush into relationships just to prove we *are* attractive to someone.

Voice Four: Religious Beliefs and Morals. For some people, including many teenagers, religious attitudes about sex are very important. Many religions tell us that sex outside marriage is sinful. Their voice in your head may be saying, "Wait, wait, wait! Sex belongs only in marriage." Or "Homosexual feelings are a sin." Or "Don't masturbate. It's wrong." For many teens, that gives them the guidance they are looking for. Susan, a young teenager from Des Moines, told us:

I've never been in an experience where I might have to compromise my morals, because the people I hang out with all want to be virgins until they get married. That's all there is to it.

But other teens say the great, big *"No!"* they hear from religion doesn't offer them any options. Their sexual feelings are intense and immediate, so they reject that voice. This is a loss, because the religious voice can be a positive one. Religion helps us see and value the importance of *love* between two people. Religion tells us, "Treat other human beings with respect" or "Love your neighbor as yourself." It helps us recognize that we are hurting someone else by pushing that person to have sex with us before they're ready.

Voice Five: Your Own Feelings. If you find yourself listening only to the other voices in making decisions about sex, then try to figure out what your own voice is saying. Your needs may be contradictory. One voice may be saying, "I'm horny and I need some sex" or "I'm lonely and I need some affection" or "I love this person and want to express my love sexually." But another voice may be saying, "I'm feeling uncertain. I should wait" or "I'm freaked out about getting AIDS" or "We can't do this. I don't have protection" or "I don't know enough about safer sex" or "Will I be able to face myself tomorrow?" It's confusing. The best advice is to try to balance what your feelings are telling you with what you think will be good for you and the other person in the long run. Think of the consequences!

Voice Six: Your Own Standards. The voice of your standards may say, "Remember what you decided about not ever pressuring anyone into sex?" or "Do you know this person well enough to do X or Y or Z with them?" One fourteen-year-old girl from Michigan reported:

> When I was with my boyfriend and we were making out, I was feeling so good and so close to him, but also, another person inside me was saying, "Just don't get undressed, don't make love." So I think that means I have some control. I'm even kind of disappointed that we went as far as we did, because I wonder if he's going to try to get me to go on and on and on. I said to myself I definitely would not go all the way until at least my senior year.

Although our standards change with experience, there is always a wise voice inside. Listen to it; trust it.

she has it. Since one of the ways HIV is passed is through the exchange of body fluids during sexual activity, if you have unprotected sex with an infected person, you are very likely to become infected yourself. The best way to protect yourself is with latex condoms. If you are sexually active or planning to be sexually active, we advise you to get latex condoms and use them.

Inform yourself and educate your friends. Keep yourself healthy to be able to enjoy sex with the person you love. There are two chapters in this book that should be particularly helpful. One is called Protecting Yourself: Birth Control and Safer Sex, beginning on page 279, and the other is called Sexually Transmitted Diseases, beginning on page 253.

BLURRING THE VOICES: DRUGS AND ALCOHOL. One sure way to confuse your decision-making processes is by adding alcohol or drugs to the equation. Alcohol and drugs drown out your inner voices, leaving you at the mercy of the moment. Nell, a junior from Iowa, told us how this got her in trouble:

> The decision comes at the start when you get high. Once you are past a certain point, you can't make decisions anymore. A lot of girls I know only have sex on weekends, when they are drunk or stoned, and I was the same way. Until I got pregnant.

> *Lonnie said:* I used to get drunk just so I'd feel okay having sex. But one morning I woke up naked next to some guy I didn't even know, and that's when I realized I needed help.

> *Seventeen-year-old Jeff told us:* Last summer my girlfriend and I got crazy on beer and dope at this beach party. I had a package of rubbers in my pocket, but when we rolled off into the dunes, they stayed in my pocket. It was wild at the time, but not in September, when she told me she was pregnant.

> *Suzanna, a senior, explains:* It's happened to me. Guys will try to get you to drink or have a toke or whatever, and if you're not used to it, you feel more relaxed and what they're saying to you doesn't seem as crazy. You don't say to yourself, "Oh, I don't want to do that," like you would if you were sober or playing with a full deck. And they start talking to you and you start thinking this guy really likes me—he really wants to be with me. And you're just not as careful as you would be otherwise.

It's very hard to be careful about sex when you're high. Some people drink and do drugs exactly for that reason—because when they're high they feel less inhibited. But when you're not thinking clearly about the consequences, you're less likely to use protection, and that can be extremely risky. Please be careful. Your life could depend on it.

FEELING PRESSURED. Fourteen-year-old Elsa had this experience:

> The first time I was with this boy, we were at a party together, and we started making out. And then, all of a sudden, there were his hands on my chest. I felt really funny about it, because it wasn't my idea, it was his idea, and he sort of rushed into it. Since it was the first time we were ever together, I felt like it was too fast, but I let him do it because I didn't exactly know how to tell him not to.

Two other teenagers found that they had had similar experiences:

Jenny (sixteen): If I'm out with somebody for the first time and we double-date with two people who are boyfriend and girlfriend, of course they're making out, and I feel like, God, I don't want to make out with this guy. I don't even know him. But then he wants to, because the other couple is doing it, and so I end up either doing it and not wanting to or feeling like I'm a dork or something.

Jake (fifteen) agreed: You're at a party and you're making out and she wants more. You know what I mean. And you're thinking, Wow, what is this going to get me into? I don't want to have a relationship with this babe. But if you don't go for it, she thinks you're really weird, and the story gets out that you're queer or something.

You can't help but feel torn when someone is luring, coaxing, seducing, pleading with, or even manipulating you into going further than you feel like going

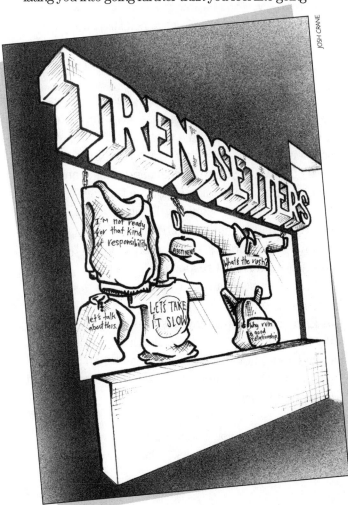

sexually. A sophomore from Iowa wrote: "This confuses the hell out of my inner voice." Boys use lines like:

"You would if you loved me."
"Why can't you just loosen up and enjoy life?"
"What are you, queer?"
"I'm too far gone. Don't be a tease."
"I'll ditch you if you don't."
"Don't worry, I'll pull out before I come."
"Everybody does it."

Girls use lines too, like:

"Oh, come on, it'll feel so good."
"Don't worry, I'm on the pill."
"You're not still a virgin, are you?"
"What's the matter? Don't you like girls?"

You have to feel pretty sure of yourself to be able to resist that kind of pressure. Mary Beth, sixteen, had an effective answer for the line her date used on her:

The guy I was out with the other night was coming on pretty strong and, like, he was getting real excited, but I wasn't really into it. He kept trying to get me to rub his penis; he even told me he had blue balls and wouldn't I do something to help him out. I was so pissed. I couldn't believe he actually used that line on me. So I said, "I'm sorry about your problem. Why don't you masturbate?" I think he was embarrassed by that, because he just sort of dropped the subject after I said that.

When both people involved want to move at the same speed sexually, no one ends up feeling pressured or used. But a lot of teenagers told us that when one person really wants to do something and the other isn't sure, it can be hard to say no. Many of us have gone further sexually than we want to at one time or another just to please the person we're with, or to keep our "cool" reputation, or not to make a scene. If you do get pressured into something, as one girl said, "Afterwards, how you feel will tell you what you really wanted." The next time maybe you'll do it differently.

When a person is being physically coerced into going further than he or she wants, sex crosses the line and becomes violence. It happens mainly to girls, but it can happen to boys too, and it may involve an acquaintance, a stranger, a boss, a relative, or a close friend. See the sections about Sexual Abuse (page 227) and Rape (page 233) for more on this subject.

SAYING NO: Let's say you like someone a lot, but you don't want to be sexual with him or her, or perhaps you just don't feel like being sexual at all at that moment. Maybe you don't want to do a particular thing, or you aren't feeling turned on. If it's intercourse, maybe you have no birth control, or you're worried about catching a disease. There are a lot of reasons for saying no in a sexual situation.

When two people are just starting to be sexual together, they may experiment until one of them says, "Stop. That's far enough!" If nobody says anything, either one of them may assume there's no problem. We recommend saying "No" and "Stop" loud and clear if you are not sure you want to keep going. Then at least you can talk about it. If you don't speak up, you may end up feeling very used and unhappy with yourself.

Of course, many teens who met with us explained that "No" and "Stop" are two words they find challenging. For instance, some of them asked, "How do you say no gracefully and still have the person believe you?" Jade said:

When I tell a guy that he can feel my breasts but not my vagina, because that's my limit right now, he acts like I'm talking about the weather or something and he just keeps on going as if I didn't mean what I said.

Jade wants to know if it's possible to say no clearly without shouting it. Rob answered her:

It's like a game. My friends told me that when a girl says no, she doesn't really mean it. So if a girl tells me quietly to stop and doesn't yell out loud about it or hit me over the head with it, I'm not supposed to listen. It's a game to find out if she really means it.

There's the double standard again: Girls are expected to say no whether or not they mean it. So

girls like Jade end up having to say it *loud* in order to be believed, and then it often becomes more of a scene than they want it to be. Dylan said:

Why can't my boyfriend just understand that even though I like making out with him as much as he does, I just have my limits and I don't want to get too heavy into sex. I'm only fifteen and I'm just not ready to go all the way. I don't even want to think about it yet.

Brad, too, has the same problem:

If I tell a girl I want to stop, or I don't want to get into sex right now, some girls are cool, but some can't believe every boy isn't a sex maniac.

Another question is, how do you say "Stop" without feeling like a jerk or hurting the other person's feelings? Matt said:

My girlfriend and I went through this whole thing last weekend because we were getting pretty carried away and I wanted to slow down and she thought that meant I didn't like her. Like I wanted to break up or something, when all I said was "Let's cool it and go out for a walk."

Many teenagers have found that it's all too easy to get carried away with the passion of the moment and forget their limits. In a way that's exactly what's so exciting about sex—you *can* get lost in the pleasure of it. When you're hugging and kissing and touching and the passion is flowing through you, things can move very quickly. If you have talked to each other about limits and desires beforehand, when the time comes, you're more likely to be able to say no and have it respected.

And that's still another question: *When* do you say no? If you say it too far in advance, you may feel as if you're not allowing yourselves to have any fun. If you say it too late, you're called a tease. Boys talked about how frustrated they get when a girl waits until the last minute to say no. Sixteen-year-old Will put it this way:

I wish my date would let me know that she's not planning to touch my cock if she's not, because I get incredibly turned on just imagining it about to happen. Here she is all passionate one minute, rubbing my legs and pressing herself into me, and then it's "I've got to go home now," just like that, and I'm left panting.

Ron had a similar complaint:

They say guys push sex on girls. But when my girlfriend is making out with me real hot and heavy and I'm getting turned on out of my mind, and then she says, "That's it," I could go through the ceiling. I'd be crazy not to try to keep her going. Is that pushing? Or is she teasing me beyond my endurance?

What Will and Ron don't realize is that the girls they were with weren't consciously trying to tease them. They were waiting until the last minute because they were probably having a wild debate with themselves: "Yes!" "No!" "Will I be sorry?" "What will he think of me?" "I'm too young." "I'm not ready." "This feels great." "Just be sure," and so on. The boy can't hear that inner argument, he only feels the results. Michelle, a junior from Illinois, said:

I don't know how many times I've been called a cock teaser, because when it gets right down to intercourse, man, it's negative—no way—I won't do it. I might get as far as taking my pants down, and then I'll chicken out. Because when it gets right down to it, that's where you start getting scared. These rushing emotions go through your head, like, "Oh, my God!" and maybe you're feeling guilty and maybe you're hearing your mother's voice in your head saying, "Don't do it. Keep your reputation!" So many times I've gotten right down to it and just left.

Holly, nineteen, had a different reason for saying no at the last minute:

It's a kind of scary thing right now because of HIV and everything. I've had sex before, but when I'm with a guy and it gets down to doing it and neither one of us has a condom, I say, "Sorry. I'm not going to do this without protection." I think it's a lot

more socially acceptable these days to say no because everybody's freaked about HIV. (For more about HIV, see page 256).

Lisa, an eighteen-year-old we met on the West Coast, said she's given it a lot of thought, and she's decided there's only one right time to say no. That's whenever you realize you've reached your limit:

Girls think they can't say no because they think they'll be considered a tease. You get drunk, and then one thing leads to another, and all of a sudden you're in bed and then you go, Hey, wait. No. I don't think so. Go away. Or you say beforehand, We can do this, this, and this, but we're not doing that. A lot of girls cannot make that boundary, because they think the guy will look on them as weird. But why do they care? If that guy doesn't want to respect your boundary, well then he's not even worth the time worrying about what he thinks.

Lisa went on to say that although she's sympathetic with a guy who might be frustrated as a result of her saying no, she feels that being true to her own feelings and limits is more important.

Ron, who was quoted above, expressed a frustration many boys told us about: When a girls says "Stop," he sometimes feels like pushing her to go further by persuading her or begging her or getting angry with her. Pushing any kind of sex on someone is wrong and in some cases even criminal. A better way to deal with this issue is to talk to each other before things get out of hand. It can be awkward if you don't know each other very well—which is why we advise not having sex with people you don't know well. And it can be hard if you're shy or feeling guilty about your sexual desires. But it's worth the effort. Getting rid of double-standard thinking would help too! If boys and girls didn't feel that they had roles they were "supposed" to play, talking honestly about sex would certainly lose some of its stigma. Peter, sixteen, is from Los Angeles. He said:

You know, I think so much bad communication goes on between guys and girls just because everyone expects the guy to move first. He's supposed to call up for a date, and he's supposed to initiate all the sex, and he's supposed to know what to do. That's such a drag. Like, I'm not into coming on too strong, that's just not my style. I don't believe in pressuring people into things, and I don't want to pressure my girlfriend. But she doesn't think the girl's supposed to be aggressive, especially not in sex, so she's always waiting for me to make all the moves. And since I don't want to pressure her, I usually hold back. I would feel a whole lot better if she'd let me know what *she* wants some of the time.

What Do People Do?

The things that people enjoy doing together sexually are limited only by human imagination and ingenuity. What *you* do will depend on what you're ready for, who the other person is, what he or she is ready for, and what you both decide is okay. But whether it's kissing or making out or having intercourse, when we feel pressure about doing it "right," it's no fun. Hannah said:

> When I'm making out with my boyfriend, I feel like a part of me is watching from the outside and saying, "How's your technique tonight? Are you turning him on? Are you doing it right?" When that voice shuts up, I have a much better time.

Pablo, seventeen, advised:

> I think you should stress in the book that sex should be an enjoyable thing and partners shouldn't worry about performing. I want to forget about what I "should" be doing and just enjoy it.

So the theme of this section is Sex Is Not a Performance! You have no audience, no judges. There is no "right" way. Once you're both sure that you want to be doing whatever you're doing, and once you've discussed limits and protection and each other's feelings, the point is to explore what makes you and the other person feel excited, close, and satisfied. People aren't born knowing how to be in a sexual relationship, so you have to learn with each other. Feeling that you ought to know what to do and how to do it

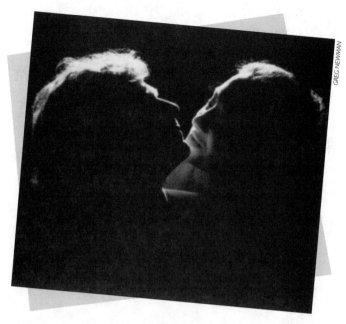

keeps you from enjoying what you *are* doing. As David, a seventeen-year-old from Oregon, said, "Everything's okay with me. Whatever we do is great as long as we're doing it together."

The best way to learn what's "right" for the two of you is to tell each other about what feels good. It's a matter of learning to relax with each other and giving yourself permission just to be yourself. Of course, this is much easier when the two of you really care for each other and have a history together.

KISSING: There's kissing: like kissing a relative hello, kissing your parents goodnight, or kissing a rabbit's foot to bring you good luck. And there's *kissing:*

> *Annie (fourteen):* The first time I kissed my boyfriend, we didn't have to say anything to each other, we just felt this thrill run through us. Just being so close to him, holding him, it was like we were part of each other.

> *Ben (thirteen):* When we were in the sixth grade, we'd play Spin the Bottle or Post Office, and you'd always hope that you got the girl you liked. Then you'd take her into the closet and kiss her, and that was about the most exciting thing you could imagine. It was amazing.

Because lips are so sensitive, pressing your lips against the lips of someone you like can be a thrill.

As with everything else in sex, however, sometimes our expectations are too high. Peter, fifteen, warned:

> Somebody should tell you that fireworks aren't going to go off on your first kiss. At least they didn't for me.

A lot of people enjoy opening their mouths while they kiss, and using their tongues to touch the other person's mouth and tongue. This is called French kissing, or Frenching, or in some places, tongue kissing. It is a more intimate way of kissing. Laura, sixteen, told us:

> I used to think there was some special trick to French kissing, like you had to know what to do with your tongue, and since I didn't know what to do, I never wanted to French-kiss. Even after I was going out with someone for a long time, I always avoided that. Then my boyfriend told me to open my mouth while I was kissing him—you know, not a lot, just with my lips parted a little—and he sort of slid his tongue into my mouth and started touching my tongue with his tongue. I liked it. I mean, it was really sensual.

Evan's introduction to French kissing was a little more of a surprise:

> At camp last summer, I met this girl who was a little older than me, and we started liking each

other. The first time we kissed, she stuck her tongue all the way in my mouth and I threw up all over her.

Like any other sexual activity, kissing feels good when you want to do it. When you don't want to do it, or when you are with someone you don't want to be with, kissing may not be so pleasant.

> *Andrea (fourteen):* I rinsed my mouth out the first time somebody French-kissed me. I was kissing this guy goodnight after our date, and he just stuck his tongue in my mouth. Just like that. It took me totally by surprise, and I didn't like it one bit. I never went out with that guy again!

Kissing is intimate, and sometimes you just may not feel like doing it. That's okay. It's not your obligation to kiss anyone, no matter what the circumstances.

MAKING OUT: Making out is more than a kiss. Jennifer, fourteen, from the Midwest, told us about the first time she and her boyfriend made out:

> When I was with my boyfriend and we were all alone for the first time, we were making out. We were out in a park where it was real private behind a bunch of trees, and I was feeling so close to him. We were French-kissing real long kisses, so sometimes I had to pull away to catch my breath. He was rubbing my back and I was rubbing his. We must have stayed there for an hour, just hugging and kissing and rolling around, but then I had to get home, so we had to stop. When I got to my house, my lips were all red and swollen from so much kissing, so I went in and washed my face with cold water. I don't think my mother noticed, because she didn't say anything.

Gloria, a fifteen-year-old from Texas, said she and her boyfriend would get silly with each other before they'd start making out:

> When we first started going out, we would flirt and make eyes at each other, but he didn't touch me, and I didn't want to start anything. This would go

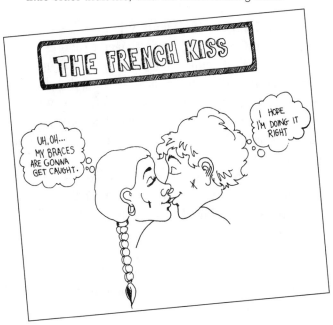

on until it was almost time to go home. I was so excited I wanted to jump him at this point. Finally, we would start laughing and tickling each other and then start making out. We'd always have this embarrassing moment before we would fall into each other's arms. He always got home late and got in trouble.

Bob, sixteen, said:

Making out feels terrific, but the hickeys stay with you to let the world know what you've been up to.

DETOUR

arms to legs
grasping
making cups
with our bodies
we roll
like one ball
following
the stains
of sweat

each crease
explored
with tongue
with touch
and mapped,
coded, diagramed,

we missed
the correct exit
followed
the wrong trail
and now
stumble
into uncharted
territory

this new land
lay fallow
and we
exhausted
can't find
the road back.
        —AMY C. ROSEN

Some guys strut around like they're great, but I get embarrassed when my family kids me about them.

(Hickeys are red spots, usually on your neck, caused by sucking the skin.)

Barry, seventeen, is gay:

I remember making out with a guy for the first time. We used to play basketball in the lot down the street and then come back to my place for a soda. This one time we were clowning around with towels drying off each other's sweat, and we started leaning up against each other. It was real exciting and real tender. We hugged and kissed for a while, then we went for a walk to get used to what had happened.

Barry and his friend went out for a walk, but when you're making out, it's not always easy to know when or how to stop. Mary Ann, fifteen, told us:

I was rubbing his back and then his stomach, and he took my hand and put it down between his legs. I felt this hard thing there under his pants. My God, it must be his penis, I thought. This must be what it feels like! I could tell he wanted me to touch it, but I didn't want to yet. Just then my parents got home, so we had to stop anyway.

FOOLING AROUND (PETTING): When you're feeling really excited, one thing seems to lead to another. If you go beyond hugging and kissing to "feeling up" (touching the girl's breasts) or to rubbing the other person's penis or clitoris, you are moving past what most people call "making out" into what some people call "petting" or "fooling around." You may or may not want to do that. *You certainly don't have to, no matter how much you like the other person.*

Billie, fifteen, was ready to go further. She told us about the first time her boyfriend touched her breasts:

He put his hands on my back and pulled out my shirt, and then he put his hands underneath. He was rubbing me all over and then, like, he was on my chest. It was so nice, because he was really gentle and I could tell he was really into it. So I didn't mind. In fact, I have to say I was into it too.

Jerry, a sixteen-year-old from Washington, described how it was for him:

I was feeling my way slowly, trying to catch on, wondering what was going to happen next. My girlfriend was more experienced than I was, so there were times when I felt like she might be wanting me to do something more than I was doing. But it wasn't like she was sitting there waiting for me to make all the moves. That was a relief. She took my hands and sort of led them around to her chest. I went under her shirt and put my hands on her bra. Then I unhooked it and put my hands on her bare skin. It felt incredible.

Reading about Billie and Jerry, you might be saying, "Things don't go that smoothly for *me* most of the time." The chances for misunderstanding what someone wants or doesn't want definitely increase when you begin to get into what some people call "heavier" sex. Anxiety about "performing" may also increase. Remember, sex is not a performance. For sex to be comfortable and pleasurable, the people involved usually need to know each other well and have each other's best interests at heart.

Some couples experiment with touching each other's genitals, which is called "mutual masturbation" when they bring each other to orgasm that way (see page 99). It is one way of sharing the pleasure of lovemaking without having to worry about pregnancy.*

Brian, eighteen, described a time with his girlfriend:

She put her hand down my pants, and I just about couldn't control myself. But I held back for a while, because it was feeling so good I wanted it to last. She started masturbating me and I couldn't hold back anymore. After I came, we held each other really tight for a while, just lying next to each other.

* Make sure none of the fluid from the boy's penis gets near the entrance to the girl's vagina. Sperm can swim, and pregnancy can happen without penetration if the boy ejaculates near or on the vaginal lips.

Then she took my hand and put it down her pants, and after a while she came too. It was great.

Most people find that having an orgasm with someone else through mutual masturbation is very intimate. Making love that way can be very tender and pleasurable, and it can make you feel more emotionally involved with each other and more vulnerable to each other. You have shared something very private.

ORAL SEX: A group of New England teenagers who helped us on this chapter were talking about what it should include. Ellie said:

I think you should have some stuff about oral sex, because a lot of people think, Oh, that's gross, or It's not good for you, or whatever. Some people feel that oral sex is bad or dirty.

Oral sex means using your mouth and tongue to stimulate someone sexually, usually by kissing and/or sucking his or her genitals. As with almost every other sexual act, some people find it unimaginable, while other people love it. Here's what Taylor had to say:

I could come just thinking about a girl going down on me. But to tell you the truth, I don't think I'd want to do it to her.

Angie had this opinion:

I nearly choked when my boyfriend shoved his you-know-what in my mouth. It was gross. I gagged and almost threw up.

Sherine said:

As a kid I was always brought up—you don't put things in your mouth, not your fingers, not pencils, not anything except food and your toothbrush. So to all of a sudden be asked by a guy to put his penis in my mouth makes me feel gross. That's why I won't let a guy do it to me. I always feel like it's smelly and dirty down there.

It may be hard for you to imagine that someone else could enjoy having his or her face so near your genitals. Girls seem to wonder about this more than boys do. Girls who have seen all the advertisements for vaginal deodorants may worry that their natural body smell is offensive. "Does he really think it smells good down there?" one girl asked. Boys wonder about how their genitals smell too. You may not want to have oral sex at all, and that's fine. But if you are worried about smelling bad, as long as you and your partner keep your bodies clean, you may find you actually like the natural aromas. Monica told us her story:

> I was with this guy who said, "Let me do something to you that I think you'll really like." And that was when he went down on me and started licking me. I was really kind of embarrassed at first, because I didn't really know what he was doing. I thought, This is sort of gross to be doing that. It must smell bad. But it felt really, really good, and I relaxed and just got into it.

Oral sex is a kind of lovemaking that many people find very pleasurable and exciting. Unlike sexual intercourse, it won't create a pregnancy, but like intercourse, it does leave you vulnerable for many sexually transmitted diseases (see page 253). You will see in the Protecting Yourself chapter that health educators recommend using condoms and other barriers during oral sex, because many diseases, including HIV, can be passed orally.

Lots of people don't feel at all comfortable with oral sex, and if they have oral sex, they don't enjoy it. As with all things in lovemaking, if you don't like it, if you don't feel comfortable doing it, and if it doesn't feel good, don't do it. Making love means creating a field of love between you. It isn't loving to expect or ask someone to do something he or she doesn't want to do.

Fellatio: Licking or sucking a man's penis is technically called fellatio (fel-*lay*-she-oh). Slang terms include sucking off, giving head, blow job, going down on, creaming. Johnny, who's sixteen, told us:

> I think there are lots of ways of making love. Me and my girl aren't into chancing a pregnancy—we don't want to have to deal with that. So we find

other ways to get each other off, and for me, when she goes down on me, it's great. I've had intercourse before, and I think this way is just as good, maybe even better.

If the boy has an orgasm during oral sex, his semen (the fluid that spurts out of his penis during ejaculation) will end up in the girl's mouth unless he is wearing a condom or one of the partners pulls away at the last minute.*

Many girls we talked with who had tried fellatio said they didn't like the taste or the feeling of semen in their mouth. They were relieved to hear from each other that the boy doesn't have to come in their mouth, and that if he does, they don't have to swallow the fluid; they can spit it out or let it flow out of their mouth. Boys can also pull out before they start to come, and they, or their partner, can bring them to orgasm manually (with their hand).

Some girls spoke of feeling as if they couldn't breathe while performing oral sex on a boy. They didn't like that feeling at all. Even though some boys put a lot of pressure on girls to perform oral sex, these girls gave each other support for feeling okay about saying no.

The girls thought that on the whole boys want oral sex done to them more than girls want to do it. "Hey, baby, will you give me a blow job?" one of them imitated. "Finish me off, will you, honey?" someone else said. From the resentment in their voices, we could sense that they sometimes feel pushed to have oral sex when they don't want to do it. Henry was sympathetic. He said, "If my girlfriend's not into it, I don't really dig it much anyway. It's not as good if she's just doing it to please me."

Cunnilingus: Licking or sucking a girl's clitoris and/or vagina is technically called *cunnilingus* (cuh-nih-*ling*-gus). Slang terms are eating, eating out, going down on, muff diving. Since a woman's clitoris is the most sexually sensitive part of her body, and since intercourse doesn't always stimulate the clitoris, cunnilingus is, for many women, the way they feel the most sexual pleasure. Hilary is a nineteen-year-old college freshman; she said:

---

* Some semen escapes before ejaculation, and germs can be transmitted that way too. That's why we advise using condoms for greater safety.

I had intercourse once in high school, and basically it wasn't all that thrilling. But this year I'm in a really great relationship with this guy who isn't into intercourse. He goes down on me, and I get lost in the feeling. It's truly amazing.

You may have heard of the slang term "69." This refers to a couple turning their bodies so that each can do oral sex with the other at the same time. Some people like this; some prefer to take turns. There is no "right" way in lovemaking between people who are freely choosing to do what they are doing.

SEXUAL INTERCOURSE: Sometimes as part of a sexual relationship, a boy and a girl will want to have sexual intercourse. If you do choose to have intercourse, we hope you will consider the decision carefully. We also advise you to prepare yourself by reading the chapters Protecting Yourself (page 279) and Sexually Transmitted Diseases (page 253) to learn how to protect yourselves from both unplanned pregnancy and sexually transmitted disease. Make sure you use protection *every time* you have sex.

NOTE TO READERS WITH GAY AND LESBIAN EXPERI-ENCE: Although some gay men who have anal sex refer to it as "intercourse," in this chapter we are using the word "intercourse" to mean vaginal intercourse (between males and females).

Deciding About Intercourse: In one sense, the only difference between intercourse and all the other things people do in sex is that in intercourse a boy's penis goes into a girl's vagina. But that simple difference is a major one for most teenagers. The decision about intercourse is bigger, tougher, and often more confusing than any of the others. If you are considering having intercourse with someone, we suggest reading When and How Far on page 107 for a discussion of the basic issues in deciding how far you want to go with someone. Here we will present the extra issues that teenagers told us have special significance to the decision about intercourse.

Having sexual intercourse means risking pregnancy. As Tyler, a sixteen-year-old from Boston, said:

My girlfriend and I do just about everything but actually screw, because neither one of us wants to get into that, since we're not ready to deal with the possibility of her getting pregnant. I don't know what we'd do if that happened.

If there's even a chance of your having intercourse with someone, it's time to think about getting protection (see page 279). Latex condoms used together with a spermicide like contraceptive foam are the best protection for teens and the easiest to obtain. But nothing is 100 percent safe or 100 percent effective except abstinence (not engaging in sexual activity). That's why many teens are choosing to postpone intercourse until they are married or at least older and in a more committed relationship. Couples who, like Tyler and his girlfriend, would not consider abortion as an option, want to protect themselves from even the remotest possibility of an unplanned pregnancy.

Intercourse also means an increased risk of sexually transmitted disease. HIV is spreading fast among teenagers, and one of the reasons is that teenagers are less likely than older couples to use protection every time they have intercourse. As we've said before, the more sexual partners you have, and the more partners they have had, the higher your risk of catching a disease. Here's what eighteen-year-old Holly told us:

It's a really scary thing right now. If for some reason you're not careful or you forget to use protection, you're like paranoid for a long time, until you get tested. Nobody that I know has it (HIV) right now, but everybody's scared about it. You never know for sure. There's this one guy in town who I know has slept with lots of girls, and he supposedly gets tested all the time. So I stay away from him, because he really scares me. Anybody who's been with that many people is like playing with fire.

Emotionally, having sexual intercourse often means making yourself more vulnerable, more open to intense feelings of both joy and hurt, closeness and distance. Andrew, seventeen, remarked:

When my girlfriend and I started making love, our relationship changed somehow. We were closer, but not completely. In fact, when we had fights we felt further away than ever, and things she did hurt me more easily. We started thinking about the future too. It was like crossing a bridge to another shore.

Ellie said:

I've always heard that having sex either brings you closer together or pushes you further apart, and in my case it was true. My boyfriend and I split up very soon after we started having intercourse. I think our relationship just got too heavy.

Some people don't feel ready for that extra vulnerability. Molly, fourteen, explained:

Breaking up after you've had intercourse is much harder, I think especially on girls. How could you face the guy afterwards, knowing that you'd done that with him? I don't want to have intercourse until I really fall in love with a guy and know we won't break up.

Molly will probably find that you can never know for sure that you won't break up, but there is a kind of commitment and closeness that most people want to feel before having intercourse with someone.

Traditionally, people have saved intercourse for a long-term, committed relationship—usually marriage. Many teenagers we met as we were interviewing for this book said they believed that waiting is right for them. Marilee, a ninth-grader from Detroit, put it this way:

Making love means something to me. It means really loving the person you're doing it with, and it means not feeling bad that you did it even if the two of you break up. I'm just not ready for that yet. I'm only fifteen, and I think that's way too young to be getting so involved with somebody. I just can't see myself handling that kind of relationship.

Dexter, a sixteen-year-old from the same school, added:

Before I'd do it with some girl, I'd want to know her really well. I'd want to respect her, and I'd want her to respect me. If you're going to be that close with someone, then you really want to feel something between you, you want to care for each other.

Greg, a gay seventeen-year-old who read over this chapter while we were working on it, said:

Bars are one of the only places that gay guys can meet, because usually we can't be open in school or at work. At this one bar I go to sometimes, there's a pickup scene that I hate. After one evening of conversation and some dancing, I feel pressured to go home with some guy and go to bed with him. But I don't do it, because what I'm looking for is a good relationship. Then I'll get into making love. That's the order I want it to go in.

Casual sex can be superficial and demeaning if the people involved are just using each other. It can also be life-threatening, because when you don't know your partner well, you don't know his or her sexual or health history. You don't know if he or she might be carrying HIV or some other incurable sexually transmitted disease. You don't know if that person can be trusted not to become violent while you are together. Greg is smart to be patient. When a "good relationship" comes along, one of the factors that will make it good is the mutual respect and caring he will feel in it. At that point, he and his partner will decide together how far they want to go and when.

Virginity: A girl's virginity has traditionally been seen as a sign that she is pure, "untouched," virtuous. In many cultures and ethnic groups, it is considered a disaster for the family if a girl loses her virginity before she marries. One Hispanic girl from Los Angeles told us:

My father was just about ready to beat up my boyfriend, because he thought he was taking advantage of me. He thought we were going to "go all the way." He saw us making out in the backyard, and he won't let us see each other anymore. So now we have to sneak behind his back to be together.

A sixteen-year-old boy from the Midwest said:

> My parents were pretty serious with me about sex. They really tried to get me to see that my girlfriend's reputation would be at stake if we had intercourse, that if anyone found out, she would be considered "damaged property." Can you believe that—"damaged property"?

First her father's to protect, then her husband's to take, a woman's virginity symbolized that she "belonged" to someone else. That is a difficult idea to accept these days, when we are working so hard for equality between women and men. (By equality we don't mean that men and women are the same, but we do mean that no one belongs to anyone else, and that women's and men's and boys' and girls' actions should be judged by the same standards.) Girls and women are *not* the property of their fathers or husbands, just as boys and men are not the property of their mothers or wives. We are people, not property, and we are responsible for our actions. If a girl or a boy chooses to remain a virgin until marriage, it is a choice to be made freely and for one's own reasons.

These days many parents stress virginity not so much for family honor as for fear of unwanted pregnancy, concern about sexually transmitted disease, and the desire to keep their child from getting too deeply into a sexual relationship at a young age. In making your decision about whether to keep your virginity or not, you will undoubtedly be influenced by your family's values, especially if they have taken the time to discuss these issues openly with you.

Having sexual intercourse with someone is a big step. The idea of virginity can remind you to respect this step. Seen this way, virginity isn't so much a matter of "protecting the property from damage" as guarding your sense of yourself and what you want for yourself.

Waiting:

Angela, a twenty-year-old from Oregon, helped us edit this book. She said:

> In the eleventh grade, I became aware that everybody I knew was having sex, and I hadn't yet. All my friends, even the holdouts, were starting to talk about doing it with this guy or that, and I thought, Oh, my God, I'm so backward. And they would say to me, "You're not worldly; you're not a woman; you can't understand what we're talking about because you're still a virgin." In my head I could say, That is such crap. How can they say that about me? But underneath it was hurting me and I was thinking, What's wrong with me? I spent a lot of time the next few years thinking about what it would mean to me to have intercourse with a guy. I just knew that I couldn't make love with someone I didn't love. So I waited. Then this year, my second year at college, I started going out with someone I really care about. We have fun together, we like the same things, and we respect each other's opinion about things. We've started talking about making love, and it feels okay to me. I feel ready. Even though we aren't thinking about getting married or anything, I feel good about us making love.

When Candy decided she wasn't ready to have intercourse, it meant losing her boyfriend:

> I was going out with this guy, and we were having fun together, but he really wanted to have sex and I really didn't want to. I just felt like I wasn't ready—like I wasn't in love with him the way I wanted to be before I'd do that. I gave it a lot of thought. I talked to my mom about it, and she really helped me to feel good about my decision. So all of a sudden this guy stopped calling me— this guy who had been all along telling me how much he loved me and everything. I didn't really feel bad about his not calling me anymore, because I knew that if sex was all he wanted, then I didn't really want to go out with him.

RICK COHEN

As we said at the beginning of this chapter, lots of us make mistakes in sex; we end up doing things that later we wish we hadn't done. Just because you've had intercourse (or any sexual activity) before, that doesn't mean you have to do it again. You can wait until you are older or in a more committed relationship or until you are married. That's what Tony, a seventeen-year-old from Kansas City, decided:

> I feel this way about it. I'm just not into making love anymore. I did it a few times when it was the thing to do, you know, but I didn't really like it. I don't need that, man. But all my friends are telling me, Hey, what's wrong with you? You weird or something? They say, Oh, that's why you're breaking out in pimples (ha ha ha). You don't get enough sex. But that has nothing to do with it. I haven't done it now in a couple of years, and I'm not planning to do it again until I want to.

And seventeen-year-old Emily added:

> I always felt after I had broken up with the guy I had sex with the first time that it was just sort of expected that every time I went out with somebody I was going to have intercourse. And especially if it was an older guy. Every time I was with an older guy they've always said, "Well, if you've already had sex anyway, why wouldn't you want to do it now?" Like once you're not a virgin anymore, what's the difference? Once you've had it, you're automatically supposed to do it all the time from then on. I felt like that for a long time, until I realized that it's up to me. I mean it's up to me not to do it if I don't want to. You have the right to say, "Hey, I don't feel like having sex with you."

Choosing to Have Sexual Intercourse:
Like so many things in sex, intercourse can be great if you want to be doing it and if you're in a relationship with someone you love and trust. It can be awful if you are just doing it to please someone else or if you allowed yourself to be talked into it.

Sometimes intercourse is passionate, sometimes awkward, sometimes funny or playful or tender or frustrating or just plain boring. When it is done quickly or casually or with someone you don't care about, it can be very disappointing. It's something

people tend to enjoy more with experience and with a partner they love and respect.

We have so many expectations, so many fantasies about what IT will be like. It seems as if everything we've heard or seen or learned about sex is all pointing in one direction: toward sexual intercourse—which, in slang, people call fucking, humping, screwing, home base, going all the way, making it. The importance of intercourse has been so exaggerated in books and magazines and on TV and in the movies that people tend to forget that it is only one part of sex. It is only one way to make love.

Teenagers get so little real information about sexual intercourse, they often don't know what to expect. An eighth-grader named Mike told us:

> In my sixth-grade class it seems like we talked about everything. I mean like we talked about rubbers, birth control, diseases, everything. The teacher told us a lot of stuff. But then a little later on I saw some people actually doing it, you know, making love, and I thought it was pretty weird-looking.

In sexual intercourse the man's erect penis goes into the woman's vagina and moves in and out in a way that in the best circumstances stimulates both of them. The couple can be lying down with the man on top, with the woman on top, or both on their sides. They can be sitting, one on the other, or they can be standing up. Any position that is comfortable for both of them and in which the vagina and the penis can fit together is a good position for intercourse. Because people come in all different sizes and shapes, each couple will find the position or positions most stimulating and most comfortable for them. It is especially important to find a position in which the woman's clitoris gets good stimulation. Usually the penis gets enough stimulation just from the act of moving in and out of the vagina.

In the best instances, a lot of kissing and stroking and licking and hugging goes on as the couple builds up to intercourse. This is sometimes called foreplay, but we don't like to use that term because it implies that kissing and stroking and so on aren't as good if they don't lead to intercourse, and that just isn't true. Many couples who used to enjoy making out for hours stop making out at all as soon as they start having intercourse. Intercourse becomes what one girl referred to as "Wham, bam, thank you, ma'am." In most people's experience, lovemaking is much better when you build up to it and when it comes about as a result of your being close to each other emotionally as well as physically.

Pre-intercourse stimulation usually makes penetration itself more enjoyable since the walls of the vagina will become lubricated during arousal, making it easier for the penis to slide in. If the vagina is not lubricated or if the vagina is tight, there may be pain on entry (see page 127 for more on this).

When both people are ready for intercourse, and after birth control/safer-sex protection is in place (see page 279), one of the partners usually reaches down to guide the penis into the vagina with his or her hand. "Ready" for a man is when he is excited enough to have an erection. A woman is really "ready" only after the lips of her vagina get wet, and when her whole pelvic area is feeling full or swollen and aroused. Couples who care about each other's pleasure take the time they need before intercourse to build arousal and excitement. They also take the time they need to make sure entry is not painful for the woman.

Once the penis is inside, the couple moves their hips and lower bodies so that their pelvic areas rub against each other, and so that the penis pushes into the vagina and then pulls partly out again (sometimes called thrusting). This moving together can lead to orgasm (coming) for one or both of them if it lasts long enough, or they can decide to stop before orgasm is reached.

You might come almost immediately, shortly after the penis enters the vagina, or you might go on for five, ten, fifteen minutes or longer. Generally it takes a man a shorter time to reach orgasm than it does a woman, since his penis gets direct stimulation from the movements they are making. The woman's clitoris gets only indirect stimulation from the thrusting of the penis in her vagina: the penis moves the swollen inner lips around the vaginal opening; these inner lips are connected to the hood of skin over the clitoris; the hood moves, rubbing the clitoris. Some women use their hand to give their clitoris direct stimulation during intercourse. Or a woman may

enjoy being on top of her partner so that she can control the movements and give her clitoris maximum pressure and rubbing.

When she heard about this difference in men's and women's body design, one girl exclaimed, "That's not fair!" Actually, it's not fair only if people define lovemaking as involving *only* putting a penis into a vagina and assume that what satisfies a man will satisfy a woman too. Many women find that they do not have orgasm during actual intercourse, and prefer to reach orgasm by oral sex or other kinds of touching before or after intercourse. There's no one right way to reach orgasm. What works is what's right for you.

Even though a lot of media space is given to the thrill of "reaching orgasm together" (simultaneous orgasm), this almost never happens, and even when it does happen, some people say its reputation is overrated. Usually, one person will come before the other and that's just fine. If possible, the man will try to wait until after his partner comes, because when he reaches orgasm, his penis will lose its erection. If that happens and they cannot continue to have intercourse because of it, they can find other ways (like oral sex or hand-clitoris stimulation) to satisfy the woman. Or they can wait until the man gets aroused again and reinsert his penis.

During intercourse a couple may experience great closeness as they share each other's rhythm and excitement and find ways to move that stimulate each other and themselves.

After the man ejaculates, if he is wearing a condom, he should hold onto the open end of the condom as he pulls his penis carefully out of the vagina. Otherwise the condom might unroll and release its contents. When his penis is completely out of the vagina, he unrolls the condom off his penis and throws the condom away. If possible he washes off his penis and dries it before lying near his partner's vagina. (If water is not available, drying the penis thoroughly will suffice, as long as the uncovered penis doesn't touch his partner, to avoid disease.) Most couples enjoy spending quiet, intimate time together after having made love; while their bodies relax and return to normal, they may dream together or talk about private thoughts. Serena is nineteen. She remembered:

When I had intercourse for the first time it was because I really wanted to do it. We talked about it and sort of planned when we would do it. We tried to make it romantic—you know, with candles and everything. I went out and got myself a diaphragm and I practiced putting it in, and my boyfriend had condoms, which he let me put on him. The actual intercourse wasn't as great for me as I thought it would be, but the part leading up to it and the part being together afterwards was really nice.

Morgan, a seventeen-year-old from Hartford, spoke for many teens:

My first time definitely lived up to my fantasies, not so much the physical fantasies, because it was so much faster than I thought it would be. I was so excited that I came right away, so it lasted just a few seconds. But it was everything I wanted in terms of the emotional fantasies. The best part was being together afterwards and not being uptight about it. My girlfriend was really understanding. It was totally emotional, much more emotional than I had expected.

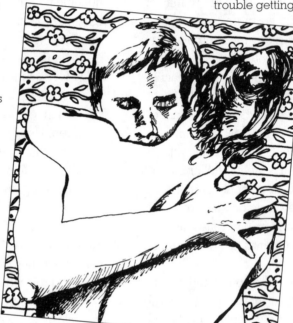

Intercourse doesn't automatically feel wonderful for many couples, and the first time, especially, can be painful and awkward. Here's what a few teens had to say about it:

Francie (seventeen): When we went to have actual intercourse, it wasn't exciting anymore. My legs were starting to shake, and he couldn't get in at first. I was just lying there going through this pain. Finally I just said, "Let's go. Do whatever you have to do, just go all the way in, because I'm getting tired of this. Maybe it will go better once it's all the way in or something." It just wasn't great. Then afterwards we were lying there, and that felt better than intercourse—hugging and kissing each other. I didn't like intercourse at all.

Ron (sixteen): The fantasies that I had about it were way off. I imagined real vivid things like heavy body sensations and getting lost in passion and feeling like we'd love each other forever after experiencing this together. And what really struck me was how different the reality was. Somehow I had the idea that things would just happen, like you'd just do everything real smoothly without much effort. But that wasn't the way it happened at all. In the first place it really seemed to hurt my girlfriend. She was really tight, and I had a lot of trouble getting in. And once I did get in, it wasn't like we were carried away with passion. I came and it was over and that was that. I have to say, it wasn't at all what I expected.

Sheri (seventeen): The first time I had intercourse, I was lying there thinking, you mean this is *it*? Am I supposed to be thrilled by this? It wasn't that it hurt me or anything, because it didn't. It just didn't feel like anything to me. I figured there must be something wrong with me, so I didn't say a word to him.

Since for so many of us intercourse has been built up in our minds to be the most fantastic part of a sexual relationship, if it doesn't feel as great as you expect—or as Sheri said, if it doesn't feel like anything at all—you might be confused and worry that you are unusual. You might think that you are the only one who doesn't enjoy intercourse. And you may worry that you never will. Girls, especially, may see that the boy is enjoying it and wonder why it isn't feeling the same for them. Kelly made us promise that we would let readers know that people don't always enjoy intercourse or other sexual acts, but that doesn't mean you'll *never* have enjoyable sex. She said:

> Kids always think, I'm *supposed* to be feeling this way or that way, and they feel bad if they don't. So you have to tell people that there's no one way to feel in intercourse.

Nineteen-year-old Joel said:

> Everyone's going around wondering why they aren't having the greatest sexual experiences in the world, and nobody's saying anything about it.

And Amy, who is seventeen, said:

> I don't like it when we are always all caught up in trying to get each other to come. Sometimes I just like to be with my boyfriend without being sexual that way. We just lie with each other and talk to each other. We spend a lot of time talking about things that are important to us and about ideas we have. Mostly we end up making out even then, but it's a different kind of feeling. It's not just that purely physical thing. It's more loving.

TALKING ABOUT SEX: In sex, a lot can be learned over time, like what feels good to you and your partner, which positions feel best, how lightly or hard to kiss or rub or squeeze or press. Generally, it's different for every different person. There aren't any rules, except to be honest with yourself and your partner about what you like and what you don't like. People can teach each other what to do both by showing each other and by talking to each other about sex. Mack, a fifteen-year-old, had this experience:

> Me and my girlfriend were making out, and for the first time she let me put my hands under her bra. I felt like I just wanted to squeeze her, but I was worried that that might hurt her. It felt so good to me, I didn't know whether to let myself get carried away or not. She told me to stop when I pinched her nipple. She said it didn't feel good, but it felt great to me.

Sam, a sixteen-year-old from Kansas, told us:

> The other night Donna kept rubbing me after I came. It had felt so terrific, but all of a sudden after I came it hurt like crazy. I shouted "Ouch! Stop!" But then I thought, Uh-oh, kid, you maybe made her feel bad. She was just trying to do something nice. When we talked about it, she said it was cool—how was she supposed to know unless I told her?

When you are learning something new in sex or learning about a new partner, it helps to be open and let each other know how you're feeling. Even people who have been married to each other for many years talk about their sexual relationship, to keep making things better. And like almost everyone else, often married people find it embarrassing and awkward to talk about sex.

There are so many movie images of people just flowing into the most fantastic, passionate, *silent* sex in the world, so we think that sex should just come naturally, without any knowledge or experience or planning or talking. We may even think that talking ruins the romance, because we never hear people talking to each other in those celluloid scenes. In the real world, however, a good sexual relationship takes work, and it takes courage to open the conversation. Louise, a seventeen-year-old from Idaho, said she doesn't think she has that much courage!

> Can you imagine making out with a guy and saying, "Oh, I don't like that. Oh, I wish you would do this." I'm not comfortable enough with myself to be able to say those things.

In lots of ways Louise is right. You may worry that what really turns you on is weird or different from what you think turns everyone else on, so you don't say anything. Or maybe you think you *ought to* be enjoying some sexual activity that doesn't do anything for you. Because of that, you may pretend to be loving it when really you don't feel anything at all. Pretending isn't very productive, though, because what's the point of having sex if it doesn't feel good to you? Iris, who's seventeen, found this out:

I told my boyfriend the other night that I wasn't really getting off on our sex together. I was pretty tactful and gentle, but he just about freaked out. I could tell he was more embarrassed than anything else. He sort of got angry with me and said, "You mean you've been faking it all this time?" And so I said yes and we argued for a while, but then we got to talking about it. He really wanted it to feel good for me. He felt bad that I'd been keeping that a secret from him, and he felt kind of dumb that he hadn't figured it out—but I was a real good actress about it. Now we feel like this weight is off our shoulders, because we have it out in the open and we're going to try to do something about it.

As Iris said, it might be awkward at first to say what's really going on, but if you don't, there's no way things can change. She understood that her boyfriend might feel vulnerable and embarrassed about what she was telling him, but she also understood that for the sake of their relationship she *had* to say something. There's no way your partner will ever know how to make things better for you if you don't tell him or her what you like and need. Robert, a senior from Iowa, said:

It takes so long for things to happen, just because each person's waiting for the other one to say something. It's so stupid. You keep wondering, Well, should I do this or should I do that? Or, Will she like this or doesn't she want me to do that? All that time wasted when if we could just talk to each other you could clear it up in a minute. But it's so hard to talk. I have this image that sex is supposed to be silent, just lovers looking into each other's eyes and knowing exactly what to do. Well, that image really messes me up a lot, because I hardly ever feel like I know exactly what to do.

Sixteen-year-old Linda told us of an experience that shows how unpleasant and alienating it can be when partners don't talk to each other:

I was over at my boyfriend Mike's house, and we were lying on his bed kissing and everything, and he took my hand and put it down his pants so I could feel his penis. But I didn't know what I was

supposed to do. I had never done that before. So I was just touching it lightly, sort of tickling it. Then he started moving my hand up and down, so I figured that's what he wanted me to do. But I was afraid of hurting him. He was totally quiet through the whole thing. He didn't say a word, so I didn't know if I was doing it right, but he got really excited and closed his eyes and had an orgasm. The weirdest thing was that afterwards, he just got up and didn't say anything about it. I wanted him to say something. It was new to me. I wanted to talk about it; I wanted to know, did I do it right? But of course I didn't say anything because he didn't say anything. So right after, we acted as if the whole thing never happened.

Lots of people say, "If we can't talk about sex, maybe we shouldn't be together," and in a way this is really true. If you don't feel close enough or trusting enough to share your feelings and your concerns with someone, then in this day of HIV and other dangerous, incurable sexually transmitted diseases, it's probably not a good idea to be trusting that person with your life. Maybe it means you need to become better friends before you go any further into sex, so that when you have something important to say, you'll be more willing to take the risk and say it. Sarah said she's really glad she and her boyfriend felt close enough to talk:

The first few times we did it, I didn't feel very much. He used to come real fast, before I would even start to feel turned on. Before we started having intercourse, we used to have really great sex together, so we talked a lot about what we could do to make intercourse better too. We decided not to rush into it but to spend time with each other first—you know, kissing and making out and everything, like we used to. Now I get turned on before we do it, and my boyfriend tries to make himself last once he's inside. He holds himself back until he feels like I'm really into it too. I think it's really important to him to make it good for me too.

By talking about their lovemaking, Sarah and her boyfriend have discovered one of the most valuable lessons to learn in sex: not to rush into it.

Another reason you want to feel close to your sexual partner is so you can decide together about birth control and safer-sex methods. To protect yourselves against pregnancy and STDs, you *both* need to be committed to using protection. Many birth control methods that girls use—like the Pill, Depo-Provera, and Norplant—work to stop pregnancy but don't protect at all against disease. You and your partner might want to read the chapter that begins on page 279 together and discuss the pros and cons of each of the methods listed. Barrier methods, like latex condoms, protect against STDs, but hormonal methods, like the Pill, don't. If you're not in a relationship, it is even more important for you to use safer sex methods each time you have sex with someone, because no matter what the other person says, only by using protection yourself can you be sure you'll be safe.

Sex with strangers or people you don't know very well is downright dangerous. And even your best friend may be carrying an STD if he or she has had unprotected sex before or has used injection drugs. Leon, a sixteen-year-old from Chicago, said:

> The first few times I did it, I didn't use nothing. Then my brother got hold of me and said I was stupid, because didn't I know that I could get AIDS? One of his best friends came down with it, and now everybody around here is walking scared. So I got some and now I keep them with me, because you never know when you're gonna need one.

Coping with Problems in Sex

Nearly everyone has a problem with sex at some point, though when *you* have one, it may not be much consolation that millions of other people have had it too. Most of the problems that teenagers have in sex go away pretty easily with time and experience, especially if they don't get too upset about them and are willing to talk with their partner about them. We will discuss a few of these problems here.

First, it is important to remember that *you don't have to put up with pain or frustration or lack of communication in your sexual relationship.* Lots of people, even married people, keep their sexual

problems to themselves for months or even years, and do nothing about them, because they feel embarrassed or undeserving. It is possible to make most sexual problems better, however, so if something hurts or bothers or frustrates you in sex, bring it up. Talk about it with your partner or with a friend or with a professional nurse or sex educator. Deanna, nineteen, gave an example of why it's important to get the problem out in the open:

> When my boyfriend and I started having sex, he would come right after he got in me. It was a real problem for us, because he was so embarrassed about it. He acted like he failed or something. He never really talked about it, but I could see how humiliated he felt, because he wouldn't look at me afterwards. It happened a couple of times, and then he just stopped calling me. It wasn't nearly as bad for me as he imagined, so I didn't understand why he didn't want to go out anymore. Finally, I saw him on campus and asked him why he had stopped calling me. He was shocked that I didn't understand. He said he felt so embarrassed and uncomfortable about it that he never wanted to see me again. I told him that I didn't mind that he came fast. I knew we could figure a way to make it work for me too. He was really relieved.

Deanna was willing to ask her boyfriend what was going on because she really cared about him. Unfortunately, if someone doesn't bring up the problem, it usually doesn't go away by itself. Our hope is that as more people learn how to communicate about sexual issues, and as more teenagers realize that sex is not a performance but a part of learning how to love someone else, this kind of embarrassment and humiliation will disappear.

There are a few specific problems that we will discuss here, because they are so common.

PROBLEMS FOR GIRLS

Pain with Entry of the Penis: Some girls do not experience pain even the first time they have intercourse. Others do. Some bleed as their hymen gets stretched. You can help yourself and your partner have an easier time by stretching the vaginal opening for several weeks before starting intercourse. This can be done by putting a clean finger into the vagina and gently pushing it from side to side. Also, when you do start to have intercourse, go very slowly.

Pain when the penis enters the vagina usually has one of these causes:

➤ The girl's vaginal opening is not stretched open enough. If it is the first time she is having intercourse, her membrane may still be unstretched. Even if she has had intercourse before, she may still be tight. It is important to tell your partner you are hurting. A sensitive partner will not try to force his penis inside. Please note: Pain is *not* an indication of a girl's virginity.

➤ She has a vaginal infection. If a girl is suffering from a vaginal infection, she may have a variety of symptoms, including pain during intercourse. See page 273 for a complete discussion of this problem. You should *not* have intercourse when you have an infection, because it will spread to your partner and it may make your own symptoms worse. If you are having pain that you can't attribute to another cause, go to a health practitioner for diagnosis. Most infections can be treated. If you don't have them treated and cured, they may lead to serious gynecological problems in the future. So don't take a chance. (See page 246 for a discussion of what to expect at the clinic, and see Chapter 9, beginning on page 253, for a discussion of vaginal infections.)

➤ The girl is not yet sexually aroused enough to lubricate, so the vaginal entrance is not lubricated enough for easy penetration. If the lips of the girl's vagina are too dry for the penis to go in easily, it probably means she is not ready, not sexually aroused enough for the natural lubrication of her vaginal walls to take place. Love play involving direct clitoral stimulation will probably help the girl become more relaxed and more aroused. Also, if you take the pressure off by not making intercourse the "goal," you may both relax a little more. Using a lubricated condom and applying contraceptive foam inside the girl's vagina helps too. Special lubricants for sexual intercourse—like K-Y jelly, Astroglide, or Probe—are available in drugstores throughout the country. Do not use Vaseline, because it is an oil-based

product and as such can be irritating; it can also damage safer-sex/birth control barrier methods, like latex condoms (see page 288).

➤ She is so anxious about sex that the muscles around her vagina are tightening. Some girls feel real pain at first, but then it goes away. Sometimes, however, the muscles in the opening of the vagina get so tight that it's just about impossible to get a penis or even a finger inside. It may be your body's way of saying, "I'm not ready or willing to have intercourse right now." Maybe you don't really want to have intercourse with this particular person. Maybe you don't feel like having sex at all at this point in your life. Perhaps you have some bad memories about intercourse or sex in general that are keeping you from opening yourself up to it. Maybe you are afraid of getting pregnant or catching an STD. Whatever the reasons are, they are important to take seriously. If your body says to you, "I don't want to do this," listen to your body and try to discover why it's giving you such a strong message. If this problem persists, it might be beneficial to discuss it with a counselor.

Not Feeling Much During Intercourse and/or Not Reaching Orgasm: More girls than you might guess experience this problem. A number don't feel sexual pleasure during intercourse because they don't really want to be doing it. Many others simply don't get the stimulation they need from the act of a penis going in and out of their vagina. Read the sections on orgasm and masturbation. It could be that other sexual activities will help you enjoy more pleasurable feelings.

Timing can play a big role. A girl usually needs to have stimulation until her whole pelvic area feels full and aroused. If the boy puts his penis in too early, he may come and lose his erection before the girl is aroused enough to come herself. Here's how Jessica described her situation:

You get your images of what sex is like from the movies, where it's always so romantic and it always takes so long and seems so passionate. That's not the way it's been for me. If it takes my boyfriend two minutes to come, that's long. I don't think I've ever had intercourse that lasted five minutes, and it takes me longer than that to get turned on.

Orgasms can feel wonderful, but trying too hard to have one (or for your partner, trying too hard to help you have one) can get in the way of enjoying being together. Evie said:

When my boyfriend and I are together making love, every five seconds if I make a sound he'll say, "Are you going to come?" Then he'll say, "What if I do this, does it feel better?" I know he is really concerned about making it good for me, but I get the feeling that I'd *better* come or he'll feel like a failure.

Evie is describing a situation that tempts many girls to pretend to have orgasm, just to get it over with and give their boyfriend "success." In the long run faking doesn't lead to making sex better. The only way to get over the problem is to talk about it with your partner and to try to find other sexual activities that do lead to orgasm if that is what you are going for.

PROBLEMS FOR BOYS

Not Getting or Keeping an Erection: Not being able to get an erection at a critical moment is one of the things that the boys we spoke with worry about most. Tony gave an example:

I was out with this girl, and it became pretty clear to me that she wanted it, and I wouldn't have minded obliging her, but I couldn't get it up. I thought about every sexy thing I could think of and nothing did it for me.

Many boys feel their reputation for manliness is on the line when it's time to have an erection, but of course erections have nothing to do with how manly you are. Almost every male has been unable to get or keep an erection at one time or another. It is very common and absolutely normal.

Sometimes not being able to get an erection is your body's way of telling you that you don't really want to have sex at that moment. These days, there are many reasons why boys don't want to have sex. It can be dangerous to have sex with people you don't know very well. Sexually transmitted diseases are epidemic, and it is very easy to catch one. Also, pregnancy is a serious concern for many boys; they don't want to be in a situation that can lead to an unwanted pregnancy. Many boys want to be in a committed relationship with someone they care about before getting involved sexually. Sometimes boys don't have erections or can't keep an erection if there's no privacy or they feel embarrassed or shy about "doing it right," or if they are nervous about being with someone for the first time or thinking about the morality of their actions.

Once you have trouble with an erection, that might make you worry so much, you end up with the same problem the next time too. The more you can relax and get your mind off worrying, the easier it will be. Remember, sex is not a performance. Lee told us:

I couldn't get it up the first few times we tried. After that, when we were together it was pretty tense between us, and we didn't talk about it. Finally I said, "Let's try again and not worry about whether we can do it or not. Let's just go slowly and try it." We had some trouble that time too, but by the third or fourth try, we really started to get into it.

There are a few purely physical factors that can inhibit erections. Drinking too much alcohol or using some kinds of drugs may keep you from getting erections. Or perhaps some disease or health condition may be the cause. If you *never* get erections, even when you're alone, it would probably be a good idea to check with a health practitioner.

Reaching Orgasm Too Quickly: The other problem that boys worry about is reaching orgasm quicker than they want to. This happens to guys all the time, especially when they are young or with a new partner. Freddie, who is gay, said:

I was so excited the first time I had sex with a guy that I came just taking my pants off. He hadn't even touched me yet.

The boys in a discussion group in Boston got to laughing about "endurance records—like screwing for six hours." Stories like these set up an expectation that a "real man" has perfect control over when he comes and can last for hours. This expectation makes the rest of us feel lousy if we come in two minutes—or two seconds.

Coming "too fast" is a matter of what is too fast for you and your partner. If you would like to last longer, there are some methods you can use to practice slowing down. First, if you masturbate, practice taking longer to reach climax. Also, during intercourse, when you feel yourself about to come, stop thrusting for a few moments, until you feel yourself getting in control again. If the girl is on top and controlling the movement, ask her to stop for a minute or to move more slowly. Just breaking the rhythm a little or changing positions can forestall orgasm but still keep the stimulation going.

Another way to stall orgasm is described by this twenty-year-old from Providence:

I force myself to think about something totally unsexy—like baseball or my job or something like that. My cousin told me about that, and the first couple of times I tried it I just about lost my erection altogether, but pretty soon I got the hang of it. Just when I feel myself getting to the edge of out of control, I switch into a different gear and think about something else, just for a few seconds and that's usually enough to slow me down.

A third way to keep yourself from coming sooner than you'd like is to have an orgasm through other kinds of lovemaking first, before you have intercourse. Wait to have intercourse until you feel aroused again, and this time you will probably be able to hold off your orgasm for a longer time.

Pain with Intercourse or Ejaculation: If your penis or testicles hurt during any kind of sex play, you may have an infection or a disease that needs treatment. See a health practitioner.

If you experience pain after intercourse, you *may* be allergic to the particular brand of birth control foam or jelly your partner used or the lubricating fluid on the condom you used. Try changing products—but of course, always use safer sex methods. If the problem persists, see a health practitioner.

Sexuality is a subject about which we are always learning new things—as we get older, as our interests change, as our lives change. We hope after reading this section you'll realize that you don't have to experience everything right now. There's no rush. Your sexuality will be with you for as long as you're alive.

EXPLORING SEX WITH SOMEONE OF YOUR SAME SEX (HOMOSEXUALITY)

Perhaps you have at some point felt attracted to someone of your own sex. Many people do. Lots of us have had same-sex (homosexual) fantasies or dreams. Some have had one or a few homosexual experiences—anything from kissing to making love.

Quite a number of people—most estimates say about 10 percent of the population—are *mainly* attracted to people of their own sex. That's hundreds of millions of people whose deepest and most emotionally satisfying relationships for part or all of their lives are homosexual. These people come from all walks of life, all religions, all professions, all ethnic groups. They include up to one in ten of our friends, relatives, teachers, doctors, clergy, bank tellers, nurses, entertainers, athletes, plumbers, electricians, writers, business owners.

Homosexual men are often called *gay;* homosexual women are called *lesbian.* When we talk about homosexual people as a group, we usually use the word "gay." Some gay or bisexual people choose to call themselves "queer" as a way of refusing more traditional labeling and taking the power out of discriminatory remarks from the heterosexual community.

In this chapter, teenagers who have mostly gay and lesbian feelings and experiences will talk about their lives. They are in a minority in our society, and like other minorities they have some special issues to deal with—in particular, other people's prejudice against them. So before we begin our discussion, let's put this topic in a little perspective.

If you've ever had a crush on or felt excited by someone of your own sex, chances are that it felt nice in some ways but a little frightening too. "What does this mean?" people ask themselves, "Is there something wrong with me?" We have this response because our society has a negative attitude about homosexuality (called *homophobia:* hoe-moe-*foe*-bee-uh). We are taught that two people of the same sex loving each other in a romantic and sexual way is bad, sick, sinful, weird. We learn insulting words for homosexuals: fag, dyke, queer, butch, fairy, pervert. Many jokes make fun of gay people. We hear scary rumors that homosexuals "seduce" children, when in fact most people who abuse children sexually are "straight" (heterosexual) men. It's hard to feel comfortable with, much less enjoy, our own same-sex feelings or our relationships with homosexual friends when we have been taught all these negative things.

We learn, wrongly, that if you have even one homosexual feeling or experience, that means you are "gay." This isn't true. We're also taught that a person is either all heterosexual or all homosexual for life, and that isn't true either.

Most people are neither "all straight" or "all gay." It helps to picture a line with "gay" on one side and "straight" on the other.

Gay ———————————————— Straight

Most of us fall somewhere along the line. Maybe a boy will have a passionate affair with a girl in his senior year in high school and find out when he gets to college that he mainly loves men. A girl may make love with her best girlfriend for a year or so while dating boys all the time, and later have a long married life with a man. A girl or boy may have sexual fantasies of both sexes. Or someone will go into a one-sex environment—a prison, a single-sex school—and find his or her emotions and natural sexual urges coming out toward the people closest by. Each of these people would be somewhere in the middle of the gay/straight line. There are also many people who find themselves able to enjoy loving rela-

tionships with people from both sexes throughout their lives. They are called bisexual.

At either end of the line are the people who feel they are exclusively gay or straight. More people would be on the "straight" end—but many would be on the "gay" end too. Looking at a line like this can help those of us who fear that a fantasy or a kiss or even making love with someone of our own sex means that we are "gay." It's more likely that at different times of our life, we will find ourselves at different points along the line.

You may never have a single homosexual thought or fantasy. You may never have a single heterosexual thought or fantasy. That's fine. There's no point in trying to feel anything that doesn't come naturally to *you,* but if you think you are "more gay" than not, it is important for you to know you are not alone.

Teenagers who stretch beyond the sexual boundaries taught by our society do so with courage. Their homosexual or bisexual lifestyle sets them apart from the mainstream in a heterosexist society, a society that assumes "normal" people should be heterosexual. For gay teens and adults, their choice of sexual partners means they may be ostracized from housing, work, friendships, and family. But as one teen said:

> It's not something I'm choosing, it's who I am, and to try to be something else would be worse. It would be like being in prison.

Some people believe that same-sex feelings and experiences are wrong—for anyone—and may just not be able to accept the idea of homosexuality. Here's how Robert put it:

> Look, I think it's weird for two guys to French-kiss each other or to screw. Being in love is for men and women, and any other way is just unnatural. I read all this stuff about being open-minded, but you have to draw the line somewhere.

Miriam, a sixteen-year-old from the East, said:

> I live in a city where there are gay couples walking around. The women are okay, but when I see two men arm in arm looking lovingly into each other's

eyes, I go to the other side of the street. I don't know, I just can't handle it.

John is from Illinois. He said:

This friend I play basketball with a couple of nights a week told me he's gay—you know, he digs guys. He didn't come on to me or anything, just told me. But I freaked out, man. Here I've been playing ball with this guy who's a queer. He wants to stay friends, but I say no way.

Finding out that a friend has had gay experiences may make you fearful or uneasy, especially if you have been taught that same-sex loving is bad. You may worry that your friend will try to seduce you, although that rarely happens. So much of your identity is in transition during the teen years, and sex in general is such a confusing mix of urges, feelings, needs, and worries anyway. Feeling sure of your sexual identity may seem especially important to you. You may worry that if you are accepting of someone else's homosexuality, you may become homosexual yourself. These worries make it harder for teens who do feel closer to the "gay" end of the line to be open about their feelings.

Fear of seeming to be gay puts a lot of people on guard about themselves. Boys, especially, talked to us about being afraid that people would think they were gay if they weren't always trying to get sex with a girl. Roy said:

If I'm not in bed with some chick on the second date, they're going to think I'm a fag or something.

Much of our society has specific and very rigid attitudes about gender. In the extreme, boys prove their masculinity by acting tough and being aggressive and athletic. Girls are supposed to be the opposite, acting sweet and understanding, wearing soft colors and makeup. They're not supposed to be angry or aggressive or strong. When people cross those gender lines, they risk being called names. Boys said they were afraid of being called gay if their body was soft rather than muscley or if they had long hair or if they were not into sports or working out or if they had a close relationship with another guy or if

they expressed themselves in a more "feminine" way than the other boys their age. Girls said they worry they'll be suspected of being lesbians if they have a muscular build or a deep voice or a hairier body or more of an interest in sports or mechanics than their friends. Even so, because society attributes openly affectionate and emotional expression to the female gender, many girls said they felt freer than boys to have affectionate friendships with their friends.

Fear of gayness makes people suspect anything in their personality that seems to be more like that of the opposite sex. Being on guard this way keeps people from being their whole selves and limits their enjoyment of life.

The best way to combat the fear and prejudice many people feel about homosexuality is to meet some open homosexuals and get to know them. Jerry, sixteen, is in a teen rap group with a boy named Ed, who is openly gay. Jerry said:

When Ed first said he was gay I thought, Let me out of here! But I knew this guy; we were friends already; I knew what he did in his spare time, what kinds of fights he had with his mother, what kind of movies he dug. I mean, he's a person. So by now his being gay is just something else I know about him. I never thought I'd hear myself saying that.

In the rest of this chapter you will hear from gay and lesbian teenagers and find out a little about their lives. We hope that will help dispel some of the myths that contribute to the prejudice and discrimination against gay people.

Sexual Orientation

DO I HAVE TO CALL MYSELF ONE THING OR THE OTHER? There's some pressure these days to "decide" whether you are straight or gay. The main pressure, of course, is toward deciding you are straight. But many teenagers with one or two homosexual experiences feel they should say they are gay. Some feel the need to label themselves gay in order to give support to other gays, because it's so hard to be part of a disparaged minority. Some feel the urge to "come out," to be honest about the homosexual feelings they have. Here's what fifteen-year-old Beth wrote to us:

> I've been bombarded with the message that it's impossible to know whether you're straight or gay or bi or whatever before you've had relationships (of the romantic and/or sexual kind) with at least one if not both sexes. I've just recently convinced myself, with the help of a bunch of e-mail pen pals that yes, I can know without having had "experiences." Because I've known for a while but I keep having this nagging voice in the back of my head saying, "Beth you're labeling yourself without ever having had any experience! You can't know!" Which I really don't think is true. I think I can know.

Terrie has this opinion:

> I came out to myself before I had had a sexual experience with anybody. I don't think you need to have experience to know who turns you on. I just knew what I wanted and didn't want: I didn't care for boyfriends, I preferred my best girlfriend and that was that.

Dan, seventeen, said:

> It's funny, because nobody says to a hetero, don't worry, you don't have to declare your sexual preference until you're older, until you know for sure. In fact, parents want their kids to declare that they're hetero, the sooner the better.

Erin agreed with Dan. She's fourteen, and her mother gives her a hard time for saying she's gay:

> My mother thinks that I'm too young to know what my sexual preference is, and even though she insists she'll love me no matter whether I'm straight or gay or bi, I know she hopes this is just a phase. I have a good friend who's a guy. He's one of my best friends, and I really love him so much. But when I talk about him to my mom she says, in a hopeful voice, "Do you have a crush on him?" And I keep having to tell her, "No, Mom, I don't. I'm sorry but I'm just not attracted to guys."

The teens quoted above say they know they are gay because they feel attracted exclusively to people of their own sex, and when they fantasize about sex, they have homosexual fantasies. For many other teenagers, however, there are years of living and loving ahead before they will know what their preference is. You may never want to say you are finally or exclusively gay or straight. Some people believe that bisexuality, an openness to sexual relationships with both sexes, is many people's true nature. A number of bisexuals we met say that as teenagers they felt pressure to be either straight or gay, and it wasn't until they were older that they felt comfortable admitting their bisexuality. Here's how one twenty-year-old male spoke about it:

> Some people assume that if you're bisexual you are equally attracted to each sex, which is not true for everyone. And many people assume that if you're attracted to both sexes, you must have a boyfriend and a girlfriend at the same time, which is no more true than straight people having more than one partner at a time. I know for me, I feel mainly attracted to females now, but when I was younger I had most of my relationships with males.

It's a good idea to resist the pressure to label yourself. Decide in your own time. There's no need to rush into it. Make your choice when you are ready—or never make a choice. That's okay too.

What follows is a discussion of homosexuality based on conversations with many teenagers who identified themselves as gay or lesbian at the time—that is, their sexual feelings and romantic loving relationships mainly involved people of their own sex.

SAME-SEX EXPERIENCES WHILE GROWING UP: It's quite common for young children to have lots of different kinds of sexual feelings and experiences. Some of our early sex play may have been with girls, some with boys, and some with girls and boys. Unless they are caught and punished, or somehow hurt, most kids enjoy this kind of sex play and exploration. Here's what a young woman from the Midwest remembers:

I can remember experimenting with sex as early as age four. It made no difference to me whether it was a boy or a girl. And that went on for years.

Eighteen-year-old Scott said:

I used to have sex with my best friends who were guys all the time. This was until I was about fourteen or so. And I never thought it was wrong or anything like that.

As children get older, their attachments to same-sex friends become deeper and may represent the first time they feel romantic love. Evan, who's fifteen now, said:

I remember when I was in the seventh grade and I got really attached to a friend at school. When he moved away, I remember being really upset and crying over it. I guess I must have been in love with him, in whatever way I could as a thirteen-year-old.

Sandra, a nineteen-year-old from California, said:

I had a really close friend when I was younger. We had pet names for each other and everything. I'd give her a little stuffed bunny because she was a Thumper and I was a koala bear, and she'd give me a bear or a card with a bear on it. It was like she was my sister, you know, and we'd write each other poems about how much we loved each other. Sometimes I wondered about that, but it felt okay, it felt good.

What starts out as friendship may gradually and naturally lead into being sexual together if both people are open to that. Anna, sixteen, is from New Hampshire. She told us:

I was with my friend, just the two of us together. We were kind of partying and had drunk a little too much. We were listening to a record, and she started to stagger and I caught her, and she held me and we started slow-dancing together. She started kissing me. And through it all I kept thinking, What's wrong with this? You know, it feels good, I love to kiss.

As you can see from these accounts, it's pretty common for people to have homosexual attractions, feelings, and maybe even experiences when they are younger. This doesn't actually predict whether we will choose homosexual relationships later on. It's a part of learning about our sexuality.

GENDER IDENTITY: Have you ever wondered what it feels like to be a person of the other sex? Even though most of us mainly identify ourselves as either male or female, depending on which genitalia we were born with, sometimes boys like expressing their softer, more tender "female" qualities and girls enjoy acting in ways that are called "masculine." That kind of cross-gender expression of feelings is common.

For a number of people, however, cross-gender feelings happen more than just occasionally. Some teens feel imprisoned by the gender into which they were born. They say they have always identified with the other sex and prefer looking like, dressing, and acting that way. Girls may bind their breasts, cut their hair really short, allow their facial and body hair to grow, and wear men's clothing because inside themselves they feel more "male" than they feel "female." Boys may enjoy wearing jewelry and soft, feminine clothing, or they may speak and walk in a style that is usually called feminine, because they identify much more with the female in them than they do with the male. These teens are called transsexuals. The definition of a transsexual is someone who feels that he or she is or ought to be the opposite sex.*

Identifying with the opposite sex can be dangerous in a society that has little tolerance for people who step outside the norm. Girls who dress and act like boys and boys who dress and act like girls frequently spark violent reactions in others who don't understand their behavior. They may be harassed, humiliated, and even physically abused, all of which is against the law. See page 221 for more on this.

Transsexual teens sometimes decide to have operations to change their genitalia and "become" the other sex. Or they may decide instead to take hormones to give themselves the outward character-

* An excellent book on this subject is *True Selves*, by Mildred L. Brown and Chloe Ann Rounsley. San Francisco: Jossey Bass, 1996.

istics of the other gender. Mainstream society calls their condition a gender identity "disorder," but people who feel trapped in the wrong body don't see their actions as a disorder. They experience cross-gender identification as the only way to express their true feelings about themselves. While that may be difficult for many heterosexual teens to understand, one girl we met said she is trying:

I always thought I was so open-minded and everything, but then I saw the movie *The Crying Game*, and as soon as I found out this one character was male, not female, my whole attitude about him changed. I was really liking him as a girl, but then I thought, Wait a minute, this is weird, he's really a boy. I thought about that a lot. After a while I realized, What's the difference? Why should it matter to me? If he feels like a female and he acts like a female, and if a guy falls in love with him as a female, well, who am I to say on some level he's not female?

BECOMING AWARE OF SAME-SEX FEELINGS: Adolescence is the time when many of us who are mainly attracted to people of the same sex begin to notice it. For some, that self-awareness and understanding is a natural and positive thing. Laura, a seventeen-year-old girl from Boston, describes it this way:

I never went through a thing like, These feelings I have are gay feelings, so I better go talk to somebody like a shrink about them. I always thought that it was natural. I just followed my feelings and went along with them, and everything was fine. I never had any head problems about them.

Eighteen-year-old Ben said:

When I realized that I was gay, I was about fourteen. I was dating a girl—really, the only girl that has ever been in my life—and I was with this guy. There was some conflict there. You know, I liked them both. But then I realized that I was more attracted to the guy. Every weekend I'd go over to his place, and his parents weren't around much. We'd go horseback riding in the woods. We really had a great friendship, including sex.

For other teens, this discovery can be unsettling and even frightening. For instance, this fifteen-year-old boy from Washington State remembers:

When I was growing up and I realized that I had emotions for other guys, I didn't know that that was anything different. But then I started to hear words like "faggot" and "queer," and I began to have second thoughts and questions about my feelings.

Jonathan stated it this way:

I was messing around with boys—you know, like two buddies experimenting with something. It was really no big thing. By the time I was twelve, though, I began to get a social awareness that you can't continue to enjoy these feelings with people of your own sex, because it just doesn't fit in with our society.

George, from Boise, recalls:

In junior high, I was actively interested in sex with other guys, almost any guy. I remember sweating it out in gym class thinking, God, if I get a hard-on in the locker room, everyone will have a field day with me.

Where sex is concerned, lots of people have very definite attitudes about what is right or wrong. If our behavior or feelings don't fit with their attitudes, they may call us names or laugh at us or put us down. If you stop to notice, when two people are loving or caring for each other in the media—on billboards, in magazines, on TV—it's almost always a man and a woman. It's rarely two women or two men together. Gradually more gay characters are appearing on TV and in the movies; their portrayal is not usually realistic, however, as a fourteen-year-old girl in Arizona notes:

There's a lot more openly gay people in the media today, but some of the characters are real stereotyped, like the butch dyke lesbian truck driver or the effeminate gay hairdresser. So those kinds of characters reinforce all the old prejudices. But there're also celebrities and entertainers who people may not know are gay, and they like them and then later find out that they are gay and then think, Oh, okay, it's no big deal.

Because we have so little information about homosexuality and so few models of regular, everyday gay relationships, most of us grow up with dreams and expectations for the future that are based on heterosexual lives—like falling in love with someone of the other sex, getting married, and having a family. Discovering that you are mainly attracted to people of your own sex can initially give you a sense of disappointment and loss.

But gay people fall in love too and stay together for years and years. Many gay people are mothers and fathers. They raise families together. Sixteen-year-old Elizabeth said:

> When I was thirteen and just beginning to realize I wasn't straight, I got a babysitting job from this lesbian couple who had a one-year-old daughter. That's when I started really recognizing that gay people live very normal lives. They were the nicest family, and their daughter was so well loved.

These days, gay *and* straight people are building alternative emotional-support networks in order to live lives that are not based on the traditional nuclear family. The bumper sticker "Love is what makes a family" says it all.

DENYING AND HIDING THE FEELINGS: Some people may try to deny that they have any homosexual feelings and attractions. Julie, a seventeen-year-old from Georgia, said:

> Well, at first when I was just kissing other girls, it wasn't hard for me to face up to kissing, but I wouldn't admit I was gay or bisexual or anything like that. I just said it was fun, and it just happened to be with a girl. But so what? There was no such word as "gay" or "homosexual" in my life. Later, as I got involved with more sexual activity with girls, I thought, Now maybe I'm bisexual or something, but that's it. I'm not a lesbian! Oh no, not me!

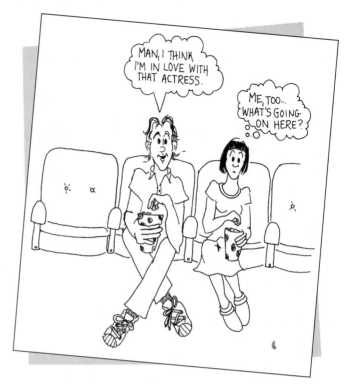

Joel, an eighteen-year-old from the Midwest, remembers how he tried to deny his feelings and attractions:

> By the time I was twelve, I realized that men were part of my sexual fantasies. I liked guys, you know? And once, around the same time, out of the clear blue sky, someone said to me, "Hey man, if you don't watch it, you're going to be a homosexual." And I said to myself, Nah, not me. That's the last thing I'll ever be. I'll never be a homosexual. So from about the age of twelve to sixteen, I squashed those feelings whenever they came to me.

Many teens who have strong same-sex feelings decide to date people of the other sex, trying to be interested in them as sexual partners. Usually they get encouragement from parents and friends to do this. Devon told us it doesn't work that way:

> In a straight person's mind, getting a homosexual guy in bed with a girl is going to be all he needs to make a miraculous change into being a heterosexual. It's funny. Some people think that the only reason that you are gay is because you had a bad experience with a woman. Like a woman laughed at you or something. So they think that all you need is a good experience to turn you straight.

Some teens themselves believe straight dating may help them become heterosexual. Merry, a nineteen-year-old from Louisiana, told us:

I had a boyfriend long after I knew that I was feeling these feelings towards other girls. I knew that I really didn't get anything out of being with a boy. The sex was okay, but emotionally there was always this wall that was never there with the girls I was attracted to. I kept seeing my boyfriend, though, because I thought maybe things would change.

Here's how Pete described his experience:

I would try to talk to all these girls and we would pick up girls in the street. I had no problems having sexual thoughts or erections over girls. But what really bothered me was that the more I pressed myself on them, the less success and satisfaction I got. I began to get a lot of anxiety over that. Pretty soon I couldn't get an erection over girls and my fantasies became totally male.

Many gay teens say they don't want to deny their feelings and attractions, but they have to be realistic about what that means in our society. There are people who consider them bad or sick. Some religions consider homosexuality a sin, and many followers of those teachings try to "outlaw" homosexuality in their communities.

Gay people may be called disparaging names like "dyke" or "bull dyke" or "faggot" or "queer" or "fairy." People use those words to hurt others whom they perceive as different from themselves. Those names and labels are based on "stereotypes"—that is, false generalizations, which are nearly always negative and destructive and ignore the fact that whatever our sexual preference, each of us is unique. Stereotypic thinking keeps people ignorant and afraid of one another.

In reaction to the negative, stereotypic labels, some gay people are using those same names as the way to identify themselves. Beth helped us edit this chapter. She had this to say about language and labels:

Lesbigay (lesbian, bisexual, and gay) people, particularly young people, are starting to use the word "queer" more and more as a general word describing anyone who is not straight. Part of using that word, which in the past has been so derogatory, is that by reclaiming the language and converting it to a positive, even affectionate, usage, it can no longer hurt us.

For most teenagers who have homosexual feelings, however, the message from society is full of anger and prejudice. Gay teens can't help but learn that to much of society their feelings are considered bad or wrong. A seventeen-year-old girl put it this way:

When you first find out that you're gay, it's a real shocking experience for a lot of people. Like, I called myself sick. It was like I was mentally disturbed.

Bill, a senior in college, said about his high school years:

I had more enjoyment with guys than I did with girls, and it just confirmed what I had already been thinking. I cried about it a lot. I said to myself, You're a homosexual. And I didn't want to be, not then anyhow. I called myself all sorts of names: You're a fag, you're a freak. Where was my belief in God? Where was my future with a wife and kids? All this was going through my mind.

Three members of a young lesbian support group in Providence, Rhode Island, talked about having to hide their feelings:

Tina (nineteen): In junior high I would look at girls' bodies and they'd be aware of it, so I'd look down at the floor and try to control it. I did a lot of strange things to cover my impulses. In the locker room I'd take a shower way down at the other end, away from everyone else, to make it clear I wasn't looking.

Alice (twenty): I got so I avoided touching my friends, I was so afraid my feelings would show. One time a friend asked me to zip up her dress and I remember my hand shaking.

Brenda (eighteen): When a rumor leaked out in tenth grade that I was gay, this group of girls would tease me by coming up and hugging me all the time, and I'd have to push them away and say, "Oh, gross!" It was awful.

Alice: What makes me so angry is that I held the feelings down for so long that now when I get with someone I love, I can't relax and touch her. There's this tightness inside me.

One of the reasons why some teenagers feel they have to deny or hide their homosexual feelings is that they may not know other people who feel the way they do. Jason said:

There aren't that many people out there who you can talk to about sex, and especially about being gay, who don't lecture you, and you think, What do they know about what I'm going through and how I feel?

Penny, an eighteen-year-old from Minnesota, said:

I knew one gay guy in junior high, but in high school I didn't know anyone else who was gay, especially any lesbians. It was pretty lonely. Gradually I got to know more gay kids in school, but not a lot. Sometimes it takes a while for people to decide that they're gay, and some people just aren't ready to come out.

And this seventeen-year-old remembers rather painfully:

For me it's been a real lonely experience. I can never show the real me, especially that part of me, to anyone because that would mean that no one would want to be with me. If I told them about my homosexual feelings, no one would care about me. It's awful.

Most gay teens say they don't grow up with many positive models of gay people. Jimmy, nineteen, remembered:

The homosexual stuff I knew about was dirty. You know, dirty old men who grabbed you and did things to you. Or very effeminate guys. I grew up in a very proper town, so I couldn't find anybody

else my age who was feeling like me. I didn't want to have to act like a "fem" [effeminate, like a woman]. I wasn't a "fem," and I definitely was not a dirty old man.

Jimmy said there were probably other gays in his community, but he didn't know it, because for the most part, you can't tell if people are gay or straight just by looking at them. A more effeminate seventeen-year-old reported being lonely too:

The only other gay guys I know in school are both jocks—real macho, on the football team and all that. I look more like the stereotype people have of homosexuals. It's one thing to be gay and macho. It's another thing to be fem. It's really isolating, but it's who I am.

Coming Out

Tony, sixteen, said:

When I feel like I'm the only queer teenager around, I think about the fact that if one in ten people are gay, that means out of the eight hundred people in my high school, about eighty of us probably are or will be gay or lesbian in our lives. This is really encouraging, even though no one is out yet as far as I know. It even makes me think that maybe I should come out at school, so that some of the other people will come out and we can support each other.

The process of feeling more open about yourself and gaining strength and pride as a gay person is known as the coming-out process. It refers to coming out of "the closet." Being "in the closet" means hiding from others, and sometimes from yourself too, that you have same-sex feelings and would like to act on them. For many people, coming out involves a series of steps—first, admitting to yourself you're gay; then coming to know other lesbians or gay men; next, telling your friends and/or family; then finally, marching in a demonstration for gay rights or joining a gay organization or social group. The process of coming out means leaving some of your old feelings behind—giving up feelings of shame, guilt, or self-hatred. It means coming to have a good sense of yourself and standing up to people who may not react positively to the fact that you are openly gay. Gina said it this way:

Coming out is a continual process—lifelong, in fact—since you have to come out to all the new people you meet throughout your life. It's not something you do and then you're over with it.

And this eighteen-year-old boy said:

When you do finally come out, it makes you want to try to help people know you and understand you, so they won't be so ready to stereotype you.

David now lives in Seattle, but he remembers:

I grew up in a big city in the East where there were lots of gangs. Like, my brother is in a gang. So I used to watch all these gangs beat up people, beat up fags. I used to watch. I even watched someone get beat up so

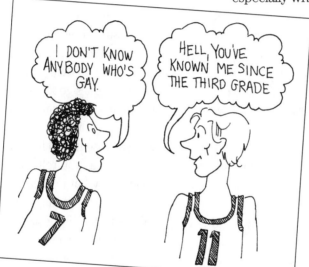

much he was bleeding all over. One guy even was murdered. And I was just watching, deep down knowing that I was a gay, but I would say to myself, "They're fags. I'm not." Finally, I couldn't stand just sitting back and watching these gangs beat up on gays. One time, I started beating up some of the gang members. And I told the gay guys to stay out of my neighborhood, because it was too dangerous for them there.

David's actions took a lot of courage and helped him realize that he was beginning to accept his homosexuality from a position of strength and pride deep within himself. It was the first step in his coming out.

To define themselves openly as "lesbians" or as "gay males" is an important step for many of the teens and young adults we interviewed. They feel that using these words helps them identify their true feelings—that they are boys who love boys and girls who love girls. Since most of them have spent a long time hiding and denying this part of their identities, the new openness offers them a kind of peace of mind.

Of course, some teens may not want to consider themselves homosexual, heterosexual, or bisexual until they are older and have had enough experience to know what they enjoy and what kinds of relationships are meaningful to them. Many teenagers are choosing to abstain from any sexual experience with another person until they are out of high school at least. So for a lot of reasons, it may not suit you personally to try to categorize your sexual preference, especially while you are still young.

If you have questions about your sexuality, you are not alone. You may wish someone could tell you how to determine if you are gay or straight or both or neither. Time and experience, reading books from the suggestions on page 150, talking with trustworthy people in your life—all these can help you while you are questioning. But remember, there is plenty of time to choose a preference or not. It's up to you.

COMING OUT TO YOURSELF: This is the first step. Alana, an eighteen-year-old from New England, said:

Before I came out to myself, I wasn't honest with myself. I didn't trust myself or respect myself in many different areas. And when you first come out, it's like you're telling yourself something you don't want to believe. "You kissed that girl, didn't you? It felt good, didn't it? So what's wrong with it?" You finally begin to relate to yourself. After that, it's like the rest of your life opens up and you stop blocking things. You start asking yourself, "Hey, what's going on?" It's made me a lot more honest with myself.

Gabriel, who's sixteen, told us:

> After I came out to myself, I kept finding pieces from my past that made more sense. A lot of my actions when I was younger became clearer. Like, I'd always kind of wondered why I never wanted to go out with girls, and now I knew.

Some teens told us that admitting they had homosexual feelings and attractions helped them discover that they did have sexual feelings after all. Josie, twenty, from Arizona, said:

> When I was with guys, I thought I was not sexual at all. I thought I just didn't like sex. I always seemed frustrated, and I didn't know why. And it was embarrassing to tell my friends. They would say, "Gosh, I haven't seen you go out with anyone for eight months, you know? What's the problem?" And I would say, "Well, I can take or leave sex." I would always say that. Matter of fact, when I got my first gay lover, I told her the same thing, "I can take or leave sex." But then, after the first time we made love, I loved it. I loved sex.

Brianna, twenty-three, looked back over her earlier years:

> For years I had been holding my sensuality down as hard as I could, because I was so scared my lesbian feelings would take me over. A month after I said to myself, Okay, I'm a lesbian, and had my first female lover, I suddenly started to go dancing a whole lot, to take bubble baths, swim nude at night, wear soft slinky shirts.

A nineteen-year-old California man described the rewards of coming out to himself:

> Finally, just about when I was graduating from high school, I looked at myself and just accepted the fact that I was gay. I looked in the mirror and said, not "You're a homosexual," but "I'm a homosexual." And from that point on I could admit to myself who I was, and that made me a man in my own feelings. It's funny, because a lot of people think that being a homosexual robs a guy

of his manhood. But for me, admitting my own homosexuality gave me my manhood.

COMING OUT TO FRIENDS: When you first realize you are gay, you may want to shout it from the rooftops and let everyone know about it, or you may want to keep it a secret from most of the people you know. It's important to take the time you need to get ready to tell your friends and family. Don't let anyone or anything push you into coming out before you're feeling strong enough and good enough about your identity to be able to deal with the mix of reactions your announcement may evoke.

Only you can decide when the right time is to tell the people who are important to you. If you are in a period of being very angry with your parents, you might be tempted to come out just as a kind of rebellion. Occasionally, teenagers do this even when they are not sure they are gay. It isn't a very good idea. Coming out can bring some big changes in your life, and it's best to take your time about it to be sure.*

Usually, it's good to begin by telling people who like you and who you think are the most likely to accept you. You may want to test the situation by telling a close friend first and then using that person for support as you tell others. Remember, not everyone knows what homosexuality is all about, and most people have been taught that it's bad. Be ready to deal with a lot of questions, and with reactions of ignorance, confusion, and perhaps hostility. Remember, too, that people may have lots of stereotypes and need the information that you can give them to dispel their false notions. One teen explained it this way:

> Everything we see about homosexuality is so sensationalized! People don't have a sense of what it really means to be gay. How many nice, normal people are gay.

Another teen had this advice for people:

> If a friend comes out to you, don't see it as them changing. Don't think that they're any different,

---

* There is an excellent pamphlet published by PFLAG (Parents and Friends of Lesbians and Gays) about coming out to your parents. It is available on the Internet and also by writing to them. See the Resource section of this chapter, on page 150, for information on how to find this brochure.

because they're not different. They're sharing a part of themselves with you because they trust you, and most likely they need your support and acceptance.

When friends do change their feelings about you after you come out to them, it hurts. A young man from New York City wrote to us:

Friends, that is, people I thought were friends, turned full-fire against me, but used other reasons for their constant verbal attacks.

Gretchen, a nineteen-year-old, from Los Angeles, related this experience:

Most of my friends that I've told have accepted it, and me, more or less. It's funny, the only person that has turned completely against me is my closest friend. We were best friends for the first seventeen years of my life. Actually, she was the first person I had sex with, when I was seven years old. Anyhow, she's the only person that has turned away from me for good. You have to be careful, because it's easy to get hurt.

Jamie, a seventeen-year-old from Wyoming, said:

After people at school found out I was gay, a lot of them kind of kept a distance from me. I think they were scared that I was going to do something to them. You know, the old fears about gay people attacking you and that junk. I guess that was one of the reasons why I didn't come out sooner, because I was afraid that they would be scared of me. It's stupid and crazy, but a lot of people feel that way.

You may be thinking that a friend who can't accept you once you come out isn't such a good friend after all, but remember, it may take time for him or her to incorporate and digest your announcement.

Beth wanted us to be sure to say that it takes a lot of courage to come out:

When somebody finally does decide to come out, they've probably agonized and thought about it for days and weeks, maybe even months. They've made a decision to tell you that they're gay or lesbian because they feel that without you knowing that about them, you can't fully know them at all.

You can tell your friends that you're still the same person you always were, the same person you were yesterday! You can explain that just because you have come out doesn't mean you're going to attack them or seduce them or require that they become homosexual too. You can explain (to family in particular) that although some of their expectations and hopes for you are disappointed, other hopes—like those for your happiness, self-acceptance, and pride—can now be fulfilled. Maggie, who's fifteen, said:

When I told my sister, she cried, and then she started calling me names and telling me I was sick. I told her, "Damn it, I haven't changed! I'm still your sister. I'm still the same person I was. Have I changed physically? Have I changed in any other sense? And if so, have I changed for the better or worse?" She said, "You've changed for the better from the last time I saw you." And then I said, "Only I'm gay, and it hasn't made me any different, has it? Has it changed your and my relationship?" And she said, "No, not really." And I said, finally, "It's just my sexuality preference. That's it, that's all. It's my life preference. It doesn't change me as a person, personality-wise. It just changes my lifestyle a little. And I'm happy. You should be happy that I'm happy."

Brian remembered:

I was telling a friend and she said, "I can understand how you can have close male friends, but to be sexual with them, that's sick!" And I said, "It's sick when a guy isn't attracted to women and won't face up to loving men. That's what's sick. It's not sick when you face up to who you really are."

When you come out to others, in a way you're educating them. You're saying, See. I'm still the same person I was, the same person you liked (or loved), and I'm gay.

COMING OUT TO PARENTS: Because parents and family are so important in everyone's life, there will probably come a time when you'll want them to know who you are and how you feel. Bridget, eighteen, said:

My mother said, "You didn't need to tell me. I knew it all the time." But I wanted to tell her, because it was coming from me. I *needed* to tell her, even if she already knew.

Your family members *may* already know. They may have felt awkward about bringing it up, and perhaps relieved to have it out in the open. Here's what Leon told us:

The term "gay" or "faggot" never came up in my house. But my father got a hint that I was gay because he heard one of my friends talking about being gay. One night he took me out to dinner, and he told me about all the girls he's had, and then he told me about all the guys he's had. That was a real shock for me! He was trying to get around to asking me if I was gay. He never really did come right out and ask me, but I'm pretty sure he knew and knows now.

John, a sixteen-year-old from Michigan, had this experience with his family:

My sister was the first one I told. Really, she asked me. I think she suspected it for a long time, and she finally asked me straight out. And I told her. She accepted it without any hassle. Then about two weeks later, my mom asked me if I was gay, and I told her too. She started crying, and we sat around and talked. She wanted to know if she had been too domineering or something like that. We ended the conversation hugging each other and saying that everything will turn out okay. My mom told my dad, and he was real understanding too. But he kept thinking and hoping that I would change, and he keeps influencing me to see girls.

For many gay teens, coming out to parents is much more painful than what has been described above. Some parents react with extreme anger, some

with blame and hostility. Sixteen-year-old Peter, from Ohio, said:

My mom wouldn't accept the fact that I'm gay. She threw me out of the house. She's prejudiced against gays and thinks I'm choosing to be gay to get back at her or something. She doesn't realize that it's not my choice, it's who I am.

Some parents react by becoming extra strict and trying to keep you from seeing any gay or bisexual friends. They may be so angry and blaming that family life gets impossible for everyone. Jenny said:

When I told my folks that I was a lesbian, they totally freaked out. It was so against their religion, their lifestyle and friends, that they just couldn't deal with it. I'm not living at home anymore, and I hardly ever talk with them. I hope after a while they'll mellow out about it.

Jenny went to live with a friend's family in a nearby town. If this kind of alternative is available to you, it can help cool down a hot family situation. But some gay teens, like some straight teens in other kinds of family battles, end up leaving home on their own, hoping to find a more accepting place elsewhere. Unfortunately, in our world it can be extremely dangerous for a teenager to be out on his or her own. To move to a new place with no resources and nowhere to stay puts you at the mercy of the street. We urge you to consider your choices very carefully. Before taking off, discuss your situation with an adult you can trust, a relative, a counselor, a minister, a pastor, a rabbi, or a respected teacher. Or call the national hotline for teen runaways, Covenant House's Nine Line: 1-800-999-9999. They may be able to help you find a placement.

On hearing that their child is gay, some parents insist that he or she see a psychiatrist or psychotherapist. These parents believe that emotional problems have made their child think he or she is gay. Working with a good therapist is sometimes a great help in sorting out feelings and problems (see page 179) as long as the therapist listens to what *you* want and how *you* see things. Sometimes it's especially helpful to attend family therapy sessions together with your parents. But therapy will not "cure" a person of being gay if that's the preference he or she feels most strongly, because being gay is not a sickness.

Perhaps after reading this, it's easier to understand why the rate of depression and suicide among gay and lesbian teenagers is so high. If you feel so much anger and rejection from your family and friends that life becomes unbearable, the chapter Emotional Health Care, beginning on page 153, may be of some help to you in finding ways to deal with your frustration and isolation. There are many organizations set up to help gay young people in trouble. They are listed at the end of this chapter (page 150). Don't hesitate to call one for advice and support.

What It's Like for Parents: A teenager's coming out can be a painful and challenging experience for parents too. Listen to this forty-year-old St. Louis mother of three:

> When our oldest son, Ted, told us he was gay, it was a very hard thing for my husband and me to handle. First we blamed ourselves, because we thought that we had made some mistake or something. We also felt a lot of strong, kind of crazy feelings toward Ted: we were angry, disappointed, and we felt sorry for him. It was a real difficult time for all of us, and we began to worry about our other kids too.

For religious parents who strongly believe that homosexuality is a fundamental sin, there are few choices. To accept your lifestyle goes against everything they consider true and moral. They see your life choice as being influenced by the devil, and they will undoubtedly do everything in their power to try to get you to repent.*

Many parents need to learn more about what being homosexual means before they can open their minds and their hearts to you as gay. They may be thinking of the stereotypes of how gay people are portrayed, and they may worry that you will have a difficult life. Parents may also fear that they will be blamed by society, as is often the case when children

turn out to be unusual or nonconformist. They may feel they have done something wrong in bringing you up or worry about how their friends or their business associates or their own parents will react. And they may be disappointed to think they won't have grandchildren, even though many gay people these days do start families. Parents may worry, too, that being gay will make you drift away from them, into a world that is alien to their own.

In addition, they may worry because they know that some people will try to make life harder for you just because of your sexual preference. They know that you may have trouble getting jobs or housing, for instance, because of discrimination against gays. They may think that you are trapping yourself into an identity that you won't be able to get out of if you want to later.

Perhaps their greatest concern will be about your health, since many people immediately associate homosexuality (especially for males) with AIDS and death.

Some of these concerns are legitimate, and you and your parents need to take time to discuss them and work them through. One father said:

> I disapproved of my daughter's lesbianism not because I had any moral problems with it, but because I felt it would make her life too difficult. My overwhelming concern, though, was to let her see that none of this had anything to do with my love and continuing support for her. I was terribly afraid that because I was so hurt and upset, I would push her away from me and jeopardize our relationship.

It is a great relief on all sides if parents can come to accept their son's or daughter's gayness. A father from Los Angeles said:

> My wife and I were really shocked at first when our son told us about his homosexuality. I felt betrayed and angry, and we had some ugly fights. But he finally convinced us that he was happy and pretty well adjusted. He kept saying to us, "Do you want me to lie to you, to pretend that I'm someone I really am not to you?" So after a year or so we finally began to accept his being gay.

---

* Jeanette Winterson, an author who was raised by a fundamentalist family in northern England, discusses this dilemma in her novel *Oranges Are Not the Only Fruit*. See the Resource section for details about this book.

The following is a letter written by one young woman to her aunt, with whom she has been very close throughout her life:

Dearest B.,

There are so many things to say, and at the same time very, very few. I'm not sure whether I'm really ready to send this, but since I love you very much and since you've heard from someone else, I would like you to understand a little more if you don't understand already.

With regards to my relationship with women . . . my strongest role models have always been women. The people who inspire me and make me feel strong and joyful to be alive and proud to be a woman have always been other women. And you can imagine, I have always had several wonderful mother figures around as well as my own wonderful mother and grandmothers and aunts. And I have had some very strong mentor-like relationships with teachers and family friends who are women. I have close male friends, but on an emotional level, my friendships with women have always been most satisfying to me.

I find women beautiful and think that we have an incredible capacity for mutual love and respect. I cared very much for the boys I dated in high school, but the relationships I have had with women have been more fulfilling—emotionally, intellectually, physically, spiritually—than I ever imagined a romantic relationship could be for me. And I do realize that this could have something to do with the level men are at, in terms of emotional maturity at my age (which is why I'm not ruling out any romantic interests with men later on). But for the moment, this is why I am and have been involved with other women. . . . I may end up with a man later on in life, but I very well may not. I most definitely want to have children and a family and love and affection and warmth. These are the things that are most important to me.

. . . I don't believe that sexuality is static. I don't believe that you ever have to know or decide on an identity. I certainly haven't, which is why I haven't spoken with you about it. I don't have a "sexual identity" to present to you. I know that you are concerned for my happiness and my safety, and I believe you would not wish for me anything that would make my life hard. But part of what makes life hard is having to hide from other people or from yourself. I realize that the world at this moment is not particularly open to homosexual people and so if I choose to spend parts of or all of my life with another woman, I may have to be discreet at times to protect myself. But at least I won't be hiding from myself. At least I won't be denying something I suspect about myself but don't accept. This helps me to love myself more. And heaven knows that deep down we all need all the help we can get in that department.

. . . I don't know if it ever crossed your mind that this might be a possibility for me, in terms of a life path, but now it's out there. . . . I do want you to know that I celebrate my life. I am glad to be alive and to be living the way I do. I feel strong and self-respecting, good about honoring my choices and feelings. Unquestionably this is due to the incredible women who have touched my life . . . and I am so proud to be a part of this long tradition of wonderful women.

I love you dearly, and it's important to me to remain close with you.

Be well,   M.

Parents may find assistance and support in special groups and organizations set up around the country for people whose kids are gay. These groups are active in most major cities and many smaller ones. They offer a chance to meet other parents who are wrestling with similar feelings and concerns; they also provide a forum for learning new information about what homosexuality is and isn't. A mother from Oregon reported:

> I think we were mostly worried about our daughter's happiness, about her life. We thought all lesbians were big, fat, mean truck driver types. The Parents of Gays group taught us that homosexual people are as varied and individual as the rest of us, and let me tell you what a difference that made!

Interested parents and friends can contact Parents and Friends of Lesbians and Gays (PFLAG). Look in the phone book for a local chapter. Many of these groups meet regularly and are always open to new members.

Meeting Other Gay People

Gay teenagers need to meet other gay people for friendship and support, but this can be difficult. With the expansion of computer networking, many gay teens are already "plugged into" the Internet, where they can carry on conversations with other gay teens throughout the world. This is helpful, as Brent explained:

> I've met lots of gay teens through Internet Chat Rooms, though most of them don't live anywhere near me. But still, it's nice to be able to talk to people who think like I do.

Robert said he appreciated the Internet because:

> When I first asked myself The Big Question—"What if I'm gay?"—I found that the Net had so many resources for young queer people, it was easier to say to myself, Yes, I'm gay. Yes, I can live a happy life. Now I'm at the point where it's not an issue for me.

The Internet's World Wide Web is an excellent resource for teens who have access to computers with modems. Like a cross between the business pages and an encyclopedia, the Web is full of information on any topic in which you might have an interest. There are dozens of sites for lesbian and gay youth and gay "chat rooms," where people from all over the country (and the world) can "talk" to one another. By doing a search on the Net for "lesbian gay youth" or "queer youth" or "homosexual teenagers" or any number of variations on that, you can find resources and people to chat with. Most teens want real face-to-face contact with other people who think and feel the way they do, however. Friends on the Internet are great, but they may not be enough.

Many teens we interviewed were surprised to find that once they came out, new friends appeared. That's what happened to Brian:

> I met this kid in my school who seemed really insecure. It turned out he was bisexual, and I told him that I had a lot of feelings about guys and that I looked at guys' bodies in the locker room too. He saw that he wasn't the only person having those feelings. It feels good to have an ally now, because our school is a tough place for gays.

Gay teens meet in organizations set up for gays, like gay clubs or gay rap groups. A sixteen-year-old from the Northwest said:

> Since getting involved with the gay teen group at our local Health Center, I've felt a lot less alone.

Sometimes lesbians meet each other through shared political work in the women's movement. Other gay and lesbian teens find friendship in rap groups. Emily, a seventeen-year-old, joined a gay youth group in New York through her sister's college. She said:

> The group was great for me. I met other gay kids, and they weren't outrageous or awful—they were just like the kids at school. It was just like a Y program: we hung out, played sports, talked a lot, had dances. I met my first girlfriend in the group.

An eighteen-year-old girl from the Midwest said:

I remember what an incredible feeling I had when I went to my first rap group meeting at the gay community center. I couldn't believe that there were so many people who had the same kinds of feelings that I had. It was a fantastic relief. Some were like me, and others were very different from me. So I felt I could just be myself and be accepted.

To find a local rap group in your area, try calling a local sexuality hot line or a local social service agency, or if you live near a college or university, try calling the student services department at the school. Check at the end of this chapter for some national numbers that might also be able to lead you to local groups.

Patrick said he could have used a rap group when he was in high school:

All through high school—four years of personal struggles, dealing with extremely homophobic classmates and teachers, parents who were in denial, and a lot of frustration—I kept telling myself, "It will be different when I get to college." I knew from friends that most colleges have strong gay alliances and groups, and that students and teachers tend to be a lot more accepting. So despite depression and family problems, I managed to keep my grades high enough to get a scholarship. And now I'm at college, hundreds of miles from my redneck hometown. And I have a wonderful boyfriend and lots of supportive friends both gay and straight.

Gabriel said:

It's important to be hopeful and to know you have options. Even if you live in a very conservative, close-minded little rural town in the middle of nowhere, that doesn't mean you are condemned to live your whole life in the closet.

Gay bars are one place teens go to meet other gays. Unfortunately, bars are more problematic for teens than clubs or organizations, because of the drinking that goes on there and the fact that so many of the clients are older. You don't know who you are going to meet, and that can be dangerous, especially for someone young and inexperienced. Now that there are more resources available for gay teens and the bar scene is not the only place to find other gay people, many teenagers prefer meeting other gay teens in safer settings, like those we have already mentioned.

Another way gay men have traditionally met each other is through something called cruising. This involves making eye contact with someone—usually a stranger—on the street, or in a park, or at a store or bar that is popular with gay men. People who connect in this way may have a conversation, flirt with each other, go for a walk, go dancing. Many end up having sex. Afterward, they may become friends or never see each other again. Some people make the contact mainly for sex, but for others it is simply a way to meet gay men who might become friends or lovers.

Cruising is, and has always been, very dangerous. You can never know who the people you meet are—whether they are psychopaths, undercover police trying to entrap you, people with AIDS or other contagious diseases, or nice guys just looking for someone else who's gay. Derrick, a seventeen-year-old from Chicago, told us what happened to him:

After I realized that gay men cruised in part of the park near my house, I started going there a lot to get some fresh air and some fun. One evening, this good-looking guy in his twenties started talking to me, and I could see he wanted more. But something about him didn't seem right to me, so I went on my way. Later I heard that undercover cops had arrested nine people in the park that night!

In "entrapment," a policeman who is out of uniform will approach someone and try to get him to do something against the law—this could be talking about going home to have sex, or having sex in a public place, or even making a move that could be interpreted to mean that's what you intend to do. If the gay man does any of these things, he will be arrested. Victims of entrapment are often young. Although many people believe that the police ought to keep out of people's personal affairs and focus on combating violent crimes, many cities still have a vice squad that harasses gay men in this way.

There have been too many news stories about psychopaths and serial killers who pick up and harm young gay teens for *anyone* to feel comfortable hooking up with a stranger in an isolated setting. But above all, homosexual men and boys who pick up strangers are placing themselves at extremely high risk for catching HIV/AIDS, which is epidemic in the gay male community. The more partners you have, the higher your risk. The more partners your partners have had, the more likely it is that they have been infected. Some people you meet may have HIV and not even know it. **Using latex condoms and other safer-sex practices lowers your risk; however, there is no method that affords complete safety from infection if your partner has the virus.** Read both the chapter called Protecting Yourself, which begins on page 279, and the Sexually Transmitted Diseases chapter, beginning on page 253, for more information on this subject.

Female homosexual encounters are generally safer, but lesbians can contract STDs too, including HIV if one of the partners has been bisexual or has used injection drugs, or has had sex with another woman who was bisexual or used injection drugs. Find out as much as you can about ways to protect yourself from catching HIV and other dangerous sexually transmitted diseases by reading Chapter 9.

Remember, people with violence in mind often look and sound like everyone else. People with HIV may not even be aware they are carrying the virus. Whenever you are with someone you don't know very well, you are placing yourself in a potentially dangerous situation.

Homosexual Sex

Most homosexual sex is just like heterosexual sex: kissing, fondling, fooling around with someone you like or love and are attracted to, telling each other what is exciting to you, making love. The section Exploring Sex with Someone Else (page 102) talks about many of these things.

AIDS and Gay Teenaged Males

Most people who have heard about HIV and AIDS know that gay males are at risk for catching HIV/AIDS. Fortunately, using latex condoms and other protective measures can help protect you from getting this life-threatening disease.

Education and prevention programs have taught older gay men the importance of using protection. But one out of every four (25 percent) new HIV infections is reported among teenagers (heterosexual and homosexual teenagers). Even though they may know that HIV is epidemic in the gay community, many gay teens continue to take risks because:

➤ They think that AIDS happens only to other people.

➤ They're too shy to use a condom or don't want to bother to use a condom.

➤ They lack self-confidence and have low self-esteem.

➤ They have the fatalistic attitude that says, "I'm going to get HIV anyway, and nothing I do will make any difference."

If you are a gay male, you *can* help to protect yourself from HIV infection by learning about HIV prevention and by using condoms and other safer-sex practices. We hope you will. (See Chapters 9 and 10.)

People sometimes wonder what it is that homosexuals do. A young lesbian told us, "I thought there'd be something that girls did together that I didn't know about." In fact, there is nothing so different about what girls do together. Sometimes they might lie together and press their bodies against each other, or one might caress the other's clitoris and vagina with her hand or tongue. Some girls like inserting dildos into their partner's vagina or anus; others don't. There are many ways for two women to make love, which they discover together as they explore what makes the other feel good.

Gay men also have many ways of making love. They may caress each other's penis with their hand or mouth. Or one may put his penis in the other's anus. This is called anal sex, and heterosexual couples sometimes do it too.

Anal sex is a high-risk activity for transmitting HIV and other infectious diseases. The lining of the anal canal is delicate and prone to tearing and bleeding, making anal intercourse an easy way for infections to be passed from one person to another. Greg said:

A lot of straight people think every gay guy does every gay sex act, including anal intercourse. That's not true. I've only done it once. What my lover and I do depends on what we're both wanting and feeling at the time.

In a gay relationship it is just as important to know your limits, talk about sex with your partner, learn about safer sex methods and STDs, and take responsibility for your own and your partner's well-being as it is in a straight relationship. See the section beginning on page 107 for a discussion of these issues.

Issues in Homosexual Relationships

Perhaps the single most important element in any kind of relationship is communication: expressing our feelings and needs to our friend or partner, and listening to the feelings and needs of the other person. Having a partner of the same sex doesn't guarantee that the relationship will be better or that communication will be any easier. Just as in heterosexual relationships, problems do arise.

INITIATING: One of the issues many gay and lesbian teens discussed was about initiating: asking a person out, suggesting certain activities, or making the first sexual move. This can be scary, because the other person may say no or, worse yet, reject you for even asking. It can be particularly awkward for girls who have been taught to be responsive, not assertive, as this eighteen-year-old from Boston recalled:

When I met Paula, I knew I liked her, but I had always waited to be asked out. I wasn't used to calling someone up and saying, "Hey, what are you doing Saturday night?" She wasn't either, so we waited around for weeks. Later on, we agreed it was a good thing for both of us to learn that—to learn how to make the first move ourselves.

Making the first move can be difficult for guys too, according to Ben, a nineteen-year-old attending college in the South:

I thought that it would be kind of rough being single and gay. I was scared of it. I thought, Me go into a gay bar? By myself? But when I finally got myself together and got up the courage, I walked into the bar and I saw people I knew. It was easier than I thought, but it's hard for me to pretend I'm comfortable when I'm not. I can look at a guy, but I'm shy when it comes to actually approaching someone and saying, "Hi, how are you? Want to dance?"

Being the one to initiate sex can feel even more risky. A twenty-year-old from Texas recalled her first lesbian relationship:

My lover was really horny. She wanted sex on a daily basis. So for a while I didn't have to say much. But then there would be certain days that I wanted it and she would be taking time off. It was hard at first to flirt with her and let her know that I wanted sex, because I had never done this before. With men, it was always, "Okay, I'll lay here and let him do it to me." It was never something that I really wanted. I must admit I was embarrassed to face up to the fact that I was horny too. The first time that I asked for it was hard. But now sometimes it's even fun—especially when I'm successful.

COMMITMENT: Another issue that comes up a lot in homosexual relationships, as in heterosexual ones, is your commitment to each other. One stereotype is that homosexuals are sex-crazed animals who jump from bed to bed. That's not true. Gay couples enjoy long-term, monogamous relationships just like straight couples. Many raise families together. Now, because of the fear about HIV/AIDS, many more gay people choose to avoid one-night stands and sex with strangers by letting a good friendship develop naturally before becoming sexual with each other.

ROLES: If you become involved in a homosexual relationship, you may find that the main challenge is the same as it is in any kind of relationship: how to become close and intimate with another person while being true to and honest with yourself. Acting out certain roles may interfere with our ability to be our full selves. Women in our society, for example, are told that they should be passive and quiet, pretty and sexy (but not sexual), and wait for things to happen to them. In the most traditional scenario, they are expected to stay home and take care of the house and family. Men, on the other hand, are told to be strong and aggressive, to get a lot of sex but not show too much feeling, to go out and work and make a lot of money to provide for the family. To be successful in the traditional male role, a guy has to be macho and in charge all the time.

In heterosexual relationships, these stereotypes may rob both the woman and the man of half of their personalities, because we all feel mixes of these characteristics inside ourselves. In homosexual relationships, these kinds of roles sometimes get in the way too. Because you both grew up being taught the *same* role, however, usually something has to give, and you both have to learn to become more flexible about who does what, or it won't work. For example, if both of you are sitting around passively waiting for something to happen, nothing will. If both of you are trying to take charge, that will be a problem too.

Sometimes in homosexual relationships, one partner chooses the "male" role and the other partner takes on the "female" role. Annie, an eighteen-year-old from Oregon, told us about her experience:

> When I first came out, my lover was very "butch," as the phrase goes, and I was more feminine. The roles were a kind of traditional male-female. But then I realized that I don't like roles. I like women who are more butch in the sense that they like to hike and do outdoors kinds of things. But although I may dress feminine sometimes, I love to work on cars and mechanical kinds of things. I don't consider myself a butch or femme. I'm versatile. Every woman is. Actually, every person is. It's just that some people pick a role, you know?

To get stuck in a role in either a heterosexual or a homosexual relationship limits us. It is usually a lot more fun for each person in a relationship to be able to express both the masculine and the feminine side of his or her nature.

To play a role because that's what you consciously choose is another matter altogether. As Hannah said:

> I like dressing in men's clothes and slicking my hair back. I look good that way and my partners enjoy it too.

Patricia said:

> When I came out, I started acting more stereotypically for a lesbian. I cut my hair short, wore men's clothes, and acted more assertively. It was empowering, and I feel okay about it. However, most of the gay people I know are the last people you'd ever guess were gay. Girls who are really feminine, wear dresses, and have long hair. And guys who play sports and do all that typical guy stuff.

No matter whether we are attracted to people of our same sex or people of the other sex, all of us want to like and respect ourselves. Healthy self-respect is the foundation of a good relationship, and good relationships can help to nurture our feelings of respect for and pride in ourselves, whether we're gay or straight or bisexual. Stuart, a seventeen-year-old from Wisconsin, put it this way:

> I'm doing really good for myself. I smile a lot more since I've come out. The definition of "gay" is being happy, and they sure picked a perfect word to describe it. Because I do—I feel very happy.

And Ruby, a senior from Ohio, said this about herself:

> I've always been proud that I wasn't embarrassed about being a lesbian. Because people would ask me, "Well, aren't you embarrassed or ashamed about it?" And I would say, "No, I'm not." I always enjoyed being able to open up other people's minds about it. Being different for me was a way of teaching people to respect others and to open their minds.

An eighteen-year-old from Arizona put it very well when he said:

Being gay is so much more than just sex. It's a whole way of being.

RESOURCES

Hot lines

Many local areas have teen hot lines offering information and support for teens' questions about sexuality, STDs, birth control protection, rape, sexual abuse, etc. Look in your local phone book under Teenline or Helpline. Call a local health clinic and ask if they know of a teen-sexuality hot line in your area.

National TEEN HIV/AIDS Hotline, open Fridays and Saturdays from 6 P.M. to 12 midnight (Eastern time): 1-800-440-TEEN (8336)

National HIV/AIDS Hotline: 1-800-342-AIDS (2437)

National Gay and Lesbian Hotline: 1-888-843-4564

Books: General Sexuality

The Black Women's Health Book: Speaking for Ourselves, by Evelyn C. White, ed. Seattle: Seal Press, 1990. A collection of moving personal stories, poems, and essays by black women about their lives. For older teens.

The Hite Report, by Shere Hite. New York: Dell, 1987. Survey of what women really do and feel sexually.

The Hite Report on Male Sexuality, by Shere Hite. New York: Ballantine, 1987. Excellent discussion of men's sexuality.

Let's Talk About Sex, by Sam Gitchel and Lorri Foster. Planned Parenthood of Central California, 255 North Fulton, Suite 106, Fresno, CA 93701 (Phone: 1-209-488-4941). Designed to help open a dialogue between teens and their parents about sexuality.

The New Our Bodies, Ourselves, by the Boston Women's Health Book Collective. New York: Simon & Schuster, latest edition. The section on women's sexuality is very detailed and informative. For teens with advanced reading skills.

The Preteen's First Book About Love, Sex, and AIDS, by Michelle Harrison, M.D. American Psychiatric Press, 1400 K Street NW, 11th Floor, Washington, DC 20005. Written for preteens in language that is easy to understand, a discussion of sexuality, STDs, sexual abuse, and pregnancy.

True Selves, by Mildred L. Brown and Chloe Ann Rounsley. San Francisco: Jossey Bass, 1996. Open and sympathetic discussion of the issue of transgender identification. Nonfiction.

Books: Same Sex Orientation

Am I Blue, by Marion Dane Bauer, ed. New York: HarperCollins, 1994. A collection of short stories about the joys and challenges of growing up gay or lesbian or having gay or lesbian parents or relatives. Fiction.

Annie on My Mind, by Nancy Garden. New York: Farrar, Straus, 1982. The story of two New York high school students who fall in love. Fiction.

Blackbird, by Larry Duplechan. New York: St. Martin's Press, 1986. An African-American teenager's coming-out story about love and healing through the acceptance of his own sexual orientation. Fiction.

The Color Purple, by Alice Walker. New York: Pocket Books, 1982. The Pulitzer Prize–winning novel of African-American women growing up in the South in the early part of this century. Fiction.

Coming Out to Your Parents, by Tom Sauerman for PFLAG (Parents and Friends of Lesbians and Gays). PFLAG Philadelphia, P.O. Box 176, Titusville, NJ, 08560-0176. Send $1.50 for each pamphlet. An excellent pamphlet full of good information and support. Nonfiction.

Free Your Mind: The Book for Gay, Lesbian and Bisexual Youth—And Their Allies, by Ellen Bass and Kate Kaufman. HarperPerennial. Helpful information about coming to terms with being gay. Nonfiction.

Go the Way Your Blood Beats: An Anthology of Lesbian and Gay Fiction by African American Writers, Shawn Stewart Ruff, ed. New York: Owl Books, 1966. Excellent collection of stories. Fiction.

Oranges Are Not the Only Fruit, by Jeanette Winterson. New York: Atlantic Monthly Press, 1985. Story of a girl growing up in a fundamentalist household in the north of England and how she begins to come to terms with the fact that she is lesbian. Both funny and moving. Fiction.

Out with It: Gay and Straight Teens Write About Homosexuality by Youth Communication; Philip Kay, Andrea Estepa, and Al Desetta, eds. 1996. Order from Youth Communication, 144 W. 27th St., Suite 8R, New York, NY 10001 (Phone: 1-212-242-3270). Young people speak in their own voices about the ways they encounter, experience, and deal with homosexuality in themselves, their friends, and their relatives. Very moving; very honest. Nonfiction.

Reflections of a Rock Lobster, by Aaron Fricke. Los Angeles: Alyson Publications, 1981. Autobiography of a boy who took his school to court to gain permission to take a male date to the prom. Nonfiction.

Trying Hard to Hear You, by Sandra Scoppetone. Boston: Alyson, 1974. Award-winning story of a group of friends who learn that two of their friends are gay. Fiction.

Organizations

!OutProud! National Coalition for Gay, Lesbian, and Bisexual Youth. On the Internet: http://www.out-proud.org

Lambda Youth Network. P.O. Box 7911, Culver City, CA 90233. Send $1 for a list of youth newsletters, pen-pal programs, support groups, and other resources.

PFLAG (Parents and Friends of Lesbians and Gays). 11012 14th Street NW #700, Washington, DC 20005 (Phone: 1-202-638-4200).

SEICUS (Sex Information and Education Council of the United States). 130 W. 42nd Street, Suite 2500, New York, NY 10036-7901 (Phone: 1-212-819-9770). Provides information and resources about sexuality.

Emotional Health Care 4

FEELINGS

Feelings influence just about everything we do. They affect our actions and our moods. They help determine how we think about things and whom we pick for friends. It's easy to label our feelings as good or bad and wish we had only the good ones, but having a whole range of feelings is what being human is all about.

Mostly our feelings drift in and out, changing as things happen to us during the day. Sometimes they get very intense and overwhelm us. At those times, it's good to be able to identify our feelings and know how to keep them from getting out of control.

Another word for feelings is "emotions." Emotional health is the ability to recognize and manage our feelings. It's an important part of growing up.

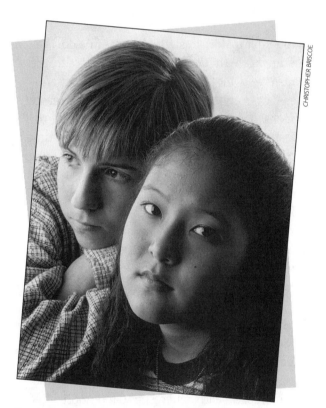

CHRISTOPHER BRISCOE

Identifying Your Feelings

As most of us have come to know, recognizing what we feel isn't always as simple as it sounds. Often we're faced with two or three different emotions all at the same time. Travis put it this way:

The problem is, most of the time I don't *know* how I feel. Am I sad, mad, or what? I feel confused a lot. Like, when my girlfriend dumped me for a guy in college, I felt horrible—empty and alone. But I also felt pissed.

During adolescence so many physical and emotional changes happen, it's hard to incorporate them all smoothly. Wild mood swings and jumbled feelings seem more the norm than the exception. Most of the teens who helped us with this book said they regularly experience two completely opposite emotions simultaneously, like both hating and loving their parents or their friends or themselves, or being both excited and scared when they're going for a job interview or entering a new school or going out for the first time with a person they like.

It's not easy to sort through emotions that are all over the place, but sometimes you feel so much chaos inside that it's important to try. At those times start with four basic emotions: mad, sad, scared, and glad. Take a minute and ask yourself, Am I feeling mad? Am I scared? Do I feel sad about anything? Do I feel glad? If you let yourself be honest, you might be surprised at what you discover. Fifteen-year-old Morgan said:

> A lot of people don't want to admit their feelings, even to themselves, because they're afraid that their problems will scare their friends away. I usually think, well, if they knew I felt that way, they'd think I was weird.

You may share Morgan's worry. A lot of us do. We sometimes have a hard time admitting our feelings, because we want to pretend to others and to ourselves that everything's just fine. Maybe the reason you feel sad is something you don't really want to think about, or the reason you're angry all the time is too painful to remember. But even though you might resist your feelings, it's not weird or sick to have them. It would be weird not to have them.

Having feelings is normal. In fact, it's helpful. Emotions are a little like smoke alarms; they warn you about your needs. If you ignore a smoke alarm, you may get burned. If you don't think clearly about the cause of the alarm, you might overreact or under-react and in the process hurt yourself and others.

Being able to slow down enough to say, I feel angry or sad or scared—and to ask, What's making me feel that way? What do I have to do to help myself feel better?—gives you a chance to see the situation more clearly and respond to it more effectively. Some people say this ability to reflect is like taking a "chill pill"; it's a necessary step toward emotional health.

Feeling Mad

Most of us are experts on what it feels like to be angry. Some people are quick to anger; they have a short fuse. Others are slower to burn, and then they explode. Still others try to bury anger inside themselves and keep it hidden. But one way or another,

---

How to Take a "Chill Pill"

Red Light	1.	Stop, calm down, and think before you act.
Yellow Light	2.	State the problem and how you feel.
	3.	Think of lots of solutions.
	4.	Think ahead to the consequences of each solution.
Green Light	5.	Go ahead and try the best plan.

---

anger has a way of coming out, and whether it erupts in an explosion or seeps out in a miserable attitude, it often causes trouble for us and for everyone around us.

If as a small child you were punished or beaten for expressing anger, you may not have learned any successful ways to manage your angry feelings. If you were shamed or abused, you may have learned to hold your feelings in and hide them. It's time to change that. It's not okay to hold your anger in so tightly that it ends up coming out as a physical illness or bad headaches or nervous twitches or substance abuse or depression or violence. It's not okay to turn anger into self-hatred, as Julie told us she does:

> Even when I was little, I've gone through times of, you know, not liking myself. And I still go through them. I have this bad way of handling it, which is to hit myself. I remember a time when I was with a group of people and I was having this bad feeling and I just kept punching myself on the leg and then I stopped because I didn't realize what I was doing. It was just my instant reaction to how I felt, and right after I did it, I was saying, "Oh my God!" I couldn't believe I'd actually done that in front of people.

Sometimes people feel so full of rage, they strike out at whatever or whoever's nearby. That's not okay either. Fifteen-year-old Lillian said:

> I used to get so mad I'd break things, smash whatever was there. Like I put my hand through the wall because I was so mad at my dad. I threw

a dish at my brother but it hit the window and broke the window. I used to break things a lot, but I don't anymore. I'm trying to learn how to control myself.

There are more effective ways to express anger than by silently simmering or fiercely attacking. The chill pill gives you a moment to ask, What's making me so angry? What's the best way to get my needs met and deal with this situation? It helps you think through what you want to do and consider the consequences of those actions.

Carlos, age sixteen, has been in trouble with the law and is now on probation:

I try and think about what will come next if I do what I'm thinking about doing. I've learned to calm myself down. I've got to watch the way I am and try to train myself not to get real angry, so that while I'm around my son he won't learn to be that way. I want him to see something different, that it's not okay to hurt people or get abusive. I think about the consequences too, you know. I've had enough.

Matt, age fifteen, has this to say:

I'm teaching myself mostly to control my anger. My mom and me are setting up a program so that when I get mad, I'll go and talk to the person I get mad at and say, "Hey, why don't we do this or that instead of getting mad at each other?" Or if I can't do that I go and punch my pillow.

The power of the chill-pill approach is that it stops your angry train of thought because it focuses your attention on how to stop feeling angry. The chill pill won't work if during the chill time you let your brain keep dwelling on what made you angry in the first place. That only triggers more anger. Teaching yourself to react calmly and even positively to a negative situation is one of the most powerful ways to put anger to rest. Fourteen-year-old Leah told us:

Writing helps me deal with my anger. If I write about it, like if I'm angry at someone and I make a list of everything I like about them, it makes the anger lessen a little bit. At first this is really hard to do, but once you remember all the good times you've had together, you don't feel as mad. Once I was in a fight with my mom and I sat down at the computer to write a list of everything I hated about her. The list was really short, so instead I wrote a list of everything I liked about my mom and of our special times together. When I showed her the list of good things, she forgave me a little bit, and we talked about the things we could both change about ourselves and our relationship.

BRUSSELS SPROUTS

*I'm like a tightened fist. Holding
back all my anger. Trying to stay
    closed
and trying not to open and explode
with anger. I can't hold my leaves
closed any longer. I'm exploding.*

*My leaves are opening. I feel like
a rocketship that just took off
for Mars. My outside leaves are green,
but my innerself is yellow with fur.*

*Now that I have been rid of my
anger, I can return to the field
and start all over again.*
                                    —ANONYMOUS

Sixteen-year-old Lucinda, who lives in a residential treatment center, said:

I cry when I'm angry and then I feel tired and go to sleep. When I wake up I almost always feel better.

Armond listens to music:

Rappers really have something to say. And Heavy Metal. I think Heavy Metal gets a lot of good messages across. For me, when I get really mad it feels so good to put it on because I don't even have to do anything. I can just lie there and listen to it, and it's like the other guy takes my anger out from me.

Seventeen-year-old Joey turns to sports:

I play a lot of basketball. For me, when I get angry or mad and I can't take it out, I like to go to a hoop or a soccer field and work out, break a sweat. Playing ball gives my mind a chance to clear and not have negative thoughts filling it up. It helps me to keep the negativity out of my mind.

Fifteen-year-old Serrie practices meditation:

The first step is to let go of your attachment to all the bad things and all the good things you have done or that have been done to you. Breathe it all out on an exhale. Then on an inhale, breathe in a deep pure breath. Any thoughts or feelings that cause you to lose track of that breath, let them pass through your consciousness. Then as you exhale, breathe it all out again.

RUTH BELL

Meditation is an excellent way to stop your mind from racing with angry and negative emotions. Try to find a quiet place to sit and breathe calmly and deeply in and out. Concentrate on your breathing. Let any thoughts that pop into your mind, good or bad, flow out of your body as you exhale. Check the resource section at the end of this chapter for some books to teach you more about meditation.

Another way to chill out is to get out of the situation that's making you angry. Take a walk. Give yourself a "time out," during which you can work on a hobby, read a book, be alone, watch a movie, play music.

For some people it helps to feel empathy for the person who made them mad. They try to figure out what's making the person act that way. They observe rather than participate. Then when they do respond, they have some perspective, and their response is often more effective.

Talking can be a positive response to anger too.

Tell a friend. Tell your counselor or your social worker. Tell your parents. Or speak directly to the person who made you mad in the first place. Bonita said:

I don't get angry much, but if I do I just look at myself in the mirror and say, "Now, why are you angry? This is so dumb. Figure out what's bothering you." Usually I can calm myself down that way and I feel better. But when somebody triggers me off and I get pissed right then and there, I just flat-out tell them. I don't hold it in at all. I just tell them.

Anger gets our adrenaline going, and sometimes we prefer that to slogging through the marsh of emotions that may be underneath. As Angie explained:

I mask my emotions with anger. No matter what I feel I act mad and then I feel tough and safe. I didn't learn what I was really feeling till I'd been in counseling for months. I learned stuff about me that I totally didn't even know by being in counseling. I started to see how sad I was about some stuff that happened in my family, and when I started to deal with that, I didn't act so mad all the time.

Talia, eighteen, was sexually abused for many years. She said:

When somebody makes you mad, at the moment it hurts you just want to grab something and throw it. You feel like you never have enough to throw. I used to smash anything that was around. There are so many things I've been through that if I didn't smash things I'd be crying all the time. But now thanks to this therapy group I'm in, I know more about what's really causing all my feelings. When I'm angry, I can control it more. I say something instead of smashing things. Or I walk away and let it go. That's a big step for me.

If you feel there's nowhere to turn and nothing matters much anyway, even little things can trigger angry outbursts. Felix told us he and his girlfriend used to fight all the time. He said:

> I used to fight with everybody, especially with Sherrie. But now that I got this job at the hospital, I can see that maybe I can have a life. Maybe me and Sherrie can get somewhere. I don't have so much anger in me anymore, and when I feel it coming out, I talk to myself and calm myself down.

Felix told us he almost didn't try for the hospital job, because he didn't think he had a chance of getting it, but one of his uncles talked him into going down for the interview by saying, "You go around looking for a fight, ready to jump anybody who blinks at you the wrong way, so now you can put that power into turning yourself around."

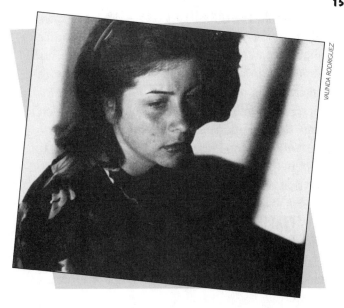

VALINDA RODRIGUEZ

Thoughts that produce anger	Thoughts that reduce anger
"It's not fair."	"Bad things happen."
"It's all your fault."	"I know how you're feeling."
"He (or she) is not treating me right."	"Let's talk about this."
"You let me down."	"Everyone makes mistakes."
"I deserve better than this."	"I forgive you."
"Everything always happens to me."	"I'm having a hard day."

Anger-Intensifying Habits	Cooling-Off Habits
Yelling.	Count to ten.
Sulking.	Sleep on it.
Plotting revenge.	Exercise/sports/walking.
Accusing the other person.	Meditation/relaxation.
Blaming the other person.	Distract yourself with dancing, movies, reading, videos, hobbies.
Escalating the argument. Hitting; violent acts.	Take a twenty- to sixty-minute break from the person you're arguing with.

Feeling Sad

All of us have times when we feel sad—we experience a disappointment, someone lets us down, we hear about a friend who's in trouble, or we feel left out. Teens say they experience the deepest feelings of sadness when something happens that is or seems final, like when a relationship ends, or someone dies, or their parents divorce, or when they have to move or live away from home, or they lose something very special.

Sad feelings are hard to live with. A number of teens said they have developed their own special ways to help themselves through sad times:

PUTTING IT ALL IN PERSPECTIVE—*Sandy (fourteen):* It helps to have something to look forward to. It gives me hope that things can change. Like, right now I'm upset because I'm stuck in middle school and I don't have many friends, so I tell myself, Okay, I've only got two more months at the middle school, then I get to go to high school and maybe it'll be better there. Maybe my life will change in a good way.

LETTING IT OUT WITH A GOOD CRY—*Sheila (fifteen):* Sometimes when I cry, I feel more upset, but it also lets out more of the sad stuff, especially if I get to cry with someone who says it's okay to cry and lets me lean on their shoulder. Then I've cried but I also know I have someone who cares for me, and that comforts me.

FINDING SOMEONE WHO CARES—*Warren (fifteen):*
After my dad moved out, I went steadily downhill for about two months. I just about quit going to school. I ended up drunk or stoned just about every day. And finally one of my teachers caught me and said, "You're not going to make it out of here if you don't start shaping up." And I really wanted to graduate with my class, so I started going back to school. I kept in touch with that teacher too. It really helped me that he cared enough to say something.

SPENDING TIME WITH PEOPLE YOU LIKE—*Kristen (thirteen):* If I'm with my friends, for the time being I can forget my problems. It's kind of like they're my chariot and they're lifting up my emotions that are down.

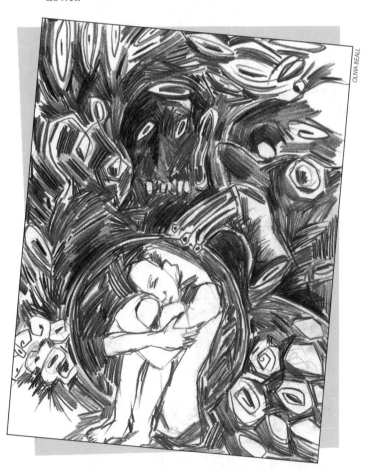

OLIVIA BEALL

Anger is an emotion that tends to give people energy; sadness drains it. When we feel sad, we move more slowly and react less spontaneously. Our heart is not in what we're doing; we may feel like it's breaking. Sometimes just recognizing what's making you feel that way—saying to yourself, "I feel very sad because . . ."—helps ease the pain. Seventeen-year-old Jenny, from California, said:

> When I wrote about my really good friend dying, it helped the hurt go away a little bit. While I was writing, I started remembering things we used to do together and I remembered how much he meant to me and how special our friendship was. It made me sad, but it also gave me something to remember about him. I kept the paper I wrote, and it helps me keep his memory alive.

Bill, a fifteen-year-old from Chicago, also had a friend who died. He said:

> I think you should talk to people when you're sad. Sad is a really heavy thing. Like, one of my best friends died in a car crash, and a bunch of us guys who knew him all got together and we just sat there and cried and talked about him. It was good.

Sixteen-year-old Paulie is missing his son:

> Being a father is hard, very hard when you're my age. I wanted a child and I wanted to start young. I wanted to grow up with my son. But now I'm locked up and I can't be with him. I'm sad about that. And lonely. But I'll get over it by not giving up. That's what I plan to do. I'm never going to give up, no matter where they take me or where they put me. Someday I'm going to be the best father to that little boy. My mother came from Mexico with us, and she used to go to work at 3:30 in the morning. She never gave up. So I figure if she didn't give up after all she went through, then I figure why should I?

Sadness is not usually an emotion that comes or goes quickly. It's one we feel deeply, and one that lasts until we have come to terms with whatever it was that caused the sadness in the first place. Don't expect to bounce right back. Give yourself a chance to feel your sad feelings fully. Try to remember that time and experience do heal most wounds and help people overcome even the most tragic circumstances, like the death or loss of a loved one.

For many teens, breaking up with a boyfriend or girlfriend after a long relationship is one of the most difficult experiences of adolescence. Glenda told us that when she and her boyfriend broke up, she asked herself, How can I ever smile again? Many other teens have felt the same way. Expressing your sadness is a way to begin to heal it. Crying is a good release. Talking to people about it is another. So is writing your feelings down on paper or putting them into music or some other art form. After Pat and his girlfriend broke up, he started drawing:

> Drawing helps me get the feelings out. Like this one is all dark and hopeless-looking. It makes me sad to look at it. But it helped a lot to do it. It helped me get some of that stuff out.

People need a period of time to mourn a loss. But sometimes sadness hangs on longer than is healthy and that's when you can help yourself heal by focusing again on something positive. James, who is unable to walk, said:

> People hurt me all the time. They say things behind my back, they laugh at me, they stare. I get sad and I feel down, just like anyone would, but I say to myself, Think of the future, James. Think about what you want to accomplish. Don't dwell on the negative. Reach for the positive. Because I know I can accomplish something great. And I know that you can't get anywhere by feeling sorry for yourself.

Annemarie has this suggestion for how to deal with sadness:

> When something really bad happens to me and I feel like crying all the time, I whisper to myself, You're a wonderful girl. You're smart and good. You'll feel happy again soon. It's like this chant that I say to myself over and over. And it works.

Feeling Scared

Many teens spoke with us about their fears. Gregory's fear is based on practical experience. He said:

> If you're a fully active gang member and you're out on the street and you got a problem with another gang member, for me, I wouldn't walk up

to them and say, "Let's talk about this," because I would get shot. I'm not trying to be funny. That's just the way it is. Fear is healthy here. It keeps you from getting killed.

Valerie's fear is based on bad memories:

> When I was little my father used to come into my room nearly every night and make me do things to him. It went on for six years, and now I can't go to sleep. I used to know that as soon as I let myself fall asleep, he would come, and the fear of that kept me awake. Even now that I can take care of myself, I'm terrified of what will happen when I fall asleep.

Valerie has become addicted to sleeping medications because of her fear. She is working with a therapist to help get over the effects of her bad memories. (See page 227 for more on sexual abuse and violence.)

Like Valerie and Gregory, many people's everyday experiences cause them fear. They live in violent neighborhoods. They are abused at home. Their parents are addicted to drugs or alcohol and unable to provide security for them. These are common situations, and because of them millions of children and teenagers live in fear all the time. Unrelenting fear like that can cause serious emotional and physical problems—for example, chronic headaches, stomachaches, poor school performance, the inability to concentrate, illness, and nervousness.

The sad fact is that there are no easy answers to eliminating some of the real-life horrors that cause young people to be afraid, but there are people who can help, and there are organizations in nearly every neighborhood that want to help. Please don't keep your fears to yourself. Find some friend or relative or religious leader or community worker to talk with about your situation. Get some of your friends together to try to find new solutions to your problems. Look together at the Chill Pill box, on page 154, for a plan to help you learn to solve problems. As a group, you may be able to make some changes happen (see Changing Things, beginning on page 369). Remember, good changes can happen when people make them happen.

Fears can also be about ordinary things. Many teens say they are afraid of the dark or of being alone or of taking tests or of flying. They may know logically that they'll be all right if they walk into a dark room or fly in a plane, but it still scares them, as Nancy, age twelve, explains:

I'm really afraid to walk outside at night. Even when my mom is standing at the door waiting for me to

take the garbage out, I get so scared I have to run there and back as fast as I can, all the time imagining someone is out there waiting to grab me.

Alison, age fifteen, said:

I stayed at some friends' house one night while my parents and the friends went out and it was a strange house for me, so even though it was summer and really hot I closed all the windows and locked all the doors till they returned. And they were like, Geez, Alison, how can you breathe in here, it's boiling, and I was too embarrassed to tell them I was scared of somebody breaking in.

Thirteen-year-old Sabrina, from Idaho, described her fear:

My entire family loves to go river rafting, and the bigger the rapids the better they like it. I'm the

only one who's terrified to go. For a long time I didn't let anyone know I was scared, and I'd just figure out a way to have something else to do when they wanted to go rafting. One time, though, my mom started talking to me about feeling scared, and she let me know she used to be scared of rafting too, and that helped me finally admit to her how terrified I get just thinking about it. What I'm really scared of is being flipped out and getting caught underneath and drowning. We decided I should start on not such a wild river. My dad said it was smart to have a healthy fear of the river, because it's so powerful, and that it was good to learn what to do in case of an accident. So now I go rafting with my family, and though I still get a little nervous, I also have a blast.

Arnie told us he's afraid of roller coasters:

There's this amusement park in town that all my friends go to, but I hate going there, because then they all try to talk me into going on the Thriller, which scares the sh—t out of me. They're all, Oh, Arnie come on. Don't be a wimp. And maybe I am a wimp. I break out in a cold sweat just going near it.

Lots of teens told us they hate to talk about their fears, because they worry that people will think they're weird. The funny thing is that almost everyone is afraid of something. Teens mentioned being afraid of driving fast, being under water, going to strange places, swimming in the ocean, climbing ladders, being alone, being away from home, making a fool of themselves. Your fears will probably lessen in intensity as you get older and gain more confidence, but for now it's important to remember you're not alone. Talking to a friend or family member about your fears can help. You may find they feel the same way you do.

The whole process of growing up is laced with feelings of inadequacy, insecurity, and fear. It's when your fears and anxieties keep you from doing the things you want to do that it's time to find ways to overcome them. That usually means figuring out some safe way to face your fear and begin to deal with it. Thirteen-year-old Jackson was afraid of talking in front of the class. His fear was so bad that every time he had to present an oral report he would skip school. His English teacher caught up with him one day and told him about a group she was starting for people who hated public speaking. She gave him the choice of failing her class or being part of the group. Jackson joined the group:

We spent a lot of time talking about how we were scared of looking stupid or sounding stupid. We must have spent about three weeks just talking about that. And then we did these exercises, like a minute of reading something from your desk. Then a minute of just talking about something from your desk. Then two minutes of standing up in front of the group and reading something. At the end we had to stand up there for two minutes and talk about a topic. By that time it was so cool, because everybody was rooting for you. It really helped me. I did great.

Sometimes fears get completely out of hand. A *phobia* is an intense fear of an object, an animal, or an experience that is out of proportion to the reality of the situation. For example, people have phobic reactions to small spaces and crowds (claustrophobia), to heights (vertigo), to leaving home (agoraphobia), to riding on airplanes, to dogs, to spiders, to doctors and hospitals, to water, to being lost. Phobias can be about almost anything. They create panicky feelings that don't go away easily, and they usually cause some physical symptoms. When faced with your fear, you may break out in a sweat, your heart may start racing, and you may feel as if you can't breathe. You may develop stomach cramps or headaches. Some people scream or run away or feel paralyzed. Some even pass out.

A number of teens we met try to adjust to their phobias by avoiding certain situations at all costs.

For example, Sid is afraid of dogs. When he sees a dog on the street, he begins to sweat and feel panicky. He may go blocks out of his way to avoid passing it. Thirteen-year-old Nonnie is afraid of swimming. She said:

Every time my friends want to go to the beach, I say, "Oh, I'm busy today." But my father makes me go when we visit my grandma. She lives near this lake, and all my sisters and my brother can't wait to jump in. But I get sick. It happens every time. As soon as we get on the bus, I get dizzy and I get these bad stomach cramps. And by the time we get there, I have to go lie down. Once I even had a fever. It's like I don't know what it is, I'm just really scared of the water.

People with an airplane phobia take trains or buses while the rest of the family flies. People who are afraid of elevators walk up ten flights of stairs to avoid being in one. A woman we know has never been to the dentist because she's so afraid of having her teeth examined.

A lot of people have phobias; having one doesn't mean you are crazy. But phobias interfere with your life. They keep you from doing things you need to do, like going to the dentist, or things you might want to do, like going swimming with your friends. And they don't usually go away by themselves. Find someone to talk to about your fear. Start by speaking with your school counselor or community-center leader or health worker. He or she may be able to direct you to a good mental health facility in your area. A few cities have clinics that deal specifically with helping people overcome phobias.

Some people experience spontaneous panic attacks. During these, your body goes through intense bodily changes; you shake, sweat, feel dizzy or faint; your heart feels like it's beating extra fast or skipping beats; you can't catch your breath. Panic attacks are very frightening experiences. Teens who have been through a panic attack say they felt they were going crazy or that their heart was going to burst and they were going to die.

A person may have one panic attack and then never have another. Some people experience them regularly, like once or twice a month, or several times a week, thus making it difficult to carry on normal activities.

These attacks can't be ignored; your bodily sensations are too extreme for you to pretend nothing's happening. Rikkia explained:

> My sister had a panic attack. Actually, she's had a couple of them. It was like, when it first happened we didn't know what was wrong, because she was walking back and forth in the room, just wringing her hands and crying. She kept looking for my mom, who was at work, and she kept saying, "When's Mommy coming home? I think she's hurt. Go call the police." She said that over and over and wouldn't let it go until I called the police. I felt so stupid. Then she'd start screaming or talking weird. Whenever I'd try to put my arm around her, she'd jump away. It lasted a whole day, but when my mom finally got home, she calmed down.

During the attack, you may be too agitated to find help for yourself. If someone is with you, that person can help by getting you to a mental health facility, where assistance will be available, in the form of both medication and therapy. When you get over the immediate symptoms and feel more in control, make sure you make an appointment to see a professional in the field and explain what you have been experiencing.

Having panic attacks does *not* mean you are crazy. It usually means that you feel threatened by something. Perhaps you are holding on to some deeply felt fear or anger or hurt that needs to be expressed. Perhaps something in your environment triggered a buried fear. Whatever the cause, you can help yourself by watching for the signs of an attack and as soon as you begin to feel them, sitting down, breathing deeply, and practicing one or more of the relaxation techniques listed on page 171. Focus on something positive in the moment. Tell yourself that this will pass.

Feeling Glad

When you're glad, you see the world in a positive way. You give people the benefit of the doubt. You feel lighthearted and generous. Glad is a nice thing

to feel when you can, especially after dealing with other, more difficult emotions. Here's how some people help themselves feel glad:

> *Hilary (fifteen):* I still sleep with teddy bears and I talk to my cat and that makes me really happy, because my cat loves me no matter what. She always accepts me totally and never, ever criticizes me or puts me down.

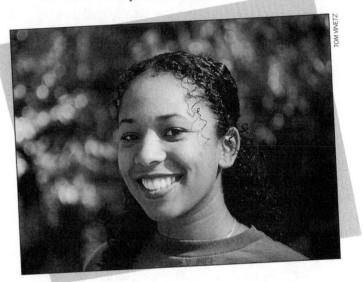

> *Rick (sixteen):* I like to be alone and listen to my favorite music, and that really makes me happy and content.

> *Tessa (eighteen):* I plant things—digging in the dirt, repotting a plant that's outgrown its container, watching the flowers bud in the little pots on the windowsill in my room. My mom told me I always used to love playing in the mud. Well, I guess I still do.

> *Aaron (fourteen):* When I'm walking home alone and stuff, I'll talk to myself in different characters. I'll just make things up and pretend I'm acting it out in front of an audience. It gives me a rush.

Like Aaron, many of the teens we interviewed explained how their lives were made richer by having a creative outlet. Reed, a fifteen-year-old, described it this way:

> I like to write. It puts me in a good mood, and I'm able to understand people better. I don't know,

maybe I just understand human nature because I write about life. It makes me enjoy life. It's fun.

Sierra, who is nineteen, has been playing the piano for years. She told us:

I know myself better, I have more of a sense of harmony with myself because of my music. It calms my mind and helps me formulate my thoughts better. It helps me focus when I'm confused.

When you're feeling glad, your body has a chance to relax, to let down its defenses. You can breathe deeply and feel good about yourself.

When people fall in love, they feel glad. In fact, that's one of the best parts of being in love—you feel glad whenever you're together, at least at the beginning. You can be in love romantically, or you can be in love with a friend or a pet or an older person you admire or a little child you care for. Love doesn't have to be romantic or involve sex to bring happiness.

One of the easiest ways to feel glad is to let yourself appreciate things. If you see a beautiful flower or bird or tree, stop and enjoy it. When you notice someone being kind to someone else or to an animal, let yourself experience the good feeling that's passing between them. If somebody says a friendly word to you and gives you a smile, smile back and show your appreciation. Denny said:

It can be tough when you're a teenager, but it can be great too. You've got to look for the spirit wherever you can find it. Appreciate it. Let it in.

For many teens, a way to feel glad is being close to people they like. Stacey, age sixteen, told us about her friends:

One night one of my friends said that she felt we were all part of the same pineapple. Now we just say "pineapple" if we need some support, and we get it.

Miriam, sixteen, had this insight:

I know lots of girls are molested, but my problem is just the opposite. Since I hit puberty, I don't think anyone in my family has touched me at all. In my family, no one touches each other, and I don't have a boyfriend. I was in this great health class at school and we hugged at the end of the class and it felt so good. So I went home and consciously made myself go into the kitchen and hug my big sister. She stiffened up at first, but I kept hugging her. Now my family does hug some. It's really weird. It's like hugging was a new concept for my family. I had to teach them how to do it.

Ronnie moved when she was in middle school. She feels glad when she keeps in touch with her friends:

I really like to write letters. I think it's because ever since I moved, I felt like there was a piece of me that got taken away. So for three or four years now, I've been writing to anyone who will write me back. Sometimes I even write to people who are in jail, because sometimes I feel so lonely I feel like I'm locked up too. Every time I write to my homies, it feels like I'm home again.

Allen said his dog is a source of happiness for him:

My dog understands me. He waits for me every day, and when he sees me, he just goes nuts. It's like I'm the most important thing in his life. We go for long walks together, just him and me, and I feel like I'm walking with a friend.

HAVING A FOCUS

Focusing on something positive outside yourself almost always makes you feel better. Brendan, sixteen, has devoted a huge amount of time over the past eleven years to his artwork:

I think it's given me something to do. If I hadn't been doing art, I might've gotten into drugs. I probably wouldn't have been able to express myself. It gives me more self-esteem, because I have something that I'm good at. Sometimes it takes me months to finish a sculpture, but when it's done I can look at it and feel really great.

Teenagers who have put time into developing their talents and interests feel gratified to see how much they can improve over time. Rachel, a seventeen-year-old who plays the oboe, began composing music two years ago:

Since I've started taking it seriously, I'm more complex. I don't know why I think it's so beneficial, because it has limited my other interests and it takes up a lot of my time. But my music represents me. How I play and the style I play is really me.

Lyle said:

When I practice my cello, I'm accomplishing something—trying to become an artist, working on a technique. It's my way of expressing myself.

Moto, sixteen, told us:

I used to hang with a gang but I got out. Now I'm in a break-dancing crew, and we're pretty good. We can do some pretty awesome stuff, because we practice all the time. You have to practice that much if you want to be good.

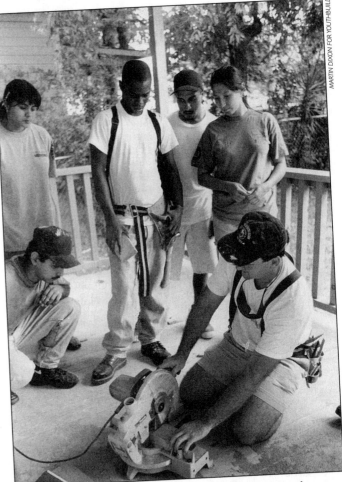

Participants in a YouthBuild program learn to use a circular saw.

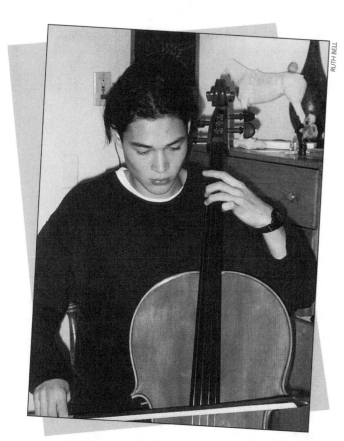

Sports are an important focus for many teens. They experience an emotional high practicing for hours, working together to make a team good and then playing their best at the game. Chelsea, fifteen, said being in sports gives shape to her days:

I guess sports have always been a big part of my life. I usually have two or three sports going on. You meet so many great people. Like this year I'm on varsity, and I've met a lot of older kids that I wouldn't have known if it hadn't been for that. And I've been lucky, because my coaches have always been great.

When I have practice right after school it kind of organizes my life. I know I have to plan, because I need this much time for practice and this much time to do my homework and this much time to eat dinner. And then you have the game to look forward to. It just works out better, because when

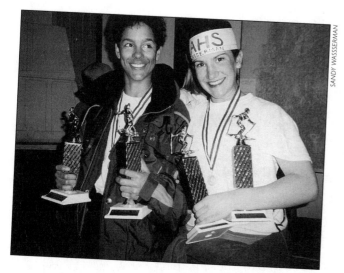

I'm not doing sports I just kind of get more lazy. There's nothing to do, and I feel kind of lost. You don't want to just go home and watch TV. So you hang out and waste time.

Roberto, age seventeen, wrote an essay to describe how important football has been in his life. This piece was excerpted from his essay.

> When I was a little kid, I had a best friend. His father and my father grew up next door to each other in Mexico. Our grandfathers were best friends, and who knows how many generations of our fathers before were best friends. We were just alike: we liked the same things; we played baseball, wrestled, boxed, played basketball, played ninjas and, the favorite sport of both of us, football.
>
> We dreamed kid football dreams, like growing up and playing for the Raiders or the 49ers. Then when he was nine and I was eight, his parents got divorced, and I never saw my friend Jaime again until this football season. I was getting ready for a football game, and he was laying in his casket, the first gang killing in our area.
>
> If I never knew before, I knew on that day what sports have done for me. To begin with, by the time the coaches have made me sweat for two or three hours, I'm too tired to go hang out

on the streets. Even if I had enough energy to go, I knew if I got into anything bad, I'd be off the team. And being on the team, well, that's important.

> Playing football this year was the greatest team experience I've ever had. I've gotten really close to my coaches; someone is always there, someone you can tell anything to.
>
> Our team is close. We had to work hard, and a lot of people thought that our team going to the playoffs was something that happened last year and could never happen again. Our team proved them wrong. Our families and community were always there for us. Where the team went, it seemed the whole town went too. Wherever we went, our town treated us like heroes. When we made a mistake or had a bad game, they told us how proud they were of us for playing so hard. When we were struggling, the cheering crowds pushed us on. We were the team. We were the Eagles.
>
> And once you've been part of the team, a piece of you stays forever. Just like a piece of my friend, Jaime, will stay with me forever. I know what playing on an athletic team has done for me, because I have seen what not playing has done for Jaime. I know all he ever really wanted to do was to play with a team. Only on his team, there was no coach to help him along, no community to make him feel like a hero, no school kids asking for his autograph, and the biggest difference of all, no next year.
>
> —ROBERTO FLETES

"I CAN'T"

Many of us fall into the trap of thinking, I'm not good at anything. We get the "I can't" disease: I'm not athletic, I can't play sports. I'm not artistic, I can't draw. I can't play an instrument. I can't dance. I can't go to college. I can't do math. I can't read so well. Lots of us with the disease don't even want to try, because we think we'll fail or look stupid. We think that if we're not automatically great at something, that means we don't have any talent or skill at all, or it means we're stupid. It's *not* true. Talent or interest in an art or music or a hobby or sport or a subject in school is only a small part of it.

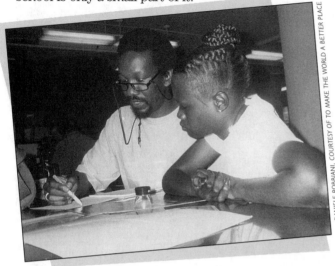

DANIELE ROBBIANI, COURTESY OF TO MAKE THE WORLD A BETTER PLACE

To become good or expert at *anything* takes work and time and patience and commitment. Benjamin rebuilt a race car motor for his senior project in high school. It took him ten months of working on it every weekend and several hours during the week. Elizabeth spent a year perfecting her Spanish enough so she could go to Mexico with her church group to help fix up houses for people that needed a place to live. It took Gretchen six months to learn how to surf well enough to be able to keep up with her boyfriend in the ocean. Zack practiced an hour every day for three years to learn to play the saxophone. Robert is a concert pianist. He practices four hours a day, every day. Lorien is making a special art project. She can only work on it a little each day, and she has already put twelve hours into it. She estimates it will take her another thirty hours to complete. Chelsea, a freshman on the varsity basketball team, practices for three hours every day after school. Lauren, Poppy, and Kirsten decided they wanted to learn how to sew. From buying the material, to redesigning the pattern, to learning to use the sewing machine, they spent nearly four months of weekends making themselves dresses.

Many teens told us their major focus is watching TV or hanging out. Those activities are fine some-

times, but they don't help you feel better about yourself. Setting your mind to a task and keeping at it until you accomplish it is one of the best ways to feel good. Then you can look back and feel proud.

STRESS

Anything that makes your body react is called stress. Stress causes strain on your body, whether it comes from something that happens automatically, like catching yourself when you start to fall down the stairs, or something you're looking forward to, like a big date or a birthday party, or something worrisome, like your parents' divorce or a big test you have to take.

There are *healthy* responses to stress, such as watching your step, breathing deeply, exercising, and taking a minute to relax and examine what's going on to gather some perspective. More commonly, people have *unhealthy* responses to stress, such as migraine headaches, twitches, eating problems, substance abuse, nightmares, chronic illness, concentration problems, or constant worrying.

Too much stress can make you feel exhausted or very nervous. It can make you fly off the handle or have accidents. These are signs that it's time to find a healthier way to manage your stress. Your body is saying, Slow down and assess the situation. Try to lighten your load. Eliminate some of your activities, or find someone to help you.

When Stress Becomes Distress

There is no such thing as life without stress, but often we're under more stress than is good for us. Before you can do anything about it, you have to be able to identify what's causing the problem. Here's a sample of things teens said cause distress in their lives:

PARENTS AND LIVING SITUATIONS: Even though almost all teenagers complain about their parents, many are lucky enough to know that their families will be there to help them when they need it. Not everyone's so lucky, however. Some teens have no adult in their life willing to assume the responsibilities of being the parent. They have to parent themselves. Leonora described her life:

When I was only twelve years old, I used to cook for my brother and sister, and do the laundry, and do everything in the house. My brother and sister could come to me, but I couldn't go to anybody. If I had a pain or anything, I had to keep it to myself. So maybe my father thought I was his wife or something, and whenever he wanted to touch me, he would.

Eighteen-year-old Amanda said:

My friend Paula was living with her mother, who was a drug addict. Paula used to have to come home from school and change her mom and put her to bed. Then her mom died. Talk about stressful.

ARTICHOKE

I build up my protection,
layer after layer
I put sharp points where their
fingers will pluck my pieces off.
Really what I'm hiding most
is my heart.

So tender it is.

Still they eat me.
It must be hard.
I must admit.
Every layer they peel right off.
Ha! Ha!
the outside's too hard!
The teeth scoop out my tender inside
anyway.
So much work for so little food.
Ohhh my h
*   e*
*   a*
*   r*
*   t*
so soft and silky
The prickles didn't stop them.
Nothing can.
Nothing will.
           —DIANE HURLEY

HOMELESSNESS AND POVERTY: Nearly a million children are living in shelters, in welfare hotels, or on the streets on any given night. Jared's family is homeless and moves from shelter to shelter. He said:

I've been in four schools in the last year. I think that's why I'm not really doing so good in my subjects. Just when I start catching on, we have to move.

Lee-Ann, age sixteen, said:

Not having a place to live really stresses you out. I was living on the streets, and every day I had to decide, you know, where I was going to sleep and who I was gonna mooch off of for the rest of my life. Basically, it's just hard. It sucks out there, especially in the winter time. It's freezing.

If you are living on the street or are a runaway, Covenant House maintains a 24-hour telephone hot line called the Nine Line (1-800-999-9999), where runaway youths or their parents can call for help. They offer counseling and places to stay; they can give you the names of resources in your area, and they provide a place where people can contact you.

RELATIONSHIPS: Whenever you care about someone, their moods, their needs, and their actions influence how you feel. Being in a relationship can feel wonderful, but it also causes stress for a lot of teens. Brenda, age fourteen, said:

Dealing with boys is stressful. Like when you have a boyfriend, worrying that he's going to cheat on you. You worry 24–7 about that.

Alex, fourteen, said almost the same thing:

If your girlfriend doesn't call that night or you hear that she doesn't like you anymore, that puts you under major stress. Then you hate going to school, because you know you'll see her there with the new guy she likes.

Paul worries about people finding out he's gay:

I haven't come out formally to anyone yet and I don't know if I can while I'm still in high school. There's so much gay bashing in this school. It would be like saying, I'm here. Beat me up.

SAFER SEX: STDS AND TEEN PREGNANCY: Teens who get involved in sexual relationships say they worry about sexually transmitted disease and pregnancy. Jack said:

I haven't always been really careful, you know what I mean. And I just found out that this girl I know was with this guy who has HIV. She's a basket case. And everybody I know is going in to be tested. Myself included.

Taryn, seventeen, said:

My period's been due for two weeks now and I'm never late. I'll die if I'm pregnant. I'm too young to have a baby.

For teen parents, the stresses can be extreme. Kim, eighteen, said:

Being pregnant and having a child at sixteen was really stressful. I wasn't ready, but I didn't want to have an abortion and I didn't want to give her up for adoption. I figured after I had her I'd be able to go out and do the things I wanted to do, not have to worry about things like where I was going to get the next twenty dollars to buy her diapers. But I do. I'm missing out on being a teenager. I always have to worry about coming home at a certain time to take care of her or I have to worry about people going, "Why do you have to bring your kid along?" because you can't find a

babysitter and you don't always want to stay home. I have to worry about finding someone to watch her for five minutes while I take a shower or walk down to the 7-Eleven to buy a Coke. I can't even go to the bathroom alone anymore—she's always there with me. I can't sleep alone—she cries so much, it's just easier to put her in bed with me. I don't resent her, but I do resent myself for not using protection and not knowing that it could happen to me.

SCHOOL AND PERFORMANCE STRESS: Worrying about getting into college, getting good grades, making the team, winning the scholarship, graduating with your class, finishing your term paper on time, having to repeat a subject, not being able to read well—all these issues cause enormous stress for teenagers. Eighteen-year-old Rachel told us:

I dropped out of school in my junior year, but then my dad and another friend talked me into going back. So I had to get twenty credits in one year to be able to graduate with my class. Fourteen credits is a full schedule, and I had to take twenty to graduate. It was a killer.

And Cory said:

I'm on the basketball team and the soccer team and I run track. But I also need to keep up my grades, because my parents said I can only do one sport if my grades fall. So I'm up till midnight every night doing my homework. It's pretty hard to do it all. Sometimes I just lock myself in my room and cry.

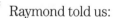

Raymond told us:

My parents go, What is this? Last year you got an A in math and this year you're getting a D. What's wrong with this picture? So they're on me all the time to study and do my homework. I know they really care about my grades, because they want me to go to college, but I feel like I'm under so much pressure. It's like every time I look at my math book I get a headache.

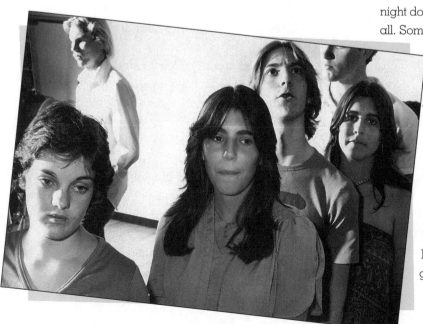

If you have trouble with reading or basic math, get help. Don't label yourself "stupid." You *can* learn to read, and you can learn basic math with proper tutoring. Many teens don't do well in school because they have an undiagnosed learning disability. It's nothing to be ashamed of—in fact, many famous people have recently come forward to say how difficult it was for them to learn in school. If your counselor or teachers can't help you at school, go to your public library and ask for assistance. There are free programs set up in many areas to help people improve their reading and math skills.

Many teens don't do well in school because they have no quiet or safe space to study or do their homework. If this is true for you, explain it to your teacher or talk to the principal. They may be able to find time and space for you to work at school after hours, or they may help you come up with another solution.

PEER PRESSURE: The teenage years are full of the pressure to fit in, to be part of the crowd, and to do what everyone else is doing or thinks is cool. Many teens worry about their appearance, their popularity, their abilities, their clothes. Shala said:

> Clothes make such a big difference. People used to laugh at me because I wore sweatpants to school in the seventh grade. They wouldn't want to stand next to me.

Thirteen-year-old Eric told us:

> It seems like kids feel they need to be in certain cliques and stuff. Like some of my friends were real jerks to me for a while, because they felt they had to avoid me. They didn't think I was cool enough.

Adam talked about the pressure to use drugs:

> A lot of kids in middle school smoke pot regularly, and in our school that's part of what it takes to be popular. If you're not into drugs, you have to really be strong to take the pressure.

For Lucy, the pressure about whether or not to have sex was the most difficult pressure to deal with:

> Guys put a lot of pressure on you to have sex. Especially older guys. When you're going out with an older guy and he wants to have sex, you feel so immature if you don't want to.

MONEY: Having a decent place to live or enough food to eat is a basic need for all teens. Wanting a particularly expensive brand of shoes or a designer-label jacket can make money issues more stressful. It's natural to want to look good, but sometimes the pressure to look a certain way or own the hottest car or the highest-tech bike gets too heavy. Lonnie ended up in a lockup center, because he stole a bicycle from someone in his neighborhood. Paula was arrested for shoplifting a prom dress from the store where her aunt works. Rico said:

> The more you see it advertised, the more you want it. That's the truth. But my mom lost her job, and it's my job that's keeping the lights on. I can't be worrying about what kind of names I'm wearing on my feet.

Consumer pressure can make us forget that simply having enough money to live is a major problem for many teens, like Laurie, who has a baby:

> I just have way too many bills. Like, I'm not even eighteen years old yet, and I have so many bills from just the well-baby checkups, and my part of the rent and the formula and diapers. It's too much.

RACISM: For minority teens, the effects of racism cause daily stress: people have attitudes about you without even knowing you; they discriminate against you; they harass and frighten you in unfamiliar neighborhoods; police stop you just because of your skin color. Racism is a gigantic subject because it is so pervasive in our society. People are different from one another for many reasons, and it's not bad to have differences. What's bad is when people are judged not for their competence or intelligence or kindness or compassion or ability to work hard or for their special, individual talents but simply on the basis of the color of their skin or their ethnic background. Fifteen-year-old Cindy talked about her experience:

I went down to apply for this job at a store near where I live. I was real excited about it, because the pay was pretty good and it was within walking distance. Well, I had the interview, and the guy told me I got the job. It was Wednesday, and he told me to start on Monday. So Monday comes, and I go down to work, and the guy comes to the door and tells me, "Oh, sorry, we hired somebody else." Since I'd lied about my age, I didn't think I could fight it, but I bet the whole thing was that somebody white applied and they'd rather give her the job than a black kid.

Racial discrimination is daunting, and it is no wonder that so many teens who have to face racism daily get disheartened and lose hope of ever being able to change people's prejudices. But there are laws against discrimination, and if you feel you have been discriminated against in terms of a job or housing or education, you may be able to fight it. You will probably need legal assistance. If your family has a lawyer, call him or her. Otherwise try the NAACP or the American Civil Liberties Union, which have branches in every state. Most big cities have chapters. Look in the phone book or call directory assistance.

We discuss some other aspects of prejudice in the chapter Living with Violence, beginning on page 209. In addition, please look in the Resource section of this chapter, on page 181, for books and films on the subject and the names of some organizations working to combat racism.

PREJUDICE AGAINST TEENS: Sometimes just because you are a teenager, people don't take you as seriously as they would an older person. Or they may treat you with disrespect that you don't deserve. Lee said he's had that experience too many times:

It's like every time I go in a store, the clerk's eyeing me as if I'm some suspicious criminal. And then when I need some help finding what I want, it's like everybody else gets waited on before me. And forget going in a restaurant. They might as well just hang up a sign saying Teenagers Are Not Welcome Here.

Poppy said:

I hate it when people say, Oh you're just acting that way because you're a teenager. It's like they don't give us any respect for being a human being with feelings. They make you feel like your feelings aren't worth anything. You're just put in this category: Teenager.

MAKING MISTAKES: As a teen, you face new situations continually, and you need as much understanding, guidance, and encouragement as you can get. That's especially true when you make mistakes, as everybody does. If you don't get the support you need, the stress can be severe. Eighteen-year-old Maria told us:

My mother is always bad-mouthing me. I can't ever do anything right, as far as she's concerned. It makes me feel like I'm a failure.

Sixteen-year-old Diana is really hard on herself when she makes mistakes:

Sometimes you just get to the point where you say, I hate myself. How could I have done that? How stupid! Or you say, I'll never be able to do anything right.

Kenny, a fifteen-year-old from Wyoming, told us:

My father's really good at fixing things. So when we're working together, he expects me to be as good as he is. Well, that isn't right. I don't know as much as he does about it. He calls me a dummy and it makes me feel like I am a dummy.

Some minority teens feel they bear a particular burden. Here's how Kendra put it:

The stakes are higher for minority teens. If you make the mistake of getting in trouble with the law or getting a bad reputation at school or dropping out of high school, you're finished. There's a lot less room for failure in a minority kid's life. White kids may get a second chance or even a third chance if they make a mistake, but minority kids, we get branded. You have to develop a stronger shell to deal with that. It's like you have to be perfect.

Stress Management

As everyone knows, many people turn to drugs and alcohol for relief from stress. Some teens say their parents are so strung-out that they can't get it together to be parents at all. And we heard from many teens who themselves abuse drugs and alcohol and have trouble keeping their lives and their responsibilities together. Janine said:

> My release was alcohol. When I was drunk, reality went away, and I didn't seem to have any feelings at all. I was slipping into a deep depression, sleeping all day long, only going out at night. You can lose touch completely with who you are. I know because that's what happened to me.

In the long run, drug or alcohol abuse is much harder on your body and your emotions than learning to deal with the everyday demands of your life. (See page 195 for more on substance abuse.)

Some people use food as a way of coping, but this too ends up creating more stress than it alleviates. (See page 185 for more on this topic.)

Since unrelieved tension can create serious health problems, it's important to learn some positive, healthy techniques for handling stress. Here are a few suggestions. Pick the strategies that fit your situation best. Or perhaps the following paragraphs will give you some ideas for inventing your own techniques.

PHYSICAL ACTIVITY: Running, dancing, basketball, aerobics, and other sports can help relieve the tension caused by stress. Many community centers and schools offer these activities. Taking a walk in the park or out in nature helps too. So does jogging. Just running up and down a flight of stairs can work off tension. Try yoga, t'ai chi, or some other form of body movement or self-defense. Physical activity is good for your body and your mind. Fifteen-year-old Tammy said:

> I try and run about five miles a day at least. It's impossible to think about anything but what you're doing, and it takes a lot of pressure off your mind.

Alvin said he likes to skateboard:

> You're free when you're skating. Your mind's on it. You're there; you're not anywhere else.

FOCUSING ON THE MOMENT: If you are someone who panics, when you feel a panic attack coming on, look around and focus on the immediate moment. Name what you see, out loud if you're alone, or quietly, to yourself, if you are with people. No one has to know you're doing it. Name everything you can see in the room: "I see the desks, I see the teacher, I see my friend David, I see the window." Do this until you've calmed down. Say to yourself, "This is the present. This is now. I'm okay now."

CLEANSING BREATHS: Take a huge breath in. Hold it for three to four seconds. Then let it out v-e-r-y s-l-o-w-l-y. As you blow out, blow out all the tension. Do it two more times. Then try deep belly breathing for a while, placing your hands on your stomach and feeling them go up and down as you breathe.

RELAXING POSTURES: Sit anywhere. Relax your shoulders so that they are comfortably loose. Allow

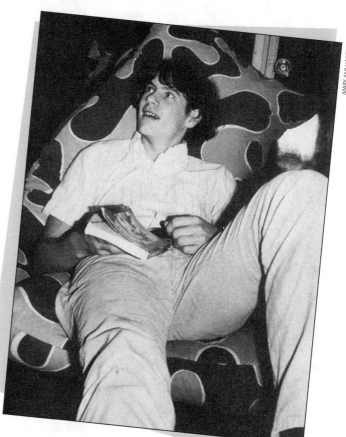

MARY ANN VIATJEN

your arms to drop by your sides. Rest your hands on top of your thighs. Extend your legs and allow your feet to fall gently outward. Relax your toes. Let your mouth drop. Close your eyes and breathe deeply for a minute or two.

MUSCLE TENSE, MUSCLE RELEASE: This takes about fifteen minutes. Lie down on a bed or the floor. Beginning with your toes, tense the muscles in your feet. Then in your legs, your thighs, your pelvic area. Then tense your stomach muscles, your chest muscles, your shoulders and neck. Tense your arms. Set your jaw. Hold the tension for a second or two, and then begin to let go. Start with your jaw. Let it drop. Then relax your neck and shoulders. Keep letting go and relaxing all your muscles till you get back down to your toes. When you are totally relaxed, take a deep breath and let it out all the way. Then breathe deeply and keep that relaxed position for as long as you can.

A variation on this exercise is to tense and then release each part separately, moving down from your neck to your toes. Some people use this technique to fall asleep.

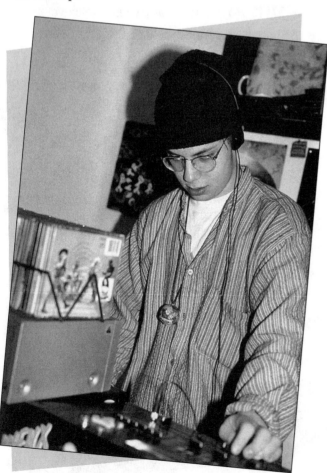

JESSE EPSTEIN

MEDITATION: Meditation helps you let negative, fearful, worrisome thoughts go. Through meditation, you can learn to let your mind rest. Check the resource list at the back of this chapter, page 181, for books that can help you learn to meditate.

DOING SOMETHING ENJOYABLE: Write poems, stories, letters, journal entries. Read a good book or magazine. Play music or listen to music. Sing; act; draw. Build something. Design clothes. Paint. See a funny movie. Get into the computer. Surf the Internet.

Jason is in middle school. He said:

> I zone into the Nintendo. I isolate myself, because I'd just rather be by myself. I do my own thing, and that helps me cope.

Alice writes poetry:

> I write a lot of poems and save them. Months later I go back and think, "Oh my God, when did I write this?" Or I try to remember what was happening at that moment that made me write that. It shows me that feelings pass. Things change.

TAKING CARE OF YOURSELF: Get enough sleep and eat healthy food. Too many teenagers skip meals or eat only junk food. Stay away from too much sugar, caffeine, and salt. Sometimes these chemicals cause stress. Eat fresh vegetables and fruits whenever you can.

TALKING TO OTHERS: Talk to people about your thoughts and feelings. Hug a friend.

WATER THERAPY: Take a hot bath or a hot or cold shower. Put your bare feet in a tub of warm water. Swim.

LAUGHING.

DOING SOMETHING TO CHANGE THE PROBLEM: Whatever is causing your stress can be addressed and changed, at least in part. First step: Identify the problem or problems. Next step: Come up with as many solutions as you can think of and then analyze

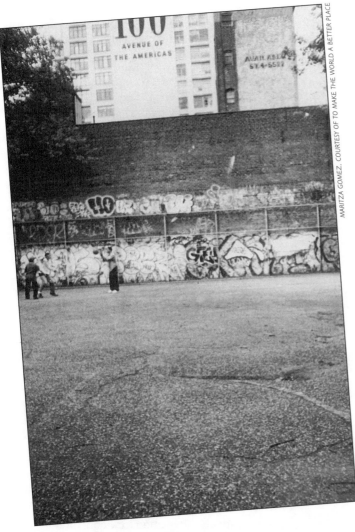

MARITZA GOMEZ. COURTESY OF TO MAKE THE WORLD A BETTER PLACE

each one. Ask yourself what the consequences are of doing one thing or another. Third step: Make a plan that helps change just one element of the situation. Don't try to do too much at once—just one thing at a time. Get friends to help you.

DEPRESSION

There are times when we just *can't* shake off our negative emotions and thoughts, when we feel we've made some terrible mistake, or when things happen that upset our lives completely. We feel so unhappy we can't imagine ever being happy again. Such moods usually last a day or two or even a week, and then we snap out of them.

Sometimes we don't snap back so easily. Our attempts to have fun or distract ourselves—to go to a movie, play sports, exercise, read, draw, talk with

friends—don't work. Sixteen-year-old Mai felt that way. She had been keeping a journal every day. She said:

> I just couldn't write anymore. My feelings were beyond writing. I couldn't even explain how I felt. I just stopped writing completely. It got pointless after a while. If I wrote down how I felt that day, it would take the whole book.

When negative feelings turn into hopelessness and when that hopelessness continues for weeks or months, we are experiencing depression. Trinity explained:

> When I'm feeling depressed, I go home and I just lie there. It feels like I've entered a black hole and am being buried alive. I don't do anything or say anything. I just lie there and stare at the ceiling.

Henry said:

> You feel like everything's crashing down on you. Everything's happening to you. Everyone else has fine lives. Everything bad only happens to you. You're the unlucky one. You can't hide from it. There's no escape.

If depression lasts so long that you lose interest in the people and things around you, that is cause for concern and a signal that you need some support. These are the signs to watch for:

Signs of Depression

A change in eating and sleeping habits.

A loss of interest in friends or hobbies.

Suddenly not caring for pets or prized possessions.

A sudden change in school grades.

Complaints of unusual stress.

Withdrawal.

A lack of interest in appearance.

Feeling hopeless or full of self-hate.

Feeling numb, uninterested, listless.

Loss of energy.

Talk or thoughts about death and dying.

DESPERATE TIMES

I'm a blighted flower.
A parrot too old to talk.
An unfinished meal.
An overfed deer.
A childhood without toys.
A boat with no sea to be sailing away.
A tamed lion.
A castrated rabbit.
A curtain that never flings open to bare
the stage.
A boring fairy tale.
A housewife with a Women's Lib T-shirt.
A child's garbaged picture.
All the neatly nailed butterflies in the
museum under the dusty glass.
A scary dream.
An expired fire of someone's heart.

I'm all I dislike.
I'm all there is in the world to hate.
I'm a leftover and a left-out.
So what a cruel irony it takes
To try to comfort me in my everyday
grief,
To soothe me, to make peace with me
And then, as a rule, to leave me.
—ANONYMOUS

If you can relate to any items on this list, find someone to talk to about your feelings—a friend, a parent, a teacher, a counselor at school, a religious leader, or a professional therapist. Call one of the hot lines listed in the Resources section beginning on page 181 or your local teen hot line. Telling someone else how bad you feel is healthy. It can be the first step toward getting out of depression.

If you're like most people, however, you want everyone to think you're just fine. Or perhaps you feel so depressed you don't want to lay it on anyone else. Or you may not know how to explain how you feel, or you don't think anyone would understand even if you could explain it. More people than you may realize walk around acting as though they're just fine when really they're in terrible pain. Sometimes, in order to open a person up, a friend has to ask "What's going on? You seem down." If you notice one or more of the signs of depression in someone you know, let that person know you care.

Counseling or Therapy

Teens told us that when they were depressed, talking with a counselor helped them. Zeke, a tenth-grader from Michigan, was getting drunk and falling asleep in class, but no one seemed to notice or care. One day he wrote this poem in class:

I'm not a big stoner
You must agree
But can't someone help me?
I don't like what I see.

I've only gone from beer to pot to
speed,
But can't you do something?
Help me. Please

I showed the poem to my health teacher and I remember she just looked at me and said really nicely, "Why don't you go talk to your counselor? She'll help you." When I got to the counselor's office, I just put the poem down on her desk and burst out crying. I must have cried for about forty-five minutes straight. I couldn't stop. I had never cried for *me* as long as I could remember. But I just sat there and cried my eyes out.

The counselor invited Zeke to join a group of other teens who were going through hard times. Zeke said hearing other people talk about their problems made it easier for him to talk about his. It was the beginning of a change, and over the next few months Zeke began to feel better.

Some teenagers say that counselors at school have such a huge work load they don't seem to have time for the students. But most counselors go into that profession because they want to help people. Give your school counselor a chance. Or find an understanding teacher, the principal, a school nurse, or a career counselor. In every school there is at least one adult who cares and will take the time to talk with you; in some schools, there are many.

You may have community resources too, such as a teen club leader, a pastor or priest or rabbi, a social worker, a health professional, an understanding relative or friend. Of course, nonprofessionals may not be equipped to deal with the seriousness of deep depression, so you may want to ask them to help you find professional therapy. (See page 179.)

Spiritual and Religious Help

Millions of people find great comfort in religion. When they are depressed, they turn to their faith in a higher being to help them get through it. Their blessing comes in the form of the strength they receive in feeling they are no longer alone. Organized places of worship offer teens a place and a path to renew their faith. Mikala is sixteen and is living in a shelter for teens:

> It's amazing how I got all the way down. I got raped. I got into prostitution. I got into drugs. I felt about as low as a person can feel. But God has helped me tremendously. Every single person in this shelter is lacking something. They don't have peace in their lives; they have no hope, the way that their heads are always down. It's sad. And I used to be just like that. But I've changed my total life around by finding spiritual healing. By finding God.

For many teens, spiritual practices such as meditation or yoga, or a deep connection with nature, offer the peace and solace they seek. On page 182 you may find some resources to help you with your search. An enormous number of books have been written on spiritual healing. Check at your local library or bookstore.

Helping Others

Teenagers from all over the country told us how helping others provides them with a way out of their own unhappy feelings. They spend time volunteering—at old-age homes, where people are lonely and eager to see a young face; in day care facilities or nursery schools, where the children look up to teenage helpers; at local animal shel-

ters or veterinarians' offices, where animals respond so lovingly to a caring person's attention. Some teens are involved in political work, helping to get laws passed that will make a difference for the environment, for animals, for children, and for human rights. Most towns have some important issue that could benefit from your help. See Chapter 12, Changing Things, beginning on page 369, for more on this.

A young woman who helps bake bread for homeless people in her town in the Northwest said, "When I hand out warm, fresh-baked bread to people, I feel good. It's really gratifying. At the end of the day, you're like, *'Yes!!'*" And another teen who does the same work says he comes back feeling all "God-blessed."

Antidepressant Medications

If you are seeing a therapist for depression, he or she may suggest using medication to get you over a diffi-

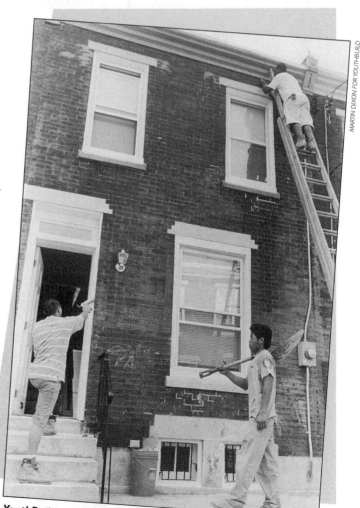

MARTIN DIXON FOR YOUTHBUILD

YouthBuild participants work on fixing up a house.

cult time. These drugs, called antidepressants, can help. They don't work exactly the same way for everyone, so before you take any, ask the therapist to tell you about how the drug works and its possible side effects.

Antidepressants may solve the problem and help you feel better for a while. Sometimes if one type of drug doesn't work for you, another type will work, so under the doctor's direction you may have to try more than one. When there are complex underlying causes of your depressed feelings, you will probably also benefit from therapy, a support group, or a change of lifestyle.

SUICIDE

Many of us have thought at one time or another, I wish I were dead. Usually we only mean we want relief. We want the situation that's causing our pain to disappear. Beth, a fifteen-year-old from the Northeast, said:

Sometimes you just get to the point where you don't really care how anyone else feels. You just want to get the hell out. You just want to escape. You feel the world is so cruel. When I felt that way, I didn't think about other people. I just thought about how much I wanted to get out, to get out of living. It's such a big pain in the ass. You feel like there's no other way out except death.

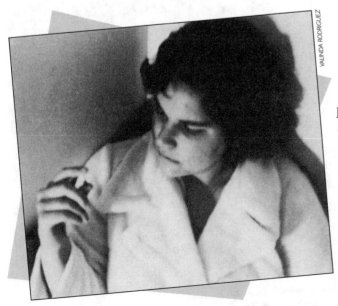

VAUNDA RODRIGUEZ

Death is final. It doesn't offer you the chance to change your mind. It doesn't give you the time you need to move past the pain into the next part of your life.

There are many reasons why some people contemplate suicide. A friendship will end, a relationship will break up, and thoughts of suicide come to mind. Donnie, a sixteen-year-old, told us his experience:

When Sandy told me she wanted to break up, I thought there was no point in going on. I loved her so much. I wanted to spend the rest of my life with her. So I started thinking about killing myself. I imagined how I could do it and what kind of note I'd leave my parents. Then I started thinking about my parents and my little sister, and I thought of them at the funeral crying and being so sad, and I knew I couldn't go through with it. I realized I didn't really want to die; I just wanted everything to be okay again. My best friend Skip helped me a lot. He listened to me talk about Sandy and how much I missed her, and he told me about how he felt when he split up with his girlfriend. And really after a while I noticed that I was actually feeling better. It took a couple of months, but now I'm beginning to feel like life's worth it again.

I would tell other kids who think about killing themselves that even though everything seems really messed up and you hate yourself and your life, there's always hope. Find someone to talk to. Find a friend who you can trust, or just find anyone who'll listen. It's amazing how much better you'll feel after a while. I would even say that going down that low gives you a better spirit for life when you come back up again.

For other teens, when a situation seems hopeless—when they flunk out of school, or don't make a team, or get thrown out of their house, or lose something precious—they fantasize about a place without that pain or shame, and death may come to mind. But remember, death is not a fantasy. Death is a stark reality.

Feelings pass. Even very intense negative feelings pass eventually, and when we make it through those intense times, we reach the other side feeling stronger and renewed.

Roger, a teen from Iowa, came out to his parents. He told them he was gay, and they had a huge fight about it. Roger said:

> I went near the bridge and I was going to jump off. God must have helped me. He told me, a voice told me, to call up my best friend, Dan. It was about 12:30 at night, but he came running over and said, "Roger, don't!" I stayed over at his house with his family, and I didn't go home for about a week.

Roger did a very wise thing: he called up his friend even though it was the middle of the night. He gave himself the chance to get help, the chance to reconsider his momentary desire to kill himself.

When Kenisha was feeling that she wanted to kill herself, she called the teen hot line in her city, where teenagers staff the phones to speak with the teens who call in for help. They talked with her about how she was feeling, and by the end of the call, Kenisha said she felt a lot stronger, a lot more in control of herself.

Ginger *had* attempted to kill herself, by cutting her wrists, but it didn't work. She was feeling pretty depressed until she listened to what one of her friends told her:

> This guy I know at school spotted my wrists at the beginning of class and said, "Don't ever do that again." And just before we left, he said to me, "Take good care of yourself." And that's what started me, right there. I said to myself, "He's right, man. You're all you've got. You may not be the most beautiful chick in the world, but you don't need that." So when that one boy said that, bingo, it just shot to my head. Yeah. That's what you gotta do. You gotta take care of yourself.

The stresses of adolescence are enough by themselves to push some teenagers into depression and thoughts of suicide. Teens who are being abused or neglected, or have been abused or neglected in the past, and those overwhelmed by poverty, discrimination, and prejudice may feel even more fragile. Also at risk are gay teens who fear coming out to family and friends or who are rejected by family and friends when they do come out.

If you yourself are a person seriously contemplating suicide, please remember: death is permanent, feelings pass. Listen to Victor, a seventeen-year-old teen, who said:

DON'T COMMIT SUICIDE. There're always ways to make your life better. Every single person in this world is supposed to be here for a reason, and even if you think it won't matter if you kill yourself, it *will* matter, and if you think nobody will care, you're wrong, because everybody is a person and everybody matters.

You deserve love and help. If you are feeling depressed or defeated, it's really important to seek out a caring adult you can trust, someone who can help you find counseling and, if necessary, help you make changes in your life. If you can't think of whom to call, pick up the phone and dial a local hot line geared to helping teens deal with problems. Try calling the Nine Line (1-800-999-9999). Or look for a local teen hot line in the phone book under Helpline, or Teenline, or Crisis Intervention services. Some areas have suicide-prevention hot lines, listed in the white pages under suicide. See page 181 for a listing of national hot line numbers.

GETTING HELP—TAKING CHARGE OF YOUR LIFE

You may need more help than this book, or any book, can give you, but it's important to begin looking for help now. What follows is one step-by-step approach to getting help:

Talking Things Over with a Parent or Relative

Aaron (fifteen): I have an uncle I get along with pretty well. He dropped out of school when he was sixteen, and he used to get in all kinds of trouble and stuff, and now he's totally enlightened. I can talk to him about almost anything. He's really cool.

Stefan (sixteen): I really like my mom a lot, and I can usually talk to her about stuff that I need to talk about. She has told me that she wants me to be careful. She never says I can't do something, she just says to be careful. Because I think she realizes that I'm growing up and I'm going to have different experiences, and so the only thing she really asks of me is that I be safe and maybe talk to her about it. And I think about that a lot. Would I tell her something that was really intimate or secret, something I might be really embarrassed about? Because she's trusted me that far, I feel like maybe I should trust her back. If she's willing to put out that much, maybe I should too.

Talking Things Over with Friends

If you can't talk to your parents or siblings, talk things over with a friend or a group of friends.

Beth (fifteen): My friends are my support system. My friends and I care about each other differently than I do with my parents. It's like having a different kind of family that can elevate you out of loneliness.

Rain (sixteen): You know how some women have their women's group and some men have a men's group, well we [teens] have our friends' group. To our parents we may just be hanging out at the mall or wasting our time helping a friend with a problem, but for us it's a time when we can talk about what's going on in our lives with people we can talk to instead of our parents or other adults. Sometime kids need to talk to kids rather than other adults because we're living it and adults aren't. Sometimes adults forget what it was like to be a teenager and they forget how hard it was.

Talking Things Over with Someone Outside Your Family and Circle of Friends

This may be a school counselor, teacher, religious leader, youth director, coach, club leader, social worker, houseparent—anyone who will listen to you and whose good sense you trust. These people are used to others approaching them for help, and they often have a different perspective from yours. They may be able to see something about your situation that you can't see because you're too close to it.

Patsy, a sixteen-year-old from Chicago, uses a wheelchair:

> The reason I can feel so open about my feelings is thanks to the teachers here at this school. They've been like a second family to me. They're always there when I have a problem, and they'll talk to me. Maybe it's lucky to be disabled to be able to have teachers like that. They're always there for you. They'll talk about anything with you.

Sasha, who lives in a group home, turns to her houseparent when she needs help:

> She doesn't hold grudges, and she doesn't take sides. You can cry on her shoulder when you need to, but if you just want to talk she's a good listener, a good adviser.

Getting Professional Help

Get professional help if you experience drug or alcohol abuse, sexual or physical abuse, suicide attempts, pregnancy, eating disorders, domestic violence, or severe depression or unresolved grief. Peter, a high school sophomore from Maryland, said:

> I never used to talk about my problems. I had to feel terrible before I'd talk to anyone. Two years ago I tried to kill myself. I was in this hospital for two weeks, and when I got out, they put me in outpatient therapy. That's where I met my therapist, and that's when I started talking.

Professional helpers are called counselors, social workers, psychologists, psychiatrists, and therapists. They provide counseling and therapy, usually for a fee. You or your family may have medical insurance that covers the cost of therapy, or you may have a medical card to cover therapy services at county mental health agencies. Some therapists have a sliding fee scale and charge you according to your ability to pay. Some therapists may see you free of charge as a way to contribute to the community. If you decide to see a professional therapist, discuss the fee and how you will pay for it. Some teens told us they get after-school jobs to help pay the cost.

In addition to individual counseling, many teens are also involved in family therapy, where members of their family or their family of friends, come to

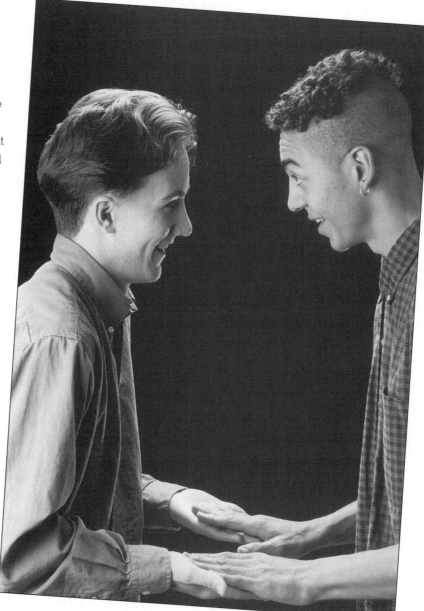

CHRISTOPHER BRISCOE

some of their therapy sessions. Other teens are part of peer groups or support groups composed of many people who have had similar experiences. Laurie-Jo was sexually abused as a child and young teen. She now attends a support group at her local community center:

> When I'm upset or think about suicide because I don't know where to go or who to turn to, I come to this group, because I found help here. People who understand, instead of judging me, people who have been there too and know that it's not your fault.

A therapist should:

➤ Treat you with respect and honesty

➤ Believe she or he can be helpful to you

➤ Be someone in whom you can develop trust

➤ Follow your lead in deciding what issues to talk about, but also nudge you to talk about the harder issues

➤ Encourage you to get to the place where you no longer need therapy

➤ Keep what you say confidential or explain the exceptions

Michael agreed:

> I've gotten a lot of help in this group. I don't think about killing myself anymore. And even though I still get depressed and my life is a mess, it's better. I think about my problems now and I ask myself, Why do I feel sad? What's happening in my life to make me feel this way? It's a process. It takes time. But it's definitely getting better.

You're Not Alone

Getting help may mean looking at yourself differently and exploring your thoughts and feelings more

deeply than you ever have before. Fourteen-year-old Wendy has been seeing a counselor for six months:

> You can change your life by changing your attitudes, by working on listening to others and not getting defensive, but you have to want to do it, and it isn't easy. Unless you want to make certain changes, your life will stay the same no matter how much people try to help you. You have to take the initiative and start trying to change your life. Maybe you're afraid people won't listen to you or believe you, so you think, What's the use of asking for help? But you've got to try anyway. It's okay to be afraid of change, but don't let your fear stop you from changing. You have to overcome your fear to change.

Sixteen-year-old Devon said:

> It was time to change when I realized I wasn't going to get the things I wanted unless I changed. It was hard to accept the help offered, because I didn't want to leave my family and live in a group home. Then after a while I got used to it and knew it was best for me to leave my family. My family was part of the problem.

Fifteen-year-old Courtney said:

> Me and my mom have a lot of problems we've been working on. I had to move out of my house because of the problems, and we've been going to counseling for a year and I'm just now being able to move back with her. We have communication problems; she does not understand me. Sometimes counseling has been helpful, but not all the time. I have counseling twice a week with my mom and once by myself. I feel sad about my relationship with my mom. It helps to talk about it.

Jason, an eighteen-year-old New Englander, gave us his reason for seeking therapy:

> They don't have a lot of preconceived opinions. They remember the things you say, and since they're objective, they can put it all together and just make it clearer. Talking to someone outside

yourself helps. It brings you down to earth. It shows you you're not alone.

The most important thing to remember about difficult emotional situations is that you don't have to deal with them by yourself. Locked inside your own troubled space, it may feel as if there's no one who cares and no one who notices. But that isn't the case. There are lots of people ready to help you. By reaching out, you can find them.

RESOURCES

Where to Call for Help

Help is available for teenagers. Help is also available for teenagers who have run away from home and feel lost and alone. Reach out by calling one or more of these numbers.

Childhelp I.O.F. National Child Abuse Hotline. 1-800-4-A-CHILD (1-800-422-4453). Crisis intervention, information, and referrals for abused kids, rape, pregnancy, gay and lesbian issues, youth services, and counseling.

STD Hotline, Center for Disease Control, Atlanta, Georgia. 1-800-227-8922. 8:00 A.M.–11:00 P.M. Eastern time, Monday through Friday. Sexually transmitted disease information only.

Covenant House (The Nine Line). 1-800-999-9999. Headquartered in New York City, this is a religious social service agency that offers shelter and services for homeless teenagers in New York City, Houston, Fort Lauderdale, Toronto, New Orleans, Los Angeles, and Anchorage. Covenant House also maintains a telephone hot line where runaway kids from all over the country or their parents can call for counseling or to leave a message.

Children of the Night Shelter. 1-800-551-1300. Established in 1979 in Los Angeles, this shelter helps children and teens who are forced into prostitution or pornography and those living on

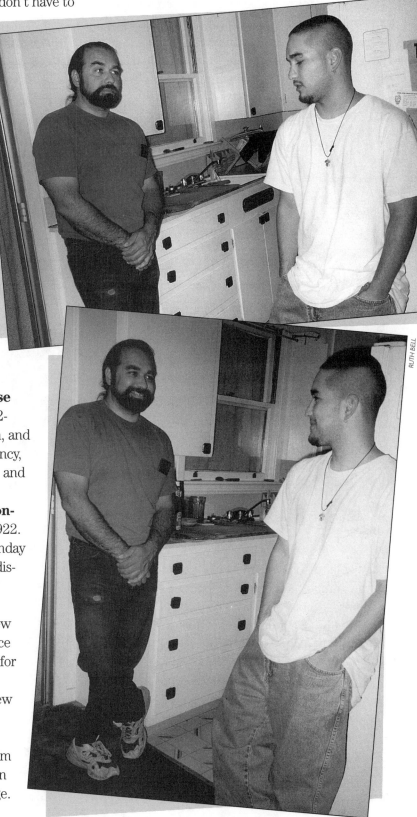

the street. There are twenty-four beds, skilled counselors, food, clothing, and emergency medical care. Call them if you are in trouble and out on the street in the Los Angeles area. If you are not in Los Angeles, they may be able to give you a referral to a shelter near you.

National Runaway Switchboard. 1-800-621-4000. TDD Line for hearing-impaired teens: 1-800-621-0391. This is mainly a service for runaways. They

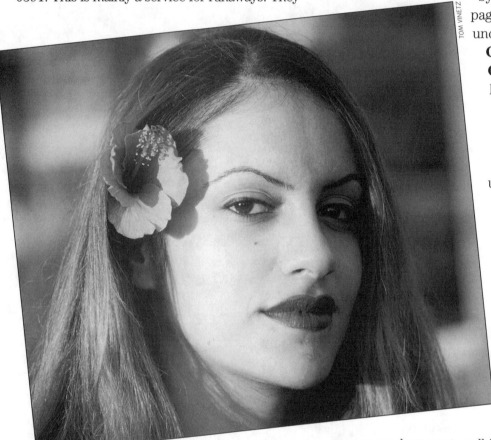

TOM VINETZ

will be able to help you find a place to stay. It's a toll-free number. You don't pay for the call. They won't hassle you.

Local Hot Lines. Check the white pages of your local phone book under one of these headings: Teenline, Helpline, Talkline, Crisis Hotline, Crisis Intervention Services, Suicide Prevention. Sometimes the name will be specific to your area, so call the police station or a teen center or community center if you have trouble finding a hot line.

If you live in a small town that has no hot line, try the phone book of the largest city in your area. You can get that phone book at the library.

County Department of Public Social Services. This number will be listed in the phone book under the name of your county. There are many services listed, so if you have a specific problem—such as child abuse, alcoholism, or drug abuse—look under those headings.

Teen Clinics. If there is a teen clinic in your area, it may provide counseling services. Call or stop by. Look in the classified pages of the phone book under Clinics.

County Mental Health Clinics. Most local mental health centers will offer teen services. Look in the classified pages under Clinics or Health Services or in the white pages under your county services.

Local Police. Your police department may provide special services to help teenagers. Call them. You don't have to give your name if you don't want to.

Churches, Temples. Your church or temple may have a youth director on staff. He or she would be a very good person to call for help.

Local Radio Stations. Stations that broadcast mainly to teenagers often have lists of teen services. If there is a talk show that deals with teen problems, that would be the best number to call. You don't have to be on the air. When you call, tell them you don't want to be on the air, you want some help.

Doctors. If you have a family doctor, he or she may be able to help you or refer you to someone who will be able to help you.

Recommended Reading

Acts of Faith: Daily Meditations for People of Color, by Iyanla Vanzant. New York: Fireside, 1993.

A thoughtful work that explores the special pressures on people of color in our society and offers insight and spiritual teaching.

Betsey Brown, by Ntozake Shange. New York: St. Martin's Press, 1985. A young black girl comes of age in a middle-class black family amidst racism and changing American values. Fiction.

The Black Women's Health Book: Speaking for Ourselves, by Evelyn C. White, ed. Seattle: Seal Press, 1990. A collection of moving personal stories, poems, and essays by black women about their lives.

Catcher in the Rye, by J. D. Salinger. New York: Bantam Books, 1964. A classic, funny, and poignant story of an adolescent boy as he searches for his identity. Fiction.

Chicken Soup for the Teenage Soul: 101 Stories of Life, Love, and Learning, by Jack Canfield, Mark Victor Hansen, and Kimberly Kirberger. Deerfield Beach, FL: Health Communications, 1993.

Confessions of a Teenage Baboon and **I Never Loved Your Mind,** by Paul Zindel. Both books: New York: Bantam, 1978. Humorous stories of teenage life. Fiction.

The Courage to Heal: A Guide for Women Survivors of Child Sexual Abuse, by Ellen Bass and Laura Davis. New York: Harper & Row, 1988. The best book we know on the subject of sexual abuse.

The Courage to Heal Workbook: For Women and Men Survivors of Child Sexual Abuse, by Laura Davis. New York: HarperCollins, 1990. Also excellent, a book to guide you through the process of healing.

Finding Our Way: The Teen Girls' Survival Guide, by Allison Abner and Linda Villarosa. New York: HarperPerennial. For young women of all ethnic backgrounds, first-person stories designed to be an inspiration to girls who are trying to come to terms with themselves and their world.

Forgiveness, by Sidney and Suzanne Simon. New York: Warner, 1990. A self-help book about how to make peace with the bad experiences you've had and get on with your life.

The Heart Knows Something Different: Teenage Voices from the Foster Care System, by Youth Communication, Al Desetta, ed. New York: Persea Books, 1996. $16.95 from Youth Communication, 144 West 27th St., Suite 8R, New York, NY 10001. 1-212-242-3270.

How to Meditate, by Lawrence LeShan. New York: Bantam Books, 1990. This book has helped many people learn to meditate.

I Know Why the Caged Bird Sings, by Maya Angelou. New York: Bantam Books, 1971. Maya Angelou, the famous American poet, writes a personal story about the coming of age of a young black woman in the South.

Listen Up: Voices from the Next Feminist Generation, Barbara Findlen, ed. Seattle: Seal Press, 1995. A collection of stories and ideas from many different women.

I Never Promised You a Rose Garden, by Hannah Green. New York: Signet, 1964. A sixteen-year-old girl's frightening experience with mental illness and the psychiatrist who helps her through it.

The Other Side of the Mountain, by E. G. Valens. New York: Warner Books, 1977. A young female athlete's heroic adjustment to a crippling accident.

Parrot in the Oven: mi vida, by Victor Martinez. New York: Joanna Cotler Books, an imprint of HarperCollins Publishers, 1996. The story of a young Mexican-American boy growing up with an alcoholic father. His sensitivity and desire to make something of his life help him to see beyond the violence and depression around him.

Push, by Sapphire. New York: Random House, 1997. Condensed from a review by Wunika Hicks in Foster Care Youth United: "Precious is strong. Although her mother is a lazy nothing and her father is simply a waste of skin, she struggles to make it—but not without a lot of obstacles. . . . I saw my life story being told in this novel. . . . Precious suffers and is hurt in every way possible, yet something inside makes her *push* her way forward. *Push* is an inspiration for those who think it's impossible to make it." Fiction.

The Relaxation and Stress Reduction Workbook, by Martha Davis, Elizabeth Eshelman, and Matthew McKay. Oakland, CA: New Harbinger, 1988. Simple, concise, step-by-step directions for progressive relaxation, meditation, coping-skills training, exercise, breathing.

Reviving Ophelia: Saving the Selves of Adolescent Girls, by Mary Pipher. New York: Ballantine, 1994. Written by a therapist, this book points out how girls' self-image declines during adolescence. Full of stories from the girls who were interviewed.

Taking Charge: Teenagers Talk About Life and Physical Disabilities, by Kay H. Kriegsman, Elinor L. Zaslow, and Jennifer D'Zmura-Rechsteiner. Bethesda, MD: Woodbine House, 1992.

Victims No Longer: Men Recovering from Incest and Other Sexual Child Abuse, by Mike Lew. New York: Harper & Row, 1988.

Wherever You Go, There You Are: Mindfulness Meditation in Everyday Life, by Jon Kabat-Zinn. New York: Hyperion, 1995. A practical, sympathetic approach to learning meditation.

The White Boy Shuffle, by Paul Beatty. Boston: Houghton Mifflin, 1996. The irreverent story of an African-American boy growing up in white America and the tribulations and successes of his life. Fiction.

Eating Disorders 5

Everyone needs food to stay alive, but most of us don't eat just to stay alive. We eat because we feel hungry; because our friends are snacking and we want to join them; because mealtimes help to organize our days and give us something to look forward to; and most of all, we eat because food tastes good. Many of us reward ourselves with a favorite taste treat after a job well done or after we've gone through something really difficult.

For some of us, eating—or trying not to eat—becomes an addiction. Regardless of what we weigh, we put ourselves on restrictive diets, check the scale many times a day, work out obsessively, count calories in our heads, or keep strict food journals in which we write down every bite of what we have to eat. Sonia is five foot seven. She said:

Maintaining and even losing weight was where I directed all my energies during my senior year in high school. I skipped breakfast every day, and lunch became a 100-calorie, fat-free yogurt. Dinner was a baked potato. I would snack on fat-free chocolate pops, vegetables, and fruit. Sometimes I would eat a piece of bread. I counted every calorie that went into my mouth, trying to stay under 700 calories a day. I weighed myself every day, usually more than once. By Christmas I was 125 pounds. "Not good enough," I thought.

We may go to the opposite extreme too, and overeat regularly and then feel guilty. Seventeen-year-old Luke considers himself very overweight. He is on a strict diet. He takes diet pills and fasts one day a week. He hardly lets himself eat anything. In the last three months, he has lost twenty pounds, but he's not satisfied and wants to lose twenty more. Sometimes, however, he can't stand not eating; he can't stand caring about his weight so much, so he gorges himself on food. He might eat a whole birthday cake and a quart of ice cream by himself when he allows himself to give in to the urge to binge. Afterward, he goes to the bathroom and vomits. That way he feels he isn't really hurting his diet.

Sonia and Luke have eating disorders. They are not alone. Millions of teenagers and adults suffer from similar conditions. Food, body image, and weight are the main and sometimes the only focus in their lives.

People don't always realize how dangerous eating disorders can be since most of us grow up hearing about family members and friends who are trying to lose weight or gain weight and we don't think much about it. But eating disorders can take over a person's life. They can last anywhere from a few months to a lifetime. They can ruin relationships with friends and family, take time away from other activities, limit future choices, cause depression and other psychological problems, and in time, ruin your physical health, even to the point of death.

Compulsive dieting mainly affects girls and women who truly believe they can't be attractive unless they are thin. Males who suffer from eating disorders are obsessed with how their bodies look too, though their goal is usually different. They also talk about their horror of being fat, but rather than just being thin, for many boys the idea is to be buff—muscular and strong. Some boys put themselves through hours of strenuous weight training and daily exercise. Some are on rigid diets. Some use steroids to help them achieve the body they want. Garth, a counselor working with males who have eating disorders, said:

> A lot of high school boys use anabolic steroids to tone up their body image. I've seen it at our school. It's not even that these guys are in sports or anything, they're just taking steroids to build up their muscles, to be buff.

Elsa told us this story:

> I was watching this talk show, and they had some guys from a football team who all had HIV because they had been shooting up steroids, all using the same needle.

Brian said:

> I was always "the fat kid." Then in ninth grade I began weight training. I still looked fat, but it was a little better. It wasn't until I was playing football in college that I started taking steroids. The fat was really still there, but with the steroids and the weight training it was getting tighter. I loved all the attention I got while I was on steroids. I never had to worry about looking fat.

When our primary goal is to slim down and look fit, it's easy to think the way Brian does and use diet drugs, steroids, and laxatives in the hopes of getting the body we want. Some people use cigarettes and amphetamines to curb their appetite. All these substances create emotional and physical dependence and they endanger our health. Steroids can cause severe mood swings, psychotic breakdown,

hormonal imbalances, weakening of the joints, osteoporosis, and liver cancer. Diet pills and amphetamines cause nervousness and irritability, heart irregularities, high blood pressure, anxiety, insomnia, and convulsions—and even death if taken in large amounts. Laxatives, too, have health risks if taken in large doses or too frequently. And we all know how dangerous cigarettes can be. But in the minds of people whose lives center around becoming and staying thin, the immediate results of taking the drugs outweigh their potential dangers.

Appearance means a lot to most of us. Almost all the teens we met put themselves down for not being attractive "enough." They examine every square inch of their bodies and dwell on how they don't measure up to some unrealistic standard. In the process, they disregard their own beauty and uniqueness. Who says you're not beautiful just the way you are? Who sets the standards anyway?

In movies, in magazines, and on TV, we see one version of what's attractive: thin and flawless. Models are thin and flawless. Movie stars are thin and flawless. TV personalities are thin and flawless. The "beautiful people" are thin and flawless. And if they're not thin and flawless, they're trying like mad to become that way with grueling exercise routines, starvation diets, and plastic surgery.

Our poor self-image bolsters the industries that sell us billions of dollars worth of "self-improvement" paraphernalia like diet books, diet drugs, exercise equipment, body toners, clothes designed to hide or enhance our figures, and low-calorie foods. Their ads feature bone-thin models to show us what we could look like too if only we used their products. What they don't tell us is that many of those models are addicted to diet drugs and suffer from obsessive exercise disorders, self-starvation, and depression.

TYPES OF EATING DISORDERS

There are three specific types of eating disorders: compulsive overeating, which can lead to obesity; anorexia nervosa, a form of self-starvation; and bulimia nervosa, the practice of binge eating and purging. People frequently experience a combination of two or more disorders at the same time. For example, they may go on an eating binge until they can't stand it anymore, then fast or exercise compulsively or purge themselves with laxatives or force themselves to vomit. Julie said:

> I would eat and eat for months. Really months of just stuffing myself with whatever I wanted. Then one day I'd just become fed up with myself. I'd feel sick and bloated. So I'd stop and go back to eating what I call more normally for myself. A couple of months later, I'd be back overeating again, and it would be this circle of eating and eating, then stopping. And eating and eating, then stopping. A lot of it was fueled by this anxiety that would just take hold of me. I would eat and eat to try to get away from it, but it would always come back.

Why do teens with eating disorders spend their days obsessed with what they are going to eat or what they are not going to eat? Some teens use eating—or not eating—as a way to take some control of their lives. Because eating and mealtimes are important rituals in so many families, these teens binge in secret, eating everything they crave, or starve themselves to the point of emaciation as a way of saying, You can't tell me what to do anymore. I'm in charge here.

Many young people with eating disorders say that being thin is an important value in their families. Taysha, who at sixteen can't remember a time when she wasn't on a diet, told us:

> My mom is tiny, but she's always talking about how fat she is. And my dad has a heart attack if I eat an extra piece of bread. It's like, Taysha, don't you know bread makes you fat? I'm not as skinny as they are, but I wouldn't call myself fat. But they make me feel like I'm a blimp. Sometimes I feel like I should just become a blimp and see what they do then.

Other teens told us that their families always comment on how they look. "Putting on a little weight are we?" Sam said, mimicking his uncle. Kyra said her family doesn't ever eat dessert or use butter because her parents are so afraid of getting fat. She

and her brothers all stash candy in their rooms so they can binge in secret at night.

Many teens who suffer from compulsive dieting say they love the attention they get from being thin. While in many cultures being thin is equated with not getting enough to eat or being sick, in our society if someone says we're thin, we take it as a compliment. Sarah, who's eighteen, said she never received any praise from her parents until she began losing weight and working out. Being thin gave her a sense of being worthwhile. Her parents showed her respect, and her friends admired her. Ellie, who at ninety-eight pounds has carried her dieting to an extreme, said she loves the way people look at her when she goes anywhere, so she tries to keep her food intake down under 800 calories a day, which is near-starvation level. Paul told us this story:

> My friend was going through a really hard time. Her parents were getting a divorce and her boyfriend was breaking up with her. And she couldn't eat. It was like she just couldn't get food down. So pretty soon she was losing all this weight. And after about two months she looked like those pictures of concentration camp victims—all skin and bones. But here are these girls in our class coming up to her and saying, "Oh Gina, you look sooooo great." It was completely sick.

One study found that 61 percent of the patients in a Florida clinic for eating disorders reported having been sexually abused before the age of nineteen. When our bodies have been so badly mistreated in a way that is completely out of our control, we may go to great lengths to try to take some control back. We may hide in obesity, hoping no one will find us attractive, or we may starve ourselves and lose so much weight that all sexual characteristics disappear as we become skinny and shapeless. (See page 227 for more on sexual abuse.)

Laurel was sexually abused for thirteen years. She blocked those memories for a long time, but when she began to remember the abuse, and the terror she had felt because of it, she turned to food for comfort. She said it helped soothe her pain and her anger:

At an early age I learned that my body was not my own. Anyone could touch it. My self-worth was so low and my anxiety level was so high; food was the one thing I could use to stop feeling so anxious all the time. So I ate and ate and I got really fat. So fat that nobody wanted to touch me anymore. And I guess that's how I wanted it.

Lots of us use food to help us cope with difficult feelings. For the moment, the good taste in our mouth soothes our pain and blocks out our fears. As Brin said, "I can stuff down a lot of anger with a good hot fudge sundae." But food is only a temporary comfort. After consuming a big box of cookies, a bag of potato chips, two turkey sandwiches, and a half gallon of ice cream, the fullness sets in, and so does the self-disgust that can cause serious depression and, in some cases, lead to thoughts of suicide. That's what Hannah remembers:

I was lying on my bed after a binge. All I could think of was how fat I was and that I just wished I could cut it all off my body. But I couldn't. I was stuck with it. I could feel the food bloating my stomach, and I knew it would be another five pounds at least. That's when I felt like I would give anything to just go to sleep and not wake up. I wanted it to all be over.

It's not surprising that many people with eating disorders are chronically depressed. It's a negative spiral: feeling bad, eating to feel better, and then feeling bad that you ate so much. Teena said she was in that negative spiral for many of her teen years:

What finally helped me get out of the negativity was realizing that everyone has a choice. Sometimes it takes hitting the floor more than once to decide to make the choice to go for help. It did me. I was almost at the point of suicide when I said, Wait a second. This is my *life*. I only have one life, and I can make it as good as I want it to be. I was so hung up on feeling unlucky, because I wasn't what you'd call classically beautiful or thin, that I was willing to throw my life away. As soon as I realized that and started seeing a counselor, my hope came back. Of course it's always a struggle,

but now it's my struggle to keep loving myself, not my struggle to keep from eating.

Amanda said she didn't eat more when she felt bad; she would *stop* eating to make herself feel better.

For me the pleasure came in impressing people with my thinness. It gave me my confidence back, since every one admires you when you're thin. I lived on that admiration and sucked it in, the way other people suck ice cream sodas from a straw.

For Amanda, denying herself food did, of course, lead to weight loss. But it also led to low self-esteem, and constant fear—the fear that if she ever did go off her diet she wouldn't be able to stop eating.

Compulsive Overeating and Obesity

Obesity (oh-*bee*-sih-tee) is being so overweight that your physical health is endangered. It can cause shortness of breath, decreased mobility, and joint pains. Obesity leads to high blood pressure, osteoarthritis, heart disease, gall bladder disease, and diabetes. Most teens we met didn't worry about illnesses they didn't yet have. Yet you should be aware that compulsive overeating puts a tremendous physical strain on your body, a strain that will eventually take a serious toll on your health.

Because fat is considered a negative in our society, obesity causes emotional stress as well. If we weigh more than we think we should, we call ourselves dumpy or ugly and we think everyone else is calling us the same names or worse. The truth is, sometimes they are. Overweight people are often blamed for their "lack of willpower" or "unwillingness" to diet. Obese teenagers are usually the last ones picked for teams, they are rarely accepted into the "popular" crowd, and they are regularly the subject of jokes and cruel remarks. Raymond described his childhood:

I was always fat, fat, fat. Never skinny! Kids tormented me constantly. I loved to swim, but I wouldn't because I was too fat and embarrassed that I had boobs like a girl. To try to cover it up I'd wear two shirts and layer my clothes so people wouldn't see how fat I was.

If you are very overweight, you might feel better weighing less than you do now, and it might be easier on your body. But trying to be thin is self-defeating for many of us who are genetically prone to putting on fat. Although all her life she had thought of herself as overweight, seventeen-year-old Lila starved herself over the summer so she would be thin when she started college:

That first month at school I fooled everyone, myself included. No one suspected that I had ever been heavy. There were three women who I hung around with all the time at first. One of them insisted that I must be one of those naturally thin girls who can eat whatever they want. I always told her that she was completely wrong. Yet I began to convince myself that maybe I *could* eat and not gain weight. This was my method for allowing myself to eat junk food—pizza, chips, cookies, etc.—along with drinking alcohol. When I started to see weight gain, I tried to stop eating, but I was totally out of control. I couldn't stop myself. I became miserable, but kept on eating because that is a very social thing to do at college. By winter break I was devastated. I swore I would take off all my excess weight during the six-week break, but I couldn't. I just kept stuffing my face. Then when I went back to school I just kept putting on more weight until I had gained thirty pounds by the time I finished my freshman year.

All bodies turn some food into energy and store fat in fat cells for times of sickness or stress. To a large extent, how our bodies do this has to do with the amount of exercise we get, the type of food we eat, and our metabolism. It also has to do with the type of body we are born with—big, small, lanky, round, wiry. We are all different, and it's absurd for us to think we should all be skinny. Some of us are just not built that way. No matter what body type we have, however, continuous, compulsive overeating or repeated binge eating will lead to weight gain, especially because overeaters usually do not binge on carrots and apples. Most crave pizza, french fries, ice cream, cookies, and other high-fat foods.

A number of teens we met say they are lucky; they have role models of proud women and men who are comfortable with themselves, adults who like the way they look and are not obsessed with being thin. Linette, a sixteen-year-old from Los Angeles, said that among her family and friends, skinny is not considered sexy. "I don't really get this thin thing," she told us. "My boyfriend likes hips, and I've got hips." She laughed as she said, "I don't want to starve myself. I like food too much!" Tawnie is also sixteen. She agreed:

I spent most of my life living down the name "skinny legs." Why would I want to go on a diet just when I'm starting to get a shape?

But for the teenagers and young adults who have bought into the American obsession with weight, who really believe that they can't be attractive unless they are very slim, being naturally big can feel disheartening. Nadine said:

My mother was constantly obsessing about her *own* weight. I used to see her trying on her clothes and crying about how fat she was if they didn't fit just right. I never understood this, because my mother was, and still is, skinny as a rail. Why this created a problem for me was because I was shorter than my mother but I weighed more than she did. How could I not feel fat when I weighed more than my mother did by the time I was nine years old! If she thought she was fat, obviously I had to be obese.

Anthony told us:

When I was in middle school, I would worry every night before bed, wondering if I would have to take a shower in gym class the next day because I was so overweight. I began dieting after failing the physical exam that you had to take to play football in eighth grade. My mother actually put me on a grapefruit diet, and I lost twenty-five pounds.

Suzanna, too, thinks of herself as obese. She told us:

I can still remember years ago when a guy in my math class told me that wearing leggings was a privilege, not a right. He thought he was being so clever, making fun of my legs. But those words just stuck to me. I didn't get mad at him, I got mad at myself and felt I just had to get thinner, make my legs thinner.

Suzanna's reaction is not at all uncommon. When others are being cruel, many of us are quick to blame ourselves for their reactions. As Suzanna said, "If I had thin legs he never would have made that comment." When she got older she told us she wished she had been able to turn her anger on her tormentor instead of on herself and say, "What's your problem? Don't you like strong women?"

The goal is to be able to love our bodies because they work and are healthy, not because they're skinny.

Anorexia Nervosa

Anorexia nervosa (an-nor-*ex*-ee-a ner-*voh*-sah) is a deceptive illness, because many teens start off thinking they'd just like to lose a few pounds. They have an idea of the body they'd like to have, and they go for it by dieting and/or exercising. Laura said:

You fit into smaller-size clothes and you get more attention from friends, from your family. You feel like you look beautiful, and you find that boys are interested in you. It's exciting. It's a real rush—knowing that you are the thinnest person in a room.

The rush Laura describes is the lure that hooks many teens into the "thin is better" attitude. But the truth is, most of the time compulsive dieters end up feeling low, not high. They have low energy, low sex drive, low self-esteem, and low emotional moods. Fearful that inactivity will lead to their gaining weight, many of them exercise compulsively too, which drains even more energy. They may take diet pills to keep themselves from feeling hungry, but they never feel thin enough. No matter how much they lose, girls and boys who spend all their time being obsessive about weight tend to have one focus only: how to get even thinner. Their dieting gets extreme and becomes a form of self-starvation, which eventually leads to severe illness and sometimes death.

Teens who have little or no self-confidence, who may not have received much praise or attention from their parents, sometimes find comfort in the "specialness" of being thinner than everyone else. Amanda, now in her thirties, suffered with anorexia in her teens and twenties. She said:

My need to impress was enormous, my need for praise insatiable. I spent all my life looking for praise and appreciation and never getting it, so I was obsessed with other people's opinions of me. And I was so lacking in identity, the only thing I felt I knew how to be was thin. To be thin and remain thin was my goal in life, because I didn't think I was capable of achieving any other goals.

Leanne, nineteen, said:

My father is totally egotistical. He never wants to know about me, about how I'm doing or feeling. And he's never satisfied with me except when I'm conforming to his expectations. I guess you could say he's very controlling. So it was pretty easy for me to give up after a while and not even try to be anything except pretty and thin. All I had to do was stop eating and I could get all the attention I wanted.

Anorexia nervosa depletes your body of the nutrients it needs. Every living thing is made up of cells, and for the cells of your body to function normally, they need a constant supply of vital nutrients: vitamins, minerals, protein, carbohydrates, and fats. Protein helps repair and maintain tissues, especially muscle tissue. Carbohydrates provide the energy cells need to work. Fats absorb vitamins and are essential to the structure of all our bodily organs. When we eat a variety of healthy foods, we get all these nutrients and our bodies thrive. When we don't eat enough, or eat only junk food, our cells begin to deteriorate.

Bodies are designed to keep nutrients in reserve—for times when we're sick, for example—but those reserves don't last very long. If it doesn't get enough healthy food, the body begins to break down its own tissues to stay alive. You begin to feel tired and run-down. Your muscles deteriorate. You may experience irregular heart rhythms (arrhythmias) and even heart attack. Protein is pulled from hair and nails, making them brittle, dull, and easily broken. Your hair may fall out. Without a normal store of carbohydrates, your temperature control is off and you feel cold all the time. Your skin dulls, dries, and becomes flaky. Minerals are leached from your bones, which become weak and susceptible to fractures. You may become anemic from low supplies of iron.

Your hormones may suffer too. In young girls, that often means a delayed onset of menstruation. If a girl has already started her menstrual cycle, it may simply stop (amenorrhea). People have these symptoms during famines. Anorexia nervosa is a self-imposed famine. You are starving your own body.

Since being thin is the only thing that matters to them, eventually anorexic teens begin to lose interest in school, hobbies, family, and friends. They spend their time obsessing about their weight and trying to make do on as little food as possible. Alicia wrote to us about her long bout with anorexia. Because she felt becoming thinner and thinner meant she was getting better and better, she didn't notice the ways her body was deteriorating:

> At 102 pounds I thought I would be happy. But when I lost another two pounds, I was even happier. By the time I was down to 98 pounds, I stopped getting my period. Actually, I didn't get my period for ten months. Also, my hair, which was normally healthy and shiny, became very brittle and dull, and it started falling out. I lost a lot of coloring in my skin. It took on a yellowish tone that on me looked sick, but I didn't care. I thought I looked better than I ever had in my whole life. People commented on how skinny I had become. Most of them, I realize now, thought I looked sick. But I was wearing a size 1–2 or 3–4 for the first time in my life, and as far as I was concerned, nothing could compare to that.

Through highly controlled eating patterns—sometimes eating precisely the same few things day after day or counting calories to an exactness usually reserved for scientific research—anorexic teens try to put order into their lives. These teens find it easy to deny that they have a problem: "I must be okay. Look how controlled and organized my life is." And since they don't think they have a problem, they don't seek help. Going to a doctor or counselor would mean giving up the idea that everything's under control.

Anorexia is a life-threatening condition, and when the pain of starving becomes great enough, many teens do seek help. Unfortunately, by then it can be too late; their bodies may have deteriorated too far ever to be able to recover. Of the people who suffer from anorexia, approximately one person in twenty will die from self-starvation.

Lydia was luckier than some people. She realized she needed help in time to do something about her condition:

> The beginning of my senior year in high school was when I began to get it. I was starving myself. I wasn't getting enough food. It was in a human anatomy/physiology class. We were studying the structure and makeup of the body and how each part functions, and I was learning the facts for the first time that I can remember. It made me realize how important it was to eat an adequate amount. It was like, My God. I'm starving. That's why I was so tired, so depressed, so low-energy. Sometimes I'd leave class in tears because of realizing all the damage I had done to myself.

If you recognize the symptoms of anorexia in yourself, please get help. Talk to your parents. Call your doctor or hospital. Seek the advice of your school counselor. Talk to a trusted friend. See the Resource section of this chapter, page 194, for other resources. Being too thin is more dangerous than you realize.

Bulimia Nervosa

People who eat huge quantities of food and then vomit it up or purge it by taking laxatives or try to work it off by compulsive exercising suffer from bulimia nervosa (boo-*lee*-mee-a ner-*voh*-sah). It is another eating disorder in which the victim becomes obsessive about food and weight. Most bulimics are ashamed of their behavior and go to great lengths to hide it. They rarely eat with other people around, because when they allow themselves to eat, they often can't stop until they are stuffed. Then they purge themselves. Kelly describes her experience with bulimia:

> I would plan times to binge and purge around my daily activities. Like, if I needed to throw up that day, I would go home while my parents were at work. They must have known something was up, because huge quantities of food would be missing from the kitchen, but they never said anything. I missed going out with my friends at times, because it meant I wouldn't be able to throw up. Bingeing for me was a way of stuffing down my feelings. The more I would eat, the more my feelings of unworthiness would be numbed. Then purging was getting them up and out of me.

Kelly said she hated her body. She felt ugly and unworthy most of the time, except when she was eating:

> I felt like I was not worth pleasing. Like with sex. How I related to guys. I would be in bed with a guy and I was thinking to myself, Why is he with me? My body is so ugly.

You can recognize an obese person because of excess of fat. You may know that someone is anorexic because they look so rail-thin. But a person with bulimia may be hard to spot. Bulimics are sometimes average weight. They act normal when they are not eating, but they think about eating all the time. They plan their day around eating, and they often give up other activities so they can eat alone. Bulimics try to be in control of their food intake by purging it afterward. Many bulimics say they feel a sense of accomplishment after they have vomited or had diarrhea or worked out for hours. Though they can fool themselves for a while by saying they are just trying to stay thin and fit, most people with this illness eventually realize that their behavior is really out of control.

As you can imagine, a routine of bingeing and purging is very hard on a person's body. Repeated vomiting is especially bad for you. When food is vom-

ited up, bile and stomach acids are vomited too. While the stomach has a naturally thick mucus lining to protect itself from those acids, the esophagus and mouth don't have that lining. After bouts of purging, the stomach acids you vomit up begin to eat away at the normal tissue in your mouth. Bile and undigested food tear holes in the lining of the esophagus, creating a direct passage for bacteria and viruses to challenge your immune system. The glands in your throat become swollen and sore. The enamel strips away from your teeth, leaving them susceptible to cavities and rotting. Your gums deteriorate, leading to gum disease and tooth decay. Ulcers may form in your stomach and your mouth.

Purging with laxatives has its own hazards, such as intense stomach cramping, dehydration, bowel dysfunction, and ulcerated colon. Nadine describes what happened to her:

> At some point I began "splurging and purging," making myself throw up after eating large quantities of food. Sometimes I'd take Ex-Lax to achieve a similar effect. And I started drinking a "Dieter's Tea," which was supposed to be a cleansing product, but really it was the same thing as taking Ex-Lax, just to a lesser degree. During all this, I started to follow a diet again. I stuck with it for about three weeks, but I was experiencing constipation. While I was dieting, I definitely didn't want to take something for my constipation, because my stomach was empty. But one night while I was babysitting, I completely binged. Cookies, chocolate, cheesecake, chips—you name it, I ate it.
>
> Brilliantly, I decided that because I had stuffed myself so much, I could take Ex-Lax without hurting my stomach. Subconsciously, I know, I wanted all of that food out of my body. So I took the normal dosage of two Ex-Lax before bed.
>
> At 5:30 the next morning I woke up with intense stomach cramping. I was in so much pain I thought I was going to die. I was afraid to wake my parents to tell them. I was afraid of my father's reaction, because he has little patience or sympathy for my eating disorder. Instead I decided to try and walk around and see how I felt. I was gasping for breath and sweating profusely.

At about 6 A.M. when my father got up to get ready for work, I went in and woke up my mother, who's much more sympathetic, to tell her that I needed to go to the emergency room.

She and my dad rushed me to the hospital, where, to make a long story short, I needed three enemas and two shots of Demerol. I was in the hospital for ten hours. I never felt so awful in my life.

Nadine's traumatic trip to the hospital shook up the whole family. After that, her parents helped her find a counselor who specialized in eating disorders. Nadine has been attending weekly sessions for over a year and feels she is gaining some control over her bulimia.

Bulimics try to keep their condition secret, so it is not something they usually discuss openly with their families or friends. But if you suffer from bulimia or one of the other eating disorders, you need help. Eating disorders are not just bad eating habits, they are life-threatening conditions. They are damaging psychologically, and they are socially and emotionally isolating. We recommend that you come out of the eating-disorder cupboard and let your parents or someone else know about your condition.

Breaking an addiction is nearly impossible to do alone, and eating disorders are addictive behaviors. However much in control you may feel, you are fooling yourself. Check the Resource section at the end of this chapter for some ideas of where to find help.

At twenty-three, Allison is recovering from bulimia. She said:

I work eleven hours a week at my local gym and go to therapy once a week. I do feel I am making progress. In the past, although I knew I had a problem with my eating habits, I never truly wanted to admit how deep that problem was. I wouldn't let myself believe that my obsession with weight ruled my life. Through therapy, I have finally come to admit that it has. Admitting to the problem is the first step, and it's probably one of the hardest things I've ever had to do. For a while I felt helpless and alone. I didn't think there was any way I could ever change my life.

I am very much of a perfectionist with an "all or nothing" attitude, and I tend to be an emotional eater. The more unhappy I am about things, the more I turn to food to ease my pain. When I am overwhelmed by a situation and feel like I can't come up with the perfect solution, I go directly to the kitchen. I get so miserable that I shut down. When this happens, I eat. Most likely I do this because since I feel like I'm a failure anyway, why not screw up my diet by getting fat? However, then I feel worse about myself, and the whole thing becomes a vicious cycle.

This all probably sounds very depressing, but I'm working on my problems and getting better. If any of it sounds familiar, just remember, you're not alone. Being concerned with weight issues does not make you a weak person. It's not a sign that you're a failure. If you think that being thin is more important than anything else and that you can't be an attractive person unless you're thin, well, most likely there's a deeper set of problems that you need to face. It's really important to speak to someone—a parent, a school psychologist or nurse, a teacher, a close friend, or anyone you trust—if you feel bad about yourself. If you have some form of eating disorder, try to admit it so you can begin to do something about it. I waited until I was twenty-three years old. There were so many years I wasted making myself miserable and missing out on all the great things life has to offer.

WHO AM I?

Who am I?
I ask myself as I reach the mirror.
I look,
Hesitate,
I find interesting dark brown eyes,
Smooth cocoa brown skin.
Before me I see a beautiful person.
I look around,
But no one's there.
I look back in the mirror,
And find me!
                    —CHANDRIA McCASKILL

This chapter was in part written and researched by two young women who have experienced eating disorders from the time they were very young. They wanted to share some of their knowledge and experience with you in the hope that they might save other teens from the suffering they have been through.

RESOURCES

Organizations

AA/BA (American Anorexia/Bulimia Association). Regent Hospital, 293 Central Park West, Suite 1R, New York, NY 10024. (Phone: 1-212-575-6200) Provides information and treatment referral, support groups, and a newsletter.

EDAP (Eating Disorders Awareness and Prevention). 603 Stewart St., Suite 803, Seattle, WA 98101. (Phone: 1-206-382-3587) Provides information and education on eating disorders.

MEDA (Massachusetts Eating Disorders Association). 1162 Beacon St., Brookline, MA 02146. (Phone: 1-617-558-1881) Offers support groups in Massachusetts, treatment referrals, education, and a newsletter.

ANAD (National Association of Anorexia Nervosa and Associated Disorders). Box 7, Highland Park, IL 60035. (Phone: 1-847-831-3438) Provides listings of therapists and hospitals, support groups, and information on a national level.

ANRED (Anorexia Nervosa and Related Eating Disorders). P.O. Box 5102, Eugene, OR 97405. (Phone: 1-541-344-1144) Collects and distributes information about eating disorders and offers national educational outreach, with newsletters and booklets. Write or call for information.

OA (Overeaters Anonymous). P.O. Box 44020, Rio Rancho, NM 87174-4020. (Phone: 1-505-891-2664) A national twelve-step, self-help fellowship offering free local meetings. Look in your local phone book under Overeaters Anonymous.

PENED (The Pennsylvania Educational Network for Eating Disorders). P.O. Box 16282, Pittsburgh, PA 15242. (Phone: 1-412-922-5922) Information and referral service. Support groups and a supportive telephone line. Newsletter and educational services.

Books

The Beauty Myth, by Naomi Wolf. Anchor, 1992.

Fat Is a Feminist Issue: A Self Help Guide for Compulsive Overeaters, by Susie Orbach. New York: Berkley Books, 1994.

The Golden Cage: The Enigma of Anorexia Nervosa, by Hilde Bruch. New York: Random House, 1978.

Heads You Win, Tails I Lose, by Isabelle Holland. New York: Ballantine Books, 1988.

Nothing to Lose: A Guide to Sane Living in a Larger Body, by Cheri K. Erdman. San Francisco: Harper, 1996.

One Fat Summer, by Robert Lipsyte. New York: HarperCollins, 1977.

Sacrificing Ourselves for Love, by Jane Wegscheider Hyman and Esther R. Rome. Freedom, CA: The Crossing Press, 1996.

The Secret Language of Eating Disorders: The Revolutionary New Approach to Understanding and Curing Anorexia and Bulimia, by Peggy Claude-Pierre. New York: Times Books, 1997.

Surviving an Eating Disorder: Strategies for Family and Friends, by Michele Siegel, Judith Brisman, and Margot Weinshel. New York: HarperCollins, 1989.

Video

Redefining Liberation, by NOW, the National Organization for Women, 1998. About women's health and self image. Also deals with substance abuse and violence. To order, send $10 to NOW Foundation, Redefining Liberation Video, 1000 16th St. NW, #700, Washington, DC 20036. (Phone: 1-202-331-0066)

Substance Abuse: Drugs and Alcohol

One of the most important decisions each of us faces throughout our life is whether or not to use psychoactive drugs—drugs that affect our mind and our emotions. Alcohol, marijuana, cocaine, methamphetamines, narcotics, and nicotine are some of the substances that fall into the psychoactive category.

While use of these substances does not necessarily mean abuse, when young people use, the risk of abuse is extremely high. The earlier you start using, the higher the risk. Some kids are smoking marijuana and getting drunk before they reach middle school. By junior high, more are using, and most teens know that drugs and alcohol are available. Nearly all the teens we met said that by high school, if they want to use alcohol or a drug, someone is always there to supply it.

The choice about whether to use is yours, since no one can supervise your actions every minute of every day, but very often teens are pushed into using by a combination of factors. Peer pressure—being around people who use—is one of the most significant reasons teens try drugs. Another is the desire many teens have to do things their parents don't know about and of which they might not approve. A third factor is curiosity. We hear about drugs and see people using them and we wonder, What is it all about?

The decision is further complicated by the fact that almost everyone in our society uses drugs of some kind. We drink tea or coffee to wake us up in the morning. We sip colas and other soft drinks with caffeine and sugar to give us a lift during the day. We use medicine to heal us when we are sick, painkillers to cure our headaches, antihistamines to clear our sinuses, and tranquilizers to calm us down. We take diet pills to slim down and sleeping pills to help us sleep. People who smoke cigarettes say it helps them relax. And many people who drink say it helps them slow down or cheers them up. It is legal and socially acceptable to use these substances, at least for people above a certain age.

Teens reminded us about how unfair it is to talk about the "teen drug problem" without mentioning these common, legal drugs that adults use regularly. But just because older people are dependent on chemical substances doesn't mean that you should do the same thing. The fact is, drugs and alcohol interfere with a person's normal physical and social development. They keep you from learning valuable life lessons, like how to cope with everyday stresses and unfamiliar or tense situations. Drugs and alcohol can hurt your mind and damage your body. They can even kill you. Many teens know this and have begun to teach their parents about the dangers of smoking, drinking, and doing drugs. Some parents are listening.

Society doesn't give adolescents a consistent message. On the one hand, you hear "Just say no!" You're told that drugs and alcohol are dangerous and bad for you. You know that smoking and drinking can cause illness and death. On the other hand, in movies and on TV you see drugs and alcohol portrayed as glamorous and exciting. You see adults turn to drugs and alcohol to relieve tension. You're bombarded with slick media advertisements that promote drinking or smoking as part of the "good life." It's confusing, and it tends to make many teens skeptical of what adults tell them about substance abuse.

In the past, drug education sensationalized the dangers of substance use. If teens then went out and experimented and found the dangers didn't materialize right away, they tended to disregard the entire message. As Paul said, "They tell you smoking kills you, but what the hey, it hasn't killed me yet."

The truth is that each psychoactive drug *does* have a major downside, and almost all drugs can cause irreversible damage. You are taking a risk when you use any drug, because drugs are powerful. That's why people use them; they *do* change your consciousness and affect your body. It's important to realize that the same drug may cause different reactions in different people, so you can never be sure how *your* body will react. Nor can you be

sure how your mind or attitude will change as a result of having used a certain drug. Furthermore, the effects of some drugs are cumulative, meaning they build up over time, like a time bomb in your body, waiting to go off.

YOUR REACTION TO DRUGS

Different factors influence how you, personally, might react to a particular drug: your environment, the chemical makeup of your body, your emotional and psychological state of mind, your age, and your level of maturity. Since each of these factors can change over time, your reaction to specific drugs may also change from time to time. Melanie, who's eighteen, said:

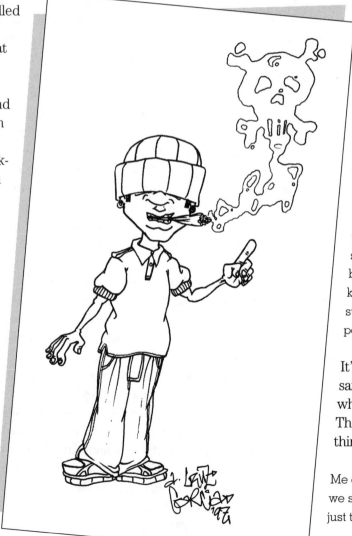

AARON CRUZ-GARCIA

I started smoking when I was thirteen. I started doing everything when I was thirteen. I wanted to be cool. I didn't really get into it until I was sixteen, though. It gives you a nice buzz when you first start and you kind of feel happy for a little while. And then you kind of get used to it, so you smoke more. But even then I wasn't a really heavy smoker. Not until one of my best friends died and I just kind of said "Fuck it" and I started smoking about two packs a day. Now I can't stop.

It's the same with alcohol. John said he started sipping drinks when he was eleven or twelve. Then last summer when he was thirteen, he said:

Me and my drinking buddy, first we started out getting a six-pack just to get a little high. Then we couldn't do six-packs, we had to get a half rack. Then that wasn't enough, so we'd get a half rack and maybe one 22 and split it. Then we had to get a half rack and each have our own 22. It just got more and more. We'd drink till we'd pass out. The funny thing is, I never thought I had a problem. I always thought I could stop if I wanted.

Egypt said she's trying to stop drinking because she's worried about herself:

> I think I have alcoholic tendencies. In fact I think I was on the verge of becoming a slobbering, disgusting drunk. I drank a fifth of gin one night. Downed the whole thing within like two hours and I was so gone I don't even remember the next day. I woke up naked in a strange place with a strange guy. But even after that, I still kept drinking. I'm afraid that my body's using so much energy just trying to clean up all the junk from the alcohol, my liver must be working overtime.

Some individuals can use moderate amounts of alcohol as adults with little apparent damage to their bodies or their lives; others may develop a lifelong addiction that will have devastating effects on their own lives and on the lives of those who are close to them. People may think that drugs and alcohol affect only the user, but that isn't so. Just ask the approximately one in three kids who have grown up in an alcoholic or drug-abusing household how painful addiction can be. One man we spoke with said his father was an alcoholic who made his family's life hell. Now this man works with kids who come from addictive households. He said:

> Every alcoholic has a negative effect on at least twenty-five other people. You don't just trash your own life if you drink, you trash the lives of your spouse and your children, and all the people they get involved with during their lives.

More than 90 percent of the teens who run away, get into trouble with the law, or become teen parents come from families in which at least one parent was addicted to drugs or alcohol. Misty said:

> My dad is a drug dealer. He's on the streets now, and I haven't seen him since I was seven. He did drugs in front of me all the time when I was little, and he used to just fall asleep and leave me to take care of myself. I was like three years old, and I'd have to make my own food and take care of my baby brother.

Eventually Misty ended up living on the streets herself. Finally, she found her way to a shelter for runaway teens, where she is getting help controlling her own drug addiction.

SAYING NO

Because they know the devastation addiction can bring, many teens whose parents abuse decide against using alcohol and drugs themselves. Mary is sixteen. Her mother continues to drink even though she has been told she will die from liver disease. Mary said:

> Alcoholism runs in my family. My mom, her mom, and my aunt are all alcoholics. My father died of a drug overdose when I was eight. Since I'm the oldest of three kids, they depend on me to take care of them. I love my mom, but I hate her when she drinks. I swear I will never put my kids through what I have been through.

Tony said:

> I've seen my friends have to fight their parents, because their parents have been high on PCP and shit. Their parents get high all the time. When they see them loaded on the stuff, it's like, Why would anybody want to be like this? So they don't want any part of it.

Crash told us about his dad:

> My dad's been using stuff for years. He gets really weird when he's high. One night when he was on meth, he almost killed my mother. I had to fight him to keep him away from her. I think you're a fool if you use drugs.

Religious and moral values also keep many teens from trying drugs or alcohol. They've made a personal decision about the kind of life they want to have, and drugs and alcohol are not part of it. Ann, a seventeen-year-old, told us:

> My life is fun without the hassle of alcohol or drugs. I have friends who sometimes use on weekends, but they respect me for being drug-free. I don't think less of my friends who use, and they don't think less of me for not using. We still have a lot in common.

RISKING ADDICTION

Even though people know about the risks of drug and alcohol use, a majority of teens end up using one or more of these substances at some time in their lives. The risk you take when you use is the unknown factor: how your body and mind will respond. You may be one of those people who can't seem to get enough, who begin to depend on drugs or drink to get through the day. Unless you can control your drug use, there's no doubt that it will eventually control you. That's the danger all users face.

Of the people who use alcohol and other drugs, about one in nine will develop a physical addiction to the substance. If you are one of those people, it means you will lose the ability to control your use and will continue to use despite many negative consequences.

Some people don't become physically addicted but keep increasing their use until they experience serious physical and emotional effects, like anger outbursts, loss of sex drive, severe depression, hypertension, slowed reflexes, inability to concentrate, loneliness, self-doubt, and self-hatred. There is no way to know beforehand how you will be affected.

The earlier a person begins to use drugs and alcohol, the greater his or her chance of developing serious abuse-related problems later on. Using chemicals before your body is fully developed interferes with the body's normal growth and development. Drugs and alcohol interfere with normal mental and emotional development too.

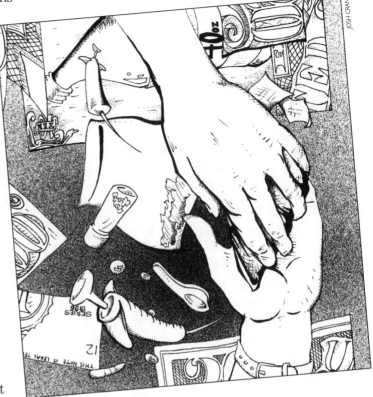

JOSH CRANE

Genetic predisposition to addictive disease is another big risk factor. If you have parents or close relatives who have substance-abuse problems, you may be genetically susceptible to addiction. You may have inherited an "addictive personality"—the feeling that you can't get enough of things you enjoy, whether it's candy or ice cream or food or liquor or drugs. If the substance you are taking is addictive—as are alcohol, nicotine, caffeine, and many psychoactive drugs—that of course makes the problem worse. So if substance abuse runs in your family, think it over carefully before getting involved yourself.

You can tell you may be heading for addiction if you have any of these symptoms: blacking out after use; needing more and more of the substance to get the desired effect; extreme behavior changes—like anger, paranoia, depression, violent outbursts. Rosie said:

> I tried quitting smoking. I actually stopped, but then I had to deal with the mood swings and my taste buds coming back and everything smelling so pretty. Smoking had completely dulled all my

senses, but when I stopped, I started going crazy. Everything was just too intense, I wasn't used to it. I just went completely loony. I was so fidgety. I couldn't sit still. So I said, Okay, just one cigarette. And then pretty soon I was hooked again.

Patrick, age seventeen, told us:

I thought it was cool that I could drink all my buddies under the table and walk away from the party while all of them were passed out. I would fight someone for that last beer and would get defensive and angry if someone told me that I drank too much.

Patrick eventually realized he had a drinking problem and sought help from Alcoholics Anonymous. But if you continue to use despite experiencing negative consequences and lifestyle changes, that is usually a sign of addiction. If you find yourself giving up hobbies and sports; spending less and less time on your homework; losing interest in friends, school, and work; avoiding important social and community functions; needing to party and get wasted regularly; getting into fights while drunk or stoned— these are signs that your substance use has become substance abuse. Drugs and/or alcohol are controlling you rather than the other way around. If you have reached the point where you are stealing or working overtime to buy your drugs and keep your habit going, you have definitely crossed the line and need help. Joanna, age eighteen, thought marijuana wasn't physically addicting. She said:

I started off using about every other weekend, and pretty soon it increased to three to four times a week. But I still thought I was in control, since I had to quit for three weeks while I went to visit my dad in California. But when I got back home, I started skipping classes to get high. I quit soccer because my coach was a jerk. My grades dropped, but I blamed that on my not being into school anymore. I had an answer for everything. Finally some of my friends cornered me and told me how much I had changed, and they said it started when I starting using more marijuana.

They came with me to see the substance-abuse counselor at school. That helped me to stop using.

People wouldn't use chemical substances if the substances didn't produce a favorable effect on them. Drugs and alcohol can become habit-forming for precisely that reason: you feel that the favorable effects of using outweigh the negative feelings you have when you aren't using. At first drugs, cigarettes, and alcohol can make people feel more sociable, smarter, cooler, braver, more exciting to be around, more attractive, less stressed. The danger is that we start to rely on the drugs to give us these good feelings, and we never learn how to achieve them on our own, without chemicals. Here's how Emily described it:

When you're drunk you're having fun. You're laughing. You're enjoying your friend's company. I mean if you're sitting there watching TV, that's not a whole lot of fun. It's a lot more fun to be laughing. You know. Booze is the conversation lubrication. The nervousness is gone. Your inhibitions are deadened. Unfortunately, pretty soon your whole body's deadened too.

Ron, age nineteen, said:

On drugs I felt like I was "all that I could be," that I was a better person on drugs, and if I used more of them more often, I would be even better. After a while I realized that I relied on my drugs just to get me through the day.

YOUR CHOICE

Drugs and alcohol are out there and pretty easy to obtain. If you want to use, you probably will find a way to do it. So the only way to stay in control of your life is to take an honest look at how you want to live it and make some decisions. What's important to you? What are your goals for the future, and how can you achieve them? What do you need to learn or to accomplish to become the person you'd like to become? Once you've given that some thought, consider where drugs and alcohol fit into the picture you've created. How does getting wasted every weekend or every day help or hinder your plans?

Maybe one of your goals is to fall in love and get married. Maybe you want to have children and raise a family. How does drug and alcohol abuse fit with family life? If your own parents are abusers, ask yourself if you want your kids to go through what you've had to go through. Relationships can be ruined by substance abuse. Friendships disappear. Michael, age fifteen, told us:

> I thought I had more friends when I was using, because stoners are open to everyone, and we instantly have something in common. It wasn't until I quit using drugs that I found out who my real friends were. Most of my stoner friends stopped hanging around with me as soon as I got clean.

Lizzie, nineteen, described her relationship:

> Me and my boyfriend, we'd get off work and start drinking and bring our friends over and drink all night. We'd pass out, wake up and go to work, and then start all over again the next night. Every night.

It wasn't until Lizzie got really sick and stopped drinking that she realized how she and her boyfriend only related to each other when they were drunk. He got mad at her for not wanting to drink with him and went off to someone else's house to get drunk. She broke up with him, and now she's in a recovery program:

> Cleaning up is hard, but it's great. You can't have a life when you're drunk all the time. In fact, that's kind of my definition of a drunk: someone who thinks being drunk is having a life.

Your health is at stake too. Serious abusers face health risks like accidents, lung cancer, liver disease, and a lot more. Alcohol-related car crashes are the *number-one* killer of teenagers in this country. Over 90,000 teenagers are injured or killed by alcoholic or drug-abusing drivers. Passengers get killed by alcoholic drivers; so do people in other cars and pedestrians. Lydia said:

> My brother was killed by a drunk. Tommy was riding his bike home, and some drunk lost control of his truck and slammed right into my brother. He was only ten years old.

Tobacco kills even more people; 430,000 people die every year of tobacco-related illnesses. Of course most of them are older people who have been smoking for a long time. Thomas, age nineteen, said:

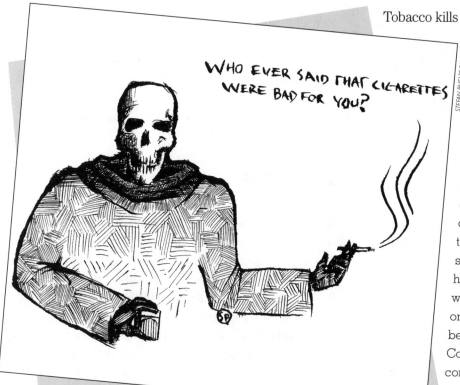

WHO EVER SAID THAT CIGARETTES WERE BAD FOR YOU?

STEFAN PHELPS RANSOM

> I've been smoking six years already and I'm still a teenager. And I sure as hell am not thinking about quitting. You don't want to quit. You want to believe you'll be that one person who can keep smoking without anything happening to you. You basically want to live in denial. I saw a picture once of some guy's lungs after he'd been smoking for thirty years. Completely black. His lungs were completely black.

Finally, it's important to realize that when you're too stoned or drunk to protect or control yourself, you may end up in a dangerous situation. That happened to Marsha, a high school senior:

> I thought it was so cool to be invited to college parties with older kids. There was lots of beer and alcohol and other drugs. It was all over the place. So I got drunk pretty fast on some jungle juice and then realized that all the guys were coming on to me. It was pretty clear that's why they invited me, to get me drunk and then have sex. Luckily my best friend was with me and she was sober and she forced me to go home with her. All I had to deal with was a bad hangover. But I could have been raped.

Tyronne, who's sixteen, had a very frightening experience:

> I was addicted to meth for about three years and I was going down. My dad used to deal, so I'd get it from him. But this one time I was up for about three days and I was like totally strung-out and crazy and my brother was talking shit to me. And before I knew what I was doing I got my dad's gun and shot my brother. He almost died. If somebody hadn't come and taken him to the hospital, he would have died for sure.

Tyronne was placed in a treatment center connected to the juvenile justice system in his state. He says he feels as if he's finally waking up from a very bad dream. Gloria, a friend of Tyronne's, said she wasn't really surprised by what happened:

> You go all weird when you're on meth. You see someone who's totally cool, totally nice, and then they're on meth and they get super negative and you feel these evil vibes. It brings out any inside evil feelings you have. Especially the stuff we have around here, because it's cut with so much bad stuff.

You never know how a particular drug is going to affect you, and as Gloria said, you never know what else is in the drug you're taking. Almost all drugs these days are mixed with other substances, every-

thing from powdered milk and sugar to talcum powder and cleanser, some of which may cause dangerous side effects, including death. Amarette said:

> I had a bad experience once with a joint treated with angel dust. My head filled up with all these negative pictures and thoughts and I really wanted it to stop. But it wouldn't. You have to keep reminding yourself every minute that it's not you, it's from the drug. I kept saying, It's not real. It's going to be over soon. It's not permanent. But I was scared and shaking the whole time.

Chuck is seventeen. He said:

> A lot of drugs are being handled by organized crime and they're not exactly into quality control.

On top of all the other negative effects and consequences of substance abuse, Jerome, age eighteen, had this comment:

> Probably the hardest thing to deal with from my constant drug use during junior high and high school was all the wasted time. I lost six years of my life that I can never make up.

THE SUBSTANCES

Every psychoactive drug has a unique way of affecting each user, but it also has certain general characteristics. In the following section we'll look at categories of drugs to see how they work.

Alcohol

Since it is illegal for teens to use alcohol, teens who drink run the risk of being arrested and fined or put in jail. That's what happened to Arthur:

> I was carrying beer in my backpack and we got stopped. When the cops opened my pack they found it, so even though I wasn't going to drink it— I was just carrying it for my friends—I still got busted on an MIP [minor in possession].

Alcohol appeals to many people because it allows emotions to override thoughts. It makes people more at ease in social situations; it reduces their fears and dulls their inhibitions. By the same token, because alcohol is a depressant, people on alcohol don't have the same awareness of their surroundings that they have when they're sober, and their reflexes aren't as keen. That's why it's so deadly to mix alcohol and driving or to drink while you are using powerful machinery or heavy equipment.

When alcohol is used regularly, excessively, or over long periods of time, the results can be devastating to the user and to his or her loved ones. Excessive use means different things to different people. For some people, even one drink can cause problems. A beer leads to a six-pack, or more. A glass of wine leads to another and another. Many teenagers who use alcohol report that they drink to get drunk. They party to get blitzed out, maybe to the point of losing consciousness. Aggie told us about her first experience with alcohol:

> I went to this party with my friend. She was twelve and I was ten, and I had never really drunk before. I remember I was drinking so much because this guy was daring people to drink this particular tequila. So I just took hold of the handle and slugged it down. You know, just to show them I could. I don't know how my little body could take in so much alcohol. Especially my first time. Everybody tried to stop me, like, "Oh my God, her heart's going to stop." They were looking at me like I was crazy. I was so wasted the next day, I felt like I was going to die.

Basically, if you don't have fun with your friends unless you drink, if you find that you can't get through the day or the weekend without drinking, if you can't sleep at night without using alcohol to put you out, you have a serious drinking problem and need help.

Some other indications of a drinking problem are regular hangovers, feeling weak or dizzy, getting depressed when you're not drinking, not wanting to stop drinking once you start. Overdoses of alcohol can depress breathing and cause a loss of consciousness or coma. In some cases an overdose can cause death, particularly when alcohol and drugs are used in combination. A person who passes out from too much alcohol consumption can choke to death on his or her own vomit.

Alcohol plays a role in many homicides and suicides; it is a factor in most traffic accidents involving teens. Drinking alcohol holds an additional risk for girls who are sexually active and do not protect against pregnancy or sexually transmitted diseases. Babies born to mothers who drink are likely to be subject to fetal alcohol syndrome and fetal alcohol effects, conditions that lead to permanent handicaps and often mental retardation in babies who would have been healthy otherwise.

Marijuana

This drug is derived from the leaves of the hemp plant. Some experts call marijuana a "gateway" drug, one that leads to other serious drug use. Other authorities say it is a relatively safe drug and should be legalized. People who believe in legalizing marijuana say it is actually less harmful than alcohol.

Marijuana's effects include a dreamy state, a distorted sense of time, a belief that your ideas are free-flowing, and an increased awareness of details. Some people say marijuana can offer relief to people suffering from conditions like glaucoma, arthritis, HIV/AIDS, and the nausea related to cancer treatments.

Other drugs may be more life-threatening and addictive than marijuana, but people who smoke marijuana regularly, just like people who smoke cigarettes, run the risk of serious lung disease and chemical poisoning. Because marijuana distorts a person's sense of reality, people who use this drug while driving automobiles or running machinery or complicated equipment are at high risk for accidental injury. People say they have experienced extreme paranoia, confusion, and panic attacks while high on marijuana.

For teenagers, the negative effects may build slowly. People who like the feeling they get from marijuana tend to use it more and more. The drug begins to intrude on their lives. It interferes with their ability to perform well in school and in other activities. Frequent users fall behind in their homework, have trouble concentrating on their studies, do poorly on tests, and lose interest in their hobbies. They may also have a hard time maintaining friendships or participating in social activities. Some people become paranoid and fearful when they're high on marijuana. And the more you use marijuana, the greater the likelihood that you will become dependent on it, unable to function without it.

Another marijuana-type drug derived from the hemp plant is hashish. Hashish, or hash, is made from the resin of the plant; it is pressed into small cakes that can be broken up and smoked in pipes. Sometimes hashish is added to a marijuana joint to make the joint even stronger.

Marijuana and hashish are fat-soluble drugs; they concentrate in the fatty organs of the body, such as the brain, the lungs, the heart, and the sex organs. Unlike water-soluble chemicals, which are eliminated from the body in one or two days, marijuana and hashish are stored in the fat cells for up to three or four weeks. Each time you use you add more. No one knows exactly what effect this accumulation of toxins has on the body, nor are they clear about what damage this may cause later in life. Some studies indicate that long-term use can change your hormone balance and increase the chance of infertility in both males and females. It may also increase the chance of miscarriage for pregnant females. Smoking marijuana or hashish carries with it the risk of cancer, emphysema, and heart disease.

Hallucinogens

The drugs included in this category are LSD, mescaline, peyote, psilocybin mushrooms, and PCP (angel dust). They produce extreme changes and distortions in your perceptions, sensations, thinking, and emotions. Some people who take hallucinogens feel disoriented, confused, and very anxious, sometimes to the point of permanent psychosis (extreme mental instability). How people react to these drugs is unpredictable. Paul, age sixteen, said:

I used LSD with no problem, and then one time when I thought everything was okay, I had a bad trip. It really freaked me out, because although it started out fine like before, it turned into this

nightmare trip that lasted all night long. I almost panicked, but I got through it. But I have to say it changed my feeling about LSD. It's like playing Russian Roulette. You may not experience a bad trip, but each time you do it, the risk is there.

Hallucinogens are powerful psychoactive drugs that may create mental distortions for up to twelve hours at a time. Using them can cause a panic reaction, or a psychotic break in which the user may act and speak as if he or she has completely lost touch with reality. Supportive friends may be able to help you handle a panic reaction by offering reassurance and constant attention. A psychotic break, on the other hand, requires trained assistance and sometimes hospitalization, because the drugs can unleash internal feelings and distortions that don't easily disappear.

Flashbacks can occur weeks or months after you use a hallucinogen, especially LSD. People who have experienced flashbacks say they often come with little or no warning and recreate the worst part of a bad LSD trip. Greg said:

I was so scared, I thought I was going to stop breathing. Charlie helped me through it. He stayed with me. I had to get out of my house because my mom would have completely gone berserk.

LSD: LSD is usually sold on the street in thin blotter paper sheets that have been imprinted with a design and impregnated with the chemicals. As with all illegal drugs, the quality or quantity of the drug in each "hit" will greatly influence your reaction to the drug. The problem is, there's no way to know exactly how much is in each hit or the quality of the drug you get. Lorie, age fifteen, said:

Some bad acid came into town and a few of my friends got really sick while frying. We found out later it was laced with strychnine. Strychnine is rat poison! They could have died.

PEYOTE AND PSILOCYBIN MUSHROOMS: These are less potent than LSD, yet they carry their own dangers. Most users experience nausea and vomiting.

Confusing these mushrooms with one of the poisonous varieties of mushrooms can cause severe gastrointestinal illness and death.

PCP, OR ANGEL DUST: This drug was developed as an anesthetic in the 1950s, but because of the severe reactions it caused, it was taken off the market. PCP can produce bizarre behavior in users. Some become extremely violent and unpredictable. High doses can result in convulsions and a coma, or in some cases, death.

Although many users claim a hallucinogenic high expands their minds, the risks of brain and body damage are serious and potentially permanent. Hallucinogenic mind expansion can be achieved through other, nonchemical activity such as meditation, chanting, and other practices that require dedication and discipline but produce greater and longer-lasting rewards.

Depressants

This class of drugs, of the sedative-hypnotic category, includes barbiturates, muscle relaxants, and tranquilizers, such as Valium and methaqualone, or Quaaludes. They are commonly known as downers. Alcohol is also a depressant. Some of these drugs are prescribed legally by physicians to calm anxious people or as an aid to sleep. They slow down your body's functions by depressing your central nervous system.

Depressants can be extremely addictive, with the user needing more and more of the drug to achieve the same effect. The body's withdrawal from depressants is an intense process, causing anxiety, convul-

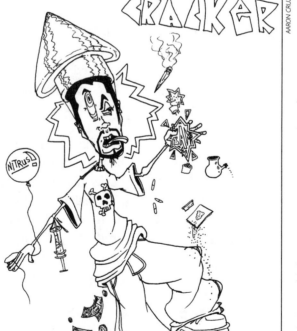

sions, or in some instances, death. When the drugs are used without a physician's supervision, the risk of overdose is very high. If you combine them with other depressants, like alcohol, the result can be fatal.

Depressants affect one's memory and judgment and should never be used before driving or before operating machinery or dangerous equipment.

Deliriants or Inhalants

These chemicals produce fumes, which when sniffed, or "huffed," give a mind-altering effect. Glue, gasoline, nail polish remover, typewriter correction fluid, and nitrous oxide are inhalants commonly used by teens and pre-teens because they are easy to obtain. At low doses they lower your inhibitions and give you a slight high. At higher doses, you can lose consciousness. The chemicals in these substances are extremely toxic; they cause damage to the liver and lungs and may cause cancer. They often make you nauseous. Some people vomit. If you sniff too much, you can suffocate or your internal organs can stop functioning.

Narcotics

These drugs (also known as Opiates) include heroin, opium, codeine, morphine, Percodan, and Dilaudid. Heroin is completely illegal in the United States; the others are legal only with a prescription from a certified medical doctor. Many of these drugs were developed for the medical market to suppress coughs, to reduce pain, and to calm the patient. The allure of these drugs on the street is that they are supposed to create a feeling that everything is fine. For people whose lives are far from fine, that is a powerful attraction. Narcotics are dangerously addictive, however. Once a person becomes addicted, narcotic withdrawal is severe, with symptoms such as sweats, convulsion, nausea, shivering, and intense panic. Users who have built up a high tolerance for the drug must keep using more and more of it to avoid withdrawal symptoms. The financial burden is extreme, since these drugs aren't free, so people in the throes of addiction find themselves stealing and prostituting themselves to keep their habit going.

Once you get used to facing life high, you temporarily lose your ability to function without that crutch. Addicts say they are powerless against the forces of the drug and can only recover with the help of recovery circles, twelve-step programs, and other committed, organized, and well-defined recovery programs. (See the Resource section at the end of this chapter, page 207.)

Narcotics can be smoked. They can be injected under the skin. They can also be administered intravenously by injection directly into a vein, called "mainlining" or "shooting up." Illegal narcotics sold and used on the street are cut with fillers, so you can't tell how powerful they are, nor can you tell exactly how much is needed to produce a particular high. This greatly increases your chance of accidentally taking an overdose and dying.

The health risks associated with intravenous drug use are extremely high. HIV/AIDS and other diseases that spread through an exchange of contaminated blood and body fluids are epidemic among intravenous drug users who share needles and neglect to sterilize their needles. Fifty percent of women and girls with HIV say they got the disease from IV drug use. Twenty percent of women and girls with HIV got it from having sexual relations with a male IV drug user. AIDS kills people, and as this book goes to press, there is no cure for it.

Stimulants

Cocaine and crack stimulate your central nervous system functions: your heart rate, your breathing, your blood pressure. Like other stimulants, cocaine and crack keep you awake and take away your appetite. People used to think that cocaine was not

addictive, but they were wrong. Thousands of users have found themselves unable to stop their habit because the negative effects they feel as they come down from the drug-induced high completely overwhelm them. What starts off as an occasional hit increases into many hits a day as the user tries to keep his or her high going. People turn to freebase cocaine or "smoking" crack cocaine for a faster and more intense high.

The cocaine user is constantly trying to avoid crashing. Margie told us how she felt when she was trying to break her habit:

> There's this moment when you know you're crashing and you panic. You don't want it to go away. You do anything to keep it going.

People "do anything" for cocaine, from prostitution to theft to spending all their savings. The drug is reported to make you feel confident, clear-sighted, and powerful; the low for many people is a panic attack full of anxiety and self-doubt, irritability, irrational speech and activity, and depression. The choice for the user is to experience these withdrawal symptoms or get high again.

Crack cocaine creates this dependency much more rapidly than straight cocaine. Crack was created with one objective: to build consumer demand. It is packaged for easy concealment; it is relatively cheap; it creates an intense high that comes on quickly. The high lasts for less than a half hour, however, and then the user is left wanting more. And more. And more. Billy said:

> You have to ask yourself, Is it worth it? Wreck your life for a fifteen-minute high? Not me. I know too many people who are hooked. I know what that's like, and it's just not worth it.

Because crack is often sold in smaller, more affordable quantities, many teens start off using it instead of straight cocaine. Then, as their addiction grows, many need to steal to keep their habit going. Some inner-city areas are full of crack houses and people who deal crack on the street. Young kids are enlisted to deliver the drugs. Gangs control the drug trafficking in their neighborhoods, creating violence and criminal activity that affects the entire community.

Aside from their devastating social effects, these drugs have severe physical effects too. Constant snorting of cocaine can damage your nasal passages. People have actually had holes form in the membrane between their nostrils. Both cocaine and crack can cause long-term depression, paranoia, respiratory failure, heart attack, stroke, and death. Smoking crack can lead to lung disease and cancer. Babies born to women addicted to cocaine or crack, "crack babies," go through withdrawal symptoms at birth and may suffer from birth defects, retardation, and severe learning disabilities. Many die from stroke or heart failure.

To recover from crack/cocaine addiction is a long, slow process that requires commitment to a good recovery program. (See the Resource section at the end of this chapter, page 207.)

Amphetamines

Known as uppers, speed, amphetamines, methamphetamines, meth, crank, tweak, and crystal, these drugs act similarly to cocaine but have a longer period of high. They have been used as diet pills and to increase a person's ability to stay awake. Some people report a temporary feeling of self-confidence and happiness. Brianna told us about her experience:

> At first it was pretty cool. Everybody was just bonding and loving each other, even people you hated, but then suddenly it turned bad and it was like, Get me out of here! It was like, I can't stand this. *Help!*

Users build a tolerance to these drugs and require larger and larger doses to achieve the desired effect. High doses of amphetamines can result in an abnormal mental state, panic, confusion, hallucinations, and aggression. In some people, use of amphetamines results in psychosis. The drug may also cause serious heart irregularities. Physical deterioration comes from weight loss, poor nutrition, lack of sleep, and neglected health care while high. People who inject amphetamines intravenously are sub-

ject to the same dangers as other IV drug users: HIV/AIDS, hepatitis, and other contagious diseases.

Methamphetamine, or crank (tweak), abuse is growing, because it's relatively easy to manufacture and cheap to buy. In fact, some people call it the poor man's cocaine. Kyla said:

> Crank is basically like the crap off the floor. It's like the really bad, overprocessed crap they can sell really fast and really cheap. The high you get from it's not worth what it does to your body. It's like really, really bad for you.

Long-term use of meth can result in depression, paranoia, and extreme antisocial behavior. Here's how Ty described his experience with it:

> I was up for two nights straight. I didn't eat. I didn't sleep. My teeth were grinding, and I chewed two holes in my cheeks and didn't even feel it. You chew on things and just grind your teeth. And you get paranoid. You don't trust anybody. It messes up your brain.

An amphetamine that has hallucinogenic properties is MDMA—Ecstasy, more popularly known as X or X-tasy. It's called this for the feeling it reportedly produces in users. This drug is widely used to produce distortions in perception and a greater sense of awareness. Prolonged or repeated use or high dosage can result in an increased heart rate and hyperactivity similar to that produced by speed.

The destructive social and physical effects of amphetamine and methamphetamine addiction are similar to those of cocaine and crack. Babies born to addicted mothers suffer serious health problems and learning disabilities.

Nicotine

The active ingredient in cigarettes and chewing tobacco, nicotine, is one of the most addictive drugs on the market. Smoking or chewing tobacco is very bad for your body and your overall health. Over 400,000 people die each year from tobacco-related illness, and smoking leads to more health complications than all other drugs combined. But that doesn't seem to stop people from smoking. Over 50 million Americans smoke cigarettes. Dan said:

> Both my parents smoke, so I'd steal cigarettes from them, and me and my friends would go out and practice inhaling and blowing smoke rings and shit. We'd just be fooling around to get the head rush. But then I'd start really wanting one, so I'd start stealing packs and hiding them under my bed and smoke in the middle of the night while my brother was asleep. I'm totally addicted now. No hope. I don't even think about quitting, because I know it's hopeless.

Babies born to parents who smoke have a higher incidence of asthma, allergies, and respiratory infections. Children who grow up in tobacco-addicted households are more likely to smoke and do other drugs when they reach adolescence.

The choice is yours. No matter how much your parents and teachers warn you to stay away from drugs or how much you read about the negative effects of substance abuse, ultimately you will make your own decision. We hope you decide to choose health.

RESOURCES

Millions of people are recovering from drug and alcohol addiction, many successfully, but it doesn't happen unless you are willing to commit yourself completely to an intense recovery program. Recovering addicts say that recovery is a slow process—one day, one step, at a time.

Once you decide to break your addiction, people will help you. Ask around. Go to some meetings. Find out for yourself which program feels right to you. Ultimately, your recovery is your choice, and when you choose it, you choose life.

National Recovery Programs for Drugs and Alcohol

Alcoholics Anonymous, 1-212-870-3400 (main number in New York City). AA is a free twelve-step recovery program, with chapters in every state and nearly every city in the United States. Look in your

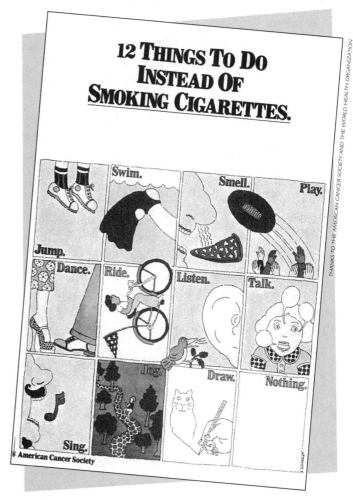

12 THINGS TO DO INSTEAD OF SMOKING CIGARETTES.

Swim. Smell. Play. Jump. Dance. Ride. Listen. Talk. Jog. Draw. Nothing. Sing.

American Cancer Society

THANKS TO THE AMERICAN CANCER SOCIETY AND THE WORLD HEALTH ORGANIZATION

phone book for the local number, or call directory assistance and ask for the number to AA. When you call, tell them you are a teenager looking for a recovery program. The people who answer the phones are generally kind and understanding and will help you.

Al-Anon, 1-800-344-2666. If someone in your family has a problem with alcohol, you may find help at Al-Anon, the program for family members of alcoholics. Look in your phone book under Al-Anon or ask directory assistance for the number.

Alateen, 1-800-344-2666. Alateen, a program especially directed to teenagers, is available through most chapters of Alcoholics Anonymous.

Narcotics Anonymous. NA is about drug addiction. There may be a specific number for NA in your local phone book, or call directory assistance and ask for Narcotics Anonymous. If you cannot find the number that way, call Alcoholics Anonymous and ask about NA.

Students Against Drunk Driving (SADD). P.O. Box 800, Marlboro, MA 01752. 1-508-481-3568, FAX 1-508-481-5759. SADD has programs for middle schools and high schools. Its goals are to prevent underage drinking and drunk driving, save lives, and eliminate the illegal use of drugs. SADD organizes peer-counseling programs and community-awareness projects. It has a manual for how to start a chapter at your school.

Local Recovery Programs

Many excellent local programs exist throughout the United States to help teenagers stay off drugs and alcohol and recover from addiction. To find them, call your local department of health for a listing, ask the drug counselor at your school, look in the business pages of your phone book under Drug Treatment or Alcohol Treatment, or check at a community health clinic or center.

We have chosen to list one local program here as an example. You can call it for information about services and for referrals to programs in other areas.

Free at Last. 1946 University Ave., East Palo Alto, CA 94303. 1-415-462-6999. e-mail: freelast@aol. com. Established to provide community recovery and rehabilitation services, Free at Last offers a drop-in center, a community meeting space, an outpatient program, an adolescent/young-adult support program, residential shelters, and street outreach programs. It is a new model of recovery: in the community, by the community, and for the community.

Smoking

For recovery programs to help you stop smoking, call your local chapter of the American Cancer Society, or check at your local health center.

Living with Violence

7

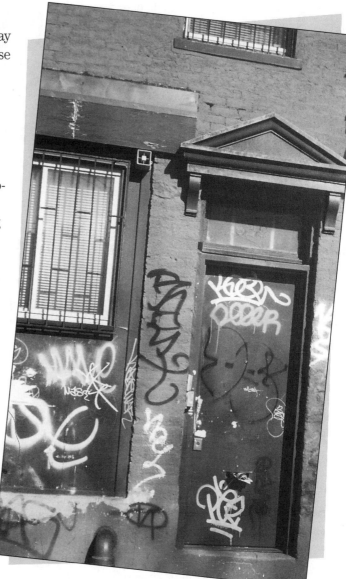

JOHN D. RAMBOW

For too many of us, violence is part of everyday life. We experience physical and sexual abuse at home. There are gang fights and random shootings in our neighborhoods. We hear about murder and rape almost on a daily basis. We witness prejudice and acts of violence against foreigners, minorities, and homosexuals.

It doesn't help matters that movies and TV programs present brutality and abuse as if it were entertainment. People get blown away in appalling detail on the big screen, and we pay to watch. In many of the most popular sitcoms on TV, characters physically and verbally abuse one another regularly while we laugh. Saturday-morning cartoons, supposedly for little children, have more violent acts per hour than any other shows on television. In music, too, singers and rappers celebrate violence and hatred and abuse—most commonly, abuse of women.

Just for one day, try to count all the violent acts you see and hear about in the popular media. Include the times people are sarcastic to one another, talk trash to one another, and show disrespect for one another with gestures and looks. What kind of messages do you think children receive from witnessing all that violence and disrespect?

The more violence and hatred we see, the more we come to think of it as normal behavior. We get used to it when instead we should be outraged by it.

If we want the escalation of violence to stop, it's up to each of us to start doing things differently. We must learn to treat others with respect and compassion even if their values or beliefs are different from our own. We must be willing to listen to our friends even when they have an opinion we don't agree with. In sexual situations, we must respect people when they say no. When we see someone acting cruelly or unfairly we must speak out against his or her cruelty. We must do what we can to educate each other against racism, sexism, and homophobia. And perhaps most important, when or if we choose to have children of our own, we must try our best to raise them with kindness, respect, and love.

In the following pages you will hear from teenagers who have experienced violence in many different forms and from some who have found ways to get help. As you read their stories, we hope you will remember that they are not just stories. They are the life experiences of real teenagers, just like yourself.

PHYSICAL ABUSE

Using physical violence against another person is illegal, but it happens all the time. It happens at school, on the job, and in the street. When it happens in our very own homes, within the confines of our family, it is called domestic violence.

Domestic Violence

In some households, violence occurs on a regular basis. Siblings have fights. They scream at one another, talk trash to one another, hit one another. Parents also scream, fight, beat each other, and beat their children. Shaquor, a twelve-year-old from Connecticut, said:

> It wasn't too good at my family. My mom used to treat me bad. Holler at me. Call me names. It was a two-story house, and when she was mad, my mom would tie me to the stairs so I couldn't get

away. Then she'd whoop me with her big ol' leather belt. If I screamed for help, she'd just turn up the TV.

We met Thomas, seventeen, at a home for boys. He said:

> My dad would hit me so hard when I was little I wouldn't be able to stand up. I had so many bruises up and down my leg I couldn't walk. He'd pull my hair. One time he bashed me into the wall so hard he almost broke my arm. That's why I ran away when I got old enough.

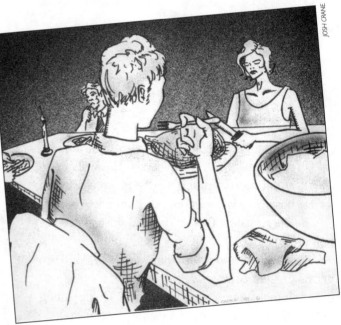

James wrote his story in the magazine *Foster Care Youth United.* Here's a condensed version of it:

> The foster mother who eventually adopted me and my siblings often told us that she took us in for the money. She always said she could care less about us, as long as her bills were paid. She beat us with any object she could get her hands on, and she never had mercy for our faces. She beat us with a thick cowhide belt which she slit into seven strips. She called the belt "Mr. Brown." My siblings and I had welts on our skin for days due to the beatings.
>
> When I was eleven or twelve, I called the Child Abuser Registry Hotline, and a man assured

me that they would look into my case. I felt relieved, knowing I wasn't alone. A social worker arrived the next day. My adoptive mother denied the abuse. The social worker then asked us—in the presence of my adoptive mother—if we were being abused. Since we were terrified of her, of course we said no. The case was immediately dismissed.*

You have a right to live in a safe environment. We all have that right. Find an adult or friend you trust who can help you decide what to do to be safe. Tell your teacher, if you have a close relationship with him or her. Tell a religious leader or a sports coach. As James went on to say, however, it's easy to say, "Find someone you trust," but finding that person and feeling comfortable enough to tell him or her about what's happening to you is not easy:

> People must realize children are terrified of telling someone that they're being abused. I went to school many days with cuts and bruises on my face. My teachers often asked what happened, and I would always say I fell or tripped over my shoelaces. I was afraid no one would believe I was being abused.
>
> I eventually left the abuse by refusing to go back home, and when I was fourteen, I was finally signed into a new placement.

Lily, fourteen, told us about what happened in her family:

> My father beat on my little sister a lot. One day he beat her up so bad I had to bring her to the emergency room, because I thought she could go blind. She had these bruises on her eyes, and her nose was so swollen it was like all over her face. So I took her to the emergency room, and I thought they were going to make us go home, but

they didn't. The doctor who took care of my sister was really nice. He took pictures of her and asked a lot of questions, and that's how he got to know the truth, because my sister was telling him that she fell down the stairs. He was like, "Tell me what really happened," but my sister didn't want to. So I got mad and I said, "Tell him. Tell him what really happened." So she did. And it was good, because they found a social worker to help us.

If you haven't experienced this kind of abuse yourself, it may not seem possible to you that parents could torture their children. Mostly, these parents are people who were themselves beaten or tortured as children and didn't get help, and as a result they have very few, if any, role models for either good parenting or controlling their anger. They are emotionally unstable. Many are drug addicts or alcoholics. When they feel bad or get mad, they lash out instead of trying to communicate their feelings in a more effective, less violent way. You can feel sorry for the hard lives these people must have led, but you can't excuse them for the way they treat children.

Battered children who don't get help are at risk of suffering long-term depression and low self-esteem, or themselves turning to violence whenever they face stressful situations. If you are being abused or if you know someone who is being abused, please follow Lily's lead and tell someone in authority. Don't give up until someone listens.

The Nine Line (1-800-999-9999) is available for support and referrals. If you have no one else to help you, call them. (See the resource section at the back of this chapter for more suggestions.)

Date Violence

A problem for many teenagers, especially girls, is date violence. Like married partners who hurt each other physically, in date violence one partner, usually the boyfriend, beats up or harasses the other partner, usually the girlfriend. What starts off as a normal dating relationship may turn into an abusive situation before you're even aware of what is happening.

It often begins with one partner accusing the other of lying or cheating or being less "in love." Excessive jealousy is common in these relationships.

---

* We printed this condensed version with permission from Youth Communication. The story, called "I Could Have Been Elisa," by James Knight, is published in its entirety in the September/October 1996 edition of *New Youth Connections*. It originally appeared in *Foster Care Youth United*, a magazine published bimonthly by Youth Communication. Teens who are part of the foster-care system are invited to submit poetry, writing, and artwork. For more information, write to them at Youth Communication, 144 W. 27th St., Suite 8R, New York, NY 10001.

While you may have been taught to take your boyfriend or girlfriend's jealous feelings as a sign of how much he or she loves you, obsessive jealousy is *not* a sign of love. Obsessive jealousy that leads to name calling and hitting is not caring; it is abusive, as Glenna, eighteen, described:

> I'd only been going out with Monroe for a couple of months when I said something to him about some other guy and he really got mad. Pretty soon he was shoving me, and I fell back and hit my head on a chair. When I got up, I said, "I'm calling the police." And I did. I called his parents too, and they came over. He'd been drinking and he just got out of control. It had happened before, and I wasn't going to take it. His parents helped him get into an alcohol program, and the police put him on a six-month probation with fines and everything. It's amazing how much he's changed. But we're just friends now. I'm not into having a relationship with someone who can't control his temper.

Helen said she and Jeremy had been going out about a month when he started telling her how much he loved her and how he wanted to be with her all the time. At first she was flattered by his attention, but

> Pretty soon it was like I couldn't do anything without him. I'd say, I've got to go home now and do my homework, and he'd want to come with me. Or he'd call me on the phone over and over. If the line was busy, he'd get all mad and say, "Who were you talking to?" One time we were out and I said hi to this guy I know from one of my classes, and Jeremy went berserk and grabbed me by the hair and pulled me out to the car. I was hysterically screaming. When I told my mom, she made me change schools, and now she answers the phone to screen my calls. I'm glad. It was scary.

Monica, fifteen, lives in Chicago:

> I was going out with this guy for almost a year, but I broke up with him. Then about a couple of weeks

after that, some guys stopped me in the street and beat me up and raped me. I found out it was my boyfriend's gang. They were trying to get back at me for breaking up with him.

This is what Dara told us:

> My boyfriend's hit me a couple of times, but I know he doesn't really mean it. Usually it's when he's been drinking too much.

Dara may think her boyfriend doesn't really mean to hit her, but she's wrong. A person who uses physical violence does mean to hurt. Many people can't deal with their emotions. When they feel angry or scared or hurt inside, they think it's all right to punch somebody; they think that's what everyone does. Magdelena is twenty. She said:

> When I married Joey, it was because I really loved him and I loved being with him. We used to have fun together. But as soon as we got married, it all changed. I think he thought that being married gave him the right to control me. He always wanted to know where I was every minute. He turned into this jealous monster. He wouldn't even let me visit my friends or go shopping without him. If I did anything that made him upset, he hit me and beat me up. I had bruises all over my arms, on my face even. Finally I had to leave him and go stay at my aunt's house in another city.

Here is a fact: Between 2 and 4 million wives and girlfriends are beaten by their partners each year in this country. Beating is *the* major cause of injury to women. Males can be battered too, by their fathers or mothers and/or girlfriends and wives. It is not as common, but when it does happen, it creates a different set of problems, since people tend not to take it seriously. Leo told us:

> People think it's funny to hear about guys being beat up by girls, but it's not funny. Look at me. I'm a big guy, and I had this little girlfriend who used to hit me, bite me. She'd throw things at me. So what am I supposed to do, anyway? If I hit her, I would have really hurt her, and I don't hit girls. It's

Signs That May Indicate Future Physical Abuse

We're going to use the word "he" because partner abuse is mainly perpetrated by men against women. In homosexual relationships, of course, either women or men can be responsible for abuse. Here are some indicators of a potentially abusive partner:

Very controlling behavior: He wants to limit your activities, friendships, and time. He wants to know exactly where you are at all times and who you're with. He doesn't want you to talk on the phone to anyone else or have any other friends. He seems extremely jealous.

Emotional abuse: He puts you down a lot and calls you names. He tells you how dumb you are or makes you feel as if you're crazy. He plays a lot of mind games and humiliates you in front of others.

Guilt: He makes you feel guilty for not being perfect and makes you feel bad about yourself.

"Male Superiority": Your boyfriend or husband treats you like a servant. He always makes all the decisions and won't let you do anything for yourself. He makes you feel that his needs and desires come first.

Threats: He threatens to use violence, as when a boy says, "If you don't stop talking to so-and-so, I'll kill you (or kill him)," or, "I'm going to kill myself if we break up." Beware of anyone who threatens violence.

Intimidation: He scares you with his anger. Or he may show off his weapons and shout about how he's going to use them. He may smash things and punch walls.

A person who exhibits any or all of these behaviors is likely to become abusive. If you are in a relationship with someone of this description, talk to a parent or a counselor and get help ending the relationship immediately.

just not something I would do. But she would be drinking and screaming, and it would just go on from there. One time she hit me with a big old metal pot and broke my wrist. It really fucked up my work, since I lift heavy things. I actually had to call the police on her once, and when they came they just rolled their eyes and laughed at me.

When Leo broke up with his girlfriend, she was very upset. She couldn't understand why he didn't want to be with her anymore. Having grown up in a violent household, that's the way she thought relationships always were.

Growing up in an atmosphere of violence is not only physically threatening, it is psychologically harmful too. When children are raised with violence in their families, they learn to think of violent behavior as normal. They may themselves become violent in their own relationships. Violence is not a part of healthy family life. Love should be caring, not abusive. No one deserves to be beaten. If it is happening to you, let a caring adult know about it and help you.

Harassment

Leeann is thirteen. She said:

> This girl I don't even know has been following me around and telling me that when she gets me alone she's going to beat me up. I'm scared even walking alone when I'm at school. I saw this girl fight and she used a knife, so finally I went and told the counselor. But all he did was say we'd have to meet with her and try to work it out. So I said forget it, and I told my mom, and she went to the police. But then I was too scared to go back to school. I was even too scared to leave my apartment until they caught the girl and put her in a different school. It turned out other people had already complained about her doing the same thing to them.

No one has the right to intimidate or terrorize another person, to disrupt that person's life so that he or she is afraid to go to school or work or walk the streets. Harassers choose as victims people they think are less powerful than themselves. Their sole purpose is to make life miserable for those people. It is criminal behavior that often does not stop until someone in authority steps in. If you are being harassed and feel afraid, tell someone who can help you put a stop to the problem, such as a parent, an older friend, a teacher, a counselor, a member of the clergy, or the police.

Much harassment and violence occurs as a result of prejudice. Out of fear and ignorance, some people harass others who are different from themselves. Miranda is gay. She says:

I came out in tenth grade and basically spent the three final years of high school hiding out in the rooms of sympathetic teachers. Most of the gay kids I knew in school either dropped out or graduated early. It's not a friendly place to be when there's the constant threat of somebody beating you up or humiliating you just because you've decided you're gay.

John told us about his experience at boarding school:

I lived in a dorm with eight guys on the same floor, and there was this one guy who right from the first week of school had it in for me. Basically, he'd get me alone and pin me down or force me into a corner and threaten to rape me whenever the opportunity arose. A couple of times he almost did it. He said he'd kill me if I told, but eventually I did tell anyway. It was the only way to keep myself from going crazy.

Lots of the teens we spoke with said they believed adults were prejudiced against them and sometimes harassed them just because they were teenagers. Black and Hispanic teens have told us they were regularly harassed by the police simply because of their race. Gary remembered:

When I was in high school, I was a good kid and I ran with a bunch of guys who were good kids too. We got good grades. We were clean—we didn't do drugs. Still, one time we were walking down the street, and this cop car cruises by, and before we know what's happening they're out of the car with their guns on us. One of them yells, "Freeze," and they make us lie down on the sidewalk. One cop put his boot on my back while another one searched my friend. I was so humiliated—and scared—I felt like crying. All I could think about was "What if somebody I know sees me?" And to

this day I don't know what it was that made those cops stop us except that we were black.

Aaron is seventeen and from Washington State. He said:

I was out with my friend and we were walking to another friend's house. The next thing I knew, I saw this spotlight coming across the trees and then voices saying, "Lay down on the ground and put your hands behind your head." And these cops came out and cuffed us and pulled us up by the chains, cutting our wrists. And they just kind of harassed us with "Where are you going?" "What are you doing?" "What are you up to?" And then we'd tell them, and they'd say, "Don't lie to us." But we weren't lying. They try to get you to admit stuff that you weren't even doing. And then they asked us what gang we were in. When we told them we weren't in a gang, they said, "Why are you wearing blue jeans and blue flannel shirts?" So I was like, "Because I don't own any brown flannels and it's cold outside." "Why are you wearing that kind of hat?" They just think if you're Mexican, that every little thing about you has something to do with a gang, even if you're not even in a gang.

Racism and hatred are behind everything some people think and do. People who are members of racist groups tell the world they are *for* the honor and perpetuation of a particular country or religion or belief system or ethnic group, but really their actions are *against* whatever and whoever isn't exactly like them. Elizabeth lives in a small town in the Midwest where her family is one of the only black families. She said:

A guy at school threw a bucket of whitewash on me right in the hall at school. He said it was an accident, but give me a break. Another time, a bunch of them put swastikas on my car. Another "accident"? Then when I started getting hate notes, I told my parents and they said, "Okay, that's it. You're out of that school." They put me in a private school in the next town. Those guys finally got expelled, but not until months after they harassed me.

Julio told us this story:

I ran into a real scary situation when I lived in Los Angeles and me and a friend of mine skipped school and went downtown. We were walking around minding our own business, and all of a sudden these three huge skinheads grab my friend and throw him down on the ground and push me up against the wall. I don't know what's going on. I mean, I'm just this little fifth-grader and there's these three huge skinheads in front of me with their little swastikas on them and stuff. So I was thinking I was dead. I didn't even understand what they were saying 'cause I was so scared. My friend's lying there on the ground crying, and I was too scared to even cry. The next thing I know this huge black hand grabs one of the guys' heads, and then a big old fist goes right across his face and these black gangbanger guys are beating the crap out of these skinheads. Right in front of us. They're telling us to get out of there. So we took off.

Bullies are only bullies until they're busted, but it takes courage to bust them. Many of us who have felt abused or have seen abuse occur do nothing about it. That is one of the factors an abuser counts on. Georgia is from Ohio. She said she found a strength inside herself to stand up to some prejudice:

I remember one incident, with some friends of mine. We were all fooling around together. Then the guys started talking about blacks and putting them down. They didn't know that my stepdad is black. And I got really upset, and I told them that they had no right to put down minorities. Because they are insulting a lot of great, kind, good-hearted people. And they all looked at me really strange. But they never said another word.

Using Violence to Solve Problems

When you're living in a violent atmosphere, using physical violence can come to seem normal. Toni said:

My life was just so much into violence. That's all I knew. My dad was real violent. And my mom, she had no choice but to protect herself, so she was pretty violent back. There were fights at school all the time, and across the street a bunch of winos fighting at the park. No matter where you went. Go to the grocery store, you don't just walk and look around and enjoy the walk, you just go directly where you're going and you don't look at nobody. Because you never know who's going to start some shit with you. And then you'd have to fight. I was expelled from both elementary school and junior high school for fighting. But it was like, that's all I knew how to do. If someone talked shit to you, you fought them.

Alexandra wrote to us about what happened to her:

When I was in seventh grade, I moved to a small town in Idaho. I had a friend who was part of a group of girls, and I was sort of absorbed into it too. They all joined the softball team, which needed members to qualify for tournaments. But once the team had more than enough members, they decided that the players who weren't good should quit. One or two girls were talked out of being part of the team, but I didn't want to quit. So they decided there were other ways of "talking" me out of it, like throwing me in the shower with my clothes on, spreading bad rumors about me, throwing fast balls during practice that would "accidentally" hit me. The worst was when about six or eight of them ganged up on me and slammed my head into a locker. They came about a half inch from spiking my eye on the door hook.

In our society we give people a mixed message. On the one hand, we tell them that violent behavior is not okay, and on the other hand we show them that violent behavior is actually admired. Emile said:

I just saw that big heavyweight match on TV. And like all those boxing matches, those fighters are really good, but the fights are so brutal. And I was watching, and I was thinking, No wonder why there's fights in the streets. It's glorified on TV.

These guys are getting paid millions and millions of dollars for beating up somebody. It's crazy.

James told us about his experience:

I was fighting this punk, and everyone comes running from all directions yelling, "You can do it." "Kill him." "Hold him down." "Kick his ass." It was like when I was on the football team. They were like fans, yelling for me to win. But the more blood I saw, the more scared I got. I wanted somebody to stop us, but I never asked for help out loud, and I finished the fight. So that made me a big hero, right? A couple of girls gave me their phone numbers. A teacher even slapped me on the back. That night, after my dad heard about it, he offered me a beer, like he was saying, "Congratulations."

That so many people have guns makes the problem far worse. What might have been a fistfight in the past now turns all too frequently into a gunfight and murder. We've all heard stories about drivers who get so mad when someone cuts them off that they smash into that person's car or get out and shoot the person. We've heard about people killing their neighbors over minor incidents like playing music too loud. A foreign-exchange student was killed as he walked up to someone's house on Halloween for trick-or-treat because the owner of the house thought he looked dangerous. In our own homes, guns can escalate the violence too, as Trevor told us:

My dad was in the Vietnam War. My older brothers and sisters told me he has always been weird ever since he came back. He has night terrors. He gets up and takes his gun and chases my mom around the house. Sometimes he comes in and makes me hide behind the bed or in the closet, because he has some paranoia about people outside. He never really explains it. And he can be mean. One night he came home high on meth, and he was accusing my mom of having an affair. It wasn't true, and she was telling him, and then I heard gunshots, so I ran into her room and he was shooting the mattress, getting closer and closer to her as she backed away to the wall. I hit him with a skillet. I had to hit him to make him stop. It wasn't the first time.

When you live with violence day after day, it's hard not to give up hope. You always have to watch your back. You never feel safe. Brian said he is on edge all the time:

I'm so paranoid. Like on the buses or subways, I just sit there and stare at everybody to see if anybody is giving me shit. You never know. You can get your ass kicked pretty bad if you're not watching. My friend was shot a month ago. He's gone. It could happen to me. It could happen to anybody.

When you use violence to deal with problems, it's hard to change your behavior. You may not know any other way to react. But it's worth the effort to learn how to do things differently. Maybe you're feeling so tied up inside that you don't know how to ask for help. Maybe you think people would think less of you if they knew you wanted to change. You build up walls around yourself. Only when you start to see things in a new way do you realize how much it takes to tear those walls down. Here is Gabriel's story:

When I was about nine years old, my father left us. He left me the man of the house with my mother and my two sisters. But the responsibility was too big. I guess it was too big for him too, or else he wouldn't have left. I felt I needed to prove that I was cool. That I was tough. I got in with the gangs, and I got to the point where I had no heart for nobody. What basically helped me change my life was being incarcerated. I was locked up at fifteen years old because I tried to kill somebody. I was in a cell by myself with time to think slower, out of pressure from the street, out of the fast lane. I was lucky that they put me in a violent-offender program, where I was exposed to people who were making the effort to change their lives. They took me from behind the cave I built up for myself and helped me break down the wall into my heart, so I could feel again, and that's the only way you can stop being an offender. You have to be able to feel your victims' pain and be sorry.

Feeling other people's pain may mean remembering your own childhood pain, an experience that can seem overwhelming if you have no support. We urge you to seek help from a counselor or therapist if your angry feelings lead to violent actions. Violent behavior will stop only when people learn how to express their anger and frustration in words, not punches. There are many groups that have started throughout this country to help you do exactly that, and in the process help stop the cycle of abuse and violence that is ruining too many people's lives. See the Resource section at the end of this chapter for some of those groups.

GANGS AND GANG VIOLENCE

Gangs and gang violence have been part of the scene in most urban areas for many years. Teens say they join gangs for the excitement, the glamour, the cars, the fast life. Some say they join for the money or the recognition. They also join gangs for a sense of family, a feeling of belonging to a group that cares, and they join for protection from the violence around them in their communities.

Teens don't usually join gangs because they *want* to get killed or kill someone else. They don't join because they *want* to put their families in danger. Because of gangs, however, community violence continues to escalate, and that does put families in danger. It seems to be another vicious circle that has no end.

The teens we spoke with about gangs had a lot of different ideas and opinions. Randy told us his story:

> I started associating with gangs in about the ninth grade, because I was being bullied around by these other kids. Then you

get in with the gang and feel like your homeboys are there for you. And you see the money, the drugs, the cars. It looks pretty good. But it's a fast life and you die fast too. Right now, I'm out of the gangs, and what's keeping me out is my parole officer and my teacher at the alternative school where I go. They care about me. They want me to make a better life for myself.

Freddie's reason for joining a gang was different:

> In my neighborhood, just walking to school and back day after day was the start. Being exposed to gangs and violence and drug deals, being exposed to everything just right there. My dad left when I was little and my mom works, so I was out there with them. Everybody who was around me was doing that kind of thing, young and old. I didn't want to be the nerd, going to school while everybody else was out on the block. I wanted to be known, and to be known I had to be in with them. It was a lot of pressure, but it was my choice to become a gang member. It started off by just basically running with the crowd, drinking, getting

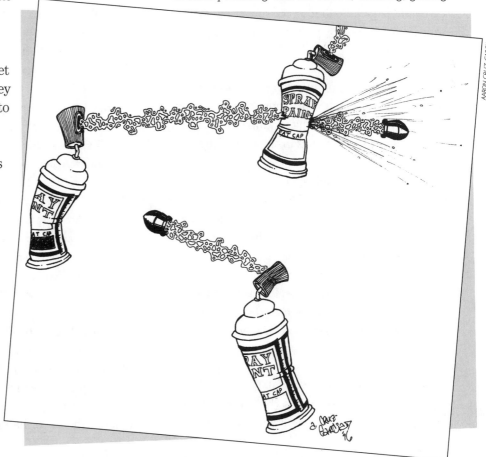

high, and after that came drug deals, came the shootings, came the crime. I was fourteen years old when I was put away. Now I'm seventeen. Now I see what that life leads to. I don't want that life no more.

Tina, nineteen, said:

There are fights all the time in our neighborhood. You have to be able to protect yourself. It's good to be part of a gang because your homies are around you and you're fighting this chick or this guy and they will just automatically jump in. Or if you say, "No, this is mine," then they'll be cool and let you handle it. They're there to help you.

For gang members, the gang becomes their family, and the leaders of the gang become their role models. Tony said:

You go with the gangs mainly to like have a family if you don't have one. Or to be part of the neighborhood. Your gang is your family. And there's a lot of respect inside the gang. A lot of love and respect. So that's a reason for being in a gang, to get respect. They're there for you, and you're there for them.

While for guys being in a gang may bring companionship and respect from other gang members, Lucas said the girls who hung around with his gang were like "slaves" of the guys in the gang. He said:

You know about the rookie days in the gang and how you have so many girlfriends lined up, just waiting to be with you. For me, it wasn't like I was loving them, it was like they were there for me to manipulate them and use them. Dis them. Because they never said anything about it. They were just there to do whatever. I felt bad for them, because I was just using them, and maybe they thought that I loved them and was there for them. But I wasn't.

Every gang has its entry ritual, how a new member gets "jumped in." For males this often involves a vicious fight to see if you can take ten minutes or

more of people pummeling you. Or you may be expected to perform some act of violence outside the gang to prove yourself, like being part of a robbery or break-in or drive-by shooting. For girls, the ritual will usually include a physical fight with other girl gang members, and also a gang rape in which you become the forced sexual partner for any number of male gang members. Girls, too, may be required to prove themselves by killing someone or participating in a drive-by or a holdup.

Cee Cee told us about her initiation:

I got jumped in pretty early. A lot of it had to do with starting puberty early. My friend had a lot to do with it too. She was always wanting to do something a little bit crazier than like what I wanted to do. She took me to my first hotel party with a bunch of guys when I was only ten. She was in the bathroom with some guy, and so I went in there, and this guy stripped me naked and was saying, Don't be a little girl. He's like, Oh, look, your friend's doing it. And I was like, I don't want to. He had no idea I was so young.

Teresa told us that for her being in a gang was about being part of a group of friends who would stand by you and help you out. She told us about the time she was jumped in:

I don't remember it too well. They hit me for about three or four minutes. Not too long, but long enough. And one other thing I remember is they wanted to give me a tattoo. The girls got like a cross on their hands, right next to your thumb. It didn't look too tacky, but I didn't want to do it. Afterwards my face wasn't really swollen, I was just bruised. I had these cuts everywhere. You got to prove that you're not just a little wannabe, but like, yeah, you actually got jumped in, you actually went down for something.

Outside of gang life it may be hard to understand why teens would choose to submit themselves to physical and sexual abuse or be willing to commit murder just to be in a gang. Even teens who are drawn into gangs say that if they lived in different neighborhoods or had more resources or felt more

Juan lives in Queens, New York. He wrote a story called "When Things Get Hectic" about gang violence. Here is an excerpt from his story:

When Things Get Hectic

Last summer, I was headed to the bodega around my block to get a hero when I saw my boy Deps step to some kid I'd never seen before. Being the nosy friend that I am, I went over to see what the problem was. "Yo, Deps, what's going on man?" I said.

"This b– –ch ass n– –ga got an eye problem," Deps answered.

"Whatever, man," said the kid. I noticed he got scared when I came over, knowing there were two of us now and this wasn't his neighborhood.

But fighting over a bad look wasn't exactly the move. "Yo, forget about that sh–t man," I said. "He don't want no beef."

"So why he trying to scope if he don't want none?" said Deps.

"I wasn't scoping at you man," answered the kid.

"Yo, man, squash this bullsh–t already so I could get my sandwich," I told Deps. "My stomach is growling."

"Aaiight, man, just don't be trying to act like you represent around here," Deps told the kid. They both gave each other the hand along with dirty looks and slow moves.

After the fake pound, I went inside the store to get my salami and cheese, and Deps tagged along. About fifteen minutes later, there we were chilling in front of my house. It was really hot and we were trying to throw girls in front of the hydrant and munching down that delicious hero, when all of a sudden a blue Corolla with tinted windows rolled up in front of us.

I knew right away this was the kid Deps was riffing to. I remember the hero losing its delicious taste. The girls were still teasing us, trying to get us to chase them, when Deps tapped my leg 'cause he knew what time it was. Before I could yell "duck," I saw the back window roll down enough for a gun to fit through. I grabbed Deps like a reflex, and we both hit the floor at the same time two bullets hit the side of my house.

The car was long gone before me and Deps had a chance to feel burnt. All of a sudden the girls didn't want to play anymore, and it wasn't that sunny. I never knew things could get to that point so fast. A dirty look setting bullets off didn't make any sense. What if they had caught us from behind? What if they had shot one of the girls? What if my mother had been standing there?

. . . This kind of thing goes on all the time: "Yo, you heard who got shot?" "I ran into some beef today." "Yo, man, bring a shank just in case." I am sick and tired of hearing it. Violence surrounds us everywhere: school, work, even in front of your crib. That's the number-one reason for deaths among teens in New York City. Kids nowadays are ready to kill each other over the dumbest things.

I know a lot of kids who are scared one day they are just going to get blasted for something stupid like that. There are so many other kids out there with guns, knives, and short tempers.

I live in C——, Queens, and when the weekends come, I feel like I am in a battle zone. . . .

—Juan Azize*

* This story was reprinted with permission in an excerpted version from *New Youth Connections*, copyright © 1994 by Youth Communication. For more information write to Youth Communication, 144 W. 27th St., Suite 8R, New York, NY 10001.

self-confident, they would not choose gang life for themselves. Ronnie told us:

> People think that you're really hot shit if you're in a gang, that you're tough and hard, and that gets you a lot of respect. But from what I saw when I was running with the gang, I saw a lot of stupid, scared people trying to cover up their fears and their insecurities.

Some teens are able to stay out of gangs even though they live in gang neighborhoods, but it's usually because they have very strong support at home. Emile, sixteen, told us:

> For me, it's my mom. I know that's why I stayed away from the gangs. My mom was strict. She let me know every minute that there was a difference between right and wrong. She really watched over me. A lot of my friends are in gangs, and I've been in some fights. But I try to stay away from it. It's no good.

Aaron, a seventeen-year-old from the Northwest, said:

> I really don't know what kept me out of the gangs. Maybe because I know inside me what's right and what's wrong. I don't know. Because there was plenty of times when I would skip school or get bad grades and I been in three different high schools so far. But my dad is a good role model. He shows me how much he cares. That's why we moved out of the city last year. He wants me to make a good life for myself. And I was lucky that when I did get in trouble, they put me in a diversion program with this person who really cares. So many good things have come out of that program.

Many families move out of gang areas if they can afford to move, because living with gangs around isn't easy. Tension is everywhere all the time, and teens growing up in that atmosphere don't often have a chance to slow down and get to know themselves. They say there's danger everywhere you go, and even inside your own home you're not safe.

Everyone knows of people who've been shot while sitting at their dinner table or watching TV.

It's possible to be friends with gang members without actually being "in." But once you are in a gang, it's not always easy to get out. Carlos used to be in a gang. He said he was tight with his friends until he decided to leave:

> A lot of the people who I thought were my friends, they say they're my homeboys and all this, but it turned out they weren't really my friends. Now that I'm out the gangs, my family's been threatened, my mom's been shot at. There's a lot of people that will threaten you. They don't want to make it easy for you to get out.

Many ex–gang members say there will always be gangs, because people need to feel respect, and they need the protection they get from their homies. They say the only way to get rid of gangs is to give people the opportunity to use their intelligence and talents out in the world, away from the gangs. Gus said:

> I think to hold a gang together it takes a really smart person, because there's so much anger within the gang, and to keep that away from the members within the gang, to focus it outside, or even to just tell your members to chill out and not worry about some guy talking trash to them, it takes a really born leader. So I mean there's a lot of people out there who could try and do some real good in their communities if they just had the right motivation.

Penny told us about her cousin:

> He was in a gang. Him and his brother were, but after his brother got shot, he got out and started break-dancing. So now he's in this breaking crew, and he is like a natural. He could be a professional dancer.

Tomas is eighteen. He used to be in a gang too, but when he was arrested, he was put into a violent-offenders program that has helped him sort out his feelings and explore his talents. He said:

Everybody is good at something in their life. For me, I like to do a lot of airbrushing. I'm very good at it, so that's something I like to do and I know I can do. I used to do it a long time ago, but as I got into the gangs I stopped doing it. Now I'm starting back up. But what I really want to do with my life is be a gang counselor. I want to help kids like me stay out of the gangs.

Manny's out of his gang now and trying to get work as an artist. He said:

There's a lot of kids that have so much potential that adults don't see. There's these guys in tagging crews out here spray-painting these huge murals on brick walls, and it's just amazing what they can do. Some guy with a brush that's doing abstract art that really looks just like what everyone else is doing, and they're getting paid thousands of dollars for it, when these other guys are here with all this talent and they're getting busted for it.

Lots of the people we met as we were working on this chapter had been in gangs and had been in trouble with the law at one time or another. We met them when they were trying to change their lives. They had some important things to say about what we can do to put an end to the cycle of gang violence. Tomas summed it up this way:

I would have to say that I could have used somebody that knows and has been through our experience. Somebody who could have thrown some knowledge to me. Somebody who could talk to me, who knows what he's talking about because he's been there himself. Don't wait till we get to jail to put us in a group. You put those groups in the schools. You put them everywhere in the community. And even if some kids won't come, you'll have some who do come and they'll spread it around. And hopefully the others will see and they'll come too. Everybody wants to have a productive life. They just don't know how to get it, so they see easy money in the gangs and they go for that. But easy money doesn't last, and it comes with a big price tag, which is usually your life.

Millions of children and teenagers live in violent homes and neighborhoods, are part of gangs, abuse drugs and alcohol, get in trouble with the law, and have little hope. Maybe they've been turned off to school and have no goals for themselves, except how to score more drugs or find the next party. These teens need support and new models for how life can be different. Angie got that when her mother moved her and her sister and brother to a small town away from the violence and drugs of gang life. She said:

No one can even believe that I'm going to graduate from high school. I'm the first one in my whole family. And now I'm working at this job I love. It's so great. None of my homies are into school at all. Most of them don't even take their GED. They're just going nowhere. I remember how much I didn't want to leave when my mom first told me we were going to move. But I've done so much growing up here, it's amazing. And when I go back and see my friends now, it's hard for me to even hang out with them. You know, but hey, they might think the same about me.

SEXUAL HARASSMENT

Sexual harassment is a form of abuse. Harassers frighten their victims by humiliating them or making them uncomfortable with sexual language or gestures or hostile sexual teasing, by stalking them, or by making repeated, unwelcome sexual advances toward them.* One reason such behavior happens is that males and females are taught to treat each other as objects, not as equals, which creates the environment for abuse. Eighteen-year-old Ellie had this comment:

I wasn't surprised to hear that a young man who sexually harassed me at the age of twelve raped a young woman at my university when he was eighteen. Because no one told him it was wrong to try to grab my breasts or make obscene comments and gestures toward me, he grew up

* Legally, sexual harassment in its broadest sense is any persistent, unwanted behavior of a sexual nature on the part of one person toward another.

believing it was okay to satisfy his urges and "have fun" at the expense of another human being.

Greg, an eighteen-year-old from Atlanta, said:

The problem may be that in our society, guys are generally made to think that it's okay to talk in a negative way about women, so they don't see the harm in saying "nice ass" to a girl or in telling an obscene joke. In some cases it is okay, but if it's done in a way that makes you feel bad or uncomfortable or threatened, it is sexual harassment and it is against the law.

Brady, a fifteen-year-old boy from South Carolina, agreed:

Sexual harassment is anything that makes you feel uncomfortable, about your sexuality or about sex in general. For example, wearing a shirt that says, "I like girls with big tits." How would guys like it if girls went around wearing T-shirts that said, "I like guys with big dicks." It's the same thing. It reduces you to a piece of meat. It's not who you are as a person, but who you are as a sexual object.

Many people, especially teens, are embarrassed or uncomfortable reporting or even discussing sexual harassment. They worry that people will think they are overreacting. Although sexual harassment may sometimes be expressed in a joking manner, it is not a joke, and it's not trivial if the victim is hurt or feels humiliated by the attention.

The most common form of sexual harassment is called hostile environment, when one person or a group repeatedly does something to make your home, your neighborhood, your school, or your work a difficult place to be. This form of harassment can include:

➤ Sexual comments, remarks, jokes, kidding, personal sexual questions.

➤ Posting or showing sexual pictures, posters, and cartoons.

➤ Persistent or repeated staring or leering.

➤ Repeated requests for dates or sexual activity.

➤ Cornering someone or getting very physically close to someone.

➤ Gestures, whistling, cat calls, obscene remarks.

➤ Touching, such as grabbing or brushing up against someone.

➤ Sexual innuendoes (statements that can be taken as sexual).

The second kind of sexual harassment is called quid pro quo. It can either be a threat ("If you don't go out with me or if you complain about how I treat you, I'll fail you or I'll fire you"). Or it can be bribery and promises ("If you go out with me or let me touch you, I'll reward you with a good grade, or a raise, or a promotion at work").

Sometimes the two types are combined. For example, a teacher may make sexual comments to a student or touch a student inappropriately. The student may not want to report it because he or she is worried that the teacher *might* give him or her a bad grade, even though the teacher didn't actually come out and say that. A girl who is a freshman in high school told us:

I had a teacher in junior high who, whenever I asked him a question, would put his arm around me and get real close to me. His arm would always brush against my chest, just slightly but enough so it was creepy. And one time he actually whistled when I walked into the room. After that, I didn't ask him for help or anything, because I didn't want him to get close to me. He did the same thing to a lot of other girls.

You may have had such experiences and thought they weren't a big deal. That's one of the major confusions about sexual harassment: What one person might consider harassment another person considers "normal" behavior or even a compliment. A high school girl in Arizona said:

For one person, cracking filthy jokes might be acceptable, but another person might be offended at the same thing. Especially when it doesn't stop even after you say you don't like it.

Joanna said:

Name calling is big in my school. Everybody calls each other slut or queen or hunk or fag. I don't think most people stop to think how that might hurt someone's feelings or humiliate them.

What used to be considered okay to do at one time may be seen as sexual harassment today. Erica has strong feelings about this:

There's been a lot of talk lately with cases in the news about sexual harassment being taken "too far." Should a seven-year-old boy be kicked out of school or taken to court for sexual harassment? This boy pulled a button off a girl's dress and kissed her against her will. He's not some professor demanding sexual favors from a student. He's just a little boy who doesn't know any better. So maybe instead of kicking him out of school, they should have sat him down and discussed why you can't always act on your impulses. Young boys need to be taught that while it's okay, maybe even normal, to want to touch a girl's body, it is not acceptable to do it whenever you feel like it. If nobody teaches that little boy to act differently now, what will happen in ten years, when he has the urge to have sex with a girl and she says no?

Some people excuse sexual harassment by saying "boys will be boys." But as Sarah said, "Saying 'boys will be boys' just gives them an excuse for acting without any sensitivity. Boys need to learn to act like people!"

The key to understanding whether something is sexual harassment or not is how the person *receiving* it feels. A guy may tell a girl that she's gorgeous and think it's a compliment, while she may feel very uncomfortable about how he said it. A girl might comment on a guy's muscles and think she's being friendly, while he's embarrassed or even offended.

The macho male stereotype in our culture "acts like a stud" and treats girls as sex objects. "Real men" are not supposed to seem soft or caring. In its own way, that's a form of sexual harassment, since it makes boys afraid to let their tenderness and compassion show. Blaine, an eighteen-year-old boy from Boston, said:

It's funny that you get called "gay" if you don't act like a sex maniac or you like to be friends with girls. I know a couple of football players who *are* gay, and they aren't so-called "soft" or nice. And I know plenty of hetero guys who, when you get to know them, are not tough at all. Why are we so hung up on stereotyping everybody? I wish we could just let people alone. Let them be individuals.

Girls, too, are pigeonholed and stereotyped by society. They're judged by their appearance. Many spend time and money trying to look attractive and "sexy." Then they get the message that says, "Wait a minute! Don't look too sexy or you'll just be asking for it!" It's very confusing. A ninth-grader from California told us how angry she is about the way this works:

You go to all this trouble to look good, and then some guy whistles at you and you're supposed to think it's this great compliment. Being whistled at is like being called a dog. Why can't guys just say, "Hi, how are you?" But instead they say, "Hey, baby, come on over here and I'll rub you down." Who taught them that anyway? *Hustler* magazine?

Because it happens to them so seldom, some guys think they would enjoy this kind of attention. A sixteen-year-old boy from the Southwest said:

You know some chicks thrive on getting whistled at and get a rush out of it. Just like some guys would get a rush out of being whistled at.

A young woman from Oakland, California, wrote a moving radio commentary on just this issue. It was produced by Youth Radio and aired on National Public Radio's "All Things Considered."

You think I like it, huh? The attention you give me when you drive by and shout out the window, "Hey, baby," when you come up to me and ask me for my number, when you watch me as I walk by. Well, I did like it . . . when I was twelve and the newness of being watched and looked over hadn't worn off, when I was still so young your stares made me think I was special. And when I got a little older, and was fourteen and fifteen and sixteen, I wouldn't say I liked it, but I didn't mind, because I thought that was all part of being a woman. And in my eagerness to be a woman I allowed the TV commercials, and the radio songs, and my brothers' snickering conversations about women, to assure me that the assault of your eyes was the recognition of my womanness, the price of being a woman.

But now that I'm seventeen, I know that your stares have less to do with my being a woman and a lot more to do with you being a man. See, when you look at me like that, or come up and ask me where we've met, you're not recognizing me as a woman, or more importantly, as a human being. All you see is a collection of parts—and that's all you've been taught to see when you look at me. As a man in our society, you've been taught to think of me as a pair of breasts, legs, mouth, butt. I don't blame you for the way society is, but I do hold you accountable for your participation in it, your perpetuation of it.

Looking back, I can see that those stares when I turned twelve were the beginning of your daily reduction of me to something less than the full, feeling, thinking me. It was my first step toward being a woman in our society, toward the violation that all women know at some point—in your history books, in your TV shows, in your bedrooms, and in your stares.
—Dana Michael King, age seventeen

By now you've probably figured out that one of the main issues in many sexual harassment situations is whether or not the harasser knows that what he or she is doing is bothering the other person. Sixteen-year-old Rochelle, from Boston, said:

I think that many people who sexually harass others don't understand that it's hurting them. They aren't educated about the fact that making gross comments about someone feels awful to that person. It makes you feel dirty. And maybe the person they are harassing can't tell them to stop because he or she's too embarrassed or afraid. So the person that's doing it never learns that it's hurting the other person. And so it keeps happening.

Sometimes the harasser *does* know the victim doesn't like it and does it anyway. It becomes a power trip, a way to say, "I have control over you." This type of focused harassment is hostile, threatening, and criminal. LaTerra told us about what happened to her in fifth grade:

I developed earlier than a lot of girls in my grade and boys would circle around me to keep me from getting away while they would try to feel me up. Usually I could push them away, but one time they really had me pinned in, and I started screaming for the teacher. She came running over and those boys all got detention.

Some heterosexual teens have viciously harassed their homosexual classmates. It's as if they think they have a right to harass people whose lifestyle they question. A gay teen wrote us to say:

Please make sure to mention the horrifying amount of antigay violence, gay bashing, and sexual harassment of gays that exists in our country (and the world). In my high school, students could shout out the word "gay" in the halls as an insult without being reprimanded by teachers who otherwise were vigilant against hate speech. Calling someone "gay" was just considered a general negative thing, sort of like calling someone stupid.

Anthony, eighteen, remembered:

In high school if you were found out to be gay, your life was hell, especially if you were a boy. You were harassed in the locker room, chased home after school, ambushed in the halls.

Brenda said:

In middle school I was taunted and harassed all the time. People called me a "dyke," and at that point they didn't even know I was lesbian. They just said it because I didn't date and I was smart and maybe just because it was the "in" insult. One time I even got beat up by some kids just because I had short hair.

Sexual harassment is based on ignorance, prejudice, hatred, and fear. Like racial harassment, it is a desire by one person or group to demean another because of some generalized, stereotypic ideas. Until we begin to change the way we relate to one another and dispel some of those stereotypes, we can't hope to lessen the violence around us. Shawnie explained:

We need to find a way to live with each other, to look past those prejudices. I mean, I've got to appreciate who you are if I want you to appreciate who I am.

What Can You Do to Respond to Sexual Harassment?

Sexual harassment is illegal. Under most circumstances, it can be stopped without having to take legal action, but if the harassment is hostile and persistent, you may decide to prosecute.

What *you* decide to do will depend on how the harassment occurs, how you feel about it, and who is harassing you. The best way to deal with sexual harassment is to let the harasser know that his or her actions are upsetting to you. Tell him or her face-to-face. If you are uncomfortable doing that, bring along a friend or an adult to support you and as a witness.

If the harasser is an authority figure, write him or her a letter. Include a record of when and where and how he or she harassed you. Explain that you don't like what is happening and that his or her actions or statements make you very uncomfortable. Be sure to *keep a copy* of the letter, so you can use it if the harassment doesn't stop and you decide to take legal action.

Confronting the harasser is, of course, much easier said than done! If someone makes a crude comment at school that hurts you, the most straightforward way to deal with it is to say, "I don't

like that. Cut it out." In many cases, that will be the end of it. In some situations, of course, that won't work, and it may even make the harassment worse. Gina said she was too uncomfortable to confront the boys who were harassing her, so she tried ignoring them. They didn't stop:

At first it was one or two boys joking around about what size bra I wore. Then I found myself on the school bus constantly ducking away from boys' hands trying to touch my breasts. I would get on hoping there'd be a seat near the front, because the farther back I had to walk, the more hands I had to avoid being grabbed by. It started getting to me. I couldn't concentrate anymore. My grades went from A's to barely C's.

It takes a lot of courage to try to stop harassment. That's why it's always helpful to have support from friends, classmates, people at work, or adults who might have witnessed the harassment or experi-

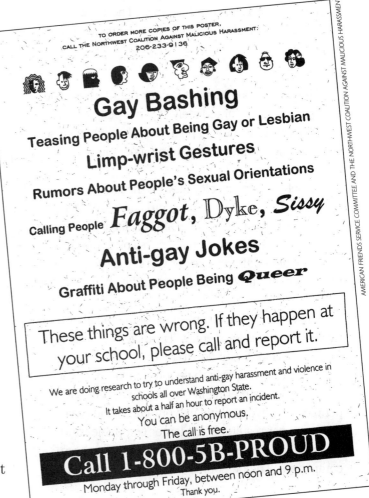

enced harassment themselves. You may be embarrassed to talk about your feelings, but doing so is better than putting up with a situation that threatens your peace of mind and could be threatening other people too.

Many victims of sexual harassment feel isolated because they think no one will believe them or no one will care. They may not want to call attention to themselves or cause trouble. They may feel they are the ones at fault or that no one will help. Gina said her teachers didn't respond to her problem:

I learned early on that when I tried to defend myself, that only escalated the situation, so I would just smile and pretend I didn't care. If only someone had said to me, You don't have to put up with this behavior, or, What is happening is wrong. Then it would have been easier to handle, but it was like even the adults tried to make me believe that just because I happened to have breasts, this was something I had to accept and live with. Like most victims, I believed that maybe I had asked for it somehow, that I deserved it because of how I looked.

You are *not* to blame. It is your right to have the harassment stop immediately. If some people you tell try to trivialize what is happening, tell someone else. Keep telling people until you find a person who will help you.

In school, a counselor may be the right person to approach for help. If you are a girl and don't feel comfortable talking to a man about this, if there is no female counselor, tell a female nurse or a friendly female teacher. If that doesn't work, tell the principal. Tell your parents. If necessary, they can go to the police.

At work, it's important to tell someone in authority about what is happening. Try to get witnesses. Keep a journal. Write down the dates, times, and types of incidents. Talk to people you know to see if anyone else is suffering in the same way. The more people you have backing up your claim, the easier it will be to get results. Some larger companies and organizations have special offices to handle these complaints. The personnel department, where you

may have filled out your application for the job, deals with sexual harassment.

If school officials or employers don't do anything after sexual harassment has been charged, they are legally responsible.

Other people may see the harassment but may be uncomfortable about saying anything. This conspiracy of silence allows sexual harassment to continue and to escalate. If you witness harassment, even if you are not the direct victim of it, break the silence by speaking up.

Taking Action

If the sexual harassment continues, or people retaliate against you for having reported it, you can complain to someone with more power than the harasser, leave the situation by quitting your job or changing schools, or pursue legal remedies. People who leave the situation figure that's the easiest and fastest way to avoid being harassed. Sometimes that's the goal of the harassment: to get you to quit or go elsewhere. Unfortunately, that means your life is disrupted, and the harasser remains free to continue his or her activities unchallenged.

The option to take legal action requires professional help. You and your parents can get a private lawyer and sue the harasser. You can go to a local women's center or a local or state gay and lesbian center, which will be able to put you in touch with a lawyer who handles harassment cases for little or no charge.

Sexual harassment is considered a form of discrimination, and most big cities or states have government departments that deal with discrimination complaints. Look in the phone book for the state department of justice or the human rights commission or the federal Equal Employment Opportunity Commission. When you call, tell the receptionist you want to file a sexual harassment complaint. If your case is of the type they handle, they may provide a lawyer.

The legal option may not be the right course of action for you. Consider it carefully and consult with an adult you can trust. It takes a lot of time, effort, and often money. If you win the case, the harasser will be punished and will think twice before creating the same problem for someone else in the future.

SEXUAL ABUSE

When anyone—an acquaintance, a friend, a relative, or a stranger—behaves toward you in a physically sexual way that hurts you or makes you afraid or uncomfortable, or if they make you behave in a physically sexual way that hurts you or makes you afraid or uncomfortable, that is sexual abuse. When that person is a close relative, we call it incest. Charlene, seventeen, explained:

> Incest is when someone from your family makes you do something in a sexual manner. In your own family! Like your father, someone related to you, someone who has power over you, and they can persuade you to do something that you don't have the capability to say yes or no to.

Sexually abusive behavior includes touching, kissing, fondling, intercourse, flashing, oral sex, and any other sexual act that is forced on you. It can appear in many different forms, like being tickled long after you beg the person to stop, or someone forcing you to have intercourse, or someone touching your breasts or your genitals without your permission, or someone getting you drunk or drugged to have sex with you while you're too out-of-it to protest. When the sexual abuse involves forced penetration of some kind, either vaginal, anal, or oral, most states call it rape. In our view, all forced sex is a kind of rape.

Sexual abusers use violence or their authority or both to exploit or control other people. By far the greatest number of abusers are heterosexual men. Many are fathers and brothers and uncles and grandfathers. Most of them know or are related to the person they abuse. In this country, one out of every three or four girls and one out of every six or seven boys is sexually molested by the time she or he turns eighteen. That's millions of people. Paula told us:

> My father started bothering me when I was like seven years old. He'd put me on his lap, and I started noticing that his thing used to get hard and he used to rub me with it. It was easy for him because my mom worked nights and we'd be

alone in the house. As I got older, whenever he wanted to touch me, he touched me.

Marilu had this experience:

> My father would give me kisses just like I was his wife or something. He used to stick his tongue all the way in my mouth. I wanted to throw up, but I was too scared.

Elisha said:

> Sexual abuse is like crossing the line in a sexual way. You feel an alarm go off inside you, and you don't feel good about it.

Given Elisha's definition, it's easy to see that sexual abuse can happen to anyone, female or male, adult or child. Billy remembered the abuse he experienced as a child:

> There was this guy who my mom had babysit me when I was little, and he used to make me put his dick in my mouth. I was only like four or something, and I didn't know how to stop him. I used to cry to my mom, "I don't like John." But I guess he was the only babysitter she knew, because he kept being my sitter.

And Greg said:

> My mother always wants me to give her massages. Like she'll be lying on the bed and she'll be all in her underwear, and she'll tell me how tense she is and how she needs me to rub her back, and mostly it's okay with me, but it got weird a couple of times when she made me massage around her chest. Guys are supposed to be all hot to get their hands on a girl's chest, but you better believe it, not when it's your mother.

Children and teens who suffer sexual abuse at home feel betrayed. Whom can they trust if not their own family? Where can they be safe if not in their own home?

Elizabeth said she was sexually abused over many years. She was terrified to stay home from school when she was sick, because she knew that meant she would be alone with her father, who worked nights:

> One day when I had such a bad stomachache, I had to go home from school, and he was there of course. He told me he was going to make me feel better. He made me lie down on top of him, and he was hugging me and rubbing me all over. And I prayed to God for him to stop, so I said, I feel much better now. But he said, No, no, no. Just a little while longer.

Marly told us how afraid she was of her brother:

> My brother used to force me to lie on his bed, and he'd climb on top of me and put his thing between my legs and hump on me. When he was done, he'd hit me and tell me he'd kill me if I ever told. I was so young I never did tell, because I was really scared. My mother was always out of it on some kind of drugs or booze or something. She probably wouldn't have done anything anyway.

When Andrea was growing up she lived in a big house in a fancy neighborhood. Her friends all thought she was so lucky and had the best family in the world. Here is her story:

> From the time I was eight years old till I was fourteen, when he died, my dad used to come into my bedroom almost every night. At first he'd come in while I was sound asleep and lay next to me. I would wake up startled. But he would say soothing things and stroke me and tell me it was okay. Then after a while he'd come in and lie on top of me. I felt like I was going to suffocate. Pretty soon I couldn't fall asleep at all because I'd know that he was going to come. I used to lay there with my eyes wide open and listen for his footsteps. It was always the same thing. When I got older, he'd actually rape me and I'd just lie there like a zombie, praying that he'd finish and leave me alone. But I couldn't sleep. I don't know how I made it through six years without sleeping.

> When he died and everybody was all crying and sad, I couldn't even pretend to cry. All I could think was, I'm free.

Child molesters generally spend time getting their victims ready for abuse. Psychologists call this "grooming the victim." The molester may leave pornographic magazines out in the open for you to discover, or he may watch sexually explicit movies with you around. All of this is intended to get you more comfortable viewing adult bodies and seeing adult sexual situations. In families, a molester might walk in on you while you're taking a bath or on the toilet. You might feel uncomfortable, but then you might think, Well, this is a family member, and it's okay to be undressed or on the toilet with a family member around. If the abuser is a neighbor, he may ask you to bring him something while he's in the bathroom, or he may take a shower and come out with just a towel wrapped around him. The molester may say he is going to teach you about sex so you won't get into trouble, or so you'll know what to expect. That's what happened to Skye:

> When I was twelve, my father told me I was old enough, and he was going to teach me sex education so I wouldn't do anything stupid with anybody. He made me take my clothes off, and he was touching my breasts and he was touching my private parts and he asked me where do I feel the most. I was so ashamed I couldn't talk.

The idea is to blur the boundaries of personal privacy, so you aren't clear anymore what is right and what isn't. A fourteen-year-old girl from Maine said:

> When I was about nine years old, my stepdad's brother gave me a short little nightie for my birthday. A couple of weeks later when he was babysitting me, he asked me to "model" the nightie for him. Then he asked me to dance for him in it. It kind of became a routine whenever he'd babysit, and he said, "This can be our special secret." One time he brought a video of a woman who took off her clothes while she was dancing, and he asked me if I'd do that for him. I told my mom what I'd done, and she freaked out.

That was the last time I saw him alone, but now I realize that he was trying to get me ready to have sex with him, and if my mom hadn't stepped in, he probably would have.

Often molesters play games with their potential victims before they begin the abuse: card games, hide-and-seek games, tickling games, show-and-tell games, all of which may eventually lead to the molester suggesting that the person who loses has to take off some articles of clothing, or touch some part of the other person's body. Since most kids make the assumption, at least at first, that an adult wouldn't intentionally hurt them, especially an adult who seems so nice, they go along. Then by the time the adult actually begins the abuse, the child has been primed to accept it as part of the play and isn't sure whether he or she has a clear right to protest.

For children and teens who are repeatedly sexually abused by an older person they know—a relative, family friend, neighbor, teacher, coach, or counselor— the situation is always fraught with guilt and shame as well as fear. They feel confused about whether what happened was their fault. Fourteen-year-old Jeannie said:

> You feel guilty if it keeps happening, because you feel like it's your fault. You ask yourself, What am I doing to make him do this? And if you didn't tell

anybody about it in the beginning, you feel even more guilty, like how could you ever tell somebody now, after all this time? But you're afraid to tell, because you don't know what will happen to you.

Carmen is devoutly religious. She said that after repeated sexual abuse, she felt guilt that she was committing a sin. When she got older and was able to discuss her abuse with others, she came to this conclusion: the victim is *not* to blame:

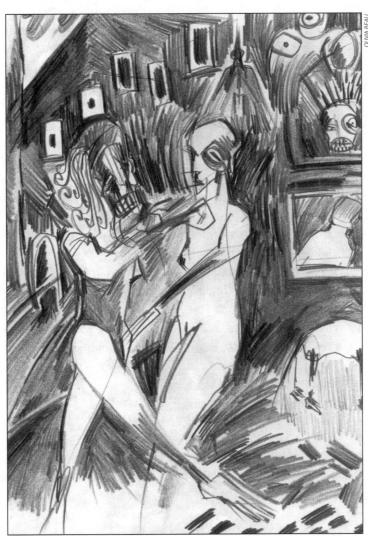

OLMA BEALL

> I believe this so strongly. Because of my personal experience I can say that this is the only mortal sin that you aren't guilty of. You can't be blamed for this sin. It wasn't your fault.

Many teens have reported feeling especially confused if the abuser is gentle, if he (or she) uses encouraging words and soft touches to get what he wants. Perhaps in the case of a father, he may be strict and gruff at other times and only tender when he is relating to you sexually. Twenty-year-old Jenny explained that her father tried not to hurt her, which in many ways made the abuse more insidious:

> Sometimes you feel guilty, because unfortunately sometimes there is physical enjoyment. And I'm not saying that you participate willingly or anything, or that you consent to it, but you find yourself thinking, God, he touched me there and it

felt nice. I mean, we're not plants, we're human, and we might react that way. It's sad, because then you say to yourself, *he's* not doing anything wrong. I'm doing something wrong, because I'm enjoying this. Then it screws you up to be able to enjoy it with someone you really love, because you feel like you shouldn't enjoy it.

David, twenty-two, remembers feeling very confused and ashamed:

My mom left when I was ten, and my dad was very bummed out and would want to come into my room while I was getting ready for bed, and then he'd lie down next to me and fall asleep on my bed. Sometimes I'd wake up in the night and he'd be there with his hand on me rubbing me and with his other hand he'd be beating off. I was like in this dreamy space and it felt good. Except I knew it was really weird.

Sexual acts can feel good even if they are forced on you. That's not because you are bad or because your body has betrayed you, it's because your body is *made* to be responsive to sexual stimulation. Girls and boys who have been raped or abused sometimes feel ashamed because their bodies responded in a sexual way. They blame themselves for feeling stimulated. But they are not to blame. The rapist is to blame. The rapist is the offender.

Many people who have been sexually abused say it is very hard for them to learn to feel comfortable again in a sexual situation. They tighten up and feel afraid, even with someone they love. Christina said:

I've seen fathers that touch their little girls in certain ways, like supposedly they're playing with you. And when you're younger, you don't really think about it, but when you get older, you start feeling strange about it. And when you try to be with a guy and he touches you there too, you want to pull away.

Bridget had this experience:

At the beginning, whenever I would have a boyfriend, I would see my father's face. If we were

kissing, I would picture my father's face, and it would be bad.

David said:

The hardest thing for me is being able to feel worthwhile in a relationship with a woman. Sex feels somehow shabby and contrived, and I can't get my brain to stop picturing my father.

Because they have been hurt so badly by someone they thought they could trust, many people who have been abused learn to distrust others. Lahkia said:

Sexual abuse has affected me in every way. It got me to a point where I just wanted to be by myself, definitely didn't trust anybody, didn't talk to anybody. It made me really depressed. I got to a point where I wanted to end it all. I didn't feel like I had anything to live for anymore. And then to think about starting a new relationship, you're afraid that that person might do the same thing to you.

Bouts of depression or insomnia plague some victims of abuse. Cleo said:

I don't sleep at night. I have nightmares where I think somebody's in the house to get me. So I don't sleep. I'm up all night.

Elisha told us:

I was having a lot of nightmares. Sometimes, yeah, it was clear. I mean, I could see him in my dreams. But sometimes it wasn't clear. It was like monsters would appear, and I would be trying to get away. I was hurting myself a lot too. I was thinking about committing suicide most of the time, and I used to get a pin and slash my legs just without thinking. I was just mad, and I didn't know how to express it.

If you have been abused, you may develop fears of going out alone, of being in strange places or in isolated areas, of being around people you don't know, or even of being home in your own bed. You may suffer from depression and avoid relationships, or you may repeatedly choose to be in relationships with people who hurt you, because that's what feels familiar to you. If you have children, you may feel especially protective of them and not want to let anyone else help you take care of them.

Healing Yourself

You *can* heal the emotional wounds caused by sexual abuse—with a lot of support, professional help, and hard work. It is definitely worth the effort. Many girls and boys say they feel so ashamed of what has happened, they don't want anyone else to know about it. But remember: *You are not to blame.* Whether it was your father or your brother or someone else you know, by telling, you will be helping to stop the person who molested you from doing it again to you or a younger sister or brother or anyone else.

Keeping others from being abused is the reason many people decide to open up about what is happening to them. But the primary reason to tell is to help yourself begin to heal. The healing process begins the moment you agree to talk about your experience and express your fears and anger. The more you talk about it, scream about it, cry about it with someone trained to help, the less likely it is to tie you up inside throughout your life.

If you are being abused within your family, it will affect family relationships whether or not you tell anyone about it. Not telling leaves you feeling alone, confused, and continually in danger. Like Elisha, you may take your hurt and angry feelings out against yourself, or you may get angry with the people around you all the time. You may fight with your parents or your sisters and brothers to the point where no one wants to be near you. Heidi is seventeen. She attends a sexual-abuse group at her local hospital community center, where they helped her talk about her anger:

> I used to go off on everybody about everything. Now I don't lose my temper so much anymore. Now I'm more open. I can talk about the rape and get mad about that but not take it out on everybody else.

Many abusers threaten their victims to keep them from talking about what happened. You may be afraid that if you do tell, the abuser will do something to hurt you or other people you care about. If the abuser is your father, you may worry that he will be taken away and arrested, leaving your family without a father and your mother without a husband. If the abuser is your only parent, it can be even more frightening. You may worry that you'll be left alone.

These are real concerns, but in order for you to begin to heal, your situation must change. You don't have to live in constant fear, and you don't have to live in an abusive household. One day sixteen-year-old Gloria decided she had had enough. She told her favorite teacher at school about the abuse she had been experiencing for three years. The teacher helped Gloria find support within her family and helped her prosecute the abuser. Gloria felt so empowered by her actions that she started a referral service for other teens in her area who had also experienced abuse.

If you decide you've had enough but don't know whom to tell or how to proceed, look in the Resource section at the back of this chapter (page 241). We list some excellent books and resources to help you.

Whom to Tell?

Whom you tell will depend on your age, your relationship with your family and friends, and your particular sexual-abuse experience. Leticia said:

> It's good to tell someone, even though you feel scared. Nobody taught me anything about sex, but once it happened, I just felt it was wrong, so I went to my mother to tell her. I couldn't confront my uncle myself, because I was embarrassed. I was only eleven, and even though I thought it would be embarrassing to tell my mother, she got so mad at that guy, it worked out good for me. I felt a lot better in the end.

Joanna said:

> It feels like a relief to tell someone. My grandfather was the one I told. When it happened, he was there for me. He trusted me. Even though

nobody else wanted to believe me, he knew I wasn't lying.

Unfortunately, some family members may not be prepared to hear the information you are giving them. They may, for their own reasons, be unwilling to believe you, especially when the perpetrator is a relative or close family friend. Patricia said:

I was living with my aunt and uncle, and when I told my aunt that my uncle was doing it to me, she didn't believe me. She said I wanted to take her husband away from her and that I was an ungrateful child. I felt like I was betrayed, and I felt useless, in every sense of the word. I didn't have anywhere to go or anyone to turn to.

Gretchen faced the same problem:

My mother didn't believe me. Lots of mothers don't. They just close their eyes and say, No, that didn't happen. It's called denial. But you have to tell somebody else if that happens. Don't give up! Keep telling somebody until somebody believes you. You have to be strong.

Gretchen told her aunt, and her aunt did believe her. Together, they were able to convince her mother about the abuse. Her father moved out, and the family is now in counseling together.

If you are close with your family, tell a parent or a sister or a brother. Tell an aunt, an uncle, a grandparent, or some other relative or close family friend. You can speak with a school counselor, a trusted teacher, a friend, or the parents of a friend. Assistance is available at local hospitals, clinics, social service agencies, mental health centers, churches, temples, teen centers, or the police. Call the Nine Line (1-800-999-9999). Look on page 241 for more information. You have no reason to feel ashamed. It is the abuser who should feel ashamed.

If you are young and have no close family to help you get away from the abuse, a professional may be assigned by the state to step in. In most cases, they'll separate you from the abuser by removing the abuser or finding you a safe place to live with another relative or family friend, or in a foster home.

Fifteen-year-old Lanita found help from a social worker at her local clinic. She said:

When I told her about what my father was doing to me, she started asking around and found a place for me at my aunt and uncle's house. My mother didn't want my father to move out, so the best thing was for me to move out.

The idea is to find a *safe* haven. If you end up in a situation that is *not* safe, be sure to let some trusted adult know right away.

Many teens decide to run away from abusive situations. This is not a good solution. Running away usually leads to homelessness and more violence. Mindy told us her story:

Things were really bad at home, and I couldn't take it, so I went to stay with my aunt, but she couldn't keep me, so I was basically staying with a friend of my cousin at his house, which was not the greatest house in the world. I got into drugs and some other heavy shit. I met a guy there, and we took off together, but then he got killed. Right in front of me. A drive-by. So I can definitely say, Trying to run away from your problems just creates more problems. The problems won't go away just because you do.

If you are so desperate you are considering running away, call the Nine Line, 1-800-999-9999, and ask for help.

Long-Term Help

Therapy provides many of us with a safe place to talk about our feelings. A good therapist will believe you and understand your experience. This may be a huge relief if you have been carrying your anger and shame alone. See page 174 for suggestions on how to find a good therapist.

Many people who have been sexually abused join treatment groups in which all the participants have been abused. These support groups allow people to share their feelings and experiences with one another. Eleanor said talking about the abuse with others who have been through similar experiences helped her a great deal:

> The first time and second time and third time I went, I felt like I could hardly hold back my sobs, but now I'm feeling like I can contribute, like I can give something back to someone else who needs help. It feels good.

Reina, in the same group, said:

> I've accomplished a lot because of this group. Before I started coming, I was not going to school. Now I have my GED. I'm enrolled in college. I have learned how to say, "No more," and I'm not in an abusive relationship anymore. That's a big accomplishment!

Luis ran away from his home because he was being sexually abused by his uncle. He called the Nine Line and found out about a shelter for teen runaways in his area:

> They help you put yourself back together here. In group, everybody has been through it too, so they listen to what you have to say and know what you're feeling. There's no bias here. Everybody's equal.

RAPE

Rape is any sexual activity forced on another person. Legally, it is commonly defined as forced sexual activity, committed against a person's will, that involves some kind of sexual penetration. Many of the teens who spoke in the previous section were raped repeatedly; what we will discuss in this section is a more sudden and unexpected type of sexual attack.

We tend to think of rape as a surprise attack on a woman in a dark alley, in an unlit park, or on an isolated street late at night. Some rape does happen that way, but most rapes are committed by people who know their victims. These "acquaintance rapes" happen on dates, at parties, at home, in broad daylight, and at night. They are most often committed by men, but rape has also been committed by women.

When the rapist is a boy or a man and the victim is his female friend or date, they are acting out the worst stereotypes of men and women. The man is taught that he is "supposed" to be aggressive and dominant, "supposed" to be sexually powerful and demanding. The woman, on the other hand, is taught that she is "supposed" to be coy and shy and passive; she must learn to flirt and be sexually attractive to men but not let them get "too far." Karen, sixteen, had this experience:

> My boyfriend raped me. When I told my best friends, they kind of acted like it wasn't that serious because he was my boyfriend. And I thought, You're wrong. It shouldn't matter if he was my boyfriend or not; I said no and I told him I didn't want to, and he did it anyway. He forced it on me.

Mike told us what happened to his sixteen-year-old cousin:

> She was dating this guy because her parents liked him—a good churchgoing guy, you know—and they were like, "Stay with him, he's perfect for you." And the guy ends up raping her.

A lot of boys have grown up hearing that they have a right to sex and that girls don't really mean no when they say it. Boys are made to feel that they have to pressure girls into having sex to maintain a "macho," "real man" image. In the case of incest rape, some fathers, brothers, and uncles consider the young women in their family "theirs for the taking." Many girls feel powerless and afraid to object; if they do object, they are often overpowered by the rapist.

Sixteen-year-old Amanda was raped at a party:

> I went to a party with a friend of a friend all the way on the other side of town, and I didn't know where I was. I got really wasted. Somebody must have slipped something into my beer, because I couldn't even move. So I went into the bedroom to lie down. And some guy came in and saw that I was totally out of it, so he came over and ripped off my clothes and raped me. When I would try to scream, he would cover my mouth. Nobody could hear me,

because the stereo was so loud. Finally, this guy's brother heard me screaming and came in and beat up his brother. I didn't tell anyone about it for a year, because I thought it was my fault, that I must have done something to deserve it.

Sexual assault is *never* the fault of the victim. You may feel that had you dressed differently or said no more forcefully or not gotten drunk or not gone to that party or not walked down that street, you wouldn't have been raped. Your abuser may try to blame you by saying he couldn't help himself because you looked so sexy. But the truth is, whether you were dressed in a sexy way or not, whether your actions were foolish or not, the person who raped you used his or her power to violate your body. This person committed an act of physical assault against you. You are not to blame. The rapist is to blame.

Rapists are cowards. Most are full of anger and self-hate. Their values are mixed-up and so are their feelings about sexuality. They often come from families in which they themselves were beaten or humiliated or sexually abused as children and were never able to get proper help.

Rapists don't think of sex as a loving act between two equal partners. Instead they generally choose victims whom they can overpower with physical force, weapons, or drugs. Some use verbal manipulation or "sweet talk." They have all sorts of lines to win their victims over. When you are drunk or stoned, you are in an especially weak position. You are not in control, and this leaves you vulnerable to attack. All drugs interfere with your ability to protect yourself. Some are so potent that even one dose can make you lose control.

There are stories about people secretly slipping drugs into someone's drink without his or her knowledge. Here's what Hannah described:

> I've been telling all my friends to be very wary about accepting drinks from anyone you don't know or trust a lot, because people are being slipped this sedative called a "roofie" and then raped. One seventeen-year-old I know was having dinner with friends, and the next thing she knew it was ten hours later and she was waking up in a strange hotel room. She has no idea what

happened to her. I say get your own drink when you're at a party.

Whether he uses drugs and alcohol, brute force and anger, or sweet talk and manipulation, a rapist's goal is to exploit his victim for his own ends. His act is an act of violence. It has nothing to do with sex, except that he uses sex as his weapon.

> *I have killed you a thousand times inside.*
> *I have gotten my revenge safely.*
> *I have seen the good in people,*
> *and the bad,*
> *but I can see no good in you.*
> *There are animals*
> *that are more human than you.*
> *Have you once thought back and regret-*
> *ted a thing?*
> *Probably not.*
> *I have killed you a thousand times inside.*
> *But you haven't died in my mind.*
> *It is a fine scar you have left on me;*
> *inside and out.*
> *I have killed you a thousand times inside.*
> *Please die.*
>
> —*Anonymous*

Why Do People Get Raped?

Anyone can get raped. It doesn't seem to matter whether you are young or old, rich or poor, short or tall, flashy or conservative. Grandmothers have been raped; babies have been raped. Boys have been raped, and many, many girls have been raped. There are some situations that are definitely more dangerous than others, however. Mikala was in one of those situations:

> I was staying with this guy I had met over the phone. That was stupid, I know, but I didn't have anywhere else to stay. Everybody was drinking and doing drugs and everything, and I was tired, so I went into one of the bedrooms to lie down. Well, this guy comes into the room, turns off the light, and locks the door. He points this gun at me with the red light right on my chest. And I was

scared out of my mind. So I pick up a pillow and put it over my chest like that would protect me, and I'm like, What are you doing? What are you doing? And he ordered me to take off my clothes and do what he said. He made me perform oral sex with him, and he told me he would beat me up if I told anybody.

There's not much you can do in a situation like that except just go along with what the guy tells you to do. You don't want to resist, because if you resist, then you're going to end up either being beat up or being dead. It's hard to say what to do. I say, the best thing is to *not* let yourself get into a situation like that if you can help it.

What to Do If You Have Been Raped

After a rape, you'll probably feel like going home and taking a hot shower and trying to forget the whole thing. You may want to be alone, to cry, to think, to try to erase the experience from your mind. But if you have been raped, you need immediate help.

First, and most important, you must get yourself to a safe place with a safe companion. If your family or friends are comforting and compassionate, ask one of them to come get you or be with you. If the rape was committed by a family member, find some other relative or friend who will help you get away from him or her.

Some rape victims call the police right away. The police will come to you and, if you are hurt, will take you to the hospital. They will ask you questions about the incident to help find and charge the rapist. But once you call the police, they will make some choices for you. If you want more control of the situation or if you are afraid to call the police because you are stoned or in any other way compromised, call a rape-crisis advocate before you call the police.

Most major urban areas in the United States have rape hot lines listed in the white pages of the phone book under RAPE, or you can ask for the number from directory assistance. Rape-crisis workers are trained to give you information and help you deal with your immediate needs. They will be supportive and caring. Many centers send people to be with you and support you as you go through the hospital and police proceedings. You may be crying and angry and

What You Can Do to Minimize Your Chances of Being Raped

Here's what a group of teens suggested about how to avoid getting raped:

➤ Don't walk alone on poorly lit streets at night.

➤ Don't walk alone or in small groups through parks or alleys, especially at night.

➤ If you feel that someone is following you, cross the street and walk fast.

➤ Don't go out with strangers; don't give strangers your address; don't arrange a private meeting with anyone you meet on the Internet.

➤ Don't get drunk or stoned in situations where you don't know and trust the people you are with.

➤ Don't go out at night if you don't have a safe way to get back home.

➤ *Be direct* about what you do want and what you don't want from any sexual situation.

➤ Don't hitchhike! *Ever!* No matter how many times you have been lucky, remember that many boys and girls have been sexually assaulted and murdered when they were thumbing rides.

➤ Take a self-defense workshop on rape prevention. Learning what you can do to protect yourself will help increase your self-confidence in a potential rape or assault situation.

➤ Don't let anyone you don't know into your home without checking their ID.

➤ When you're out on a first date or a blind date, tell someone you trust where you're going and whom you're going with and when you'll be home.

➤ Don't be alone with anyone in a house or apartment unless you know them well and trust them.

Even if you don't think you are doing anything too risky, however, and even if you are with someone you know and like, rape can still happen. The following is an excerpt from a story one teenager wrote about her experience with rape.

A Dream Guy, a Nightmare Experience

We didn't go to the same schools, but he lived in the neighborhood and was always hanging around. I used to see him in the morning, before school. He was about sixteen, kind of tall, with short, dark hair, and the most beautiful gray eyes I've ever seen. He'd say hi when he saw me, and even though I didn't really know him, I started to like him. Occasionally, I'd stop and talk to him—nothing too personal. We talked about the movies we'd seen, music, and stuff like that. I began to look forward to our little talks and was disappointed when I didn't see him around the school. I was thirteen at the time.

One day, after school, he was waiting for me. . . . When I said goodbye to my friend, I walked slowly to the end of my block. "Hello," he called out to me. I turned, slowly, and smiled at him. . . . He carried my books, and we talked all the way to the train station. When we arrived, he asked if he could have my phone number. I was so excited that I gave it to him without any hesitation.

He called that night. We talked for at least two hours. The next time I saw him, he walked me to the train station again, and we talked some more. Then he kissed me goodbye. It was just a small kiss, but it made me feel wonderful. I was convinced he was a great guy.

We were "boyfriend and girlfriend" for a grand total of five days. He called me and we saw each other throughout the week. Then, after school on Friday, he was waiting for me in our usual meeting place, on the corner by the schoolyard. He said he wanted to take me someplace special that afternoon. I was thrilled. I thought maybe we would go to the movies or something. "But first," he said, "we have to stop by my house for a minute."

It was a pretty big apartment, but it looked like it hadn't been cleaned in years. He brought me into the kitchen and got a glass of water. Then we went into the living room and sat on a sofa with the stuffing coming out of it. He told me to leave my books on the floor. Then he turned on the television and shut off all the lights and said, "We'll go in a minute. I'm tired. I want to rest for a second. Sit down with me." So I did.

We sat in the darkness and watched TV for a while. I asked him where his aunt and his brother were. He stared at me with those eyes and replied, "Out," plain and simple. He was acting kind of weird, but I didn't want to say anything, because I thought he might get mad or something. He took my hand and started to kiss me. At first it was kind of nice. But then he started getting too aggressive, putting his hands in places they didn't belong.

I remember thinking to myself, "This doesn't feel right. What's he doing?" I started getting scared and told him to stop. But he didn't. I tried pushing him away, but I was too small. He was a lot bigger than me. He forced himself on top of me and pulled my pants down. No matter how much I struggled, he wouldn't let up. He held me down by the shoulders and raped me. I was crying and screaming, "No! Stop! Please stop!" But he wouldn't. Exhausted from crying and trying to get him off me, I stared into the blackness, tears sliding off my cheeks.

It all happened very fast. As soon as I could, I fixed my pants, tried to wipe the tears away, and got the hell out of there. I walked the eight blocks to the train station and waited for the train in a daze. I kept telling myself that it didn't really happen, that it couldn't really happen—not to me. . . .

It happened almost three years ago, but I still think about it as though it were yesterday. I have to stop asking myself if it was my fault, if I "asked for it." It wasn't my fault, I didn't ask for it. I had no control over the situation. The only thing I did wrong was wait so long to get help.

Rape is a horrible thing, I know that now. You have to be aware. You have to be careful. It can happen to anyone. And yes, you can be raped by someone you know. One minute you're watching TV, riding along in a car, getting help with homework. The next minute you're fighting to get away, gasping for breath, staring off into the blackness. If it does happen to you, remember, it's not your fault. Tell someone fast. Get help. It'll really make a difference later on.

—Anonymous*

---

*Reprinted with permission in excerpted form from *New Youth Connections* (a newspaper by teens, for teens), copyright © 1994 by Youth Communication. For more information write to Youth Communication, 144 W. 27th St., Suite 8R, New York, NY 10001.

feeling powerless. Having someone to advocate for you is desirable and comforting. It's especially helpful to have someone who is knowledgeable about rape proceedings.

Rape victims need prompt medical attention. If you are a female who could become pregnant, by getting to a hospital or clinic within seventy-two hours, you may have the option of receiving an emergency birth control treatment to help eliminate the possibility of pregnancy (see page 309). Also, because sexually transmitted diseases are epidemic, you should be tested and treated for STDs. Some STDs take time to show up on a test. Ask the doctor when these tests should be scheduled to give the most accurate readings (see Chapter 9, beginning on page 253). Rape victims who are planning to prosecute the rapist or at least want that option may need physical evidence of the rape. This evidence, like hair or semen or blood samples, must be collected as soon as possible after the attack, before you shower or clean up in any way. For all these reasons, it is a good idea to get to a hospital emergency room or doctor's office as soon as you can.

Many large hospitals have someone on staff—a nurse, a doctor, or a patient advocate—who knows about rape. If she is available, she will talk to you about your experience, help you deal with your emotions and fears, and tell you what options you have. Rape victims sometimes feel that the police and hospital staff are critical of them for being raped. Because of this potential insensitivity, rape-crisis counselors suggest going with a rape advocate (from a rape-crisis center) when you report the rape.

If you cannot find a local rape-crisis phone number, you can call the Rape, Abuse, Incest National Network at 1-800-656-HOPE (4673). This is a toll-free call. A counselor will answer your call and switch you to a crisis center in your area. You can also call the Nine Line at 1-800-999-9999. This free, twenty-four-hour hot line offers resources and referrals all over the United States. They may be able to direct you to a safe place. Perry, fourteen, a boy who lives in Southern California, said:

I ran away after my brother raped me. When I told my dad, he just laughed and called me a fag. I didn't have any place to go, but I saw this sign for the Nine Line, so I called them, and they turned me on to the Children of the Night shelter.* It's a good place. They're helping me get my life together.

Rape is a terrifying experience that can be hard to forget without the help of a support group or counselor. A rape-crisis center can offer assistance and information, and it can direct you to a support group to join. Darla said:

After I was raped I couldn't go out with a guy at all. It took me about a year to get to where I could trust any guy. I started going to this group of other people who were raped, and that helped a lot. Just knowing that everyone there understood what I was going through. That helped.

Deciding to Prosecute

Deciding whether or not to take legal action against someone who has raped you can be tricky. Maybe you know the person or are afraid of hurting someone or of getting hurt again yourself. People who work with rape victims often encourage them to prosecute, because it is a way of doing something active about the problem of rape in our society. It is also a way to organize your emotions and give you an outlet for your angry feelings. Friends and family may offer advice about whether to prosecute, but you will need to make your own decision.

The sooner you start the proceedings by reporting the rape, the more details you will remember from the experience. Your description of the rapist, if he was a stranger to you, will help the police locate him, and although you may think you'll never forget his face or his appearance, time has a way of distorting images and erasing details.

The law says that you can report a rape up to three years after the incident occurred. Here is what Amanda told us about her decision to prosecute:

* Children of the Night is a twenty-four-bed shelter in the Los Angeles area that offers food, counseling, and a place to stay for abused teenagers. The shelter provides a twenty-four-hour hot line service (1-800-551-1300) to help sexually exploited teens get off the streets. See the Resource section at the end of this chapter for more information.

The sad truth is that rape is all too common in our society. But there are many other countries and cultures in which rape is not at all common. We came across a letter from an American woman who was visiting Leh, a small city in northern India. In it she describes how that culture responded to the crime of rape*:

A thirteen-year-old girl from Leh was raped by an Indian Army soldier/driver. NOTHING LIKE THIS—NO RAPE—HAD EVER OCCURRED HERE. In response, all the shops immediately shut down. This was around 2 P.M. There was talk of the shops being closed the next day too, and of a demonstration. I have no idea how the word got around since hardly anyone has a telephone. But that evening we heard that the women of the village where the girl lives were planning to meet the following morning to decide whether to walk in protest. When we arrived at the meeting place, already at least 100 people were gathered, and the men were making signs and a truck with a loudspeaker and banners that read: "NO ARMY IN CIVILIAN AREAS—ARMY GO HOME—SHAME, SHAME." The other two Western women and I were incredibly moved, as you can imagine, to see this kind of solidarity and community spirit. But this was only the beginning. Soon all the teachers and students from the largest school in town came down the road. Then came women carrying black cloth flags on sticks. We walked with the women, behind the school children, and as we walked more and more people joined us, including many students from the government schools. The women were shouting, "Shame, Shame" all the way. When we got to the polo field, there were at least 2,000 people gathered.

One of my friends who knows their language spoke to the crowd and explained that we were crying because in our countries rapes happen every minute of every day and no one does anything about it.

The people here understood that if they did not protest, it would happen again, and they were saying NO to that. It's quite a political commentary on the difference between our industrialized, "modernized" world and a so-called "primitive," underdeveloped society. Which would YOU choose?

*From Dot Fisher-Smith, as printed in *Clear Actions*, May 1997, a newsletter published by Peace House, Ashland, Oregon 97520.

About two years after I was raped, I finally decided to report the guy who raped me. Before that I was too afraid, too ashamed, and I didn't want to go through the hassle. I also thought nothing would come of it. Going down to the police station was really scary. I had to give a description of the guy, and I had to tell the story in detail. It was hard to do, and it was hard to remember all the little nitpicky things they wanted to know, but I'm glad I did it. Now that he's in jail, I'm really glad I did it.

Not all cases brought before the prosecutor are tried, however. Once the rapist is identified, it may depend on whether the prosecuting attorney thinks there's enough evidence to win. Beth said:

You know, you're more likely to get convicted for smoking weed than you are for committing rape. And even if you end up having to go to jail, rapists can end up with shorter sentences than someone who stole a stereo. It kind of makes you wonder where our values are in this country.

Speak with a counselor at a rape-crisis center before starting legal proceedings. She or he will help you sort through all the pros and cons of taking this step.

WHAT CAN YOU DO WHEN YOUR FRIENDS ARE GETTING HURT?

The teenagers who helped us with this chapter said it's hard to know what to do when someone you care about is in trouble. A friend tells you something in confidence and makes you promise to keep it a secret, but what she said shows you that she needs help. Or someone's boyfriend hits her, but she keeps seeing him anyway. Or you notice a friend's bruises and how he's acting depressed, but he refuses to say anything's wrong. Loreen asked:

What do you do if your friend keeps getting abused by his mom? My friend has a broken arm because his mom slammed the door on his arm on purpose to keep him from going out. She goes ballistic all the time, but he doesn't want to do anything about it. He says he doesn't want to cause trouble for his mom, and he doesn't want to move out. He keeps saying it will get better, that she's been like this before and it's always gotten better. I think he's just staying for his little brother's sake. I feel like I should do something.

Loreen let her friend know that she was concerned about him. She cared enough to tell him she was worried, even at the risk of appearing nosy and losing his friendship.

Intervention is when people step in to try to make a problem situation better. Teens say knowing when and how to intervene is the hard part. Is the situation serious enough to require intervention? Whom should you tell? And what do you do when the person you're trying to help tells you you're completely off base? Julie said:

My friend's boyfriend controls her. He doesn't let her go out without him, so no one ever sees her. I called her up and insisted we get together without Tim. She was real weird all evening, and I could tell she wanted to leave as soon as she could. The next day, Tim came to my job and started screaming at me that I was a dyke, a bitch who was trying to take his girlfriend away from him. He told me she said I tried to kiss her. I looked right into his eyes, trying to tell him he was all wrong, but it was like there wasn't anybody in there. Luckily, I was at work, so other people walked over and he left. But now what do I do? I'm really afraid for Jenny. Obviously, she isn't ready to leave him, so what can her friends do? Just wait till he dumps her, or kills her, or what?

Lots of teens say they want to do something to help a friend who's in trouble, but they don't exactly know how to pull it off. Gabriella, a fourteen-year-old from Idaho, said:

My friend's father was sexually abusing her for years, and now that she's living in foster care she was trying to take him to court. But he's a big man in town, and he keeps getting the trial postponed. It's been over two

years now. A bunch of us were talking one night, after the trial got postponed again; we wanted to go put a big sign in his yard "Child Abuser. Child Rapist." But we were afraid of getting caught, so we didn't do it.

Narnie, sixteen, told us this story:

My friend Carletta drinks all the time and then she gets really mad at her baby. So when I had a party, I decided it had to be no alcohol, because I didn't want her getting drunk. But she got really pissed at me, so I gave in. Now I'm mad at myself because it looks like I'm saying it's okay that she drinks, and it isn't okay at all. Especially because I'm really worried about her baby.

John decided he had to intervene:

My friend Lisa was heavy into drugs and just going completely downhill. I didn't know how to help her. You couldn't talk to her about it, so I thought a lot about what to do, and I decided the only way to get her to stop would be to tell her parents exactly what was going on. They, of course, freaked out and put her in a detox program, and she got better. She stopped using and has really gotten her life together. But she hates me for telling. She calls me a "narc." I really miss her friendship, but I would do it again if I had to. She was killing herself, and I couldn't have lived with myself if she had died of an overdose.

Abusive situations thrive on secrecy. Whether someone is abusing himself or herself with drugs or alcohol, or whether one person is abusing another, the violence and self-destruction will only stop if they are brought into the open. Unfortunately, most people don't want to talk about the bad things they're experiencing. Nina said she's learned to approach her friends with a bit of diplomacy:

It's way better to talk about something real that happened to start with—like "I heard you smashed the door in. . . . " Instead of "Why are you so mad all the time?" That way you show you care but you don't give any attitude, then you can let your friend say what the problem actually is.

Sam, sixteen, added this:

> It's better to let friends help themselves than to tell them what they should do. First, they know more about it than you do, right? Next, what you would do might not work for them. And anyway, it's their problem, they should solve it. But you can be there for them. You can ask them what they've thought about doing to solve it, and then help them see what will happen if they do that. Like, if your friend says, "I'm going over there and tell him he's an asshole," you say, "Okay, and what do you think will happen then?" You stick with them. Help them to see the consequences.

In cases of physical or sexual abuse, harassment, drug or alcohol abuse, serious illness, teen pregnancy, or some other dangerous or life-changing situation, you will probably need adult help to intervene effectively. But don't remain silent. Your intervention is important. You may choose to talk to other close friends and decide together what to do. You may decide to tell your parents or someone in your friend's family. In most states, if you tell a doctor, a teacher, a counselor, or an administrator at school that you suspect a student may be in danger, they are required to tell the authorities. This may keep you from using them as a resource, but remember, it means you can count on help getting to your friend quickly if she or he really needs it.

One place to call for help is a teen hot line or help line, where teenagers themselves answer calls from people in trouble. John, in Chicago, works the phones Saturday nights at "Contact Chicago," a teen hot line in that city:

> Once someone called about this Halloween party where a kid passed out from drinking alcohol and then inhaling paint thinner, and his friends called here first because they wanted to check how serious this was for their friend, and they wanted to know if they called 911 what would happen with the police. We ended up calling 911 for them, and got them on the phone with the hospital emergency room until the ambulance got there, and then I kept calling them back to check up on things and how everyone else was doing. The twelve-year-old who inhaled is okay now.

Another time there was a skinhead flare-up where it looked like there was going to be fight between skinheads and some black guys, and someone's little sister called in because she overheard her brother and his friends planning a drive-by.

Sarah, who works for Teenline, in Columbus, Ohio, told us:

> One time, two fourteen-year-old girls called in who had run away. They were from a small town, and they had come to Columbus, the big city. I talked to them lots of times that night, trying to help them find a safe place to stay. It can be hard. They knew I was down for them. I was one of them, because I was their same age, and I could say not to hitchhike or not to try and find a "date" to give them a place to stay, and they could hear it from me much better than from an adult. Also, for one of the girls, calling her family was not going to be the answer, because it came out that she was being abused at home and that's why she ran away. The other girl was her friend and came with her.
>
> Finally, we found them a church that had an emergency-services program, including emergency shelter. The girl who was not being abused called the runaway hot line and connected with her family. The other girl decided to talk to the authorities about her situation, even though she didn't want to. There are no easy answers when your life is a mess, and the world can really be a mess for teens sometimes. But I felt good that I could at least be there for them all during that long, cold night.

In many cases, your help will really make a difference. In other cases, it won't, because the situation will require more expertise than you can offer. Or sometimes what you thought was a dangerous scene will turn out less serious than you imagined. But if you have a strong feeling that someone you care about is in trouble, check it out. Jamal said:

> Write my sad story down so other kids will know about it. I didn't do anything, because I didn't want to look like a retard. Now my friend is dead. This is

a worse thing than supposedly losing the friendship because you talked about whatever it was. The friendship can always come back after a while. But when your friend dies, he'll never come back.

Everyone needs help putting his or her life together. Some teens are lucky enough to receive that help from their families. For those of you who don't have family support, there's no shame in asking for or accepting help from another caring person or from a community program designed to offer assistance. The shame is in our being a country that allows so many of its children to grow up surrounded by violence and abuse.

RESOURCES

Hotlines

If you are in immediate danger call **911.**
To report child abuse call **911.**

Covenant House (The Nine-Line). 1-800-999-9999. Call them for advice and help. Headquartered in New York City, this is a religious social service agency that offers shelter and services for homeless teenagers in New York City, Houston, Fort Lauderdale, Toronto, New Orleans, Los Angeles, and Anchorage. Covenant House maintains a toll-free telephone hot line where runaway kids from all over the country or their parents can call for counseling or to leave a message.

Children of the Night Shelter. 1-800-551-1300. Established in 1979 in Los Angeles, this shelter helps children and teens who are forced into prostitution or pornography and those living on the street. There are twenty-four beds, skilled counselors, food, clothing, and emergency medical care. Call them, toll free, if you are in trouble and out on the street in the Los Angeles area. If you are not in Los Angeles, they may be able to give you a referral to a shelter near you.

National Runaway Switchboard. 1-800-621-4000. A 24-hour service for runaways. They will be able to help you find a place to stay. It is a toll-free number. You don't pay for the call. They won't hassle you.

National Runaway Switchboard. TDD Line for hearing-impaired teens: 1-800-621-0391.

National Domestic Violence Hotline. 1-800-799-7233. TDD Line for the hearing impaired: 1-800-787-3224. Free call, twenty-four hours, seven days a week. A resource for people hurt by domestic violence and trying to find safety.

Domestic Abuse. To report family or child abuse, during working hours call your county's Department of Health and Human Services and ask for the department that serves children and families.

Rape. Check in the phone book under Rape for the phone number of a local rape crisis center. You may also call the Rape, Abuse, Incest, National Network (RAINN) and they will automatically transfer your call to the rape crisis center nearest to where you are. It is a toll-free call: 1-800-656-HOPE (4673).

Nonfiction Books and Publications

The Courage to Heal: A Guide for Women Survivors of Sexual Abuse, by Ellen Bass and Laura Davis. New York: Harper & Row, 1988. An excellent book. If you are female and have suffered or are suffering sexual abuse, this has been recommended by many as the *best* book to read.

The Courage to Heal Workbook: For Women and Men Survivors of Child Sexual Abuse, by Laura Davis. New York: HarperCollins, 1990. Survivors of sexual abuse tell us this book helped turn their lives around. It is a comforting, eye-opening, and very supportive workbook that teaches survivors of abuse how to heal and feel good about themselves.

Acquaintance Rape: Awareness and Prevention for Teenagers, by Py Bateman. Seattle: Alternatives to Fear. 101 Nickerson, Suite 150, Seattle, WA 98109.

Macho? What Do Girls Really Want?, by Py Bateman. Seattle: Alternatives to Fear. 101 Nickerson, Suite 150, Seattle, WA 98109. For boys, a guide to learn about how to date without being aggressive.

Top Secret: Sexual Assault Information for Teenagers, by Jennifer J. Fay and Billie Jo Flerchinger and the King County Rape Relief Staff and Advocates. Order from King County Rape Relief, 305 S. 43rd St., Renton, WA 98055 (Phone: 1-206-226-5062).

Foster Care Youth United. This magazine is subtitled *The Voice of Youth in Foster Care.* The information is up to date and important for teens in the foster-care system. Excellent articles written from personal experience mostly by teens themselves. All teens in foster care may submit articles, poems, and artwork for this magazine. Write to them or call for more information. It is published six times a year. Subscription is $10. Make checks payable to Youth Communication. Send to FCYU, 144 W. 27th St., Suite 8R, New York, NY 10001 (Phone: 1-212-242-3270).

Victims No Longer: Men Recovering from Incest and Other Sexual Child Abuse, by Mike Lew. New York: Harper & Row, 1988.

New Youth Connections. An excellent teen-written magazine from New York City, published seven times during the school year. Individual subscriptions are $10 a year. Topics discussed are all relevant to teenagers and written with the utmost honesty from people's personal experience. Sexuality, relationships, gangs, violence, abuse, book reviews, movie reviews, resources. Write to NYC, Youth Communication/New York Center, Inc., 144 W. 27th St., Suite 8R, New York, NY 10001.

Getting Free: You Can End Abuse and Take Back Your Life, by Ginny NiCarthy. Seattle: Seal Press, 1986. Self-help book on domestic violence.

Teaching Tolerance. Published by Teaching Tolerance and the Southern Poverty Law Center. This magazine is full of excellent information and ideas about how to discourage and stop violence and racism. Order it through Teaching Tolerance, 400 Washington Ave., Montgomery, AL 36104.

Teen Voices: The Magazine By, For, and About Teenage and Young Adult Women. Published by Women Express, Inc., a multicultural volunteer collective of teens and young adult women. This magazine has many articles written by teens themselves about all subjects that might interest young women. They accept articles and artwork from teens from all over the world. If you would like to write to them: Women Express, Inc., P.O. Box 120027, Boston, MA 02112. Or phone them toll-free at 1-888-882-8336. They are also on the Internet at www.TeenVoices.com

Chain, Chain, Change: For Black Women in Abusive Relationships, by Evelyn C. White.

Seattle: Seal Press, 1994. For black women who want to understand the dynamic of emotional abuse and eliminate violence from their lives.

Mejor Sola Que Mal Acompanada: Para la Mujer Golpeada/For the Latina in an Abusive Relationship, by Myrna M. Zambrano. Seattle: Seal Press, 1985. Bilingual handbook.

Organizations

Battered Women's Justice Project. 206 W. Fourth St., Duluth, MN 55806. (Phone: 1-800-903-0111 for legal assistance and advice.)

Community United Against Violence. 973 Market St., Suite 500, San Francisco, CA 94103. (Phone: 1-415-777-5500.) An organization that addresses antigay and lesbian violence and abusive relationships within the gay community.

Incest Resources, Inc. Cambridge Women's Center, 46 Pleasant St., Cambridge, MA 02139. (Phone: 1-617-354-8807.) Excellent newsletter, *For Crying Out Loud,* and other materials. Referral service.

Men Stopping Violence. 1020 DeKalb Ave. #25, Atlanta, GA 30307. (Phone: 1-404-688-1376.) They run the Violence Prevention Mentoring Project, which provides positive modeling for at-risk adolescent males and intervenes to help battering men learn how to stop their abusive behavior.

Mentors in Violence Prevention Program. Part of The Center for the Study of Sport in Society. 360 Huntington Ave., Suite 161 CP, Boston, MA 02115. (Phone: 1-617-373-4025.) This program trains men to take leadership roles in helping to combat and stop violence, especially violence against women— rape, battering, and sexual harassment.

Oakland Men's Project. 1203 Preservation Park Way, Suite 200, Oakland, CA 94612. (Phone: 1-510-835-2433.) Started by a multicultural group of men to try to stop sexual harassment, rape, assault, and battery. They offer workshops and training. They publish *Helping Teens Stop Violence* and *Making the Peace.*

VOICES in Action, Inc., P.O. Box 148309, Chicago, IL 60614. A nationwide network for men and women who have experienced sexual abuse. It provides a free referral service, and it publishes a newsletter. It can also put you in touch with local support groups.

Fiction

Bastard Out of Carolina, by Dorothy Allison. New York: Plume, 1993. About Ruth Anne Boatwright, a young girl known as Bones, because she is so long and skinny. Her mother's desperate need to get love from a man leaves Bones vulnerable to sexual abuse and violence.

Parrot in the Oven: mi vida, by Victor Martinez. New York: Joanna Cotler Books, an imprint of HarperCollins Publishers, 1996. The story of a young Mexican-American boy growing up with an alcoholic father. His sensitivity and desire to make something of his life help him to see beyond the violence and depression around him.

Push, by Sapphire. New York: Alfred A. Knopf, 1996. "Precious is strong. Although her mother is a lazy nothing and her father is simply a waste of skin, she struggles to make it—but not without a lot of obstacles. . . . I saw my life story being told in this novel. . . . Precious suffers and is hurt in every way possible, yet something inside makes her *push* her way forward. *Push* is an inspiration for those who think it's impossible to make it." (Condensed from a review by Wunika Hicks in *Foster Care Youth United.*)

The Bluest Eye, by Toni Morrison. New York: Holt, 1970. The story of a black girl who yearns to be other than who she is. The book is a deep and touching account of the effects of racism, violence, and poverty on black families.

Videos

Broken Ground, by Margaret Wrinkle and Chris Lawson. An excellent video about racism and what ordinary people can do to begin to overcome it. This video can be ordered from Broken Ground Productions, P.O. Box 131295, Birmingham, AL 35213.

"But He Loves Me," from Churchill Media. An inexperienced sixteen-year-old girl gets involved with a popular boy who has a dark side, which comes out in jealousy, possessiveness, and abuse. Order from Churchill Media, 12210 Nebraska Ave., Dept. 200, Los Angeles, CA 90025-9816.

"I Am a Man," by Bryon Hurt (who is an associate director with the Mentors in Violence Prevention Program listed above). This powerful documentary is by a black man exploring black masculinity and what it is like to grow up as a black male in our society. This video can be ordered from the Mentors In Violence Prevention Program, Northeastern University, 360 Huntington Ave., 161 CP, Boston, MA 02115.

The Shadow of Hate, by Teaching Tolerance, a project of the Southern Poverty Law Center in Montgomery, Alabama. The film shows the effects of prejudice toward Native Americans, African Americans, religious minorities, European and Asian immigrants, and other groups. Its message is tolerance and the importance of promoting peace and understanding between people. It can be ordered from Teaching Tolerance, 400 Washington Ave., Montgomery, AL 36104.

Strong at the Broken Places: Turning Trauma into Recovery, by Cambridge Documentary Films, Inc., Cambridge, Massachusetts. An intelligent, inspirational film about four people who experienced severe and continued physical and emotional trauma when they were young. Through a process of interviews mixed with still shots we learn how these people were able to begin the healing process and turn their lives around. Order from Cambridge Documentary Films, P.O. Box 390385, Cambridge, MA 02139-0004.

Physical Health Care

O ne important way to take care of yourself is to have a yearly physical examination. Just the way you'd take your car in for a regular lube and oil change, you want to take yourself in for a checkup *before* anything really serious happens. A regular medical checkup is a form of *preventive* medicine; it helps prevent you from becoming seriously ill.

WHERE TO GO FOR A CHECKUP

➤ *Family doctor.* Many of you will have a doctor you have been seeing since childhood. She or he will probably continue to serve you until you are sixteen or seventeen, if you do not change doctors. Many pediatricians these days have special training in teenage health.

➤ *Health maintenance organizations.* Many families belong to health insurance groups. Check with your parents.

➤ *Local health clinics.* You may prefer to go to a local clinic for medical services. Look in the business pages under Clinics,

Health Services, or Medical Services. Ask friends for recommendations. Check with your school nurse to see whether he or she can recommend a clinic.

➤ *Women's clinics or women's health centers.* These provide complete services for women and girls. If there is a women's clinic in your city or town, call them. Ask if they also provide treatment for males.

➤ *Community clinics.* Some areas have clinics that run solely on grants and donations. They do not charge anything for their services. If there is a free clinic in your area, that would be

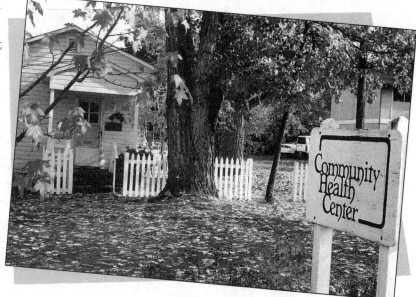

a good choice, since they are likely to treat many teenagers and they would therefore be set up to handle special teenage problems. Look in the business pages under Clinics.

Making an Appointment

You may want to talk to the people at different places before you decide where to go for your checkup. Call them and ask them about the services. Tell them your age.

Here is a list of some questions you may want to ask:

➤ Do they treat many teenagers?

➤ How many doctors and nurse practitioners do they have on their staff?

➤ How long have they been in operation?

➤ Are they affiliated with any hospitals?

➤ What do they charge for a complete physical exam?

➤ Do you need your parents' consent to be seen by a doctor?

➤ If you are a girl and would prefer to be seen by a female doctor, ask if they have one on the staff. Many places do.

You'll be able to determine by their answers and their friendliness whether you want to go to that clinic. They should be courteous and respectful and answer your questions.

Make an appointment for a time that is convenient for you. If there is a particular health professional you want to see, make your appointment for a time when that person is on duty. Once you make an appointment, be sure to keep it. If you cannot keep it for some reason, be sure to phone the clinic or doctor's office to cancel your appointment.

Ask for directions to the place. Ask if you can get there by public transportation if you need to.

We advise you to bring a parent or a friend along with you to the appointment. It's nice to have company while you're waiting for the health professional. If you prefer to go alone, you may want to bring a

book or some homework. There is usually a fifteen- to forty-five-minute wait. At some clinics there is a much longer wait.

A TYPICAL MEDICAL EXAMINATION

Lots of people put off going for an examination because they are afraid of what it will be like. They worry about shots or other procedures that may hurt or be uncomfortable. Some people don't like the idea of getting undressed in the examining room. Here we will explain what to expect from a typical exam in order to take some of the strangeness out of it and to help you to feel more comfortable.

Complete Medical History

An important part of any thorough exam is the medical history. This is a series of questions about your present and past health, and the health of members of your family. You will be asked what diseases you had as a child; what illnesses close members of your family have had; what, if any, special medical conditions you may have, such as diabetes, heart murmur, fainting spells, headaches; and what kinds of illnesses run in your family, such as cancer, heart disease, diabetes. They will ask if you have any allergies and whether you are allergic to any form of medication or whether you take any medication or drugs regularly.

Remember, according to the medical code of ethics and in some cases according to the law, the health professional must keep this information confidential unless it is about sexual or physical abuse. Medical people are required by law to report suspected sexual or physical abuse cases to the appropriate authorities.

In many clinics and doctor's offices, a trained medical professional will ask you about your medical history. In other places, there will be a form for you to fill out. This will be a checklist naming various diseases and asking you to check which you've had and which you haven't had. *Answer only those questions you understand and know the answer to.* If you bring a parent along with you to the exam, he or she will be able to help you, especially with ques-

Consumer's Rights

As a consumer of health care, you have certain rights, regardless of your race, religion, age, sex, or education. These are:

➤ The right to be treated with dignity and respect.

➤ The right to privacy and confidentiality.

➤ The right to have all procedures explained in language you understand.

➤ The right to have all your questions answered in language you understand.

➤ The right to know the meaning and implications of all forms you are asked to sign.

➤ The right to know the effectiveness, complications, and possible side effects of all medications you are given.

➤ The right to know the results and meanings of all tests and examinations.

➤ The right to consent to or refuse any test, examination, or treatment.

➤ The right to see your records and have them explained to you.

Medical professionals are human. They make mistakes. They may be very busy. They are not perfect. They can't read your mind. In order to get the best treatment possible, be sure to speak up when you don't understand something. Ask questions. Let them know if what they are doing hurts you or makes you feel uncomfortable.

If you feel your rights have been violated, talk to the clinic director or to the health worker in charge of the office. If they aren't helpful, do not use their services in the future if you are able to go somewhere else. Tell your friends about your poor treatment. You and they may be able to get together and organize a list of good medical services in your area. You can boycott doctors and clinics that do not provide adequate services to teenagers.

If you have a serious complaint—for example, if you were physically mistreated or you were lied to or misled, or if you suspect that you are, or ever have been, the subject of a medical experiment and have questions about it, or if you feel any of your rights have been violated—you can contact your State Board of Medical Examiners for physician grievances or the State Board of Nursing for grievances against nurses. Their office will be listed in the phone book of your state capital (which you can find in the public library), or you can get their phone number from calling directory assistance for your state capital. Describe your mistreatment, and give them the name of the doctors and/or health workers who were at fault. Give them the name and the address of the place where you received treatment.

tions about your past health and the health of other members of the family.

If you have trouble reading the form or if you don't know what some words mean, *don't fill out that part.* Talk to the health worker and ask for an explanation of any part you don't understand. If the whole form is confusing to you, ask for help. You have a right and an obligation to yourself to have everything explained to you so you know what you are filling in.

Time to Talk to the Health Professional

The examination should include as much time as you and the health professional need to discuss any prob-

lems or concerns you have about your development, your life, your feelings. Bring along a list of questions so you won't forget what you wanted to talk about. This time should be private, so that you can discuss things you might not want to talk about with someone else present. If a parent comes with you to the exam, ask for private time to speak with the health professional alone. Many medical people are sensitive to the fact that teens may want some time to ask questions or discuss private issues without a parent present.

The health professional should discuss with you the process of physical development and explain to you why and how your body is changing. He or she may discuss diet and health habits with you. Some medical people recommend vitamins; others believe that if you are eating well, you don't need vitamins. That is still a controversial subject in medical circles. Feel free to ask your health professional to explain his or her approach to the prevention of illness.

One important part of the talk will be about sexuality. Since your body is becoming mature sexually and you are going to be or are already capable of reproduction, the health professional should take this time to discuss birth control and sexually transmitted diseases with you—even if you have no intention of being sexually active with a partner for a long while. It's essential to know about birth control and STD prevention *before* you become sexually active. If he or she doesn't bring these topics up, you should ask him or her any questions you may have about sex. If the health professional hedges, or seems embarrassed to talk with you about these things, you may choose to find another health practitioner for future checkups. *Find a medical person with whom you feel comfortable discussing sex.* For some teenagers, this person is their only reliable source of accurate sex information.

Be honest with the health professional about whether or not you are sexually active and what kinds of sexual activity you have experienced. It's for your own protection, because if you are having intercourse or oral sex, you should have STD tests during the exam (see Chapter 9). Also, girls who are sexually active should have Pap smears (explained on page 251).

If you are having problems with drugs and/or alcohol and you want help, the health professional would be a good person to ask for assistance. You will have to decide whether you trust her or him enough to share your problem. Since the first step to ending substance abuse is admitting you have a problem, telling the health professional will be a positive move toward recovery.

If you are experiencing panic attacks, frequent headaches or stomachaches, an inability to concentrate at school, problems with family members, or any kind of abuse, tell the health professional about it. Keeping these serious problems secret allows

them to continue. Though you may feel funny discussing such intimate things with a stranger, sometimes it's actually easier talking to someone you don't know very well. Think of the health professional as an important resource person. Even if your concerns aren't medical, he or she will be able to put you in touch with other people who can help you.

The Physical Examination

After you've given your medical history and talked to the health professional about your personal concerns, the physical part of the examination will usually take place—though sometimes the order is reversed.

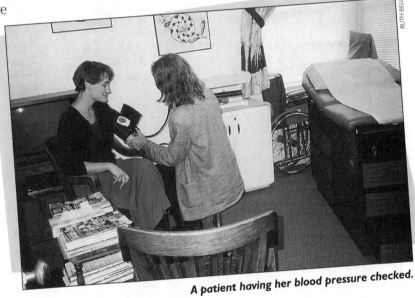

A patient having her blood pressure checked.

URINE: You will be asked to go into the bathroom and urinate into a paper or plastic cup. Let a little urine run into the toilet first, then catch some midstream in the cup. Most people fill the cup about halfway and then let the rest of their urine, if there is any, run into the toilet. Girls hold the cup under them while they sit on the toilet. Boys stand and direct their urine into the cup. Your urine will be tested in various ways to make sure your kidneys and bladder are functioning properly.

MEASUREMENTS: Then you will go into the examining room and undress. You will be alone while you undress, and there will be a hospital gown or paper robe for you to put on. A medical professional will come in and take your blood pressure and measure your height and weight. If you've never had your blood pressure measured before, don't worry—it doesn't hurt. A pressure sleeve is wrapped around the upper part of your arm and pumped up to create pressure. Your blood pressure is measured as the pressure is relaxed. (Your blood pressure may sometimes be measured before you undress.)

BLOOD TEST: Your exam should include a blood test, during which a sample of your blood is taken from your arm with a needle. The nurse will make a tiny puncture in your vein, and blood will flow into a small glass vial. Very little blood is taken. The initial puncture may sting, but the hurt should not last more than a few seconds. You can hold someone's hand if you are afraid. This is a very important part of the exam, especially for teens who are sexually active.

Your blood will be tested to see if signs of any disease are present. Syphilis and hepatitis show up in the blood, as do many other diseases and medical conditions. There is a blood test for HIV/AIDS and also a blood test for pregnancy.

If you are terrified of needles, tell the health professional.

HEAD CHECK: Your eyes, ears, nose, throat, and teeth will be checked. The doctor or nurse may give you an eye test to check your vision. This usually involves reading from a chart placed about twenty feet from where you are asked to stand. Your hearing may be tested using a machine called an audiometer. You'll be asked to put on a pair of earphones and listen to sounds.

GENERAL BODY CHECK: The doctor or nurse will look your body over, checking for swelling, rashes, or anything else out of the ordinary. He or she will feel around your neck and under your arms and along your body, looking for enlarged glands. This is the part of the exam during which the health professional may poke you a little here and there. He or she isn't trying to hurt you—it's just to check certain vital places on your body.

Your heart and lungs will be checked. The health professional takes your pulse and listens to your breathing with a stethoscope.

If you are having any pain or itching or other symptoms, this would be a good time to talk about that. These are clues to help the medical professional determine what, if anything, needs special attention.

Boy's Examination

The health worker will feel around your testicles, scrotum, and penis, checking for lumps or pain. He or she will be wearing surgical rubber gloves. Ask him or her to show you how to check your own testicles for lumps (see page 23). He or she may ask you questions about genital development and about whether you have ejaculated during masturbation or during your sleep. This is completely normal, and although it may seem embarrassing, answer honestly. It's a natural part of a boy's sexual development.

RECTAL EXAM: Sometimes the doctor or nurse will do a rectal examination—that is, feel inside your anus to check for lumps or swelling or obstructions. First he or she will put on a thin rubber glove and lubricate his or her finger with some lubricating jelly. He or she will ask you to relax your bottom and then will gently insert the finger into your anus. One doctor told us the best way to relax is to take a deep breath and bear down, just as if you were trying to have a bowel movement, then breathe out and let your body go limp. If the health practitioner is gentle and you are relaxed, the rectal exam shouldn't hurt at all. If you are tight and nervous, it may feel uncomfortable. Be sure to say if it hurts, so that he or she can slow down and be more gentle.

SEXUAL FUNCTIONING: The health professional should explain to you about the male role in pregnancy and about birth control. You can ask him or her to show you how to put on a condom.

If you have had sexual intercourse or oral sex, you should have a test for gonorrhea, syphilis, HIV/AIDS, and other STDs (see Chapter 9, beginning on page 253).

Girl's Examination

The health worker will feel around your breasts, checking for lumps, swelling, and/or pain. She or he will ask you questions about when your breasts started developing. Ask him or her to teach you how to check your own breasts for lumps each month after your period (see page 30).

The doctor or nurse will also look and feel around the groin area. He or she will examine the vulva, checking the urethra and the outside of the vagina. He or she will check to make sure there is enough of an opening in your hymen (see page 34) to allow menstrual flow to escape easily. If you have a very small opening, the health worker may discuss with you ways to ease open the hymen yourself.

MENSTRUATION: You and the health professional may have discussed menstruation during the "time to talk" part of the exam. Otherwise, this is the appropriate time to talk about when your period first started, if it has, and how often it comes. The health professional will ask how heavy your usual flow is, and how long each period lasts. Tell her or him about any discomfort you may experience during or before your period. If you haven't started your period yet, this visit can reassure you that everything is fine. Some girls don't start their periods until they are seventeen or eighteen.

We recommend keeping a menstrual record. Write down when you started menstruating, and then write down the date of the first day of each period. After a while, you will be able to see a pattern forming to help you predict when to expect your next period. Also, for medical tests and treatments, it's good to know when your last period began.

INTERNAL (PELVIC) EXAMINATION: A girl's organs of reproduction are on the inside. Unlike a boy's penis and testicles, the uterus, ovaries, and fallopian tubes cannot be seen or examined externally. In order to examine a girl's organs, the health practitioner must look inside and feel inside your vagina. She or he puts on surgical gloves before the examination.

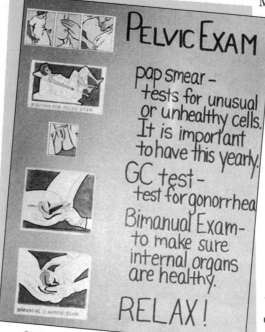

Sign in a teen clinic describing a pelvic exam.

Health professionals often choose to omit the internal exam with younger teenage girls unless there is a specific need for it, or unless the girl is already having sexual intercourse, because many girls and women feel uncomfortable about this exam. Many boys and men feel the same way when the doctor examines their genitals.

Throughout this book, we've recommended that you get to know your own genitals, that you look at them, touch them, and learn about their functions. If you haven't done so already, we hope you will read the chapter entitled "Changing Bodies," beginning on page 369, which will help you to discover and appreciate that part of yourself.

To do an internal exam, the health worker will ask you to push yourself down to the end of the examining table with your buttocks just at the edge and your knees bent and spread apart. Your feet will go into metal stirrups placed at the foot of the table. It is an awkward position to be in, but doctors and

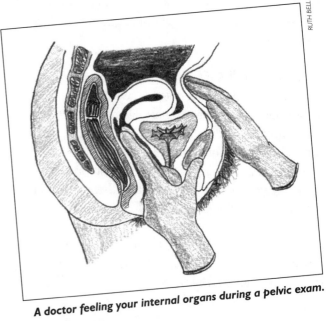

A doctor feeling your internal organs during a pelvic exam.

nurses say it is the most convenient way for them to check you. Here is how eighteen-year-old Mary described it:

I think that position is really undignified. There's something about lying there on my back with my legs up and spread open that I just think is gross. But I try to psych myself up. I tell myself, "This is okay. It's just normal. It's just a doctor. He does it all the time." I think about it that way, and then it's okay for me.

There should be a female health professional present in the examining room while a male practitioner is performing an internal examination on a girl or woman. If the practitioner is a woman, no other person need be present.

SPECULUM EXAM: Since the walls of the vagina are touching, the health practitioner won't be able to see inside without holding open the two sides of the vagina. There is a special instrument, called a *speculum* (*speh*-cue-lum) made just for that purpose.

The speculum comes in both plastic and metal in several different sizes. There is a small size especially for young girls and for women who have small vaginal openings. The doctor or nurse inserts the speculum by holding the two branches of it together and easing them gently into your vagina. If it is a metal speculum, it should be warmed before insertion. Once the speculum is inside, the health practitioner opens it and presses down to lock it in place.

Putting in a speculum can be uncomfortable for you if the doctor or nurse is not gentle or if you are nervous and tensed up. Be sure to say if he or she is hurting you. Ask him or her to give you a chance to relax.

The best way to relax the muscles in your pelvic area is to take a few deep breaths and blow all the air out after each one. Then take one deep breath and hold it. At the same time bear down on your pelvic area. Then breathe out slowly and relax your body totally. Let your mouth drop open. Relax your fingers and toes. Concentrate on opening your vagina.

Once the speculum is in place, your cervix and the inside of your vagina can be easily seen. The health professional can hold a mirror in front of your vagina so that you can look too if you'd like. It's fasci-

nating to see what you (and all females) look like inside. It helps you to understand how your body functions. (See page 33 for a description of what you'll see.)

The examiner will be looking for redness or inflammation in the vagina, which can be a sign of infection. Normally, the walls of the vagina are pinkish brown. He or she will also look for any unusual discharge and will check for cuts or tears or cysts on the cervix. He or she will also check the color of the cervix. It is normally pinkish or brownish pink, although there is a wide variation among different individuals. During pregnancy the cervix takes on a slightly bluish tint, so the color of the cervix can indicate a possible pregnancy.

PAP SMEAR: With a long Q-Tips-like stick bound with cotton at the tip, the health worker will gently scrape some cell tissue from the cervix.

The cell tissue will be sent to a laboratory to determine whether there are any abnormal cells present. This is helpful in checking for precancerous conditions. Another sample may be used to determine the presence of some STDs. You will be notified within a week's time if any abnormalities appear in your test.*

Named after G. N. Papanicolaou, the physician who developed the test, a Pap smear should not hurt, although you might feel it. As with everything else, some people are more careful than others. Let the health practitioner know if he or she hurts you.

Pap smears are recommended for girls eighteen and over, and for girls, no matter what age, who are having sexual intercourse. If you fit either of those categories, have a Pap smear once a year. If you take the birth control pill or use an IUD for birth control, if you have genital herpes or some other STD, or if you have more than one sexual partner, women's health advocates recommend having a Pap smear every six months.

BIMANUAL VAGINAL EXAM: After the doctor or nurse closes the speculum and eases it out of your vagina, she or he will want to examine your internal

* See the section on Pap smears in *The New Our Bodies, Ourselves* by Boston Women's Health Book Collective (New York: Simon & Schuster, 1992).

organs manually. He or she will put a thin rubber glove on one hand and lubricate one or two fingers of that hand with lubricating jelly. Gently, he or she will insert the finger or fingers into your vagina while placing the other hand on your lower abdomen. In this way, the practitioner can feel the size, shape, and position of your uterus, ovaries, and tubes. He or she will be looking for unusual swelling, tenderness, or growths. When the examiner presses down in certain places, it may feel a little uncomfortable, but it usually doesn't hurt. Ask the examiner to explain what he or she is feeling for. Be sure to say if you experience soreness or pain.

Try to relax during this exam by breathing slowly and deeply. Remember, if you feel tense, try to keep your fingers and toes loose and let your mouth drop open.

RECTAL EXAM: Sometimes the health worker can feel the organs better by inserting a finger into the anus. (See page 249 for an explanation of a rectal exam.)

After the Examination

When the exam is over, the health professional will leave the room so that you can have privacy while you put your clothes back on.

He or she will tell you if you should have another appointment soon, or whether you won't need to return for another year. If there is medication to prescribe or if he or she wants to discuss some part of the exam with you, the health professional will spend a few minutes after the exam talking with you.

At a clinic or HMO, they may be able to fill prescriptions on site. Otherwise, if you are given a prescription, take it to a pharmacy and the druggist will fill it for you.

If you have any questions or comments about the exam, feel free to speak up. You have a right to have your questions answered and your comments heard.

Sexually Transmitted Diseases

Everything that's alive can get sick, and germs that cause sickness are everywhere. Each time someone with the flu sneezes near you, there's a chance you'll catch the flu. Each time you share a drink with someone who has a cold, you run the risk of catching a cold. If your body is run-down or stressed, you're more vulnerable.

Lots of germs are passed by ordinary social contact—people just being around other people who are sick. This chapter is about the germs that can be caught specifically through sexual contact, the germs that thrive in people's body fluids and their moist body openings: the mouth, the vagina, the penis, and the anus.

Many of us were taught that catching a sexually transmitted disease (STD) is a disgrace, that it means you are "dirty" or "loose." A fifteen-year-old from Boston said:

Yeah, there's this feeling like, I can't get anything like that! You've got these certain kinds of distinctions in your head that say, Wait a minute, he's my friend. He can't have an STD.

Actually, it's not like that at all. *Anyone* who is sexually active can get an STD. Being clean or "nice" has nothing to do with it. Seventeen-year-old Greg told us:

I got gonorrhea from this great girl at school. She's an honor student. Just got accepted to three of the best colleges. I couldn't believe it.

Friends and strangers alike can give you STDs if they are infected when you have sexual contact with them. The more sexual partners you have, the higher your chances of catching a disease. The more sexual partners your partners have had, the more likely it is that they will have a disease to pass on to you. In fact, each year over 3 million American teenagers contract some form of sexually transmitted disease.

After the discovery of penicillin in 1928, some of the most dangerous bacterial STDs became curable. Penicillin and other antibiotics can cure most strains of gonorrhea, syphilis, and chlamydia. Unfortunately, there are a host of viral STDs that cannot be cured by antibiotics or by any other known drug. The most dangerous of these is HIV (human immunodeficiency virus), which causes AIDS. HIV kills people, and as yet there is no cure for it.

None of us wants to think that something as beautiful and pleasurable as making love can be associated with sickness and death. Yet people are dying of HIV/AIDS–related diseases every day. An estimated 40,000 to 90,000 people become infected with HIV annually, and at least one-quarter of those people are teenagers. That means each year anywhere from 10,000 to 23,000 teenagers get the virus that causes AIDS. Without treatment, all STDs can do serious damage to your body and to your future. AIDS can kill you.

We thought long and hard about how to introduce this subject without sounding so frightening that you'd find a million reasons to convince yourself why it's okay not to read this chapter. All those reasons are wrong. For your own sake, you have to read the information presented here. HIV is a killer, and about fifty new teenagers catch it every day. *Every day.* Normal, nice, smart, savvy teenagers just like you. That's why we say, *Inform yourself.* Your life depends on it.

The discussion of specific STDs starts on page 256, in the section called Facts About Sexually Transmitted Diseases. Under each STD, we talk about ways it can be prevented or cured. If you are having sex now or if you plan to have sex at some time, please read that section.

TALK ABOUT IT

Before getting into the particulars of each disease, you should know that one of the main obstacles to keeping yourself safe is lack of communication. You can't be safe if you can't talk to your partner about sex. There's a section on communication in the sexuality chapter (see page 125). In it, you'll find ideas on how to become more comfortable talking with your partner about sex in general and about STD prevention and birth control in particular.

How many times have you heard anyone in one of those movie love scenes ask his or her partner if he or she is protected against sexually transmitted disease or if he or she has been tested for an STD? Not many! That's one of the reasons it feels so weird to talk about protection with each other; we don't really know how to do it. No matter how much sexual experience you've had, when you're just getting to know someone or when you're being sexual with someone for the first time, it's pretty natural to feel nervous. There you are, alone together, and neither one of you knows exactly what to do or what to say. It's asking a lot to expect you'll be able to stop everything and talk about what needs to be talked about. But to be safe, you have to! Nineteen-year-old Alana said:

> In my group of friends, there are a lot of people who aren't in touch with being scared of STDs. I think it's a lot about not wanting to talk about sex, about really feeling uncomfortable about that and for women not feeling like they have power in that situation. Like the guy will leave if they talk about it. Most of my girlfriends think guys won't like it if they talk about using condoms. Like it will be a drag and ruin it.

In Los Angeles, seventeen-year-old Tim gave another reason:

> I think that even though AIDS is here and people know that not only gay people get it, they still don't like to talk about it. It's just a difficult thing to talk about protection and safe sex and all that, because then you have to admit what you're doing and that you're taking a risk.

LaReina, one of Tim's friends, responded:

> But if you don't use protection then you really are taking a risk.

Tim:

> Sure you are. But if you don't talk about it, you can pretend you aren't. You can just forget it for a while.

Many of us, like Tim, are simply too embarrassed, too timid, or too uninformed to speak up, so we close our eyes and pretend it doesn't matter. That's exactly why STDs are spreading everywhere, through every group of sexually active teens, regardless of gender, sexual preference, religion, or ethnic background. Remember, *everyone who has sex can catch an STD.* If you are sexually active, the only way to avoid catching one is to inform yourself, prepare yourself with latex condoms and other methods of protection, and learn to talk about safer sex with your partner.

SAFER SEX: WHAT DOES IT MEAN?

There are precautions you can take to help you avoid catching and/or passing STDs. Most of these precautions will also help you avoid unwanted pregnancy (see the chapter Protecting Yourself: Birth Control and Safer Sex on page 279). In general, covering the penis with a latex condom helps keep germs and viruses from spreading through penis-vagina or penis-anus or penis-mouth contact. It also helps protect against pregnancy. Females using a spermicide or a female condom help themselves prevent pregnancy and protect themselves from transmission of many STDs through vagina-penis contact. (We discuss protective methods in detail under each STD listing.)

Monogamy (moh-*nah*-gah-mee) is an important component of safer sex. It means two people only have sex with each other—neither one has sex with anyone else. If you are not infected with an STD and your partner is not infected either, and neither of you uses injection drugs, the two of you will continue to be safe. If one of you takes another partner, however, you are no longer safe. An STD counselor who helped us with this chapter said:

> Be careful to tell kids that adolescents are often involved in "serial monogamy," meaning they have short-term monogamous relationships and move on to new monogamous relationships. And many young women are involved with much older men, who may not be totally honest about their other relationships, and most certainly have a prior sexual history. These issues complicate monogamy. It's therefore important to stress that *any* unprotected sex is unsafe, because it's often impossible to know everything about your partner's experiences. After all, HIV can stay alive in your body with no symptoms for ten to fifteen years!

Jenny, a sixteen-year-old from Virginia, said she's very clear about what all this means to her:

> It all comes down to trust. You can be all loving and trusting and then find out your boyfriend slept with somebody else. Even if it was just one time when you were mad at each other. That's why I always use condoms even though I'm in a long-term relationship. You just never know. I care about myself too much to take that kind of a chance.

The reason we say "safer" sex and not "absolutely safe" sex is that there is only *one* way to be absolutely, 100 percent certain of not passing or contracting an STD: that is to *abstain from having sexual relations with another person*. Many teens are remaining abstinent because it is healthier and safer to do so. See page 107 for more discussion on this.

The next best way to be safe is to use protection during sexual activity and make sure that neither you nor your partner is having sex with anyone else.

HOW CAN YOU TELL?

How can you tell if you or your partner has an STD? You can't! A number of STDs have symptoms at some times but not at all times. A person with an STD may feel very sick, or he or she may have sores or a rash or strange blotches or spots on his or her body. There may be burning with urination or severe stomach cramping or a bad cough. But there also may be no symptoms at all for a very long time, and some people never notice symptoms from their STDs. For example, people can be infected with HIV for ten years or longer before symptoms start to occur, and during that time they can pass the disease on to all their partners. In the early stages of gonorrhea and chlamydia, some people don't know they have it, because they don't get symptoms until their internal organs become inflamed weeks or even months later. Genital warts and herpes may have no visual symptoms either, yet all these diseases can be transmitted to partners during sex. Here's what Marie, a seventeen-year-old from Chicago, had to go through to find out she had an STD:

> I had sex with this guy last month, and day before yesterday he called me up to tell me he caught the clap (gonorrhea) from me. I didn't know what he was talking about because I didn't know I had it. But I went to the clinic for a test, and they said I did have it and that it was already starting to infect my tubes. I remembered feeling some pains in my

stomach, but I just thought it was a stomachache. Now I think I must have had gonorrhea for about two months at least, because that was the last time I had sex. Anyway, I sure am glad that guy called me. So after I found out, I called up my old boyfriend to tell him he better get checked too, and he told me he already got tested last month. He tried to call me but my line was busy, so he just forgot about telling me. I couldn't believe it. I probably could have died and he would say, Oh, gee, I meant to call her but her line was busy.

There are now tests for most STDs that will tell if you are infected or not, even if you don't have symptoms. Many sexually active teens have themselves tested regularly, once or even twice a year. Some STDs, like gonorrhea and chlamydia, show up on tests fairly soon after infection. Unfortunately, it takes three to six months for the HIV infection to show up on a test. So unless you have abstained from sex or had sex only within a monogamous relationship for six months or more before your test, negative results may not necessarily mean you don't have HIV.

TELLING YOUR SEX PARTNERS

If you test positive for an STD, the people with whom you have had sex need to be tested too. Usually, it is up to *you* to tell them, because no one else will know. Part of caring for people is helping them stay healthy. That means letting them know they have been exposed to a dangerous disease and should be tested to see if they have it too. They need to know as soon as possible, so they won't continue to infect others and so they can get treatment.

If you simply cannot bring yourself to tell your partner/s, report their names to your testing counselor or to the Department of Health in your area, and a health worker will inform them that they have been exposed to an STD. Health workers are forbidden, by law, to give your name. They are not the police. They only want to stop the spread of HIV and other STDs.

Once you are tested, receiving a positive result means you will be faced with new concerns. You will definitely need treatment and counseling. You may feel worried and depressed. Do not leave the testing clinic before you talk with a counselor or health worker who can help you sort through your options.

By now you may be thinking, What is this? You know people are having sex all the time, and not everybody has an STD or is dying from AIDS.

No, not everyone has an STD; in fact, most people don't. But the incidence of HIV and other STD infection is growing so rapidly among teenagers, it's alarming. And it's growing so fast precisely because many teens don't use protection when they have sex. They think, It can't happen to me. Only when it does happen to them do they realize they were wrong. By then it's too late.

FACTS ABOUT SEXUALLY TRANSMITTED DISEASES

HIV/AIDS

Remember, when you have sex with someone, you are not only having sex with them, you are having sex with all the partners they have ever had during the past ten years, and all the partners those partners have had. If any one of those people was infected with HIV/AIDS, you could get it too.

—STD Health Worker

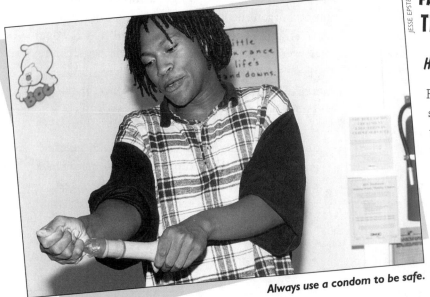
Always use a condom to be safe.

Most teenagers I know just go ahead and have sex, and they don't think about how many people are dying from HIV/AIDS. Some of them think, Oh, it can't get me. They don't understand that anyone and everyone can get this disease. You don't get HIV because of who you are. You get it because of what you do. And if you have sex and don't use protection, you can get it.

—Teenager from New York City

What Is It? Human immunodeficiency virus (HIV) is a tiny virus that gets into your body and destroys your immune system, the system that protects you from dangerous illnesses. HIV grows in the body for years, breaking down and overpowering your own immune mechanisms, until your body can no longer fight off sickness. At that point, in the most advanced stages of HIV infection, you have acquired immune deficiency syndrome (AIDS).

The immune system of a person with AIDS is so extremely weak that even a common cold can be life-threatening. He or she has few defenses to resist even the most ordinary infections, which is why diseases that attack AIDS victims are called "opportunistic." They take the opportunity to attack a severely weakened body. Opportunistic diseases frequently suffered by AIDS victims are Kaposi's sarcoma (a rare form of cancer), pneumocystic carinii pneumonia (PCP), some rare types of brain infection, candidiasis of the esophagus, and a kind of tuberculosis. It is usually these diseases that kill the person infected with AIDS, not the virus itself.

How It Is Passed. For infection to occur, HIV has to pass from the semen, blood, vaginal secretions, or breast milk of one person to the bodily fluids of another person. Small amounts of HIV have been found in saliva, tears, perspiration, urine, and feces, but not enough to allow for transmission.* In other words, casual contact with another person does not pass HIV, but sexual contact or blood contact does.

The most common means of transmitting HIV is through sexual activity. During sex, infected males

pass the virus on to their partners when ejaculating semen into the vagina, anus, or throat. Anal sex is especially risky, because the delicate lining of the anal canal tears and bleeds easily, and HIV passes through blood. An infected person can pass the disease to a woman during cunnilingus (oral sex on a woman—see page 118) if he or she has open sores or cuts on his or her tongue or in his or her mouth.

The virus does not commonly travel through the urethra (the penile opening—see page 16), so men are not as likely to be infected by women during vaginal intercourse as women are by men. But an infected female can pass the virus on to her male partner if the man has a cut on his penis or in his genital area; her secretions can enter his bloodstream through the cut. A female can also pass on the virus through cunnilingus if the partner has broken skin on his or her tongue or in his or her mouth, or possibly if he or she swallows blood or vaginal secretions from the infected woman. Menstrual blood can carry HIV. Sometimes people use their hands and fingers to stimulate their sexual partners. This, too, can transmit HIV, since the virus can be passed through a cut or an open sore. Remember, HIV, like other STD viruses, is microscopic and can pass through even the tiniest opening.

HIV is not only transferred through sexual contact. It is also passed through exchanges of blood. *Drug users sharing intravenous (IV) needles are at very high risk of infecting themselves with HIV.* Sharing toothbrushes, razors, needles for body piercing or tattooing, or anything else that breaks an infected person's skin and has contact with that person's blood can be dangerous. Exchanges of blood through "blood brother" or "blood sister" rituals, in which the blood of two or more people is mingled, can also transmit the disease. To avoid coming into contact with possible HIV contamination, you're encouraged to wear latex gloves before wiping up after a bloody accident or helping a person with a nosebleed.

Before 1985, blood transfusions spread HIV to recipients of HIV-infected blood donations. Now, as there are very careful screenings done at hospitals and blood banks to prevent such an occurrence, that is no longer considered a threat.

---

* There has just been a report of a couple who passed HIV from one to the other through French kissing. Scientists believe it was because both had cuts in their mouths and gum disease. This kind of HIV transmission is extremely rare.

Finally, HIV can be transmitted from mother to infant if the mother has the virus when she is pregnant or breast-feeding her baby.

How It Is Not Passed. HIV is not spread through casual contact. Talking, hugging, and dancing are all safe activities. You can't get HIV just by being next to someone who is infected. Fourteen-year-old Lynette said:

> I heard you could get it from a restaurant. Like if the waiter had it or if the guy who was preparing your food had it or something.

Too many people have died from AIDS.

Lynette is mistaken. Eating in restaurants, swimming in public pools, using public toilets, working with someone who has HIV/AIDS, and living with someone who is infected—as long as there's no sexual or blood contact between you—seem to be absolutely safe. There is also no evidence that HIV can be passed through sweat or through an infected person's vomit or from bloodsucking insects.

Can you get HIV infection from sharing a sandwich or drinking from the same cup as someone who has the disease? Most experts say, not likely. The quantity of HIV found in saliva is probably too small to pose a threat. It's just good sense, however, not to share food casually or pass drinks from mouth to mouth. Lots of germs are exchanged that way.

And what about kissing? Kissing is considered very safe unless you have cuts or sores on your lips. The question is really whether HIV can be passed through deep kissing (French kissing, tongue kissing). No one is absolutely sure about that. In long, deep passionate kisses, blood may be passed if either or both have a sore throat or a cut on their gums or tongues. As with other forms of intimate sexual contact, it is wise to be careful and know your partner well.

Who Is at Risk? Every single person who is sexually active with a partner is at risk. We want to emphasize that point, because when we first began hearing about AIDS in the early 1980s, it was considered to be a disease that was only passed between homosexual men. Then we learned that injection drug users who shared needles were getting it. Then some people who received blood transfusions were getting it. Then we heard about women getting it from their sex partners or from injecting drugs. And now we know that everyone who has sex or shares needles is at risk. *Don't think you can't get HIV/AIDS* because you're not gay, or you're not using drugs, or you are female, or you're married, or you're only having sex with one person. Everyone whose partner is infected can get HIV, and millions of people already have gotten it. Listen to fifteen-year-old Mandy's story:

> Last year I was away at my friend's house at the beach and this older guy started paying attention to me. He told me he was from out of state and he didn't know too many people and we ended up seeing a lot of each other and he talked me into having sex with him. It was my first time. About a month later, I heard he had AIDS. Now I'm going to die because I let some guy talk me into having sex with him.

Remember, there are ways to take precautions to make sex safer. Check the information in the chapter called "Protecting Yourself," beginning on page 279. Just because HIV is around doesn't mean you'll get it. It only means you have to be careful.

What Are the Symptoms? Although some people who contract HIV develop symptoms within just a few months, the HIV virus can stay alive in a person's body for ten years or longer before any symptoms appear. A few people may never develop symptoms. But even during this period of few or no symptoms, the virus is alive inside your body and can be passed to others. If symptoms start to appear, this is what you might experience:

Unexplained weight loss (10 pounds or more in under two months).

Extreme tiredness for no reason.

Recurring night sweats.

Recurring unexplained fever.

Chronic diarrhea.

Swollen glands in the neck, armpits, or groin.

Persistent dry cough.

Purple blotches on the skin that don't go away.

Chronic pneumonia.

Seizures.

Severe difficulty swallowing.

Many of these symptoms are also symptoms of other diseases. Don't assume you have HIV/AIDS just because you have one or two of the symptoms listed. If you have *any* unexplained medical problems for longer than a week, however, it's a good idea to have yourself checked by a medical professional to find out what's wrong.

Tests and Diagnosis. To be certain about whether you have HIV/AIDS, you must have a test. HIV/AIDS testing is private and confidential. If you prefer, it can be done anonymously, using numbers instead of names. Talk about this to a counselor where you are being tested if anonymity is important to you.

Who should get tested for HIV? Everyone who has unprotected sex with a sexual partner who has had sex with other people. Everyone who uses intravenous drugs. Everyone whose partner has used intravenous drugs. Everyone who has forgotten to use condoms and other safer-sex methods. Everyone who thinks he or she might have had sex with an HIV-infected person. If you are a young woman who is pregnant or planning to become pregnant, and if you have any of the risk factors listed, you should have yourself tested. There is a one-in-four chance that if you are HIV-positive you could transmit the virus to your baby. With medical treatment, however, your chance of infecting the baby is much lower.

Tests are offered at Department of Health clinics, hospitals, and doctors' offices. To find a public clinic near you, look in your phone book under the name of your city, county, or state. Look under Health for the subheading HIV/AIDS or STD (sexually transmitted diseases). Call that number. You don't have to give your name. Ask how to make an appointment for an AIDS test. If you are under eighteen, ask if you will need parental permission to be tested. If you do need parental permission and you are afraid to ask your parents for their permission, call the toll-free HIV Hotline (1-800-342-2437) and ask them what to do. Also, find out if there is a fee so you can be prepared with money if you need it. If you go to a public clinic for your test, the fee will probably be around $20. If you cannot afford that, let them know you are a teenager and have no financial resources. Some places are able to offer free tests. They may ask for a small donation. Tests at private doctors' offices will be more expensive.

Although home HIV tests are available, they are expensive—around $50—and you must follow the instructions perfectly for the test to be accurate. Even then, there is always a margin of error, so it's wise to repeat the test in three months. We do not advise using the home test, because you will be alone, without professional guidance or counseling. Also, waiting for the results of a home test, which may take several weeks, can make you very tense. Counselors are available at public health clinics and other health facilities. If you have your test done at one of these facilities, you will have counseling and a built-in support network.

You can call one of these toll-free telephone numbers to get general information about HIV/AIDS and HIV testing. The National AIDS Hotline is open twenty-four hours a day. It can give you the AIDS Hotline number for your state, which may have more complete local information. You will not be asked for your name.

CDC National AIDS
    Hotline: 1-800-342-AIDS (2437)
    in Spanish: 1-800-344-SIDA (7432)
    for the Deaf: 1-800-243-7889

The HIV Test.   What is an HIV test? There are now several accurate tests for HIV. The traditional test is a simple blood test. When HIV enters a person's bloodstream, it attacks certain white blood cells. Your body reacts by producing special defense substances called HIV antibodies to try to fight back. The blood test can determine whether or not HIV antibodies are in your blood. If they are, it means you have been infected with HIV. It does not mean you have AIDS, but it does mean that the virus that can eventually cause AIDS is in your system.

A newer test, the "saliva test," involves placing a special cotton fiber pad between your gum and your cheek and keeping it there for two minutes. It collects and concentrates the HIV antibodies which are present in your mouth tissue (mucosal transudate) if you are infected. HIV/AIDS is not passed through saliva, but the HIV antibodies will be present in the saliva and oral tissue in enough concentration for testing. The saliva test is 99.97 percent accurate, meaning it will give a false report in only one out of 10,000 cases.*

It takes anywhere from a few days to two weeks to get results back from your HIV test. This waiting time can be difficult, full of anxiety and tension. It's very normal to feel nervous and be worried, but don't let those worries keep you from returning to the clinic to get your results. If you're not infected, you'll be very relieved. If you use safer sex precau-

tions every time you have sexual contact from now on, you can continue to help keep yourself from becoming infected.

If you find out you are infected, the counselor will tell you about the growing number of new treatments available to HIV-positive people, treatments that can help you feel healthy and remain symptom-free for many years. As an HIV-positive person, you must use safer-sex precautions from now on because you can infect other people. Also, if you continue to have unprotected sex or share needles, you will chance continuing to reinfect yourself and further weakening your immune system.

In general, HIV antibodies will not show up on a test until you've been infected for three to six months. That is why you cannot be sure about negative test results until at least six months have passed from the time of infection. Because of this time lag, clinics suggest having yourself tested once and then again in another three months. Be sure to practice safer sex or abstain from sex completely between tests, otherwise a negative result may not be accurate.

Treatment.   At present there is no cure for HIV/AIDS and no vaccination to keep you from getting it. Of course scientists, doctors, health officials, and drug companies are trying to discover more about the illness and more about its treatment. We hope a cure will be found very soon.

There are ways to improve your chances of keeping symptoms at a minimum for many years. New drugs and treatments are being tested and approved all the time. It's not possible for us to name them here, since they change frequently. These treatments tend to be extremely expensive, but as an adolescent, you may be eligible to participate free of charge in clinical trials. Be sure to ask about that. The newest and most effective treatments require continued supervision by medical professionals.

Call the National AIDS Hotline (1-800-342-AIDS [2437]) to find out who in your area has the most up-to-date information about treatment.

To keep your body healthy longer and give your immune system the strength it needs to fight the HIV infection, consider adopting some simple health measures. Eat a low-fat diet with lots of organically grown

* This information comes from ORASURE, the company producing the only non-invasive HIV test approved by the FDA as this book goes to press.

fresh fruits and vegetables, get plenty of sleep and exercise, take vitamin and mineral supplements, and stay away from cigarettes, alcohol, and illegal drugs.

Prevention. The first thing you have to do to keep yourself from getting HIV/AIDS is to *educate yourself.* Learn how you can prevent HIV infection and tell your friends and sex partners what you've learned. If you are sexually active, the only way to avoid getting HIV is to use condoms and other barrier methods and to talk with your partner about prevention before you engage in sexual activity. Sometimes that's hard advice to follow, as David, a seventeen-year-old from California, said:

This whole thing about AIDS sucks. It's changing everybody's life. You want the facts about how to not catch AIDS, but you also want the whole thing to just go away so you can forget about it and let yourself not be so responsible all the time.

David's lament is echoed by teenagers and adults everywhere, every day. Because of the reality that HIV/AIDS kills, people all over are reexamining their ideas about "free love" and "the sexual revolution." If you care about yourself, having sex with people you don't know well, or with lots of partners, or with people who have lots of partners, is simply not safe.

Chlamydia

What Is It? Chlamydia (kla-*mih*-dee-uh) is a bacterial infection. It is the most common STD in the United States today. The government estimates that each year as many as 4 million people contract chlamydia. If you have chlamydia but do not get it treated, it can lead to pelvic inflammatory disease (PID) in females, which infects and damages the internal sexual organs, sometimes creating permanent infertility (the inability to get pregnant or carry a baby to term). In males, if chlamydia goes

---

How to Minimize Your Risk of Contracting HIV

Be responsible about sexual relationships. Your life depends on it. Follow these precautions if you decide to have sex with a partner:

➤ Know your sex partner well. Ask him or her about his or her health. If you don't feel comfortable enough to discuss these things with a partner, *don't* have sex with him or her.

➤ Limit your partners. A mutually monogamous relationship (just you and your partner exclusively with each other) with someone who is not infected is safer. But don't kid yourself: it only takes one encounter to get infected.

➤ *Always use latex condoms* (and other suitable barriers) *during penetration* whether it is penis-vagina, penis-anus, or penis-mouth. (See page 286 for complete discussion of Safer-Sex Methods.)

➤ Latex condoms along with spermicide are very good protection for penis-vagina penetration. They are also excellent protection against unwanted pregnancy. But remember, the only 100 percent effective protection is abstinence.

➤ Do not have sex with anyone who has multiple partners.

➤ Avoid kissing someone whose mouth or lips have open cuts or sores.

➤ Do not practice fellatio (penis-mouth sex) without a latex condom; if a person has HIV, his semen will contain the virus. Vaginal secretions can also carry the virus, so use a barrier for cunnilingus (mouth-clitoris/vaginal sex). (See page 288 for information about barriers.)

➤ Avoid having sex while drunk or stoned, because drugs and alcohol tend to interfere with taking responsible actions.

➤ If you inject drugs or pierce your body, *never* share needles with anyone else. Sterilize all equipment before each use.

➤ Never share enema paraphernalia or douche bags or toothbrushes or razors.

untreated, it can cause infection in the sperm-transmitting organs and lead to male infertility (the inability to produce and ejaculate healthy sperm). Unfortunately, the symptoms of internal chlamydia infection do not always become apparent until damage has already been done. That's why we recommend having yourself routinely checked for this and other STDs.

How It Is Passed. The *Chlamydia trachomatis* organism is passed from an infected person to his or her partner through unprotected vaginal or anal intercourse or through fellatio (penis-mouth sex) or cunnilingus (vagina-mouth sex). During intercourse, it is easier for a woman to catch this disease from a man than it is for a man to catch it from a woman, because ejaculate (semen) stays inside a woman's body for hours, while vaginal fluids tend to dry quickly after a man pulls his penis out of his partner's body. If there are cuts on the penis, vagina, or anal canal, chlamydia can pass during penis-vagina or anal intercourse into a person's blood and cause infection in other parts of the body. The disease can also infect your eyes, should they come into contact with penile or vaginal secretions during oral sex or if you rub your eyes after touching infected secretions.

How It Is Not Passed. Chlamydia is not passed through casual kissing or touching. It is not passed through nonsexual activities. It is not passed by sharing clothes or using public bathroom facilities. Good hygiene advises against wearing someone else's unclean underwear or sitting on a soiled toilet seat, however.

What Are the Symptoms? The early symptoms of chlamydia are an increased vaginal or penile discharge and/or pain or a burning sensation when you urinate. These symptoms usually appear within one to three weeks after you become infected.

Some people do not experience or notice symptoms at all, so they don't seek treatment. In fact, four out of every five women who have chlamydia don't know they have it. Sexually active teens should have regular tests to screen for chlamydia, even if they have no apparent symptoms, since this disease is common and spreading fast.

In females, if the chlamydial infection progresses to pelvic inflammatory disease (PID), it will cause infection and swelling in the ovaries and fallopian tubes. This can be extremely painful, and as we said, can cause permanent damage. If you are sexually active and you experience unexplained stomach cramps or internal aching, have yourself tested for chlamydia.

In males, chlamydia can cause a condition known as epididymitis, an inflammation of the epididymis, which is an important part of the male reproductive system (see page 19). You may experience pain and swelling in and around your scrotum. If you do not get treatment, this condition may cause scarring and damage to the male reproductive organs, causing infertility (inability to produce viable sperm).

Chlamydia may also cause an inflammation of the rectum (proctitis), an inflammation of the lining of the eye (conjunctivitis), and joint pains.

Tests and Diagnosis. There are two different tests for chlamydia. In the culture test, a health worker takes a small swab of discharge and cervical cells from the female, or discharge and cell tissue from the penis in a male. The swab sits in a special medium in the laboratory for about three days to see if chlamydia grows in the culture. Another faster, less expensive test is available, which also uses a swab of discharge and cell tissue from the cervix in females or the penis in males. Although this "rapid" test is less accurate, it is used in most routine checkups, since it produces results in just fifteen minutes.

Treatment and Follow-up. Chlamydia is a bacterial infection, so in most cases it responds to antibiotic treatment. The majority of clinics use tetracycline or doxycycline to treat it. However, pregnant women should be given an alternative antibiotic, since tetracycline and doxycycline (a broad-spectrum tetracycline) can harm the bones and teeth of a developing fetus. Erythromycin can be used instead. Penicillin is not effective against chlamydia.

You must take your medication over a period of seven to ten days. *Be sure to take the entire dose for the required amount of time.* Never borrow someone else's medication or give some of yours to anyone. If you stop the medication too soon, you may not kill all the chlamydia in your system and a stronger, more resistant strain may develop.

After you finish taking your medication, you will have to go back to the doctor for a follow-up exam to be sure you have been cured.

If you are infected, that means your sex partner either gave it to you or got it from you, so once you find out, tell your sex partner that he or she may also be infected and needs a test. The two of you will continue to pass the disease back and forth until you have both been tested, treated, and cured. If you have more than one partner, be sure all are tested, treated, and cured before you continue to have sex with them.

Prevention. The signs of chlamydia may or may not be obvious. To be safe:

➤ Use condoms and spermicide during penis-vagina or penis-anus intercourse. Use barrier methods on the vaginal area for oral sex on a female and a condom for penis-mouth penetration.

➤ Do not have sex with a male who has a milky discharge from his penis, or with a male or female who complains of burning urination or severe stomach cramps or internal aching.

Gonorrhea

Street names: the clap, dose, drip, morning dew, gleet, hot piss, the whites.

What Is It? Health officials estimate that nearly 1½ million new cases of gonorrhea (gah-noh-*ree*-uh) occur every year. It is a bacterial infection caused by the gonococcus bacterium, which thrives in the warm, moist areas of your body. Like chlamydia, if gonorrhea goes untreated, it can lead to pelvic inflammatory disease and infertility in females. In males, it can cause painful and swollen testicles, epididymitis, and infertility. In both males and females,

the disease can eventually cause fever, chills, joint pain, and in the most severe cases, acute arthritis and infections of the heart or the brain.

Gonorrhea has been around a very long time. There are references to it in the Bible! For thousands of years, people have died from complications of this disease. Treatment for gonorrhea was made possible by the discovery of antibiotics, although strains of the disease are resistant to some common antibiotics and require newer, more potent combinations of drugs.

How It Is Passed. Gonococcus bacteria are most commonly passed through penis-vagina intercourse and also through anal sex and oral sex. The bacteria multiply quickly in the parts of your body most congenial to their growth: the cervix, urethra, mouth, throat, and rectum in females and the urethra, mouth, throat, and rectum in males.

Eyes can be infected too if they come into contact with the bacteria. Pregnant women who are infected with gonorrhea can pass the disease to their newborn infants during delivery.

How It Is Not Passed. Gonorrhea is not transmitted by touching doorknobs, or using public toilets, sharing towels, or wearing someone else's clothes. Good hygiene advises against wearing someone else's unclean underwear or sitting on a wet or unclean toilet seat.

What Are the Symptoms? The initial symptoms of gonorrhea are vaginal or penile discharge and a painful, burning sensation during urination. These may occur within one day to two weeks after contact. Because many people show no symptoms until the disease has spread to their internal organs, however, you may not know you have gonorrhea until you feel severe pain in your groin or stomach area.

The following are some of the possible symptoms females may experience. Remember, most females (about 80 percent) show no symptoms at all at first:

➤ Vaginal discharge with an unusual odor and a whitish, greenish, or yellowish color.

➤Pain and/or a strong burning sensation during urination; inflamed vulva.

➤Sore throat and/or swollen glands.

➤Groin or stomach pain.

➤Bleeding between menstrual periods.

➤Discharge from anus.

➤Chills, fever, flulike symptoms with joint pain.

➤Painful bowel movements.

In males (about 20 percent show no symptoms until complications occur):

➤Discharge from the penis, sometimes noticed as a drip seen before the first morning urination; sometimes a continual discharge.

➤Burning, itching, and/or pain when urinating.

➤Sore throat and/or swollen glands.

➤Discharge from anus.

➤Swollen, painful testicles.

➤Pain in the groin area.

➤Chills, fever, flulike symptoms with joint pain.

➤Painful bowel movements.

Tests and Diagnosis. The health worker will listen to your description of symptoms and take a sample of the discharge from the cervix and urethra in females or from the tip of the penis in males. Even when there isn't a visible discharge, if you have gonorrhea, the tissue taken from those areas is likely to contain diseased cells. Tissue samples may also be taken from your anus and/or throat, depending on whether you've had oral sex and/or anal intercourse.

There are two tests for gonorrhea, the gram-stain test and the tissue-culture test. In the gram-stain test, which is reliable for males but less reliable for females, the technician places a smear of discharge on a laboratory slide stained with a special dye. If gonococcus is present in the smear, it can be seen. Results of this test can be given almost immediately. But sometimes gram-stain tests come back

negative even when you have the disease. That's why, especially for females, a culture test may be used too if there is reason to believe you have the disease.

In the culture test a sample of discharge is grown for several days on a laboratory culture plate. The bacteria multiply and are easy to identify 90 percent of the time. You will be asked to return to the clinic to get your results, and if your test results are negative, ask the health worker if you should have another test done just to be sure, especially if you suspect you may have the disease. Two negative cultures usually mean you are clear.

Treatment and Follow-up. Gonorrhea is a bacterial disease that can be treated with antibiotics like ampicillin, amoxicillin, and penicillin. New strains of gonorrhea have developed, however, which are resistant to penicillin and penicillin-type antibiotics, so doctors are using combinations of antibiotic drugs to treat the disease. Women who are pregnant should use antibiotics that do not cause side effects for the fetus. If you are pregnant (or suspect you might be pregnant), be sure to tell the doctor.

You may be given a shot of antibiotic, pills to take orally, or both. Follow the instructions exactly and be sure to take the complete dose of medication for as long as you're told to. *Never* borrow someone else's medication or give yours to anyone else. You need the full dose yourself.

After your treatment is over, you will return to the clinic for a follow-up test. Some gonorrhea germs are very strong and need two complete treatments before they are all killed. Be sure to return for your follow-up tests, because only then can you be sure your infection has been cured.

All your sex partners must be tested and treated if they have the disease. Do not have sex with anyone until you are fully cured, and until your sex partners have been tested, treated, and cured. Otherwise you will continue to pass the disease back and forth.

Complications. If untreated or incompletely treated, gonorrhea bacteria will continue to infect you. *Gonorrhea will not go away by itself, even if* *the warning symptoms go away.* The germs will spread and cause infection and scarring in your reproductive organs. This can lead to permanent infertility, meaning you will no longer be able to get pregnant or get someone pregnant. Untreated gonorrhea can also cause crippling arthritis in some people. If the germs infect your eyes, blindness may result.

The most common complication of gonorrhea in girls is pelvic inflammatory disease (PID). This may cause severe pain in the stomach and groin areas and swelling in and damage to the female internal organs (see page 36). PID is the leading cause of infertility among young women.

If you are already pregnant when you get gonorrhea, your baby can develop an infection in his or her eyes during childbirth, which, if untreated, can cause blindness.

In males, untreated gonorrhea may lead to chronic urethritis, which is a long-term, painful inflammation of the urethra. Problems and severe pain during urination and ejaculation may result. Untreated gonorrhea may also cause epididymitis, an inflammation of the sperm centers in the testicles. This is very painful and can cause infertility.

Prevention. Gonorrhea is highly contagious, and its effects are seriously hazardous to your health. So if you are sexually active, have yourself tested for gonorrhea regularly even if you experience no symptoms. *If you have multiple sex partners, health workers recommend your being tested at least twice a year.*

- ➢ Condoms are good protection against the gonococcus bacteria during penis-vagina and anal intercourse, and diaphragms with spermicide add further protection during penis-vagina intercourse.

- ➢ Condoms should also be used during penis-mouth sex play.

- ➢ Other barriers can be used for mouth-vagina sex play.

- ➢ After oral sex, gargling with salt water may help destroy germs.

- ➢ Look your partner over. Check for discharge. Do not have sex with a male or female who has signs of discharge.

- ➢ Do not have sex with a male or female who complains of a burning sensation or pain during urination.

Hepatitis

What Is It? Hepatitis (heh-pah-*tie*-tiss) is a viral disease that infects a person's liver, causing serious illness and even death in some cases. There are three main strains of hepatitis, called A, B, and C.

How Is It Passed? The three different types of hepatitis are passed differently. *Hepatitis A* is caused by fecal contamination—contact with the feces (body wastes) of an infected person. It can also be caught from eating undercooked contaminated shellfish and drinking contaminated water. If a person with hepatitis A wipes himself or herself after going to the bathroom and doesn't wash his or her hands, the germs can be passed to whatever he or she touches. Sitting on a contaminated toilet seat can also transmit the disease. Sexually, people can catch Hepatitis A through penis-anus, finger-anus, and mouth-anus contact with an infected person.

An infected person carries *hepatitis B* in his or her blood and body fluids. Sexual practices that bring your body openings in contact with an infected person's body openings can transmit hepatitis B. It is very contagious. It can be passed through kissing, penis-vagina, penis-anus, penis-mouth, and vagina-mouth contact. Hepatitis B can also be passed through contact with an infected person's blood. Sharing needles and other instruments used for drug injections, for tattooing, for ear piercing or body piercing, for acupuncture; sharing toothbrushes; exchanging blood through blood brother or blood sister acts; using someone else's used razor; using someone else's enema bag or douche equipment—all these activities can pass the disease from one person to another. If a woman is infected with hepatitis B, her menstrual blood will be infected.

Hepatitis C is carried in an infected person's blood. Sharing any implement that punctures the skin or comes in contact with the blood of an infected person can transmit the disease. So can sexual practices if contact skin is torn or cut. Anal intercourse is risky, because the tissue inside the anus tears easily. Menstrual blood will be contaminated in a woman who has the disease, so unprotected intercourse during menstruation can be risky.

It is uncertain whether hepatitis C is passed through semen. Everyone who has hepatitis C or has a partner with hepatitis C should use condoms during intercourse and oral sex to keep from passing the disease.

What Are the Symptoms? The general symptoms are very much like the flu: nausea, muscle achiness, fatigue, fever, loss of appetite, headaches, dizziness. People often don't realize they have hepatitis, because they think they have the flu or a bad cold. If they are having sexual relations during the time they feel sick, they can pass hepatitis on to their partner(s) without even knowing it.

Hepatitis has some specific symptoms:

1. The color of your urine darkens.

2. Your stool (feces) color lightens or appears grayish.

3. Eyes and skin take on a yellowish tint (although, contrary to popular belief, many people with hepatitis do not become jaundiced).

4. You feel tenderness in the liver area (above your stomach, mainly under your heart and right lung).

The symptoms may begin to appear within the first month after infection or they may take up to six months to appear. In some cases they are so mild you may not notice them.

Go to a health facility for testing as soon as you do notice symptoms of any kind. You are contagious to other people whether or not your symptoms are apparent. In fact, many people with hepatitis C never remember having any apparent symptoms.

Tests and Diagnosis. The health worker will listen to your description of symptoms and check for fever. He or she will look at your eyes to check for a yellowish color. When you call to make your appointment, you may be asked to bring in a fresh stool sample, which will be checked for the disease. The health worker will ask you general questions about your health and living habits. Since hepatitis is a common disease among intravenous (IV) drug users, male homosexuals, and heterosexual couples who practice anal sex, be honest with the nurse or doctor about your sex life. It will help him or her to make an accurate diagnosis.

As a blood test can identify hepatitis after the second week of infection, the worker will draw some of your blood for testing.

Treatment. There are vaccines to protect people against hepatitis A and B. Check at your nearest public health clinic. Call the STD hot line number listed in the Resource section of this chapter for more information.

Hepatitis is a viral disease, and there is no medication to cure it at this time. The best treatment is to strengthen your own immune system through bed rest, drinking lots of fluids, and eating a high carbohydrate, high protein, nutritious diet. Avoid fatty foods and stay away from non-nutritional junk foods like soda pop, chips, and sweets. Don't drink alcohol, because alcohol is a further strain on your liver, the organ most weakened already by the disease.

If you have hepatitis, you will benefit from having people nearby who care about you and can tend to your needs. Several people we interviewed said that they were so weak during their bout with hepatitis, they had no choice but to stay in bed. They could hardly move and needed someone to help them take care of themselves and feed them. Shots of gamma globulin will help protect these caretakers from getting hepatitis A, if that is the form you have. They can receive a vaccine for type B, but there is no preventive vaccine yet for type C, so caretakers have to be extremely cautious not to catch the disease from you.

If you have no one to help you, contact your local board of health or the local visiting nurse association.

Follow-up. Recovery usually takes two to three months, sometimes less than that, sometimes much longer. You must get plenty of rest until the disease has completely run its course. Avoid stress. Have frequent medical checkups, according to your health worker's instructions.

Of course it is easy enough for us to tell you to get plenty of rest and avoid stress, but sometimes that is hard to do. If you are a student, you may have to give up your classes and schoolwork for a while. If you are working, you may have to take a leave from your job. Stay away from partying. Don't drink alcohol or do drugs. *Do not have any sexual contact until you are completely cured.* Not only are you likely to pass the disease on to someone else, but you are also much more vulnerable to catching other STDs, especially HIV/AIDS, while you have hepatitis.

One attack of hepatitis generally gives you immunity to that particular strain of hepatitis, so you will probably not come down with that type again. Some people seem healthy outwardly, but carry hepatitis in their system even after all their symptoms have disappeared. These people are called chronic carriers, and they can continue to infect others even though they themselves don't feel sick.

A blood test will tell you if the disease is still alive in your body. If you are a carrier of hepatitis, you must let your sex partners, your health workers, and your dentist know of your condition and you must not donate blood.

Complications. Complications vary according to the type of hepatitis you have. For this reason, make sure you are tested for and informed about your particular type of the disease.

Liver problems are the most common complication of hepatitis, since the disease affects the liver. In rare cases, hepatitis can cause permanent damage to your liver, liver cancer, or death due to liver failure.

During pregnancy, hepatitis may cause miscarriage. If a woman has hepatitis B during the last months of pregnancy, the newborn may develop the disease and become a chronic carrier. About 40 to 50 percent of the children born to infected mothers develop liver cancer. Special injections of globulin may protect the infant, so if you are pregnant and have hepatitis, make sure you tell your doctor right away.

Prevention

➤ Don't have sex with anyone who appears sick or looks jaundiced (unnatural yellowish cast to skin and whites of the eye).

➤ Never use someone else's toothbrush, razor, enema, douche equipment, or other equipment that may be contaminated by body fluids, body wastes, or blood. Do not share needles or other skin-piercing devices.

➤ If you are living with someone who has hepatitis, keep all their food preparation and eating utensils separate, and make sure they have separate towels, bed linen, and dishes. If possible, they should use separate toilet facilities. If that isn't possible, careful cleansing of the toilet with a disinfectant after use is essential.

➤ Do not sit on dirty or possibly infected toilet seats.

➤ Wash your hands thoroughly with soap and water after using the toilet.

Extra Precautions:

➤ Wash your genital area, especially your anus and anything that touches it, before and after sexual contact.

➤ There is a product called Fleet's enema that can be used to clean the anal canal before anal sex.

Herpes

What Is It? Herpes (*her*-pees) is a viral infection. One out of every four adults is infected with the herpes virus. Common cold sores—the fever blisters and canker sores people get around their mouths and noses—are one type of herpes. Another kind is genital herpes. Painful blisters and sores appear on and in the penis, vagina, and/or anus. Genital herpes can sometimes be found in the mouth area as well, probably resulting from infection through oral-genital sex.

Before the sores come out, a person may notice a tingling, burning, or itching sensation in the affected area. Then the blisters burst out and usually last for two or three weeks. In some people, the attack is so minor they confuse it with jock itch, or an ingrown pubic hair. After the attack, if you had blisters they will disappear, but the virus doesn't die. It travels along your nerve endings to live at the base of your spine or in the ganglia, the collections of nerve cells throughout your body. When a person with herpes is under stress or run-down or has had too much sun, the virus travels down the nerves and causes the painful sores to erupt again.

How It Is Passed. The virus is passed by direct contact with the infected area. It can be passed a few days *before* the sores erupt, *during* an outbreak, and a few days *after* the sores disappear. If your partner doesn't have visible sores, that doesn't mean he or she is not contagious. The virus enters your body through cuts, genital openings, mouth, eyes, and sore-to-skin contact. You can pass the virus from one part of your body to another when you touch an infected area and then touch another body opening.

What Are the Symptoms? Symptoms of herpes usually show up two to twenty days after contact with the infection, but sometimes the virus will stay in your body without symptoms for several months or even a year or more before erupting into sores. Some people have the disease but never experience any symptoms. Even with no symptoms, these people can pass the disease on to their sexual partners when the virus is active in their body.

Symptoms of an attack are itching, tingling, burning, or achiness around your genitals. You may also feel a general achiness, as if you're coming down with the flu. You may develop a slight fever, a headache, and swollen glands.

The area becomes red and tender and sores appear. In males, the sores can appear on and around the penis, scrotum, buttocks, anus, and thighs. In females, they can appear in and around the vagina, clitoris, cervix, buttocks, anus, thighs, and navel. They can be very painful. They may crack and become blistered and ooze fluid or bleed. During this active stage, you may feel the urge to urinate frequently, but urination may be painful. These symptoms usually last from two to three weeks during the first outbreak. Then the blisters go away and may never return. Or they may go away and return at different times throughout your life, especially when you are run-down and under stress. Repeat attacks are generally less painful than the first attack.

Tests and Diagnosis. Most diagnoses occur by sight, when the sores are present, although the herpes sores can be confused with a few other diseases.

The two most effective tests should be done at the beginning of a herpes attack, when the sores are fresh. These tests are the smear test and the viral culture. The smear test involves scraping some material from one of the active sores and smearing that on a specially prepared laboratory slide for evaluation. This test is fairly accurate and cheap. The viral culture test, which involves taking some living cells from the infected area when the sores first appear, can determine which type of herpes you have. Both of these tests can be painful, because scraping the herpes sores can cause pain. Nonetheless, it is important to test for herpes, so that you know for certain what is causing your symptoms.

Treatment. There is no medication to cure the herpes virus at present, but researchers are trying to find a cure. A vaccine to help prevent the disease is reported to be due out soon. Until there is a vaccine, medical practitioners recommend antiviral drugs (like Valtrex, Famvir, and Zovirax) for extreme cases of herpes. These drugs should be used only for long-lasting and frequently recurring outbreaks.

Over the years, people have found a variety of techniques to help themselves deal with herpes. Here are some suggestions:

➤ Keep the sores clean and dry. Dry well after washing. Change underwear at least once a day.

➤ Ice numbs the area and relieves pain. If you feel an attack coming on, apply ice in an ice bag (or use a plastic bag to keep the area dry). Ice may even stop the sores from erupting.

➤ Aloe vera gel may be soothing and help dry the sores.

➤ Eat a healthy diet. Stay away from chocolate, cola drinks, and peanuts (a substance found in those foods may make herpes worse). Also, be sure to get enough vitamin C (oranges, leafy green vegetables, broccoli, berries, sweet peppers). Wheat grass may help; so may powdered chlorophyll (check for these at your local health food store). Don't eat fatty, greasy foods. Keep your diet simple and healthy—whole grains, lots of fresh fruits and vegetables.

➤ Get enough sleep. Keep your stress level down; stress often leads to an outbreak (see page 171). Relax. Try meditation or yoga or long walks or some other relaxation technique. Since many teens don't have much private time, you may have to improvise. Going to the library to listen to good music or read a good book helps a lot, and it's free.

Follow-up. If your sores do not go away within ten days to two weeks, go to the clinic for a checkup. Continue going once a week until the sores clear up. Sometimes a bacterial infection will complicate the healing process, and you may need to take antibiotics for that.

Avoid all sexual activity until two or three days after the sores disappear completely. Do not even masturbate, since your hands can pass the disease to other parts of your body.

Sexually active girls should have a Pap smear every year (see page 251 for a discussion of Pap smears). This is especially important for girls with herpes.

Complications. For males, herpes can be painful and annoying. For females, it can be painful, annoying, and potentially dangerous. A herpes outbreak can complicate a pregnancy and delivery, possibly causing miscarriage and/or premature delivery. Pregnant women with herpes need to take special care. Newborns who come into contact with herpes during delivery are in the most danger, since the virus can cause brain damage, blindness, and death. The risk to the baby is highest when mothers have their first herpes attack around the time of delivery. Pregnant women who have had recurrent herpes for a long time will pass protective antibodies to the baby through the amniotic fluid, lowering the risk of birth defects and infant death.

If you are pregnant and you have herpes, *be sure to tell your doctor.* Whether you do or don't have herpes, during the two months prior to your due date do *not* have sex with any partner who has herpes.

Prevention. Although at present there is no cure for herpes and no vaccine to prevent it, there are some ways to avoid this disease:

➤ Do not have oral or genital sex with someone who has sores on her or his genitals or mouth.

➤ Ask your sexual partner if she or he has herpes. Ask if she or he feels an attack coming on, since the virus is contagious before sores erupt and just after they disappear. Some symptoms of an attack are like flu symptoms. Sometimes there is a tingling or burning or itching in the area of the outbreak.

➤ If you fall in love with someone who has herpes, talk about it, inform yourselves, and take precautions. A lot of people who have had one outbreak of herpes never have another.

➤ Use latex condoms and barrier methods with your sex partners.

➤ Herpes can be passed when a person's skin comes in contact with the infected area. Condoms don't cover everything, so be careful.

➤ Keep yourself healthy. People who are run-down are more susceptible to viral infections.

➤ Don't get too much sun. Sun doesn't cause herpes, but overexposure seems to bring on attacks if the virus is already in your system.

Herpes is spreading fast. For excellent information about herpes, you can call the free National STD Hotline: 1-800-227-8922.

HPV—Human Papilloma Virus/Genital Warts

What Is It? Health workers estimate that over 40 million American people are infected with the human papilloma virus (human pa-pih-*loh*-ma virus), a family of viruses that cause warts. There are more than 65 different varieties of the virus, from HPVs that cause the ordinary warts many people have on their hands or feet to the ones that cause life-threatening illnesses. Human papilloma virus is responsible for serious health problems like laryngeal papillomatosis—LP* (warts growing on the larynx, which can make talking difficult and/or affect a person's breathing)—and recurrent respiratory papillomatosis* (warts growing in the lungs and/or bronchial tubes that can kill a person if they grow out of control). The HPVs we will discuss in this chapter are those that cause warts to form on and around a person's genitals. A few of these may be associated with the development of cervical and other genital cancers.

In females, genital warts show up in and around the vagina, the cervix, the vulva, and/or the anus. In males they may develop on the head of the penis (often under the foreskin if a male is uncircumcised), on the shaft of the penis, on the scrotum, and/or around the anus. The presence of warts inside the vagina may make intercourse painful or itchy for females. Genital warts may also appear around a person's mouth.

Smoking worsens a papilloma condition. Research has shown that smoking cigarettes keeps the human papilloma virus active.

How It Is Passed. Genital warts (also called venereal warts—*condylomata acuminata*) are very contagious. They are passed by direct contact between a wart and someone's skin. Two out of every three people exposed to genital warts will become infected. That's a huge number of people, about one million new cases every year.

If you have oral-sexual contact with someone who has genital warts, you may develop warts in and around your mouth area. These can then be passed to a partner during kissing or oral sex.

Genital warts may be big enough to be seen easily. As they grow they tend to spread and cluster in cauliflower-like groupings, which make them even more noticeable. On the other hand, sometimes they are so tiny they can't be seen with the naked eye. Genital warts are contagious whether or not they can be seen.

---

* For more information about treatment for LP or RRP, contact Recurrent Respiratory Foundation, 50 Wesleyan Dr., Hamilton, NJ 08690.

How It Is Not Passed. This condition is not passed by any method other than through direct contact with the warts.

What Are the Symptoms? Genital warts are hard, wrinkled bumps that appear on your skin or in your genital area usually within one to three months after contact. They are painless, but they can be irritated by rubbing, and sometimes they itch. When they are inside the vagina or anus, most are pink and wet, and they may go unnoticed.

Sometimes these warts are mistaken for syphilis chancres or herpes blisters, but warts are not filled with fluid as blisters and chancres are.

Tests and Diagnosis. The health worker will examine the warts and be able to identify them from their appearance. Sometimes vinegar is applied, which turns the warts a paler color then the surrounding tissue. If they are microscopic, a gynecologist may use a special instrument to see them. Tests are rarely done except in special cases when it is important to identify which HPVs are involved.

The virus can affect cervical cells (in the cervix—see page 35) in such a way as to make them precancerous. Over several years, this condition may develop into cervical cancer. The only way to check and possibly deter this development is with regular Pap smears (see page 251).

Treatment. Having genital warts means the papilloma virus exists in your body. There is no cure for this condition. Like many viruses, it may stay with you for life. Some people opt to have their warts removed both for cosmetic reasons and so the warts won't spread. If a wart is present, the virus can be passed to your sexual partner.

Genital warts, like other types of warts, sometimes go away on their own, although the virus may remain dormant in your body.

The following are ways to treat warts. These treatments may eliminate the warts, but they may not kill the virus.

➤ Chemical Treatment. Warts can be treated with TCA (trichloracetic acid), an acid solution that is applied directly on the wart. Often this treatment requires several visits.

Many clinics will give you a prescription for a chemical treatment you can apply yourself at home. Ask about that. It is called podofilox. Podophyllin is another chemical that has been used. These are strong and potentially harmful chemicals. Do not use podophyllin if you are pregnant.

➤ Freezing. Called cryotherapy (cry-oh-*ther*-uh-pee), this is a special dry ice treatment that, when applied to the area, freezes the warts. The treated warts die and disappear; unseen and untreated warts, however, may continue to grow. Some temporary or permanent scarring may develop where the warts were removed.

➤ Burning. Electrocautery (ee-lec-tro-*caw*-ter-ee) is used to burn the warts and kill the infected tissue. You may choose to have local anesthesia for this procedure. Electrocautery may also cause temporary or permanent scarring.

➤ Surgery. For very large warts or large clusters of warts, surgical removal is recommended. Laser surgery is considered an effective treatment. Surgical techniques require anesthetic (sometimes general anesthesia—which means you are put to sleep while the surgery is being performed), depending on the placement and severity of the warts.

Be sure to ask your health worker to explain all the possible treatments, their pain factor, their side effects, and their risks. Then you can decide together which treatment would be best for your case.

Human papilloma virus is a very frustrating disease to treat. There is no guarantee that any of the treatments listed will totally eliminate the disease from your body, and if traces of the virus are left, you may continue to pass the virus on to your sex partner(s).

As with any viral infection, enough rest, good nutrition, and relaxation techniques are important elements in supporting your body's own immune system. Also, folic acid supplements may be helpful in reducing outbreaks of warts. Consult your health practitioner for the correct dosage.

Complications. If the warts are not removed, the condition may get worse. The more it spreads, the more likely it is to infect your sex partner(s).

Babies born to mothers who have genital warts may develop laryngeal papillomatosis, a condition in which warts develop on the larynx (voice box) and can obstruct the airways, making breathing difficult. This is a potentially life-threatening disease and requires repeated surgeries.

Genital warts tend to enlarge during pregnancy, which may make urination difficult and painful. If large warts are on the walls of the vagina, they may make delivery more difficult.

Human papilloma virus has been associated with cancer of the cervix, cancer of the vulva, anal cancer, and cancer of the penis (very rare). No one knows for sure what link HPV has to cancer, because other factors such as cigarette smoking, using oral contraceptives, and the presence of other STDs may contribute to the problem. If you are a female infected with HPV, you should have regular Pap smears (once or twice a year) to test for abnormalities in your cervical tissue. This is the best way to check for cancer and treat it early.

Prevention. Since you catch HPV from direct contact with HPV-infected areas, you want to avoid that contact.

➤ Do not have sex with anyone who has visible warts on his or her genitals. Unfortunately, sometimes the warts aren't visible, so you may think you're safe when you're really not.

➤ Using a latex condom during penis-vagina and penis-anus intercourse offers some protection, but since it only covers the penis, if other areas are infected, you are not protected.

Syphilis

Street names: siff, pox, lues, bad blood, Old Joe, haircut.

What Is It? Syphilis (*sih*-fih-liss) is an STD caused by tiny spiral-shaped bacteria. The disease comes on in four stages: primary, secondary, latent, and late. At first, there may be some temporary external signs of the disease, like a *painless* sore or blister, called a chancre (*shank*-er), then possibly a rash on the body or on the palms of the hands or soles of the feet. There might also be flu-like aches, a mild fever, or a headache, all of which usually go away on their own. Even though these initial symptoms may disappear, however, the disease remains alive in your body. Without treatment, it can eventually cause major damage to your vital organs and even death. Syphilis is not as common as gonorrhea or chlamydia, but it is very dangerous.

How It Is Passed. When symptoms are present, you can get syphilis from sexual or skin contact with the chancres or rash of a person who has the disease. The syphilis bacteria enter your body through body openings and through cuts and open sores. The disease remains infectious for several years, even for a while after symptoms disappear.

An unborn baby can get syphilis if the mother is infected, especially during the first few years the mother has the disease. Syphilis germs attack the unborn baby through the placenta. If syphilis is treated within the first three months of pregnancy, the baby may be spared any side effects from the disease. All pregnant women should be tested for syphilis at the beginning of their pregnancies. If a woman tests positive, she can be treated with antibiotics to protect herself and her baby.

How It Is Not Passed. You can't catch syphilis just from being near someone who has the disease. You have to have contact with their rash or their sores.

What Are the Symptoms? Since many of the symptoms of syphilis are like symptoms of other diseases, you may not realize you have it. If you are sexually active and you notice any strange sores or blisters or rashes around your genitals or on your hands or feet, or if you have an unexplained fever or swollen glands, have yourself tested. The symptoms of syphilis come in four different stages:

STAGE 1: Painless sores (chancres) appear at the spot where the germs entered your body. Often just one chancre will appear at first. In females, the sore may be inside the vagina or around the cervix and therefore not visible. In both males and females, the chancre may be in the anus, and therefore not visible. Sometimes a rash will be present. The chancres and rash will disappear in one to five weeks, but the germs will stay alive in your body.

STAGE 2: Months after the chancres disappear, some people get secondary symptoms like fever, aches, sore throat, mouth sores, patchy hair loss, swollen glands, and other flulike ailments. A rash may appear over the entire body or parts of the body, or maybe only on the palms of the hands or soles of the feet. These symptoms will also disappear by themselves after a few months, but the disease will stay alive in your body.

STAGE 3: For months or even years after the Stage 2 symptoms disappear, you may experience no symptoms on the outside, but internally the disease may be attacking your organs: your heart, your brain, your sexual organs, your eyes, your ears, your coordination, your nervous system.

STAGE 4: This is when extreme damage becomes apparent. Twenty years may pass between your initial infection and the appearance of late-stage symptoms: blindness, deafness, paralysis, insanity, heart disease, coordination problems, seizures, and death.

Some people with untreated syphilis never experience late-stage symptoms.

Tests and Diagnosis. At the clinic, a health worker will listen to your description of symptoms and check you for fever, swollen glands, unusual discharge, and chancres.

Teens who have had any sort of sexual activity with another person should go to the clinic right away when they notice a painless sore or blister around the genitals. The health worker will take a sample of fluid from the sore and examine it under a microscope to determine whether you have the disease. You will also be given a blood test, called a VDRL, which can detect syphilis from about one week to ten days after the chancre appears. If the VDRL test comes back negative, but you definitely have or had a painless chancre, have another test taken. There may not have been enough bacteria in your bloodstream to show up the first time.

Remember, if you are pregnant, have a test for syphilis right away.

Treatment and Follow-up. *The earlier you get treatment, the less damage will be done to your body.* Long-acting penicillin injections are the treatment of choice. If you are allergic to penicillin, other antibiotics can be used. At every stage, syphilis can be cured with antibiotic treatment, but damage done to your body during late-stage syphilis can't be undone.

In some people, the antibiotic begins to work right away. Other people require repeated dosages. To make sure the disease has been completely cured, you will be asked to return for follow-up blood tests every three months for one year.

DON'T HAVE SEX UNTIL THE HEALTH WORKER TELLS YOU THE DISEASE IS NO LONGER ACTIVE.

Complications. Untreated syphilis is life-threatening. See discussion under Stage 4 on page 272. If you are pregnant, untreated syphilis can cause birth defects and even infant death.

Prevention. Never have sex with a person who has sores or a rash around his or her genitals or mouth or a rash on his or her body or on the palms of the hand or soles of the feet. Of course, not all sores or rashes are signs of syphilis, and not all are contagious. But unless you are sure that your partner's sores are *not* contagious, don't take chances.

➤ Avoid direct contact with the sores or rashes of syphilis.

➤ Avoid contact with the blood or body fluids of an infected person.

➤ Using latex condoms and other barrier methods will help protect you, but barrier devices only cover specific areas, and the sores or rash may be outside those areas.

➤ The most effective method of prevention is to limit your sexual partners. Make sure you know the person well and can talk to him or her about whether he or she might be infected.

➤ Have periodic tests for syphilis and other STDs. Make sure your partner does too. If you and your partner are having sex only with each other and neither one of you is infected, you are safe.

Vaginal Infections (Vaginitis)

What Are They? Many bacteria and organisms grow normally inside the vagina, just as they do inside the mouth. They help to keep a healthy chemical balance in the vagina. Harmful bacteria and organisms, however, can multiply and upset the normal balance, creating vaginal infections. These can cause itching, burning, discharge, and general discomfort—generally called vaginitis (vaa-gih-*nye*-tiss).

The three most common vaginal infections are *trichomoniasis* (trih-coh-moh-*nye*-uh-siss), *bacterial vaginosis* (or BV), and *candida.*

Trichomoniasis, or trich (pronounced "trick"), is caused by a tiny, one-celled parasite called *Trichomonas vaginalis.* In males it is most commonly found in the urethra; in females it is most commonly found in the vagina. Many girls have trich organisms living normally in their vaginas without any symptoms of disease.

Bacterial vaginosis (or BV) is caused by the Hemophilus bacterium, and *candida* is caused by an imbalance of yeastlike organisms in the vagina. Normal yeast may not be a problem in a healthy vagina, but when the organisms multiply out of control, they cause infection.

How Are They Passed? Infections can start in many ways, not all of them sexual. Wearing tight pants that cut into your crotch; wearing pantyhose or nylon panties that don't allow air to circulate; using bath oil or a perfumed lotion in the vaginal area that might irritate you or cause an allergic reaction; douching; taking antibiotics to cure an illness; an allergic reaction to birth control; stress; illness; pregnancy—all these factors can create an imbalance in the vagina that may develop into an infection.

Unhealthy yeast, causing candida, can be carried from the anus to the vagina when the penis or finger or tongue goes into the vagina after touching the anus.

Trich is passed through sexual intercourse or finger-genital play. If you touch your partner's penis or vagina and then touch your own penis or vagina, you can pass the organism to yourself if your partner has the disease. If your partner touches himself or herself and then touches you, he or she can infect you. Males with trich sometimes have the parasite in their semen and pass it to their partners during sexual intercourse.

The trich parasite can stay alive outside the body for up to seven hours, so it's possible to catch this disease by using someone else's towel, by wearing someone else's underwear or bathing suit, or by sitting on a contaminated toilet seat.

You can get BV through sexual intercourse and other sex play, and possibly also by sharing towels, washclothes, and clothing with someone who has the disease.

What Are the Symptoms?

➤ Yeast infections (candida): Itchiness around the genitals; heavy white, cheesy discharge that smells like yeast; pain or redness around the vagina or opening of the penis.

➤ Trich: Intense itching in the genital area (boys may have less itch); pain during urination; red, tender labia in girls; bad smelling discharge from vagina or penis.

➤ BV: An excessive creamy discharge and a foul smell after intercourse (some people say it smells "fishy"). Itching; possible pain during urination; red, tender labia.

Tests and Diagnosis. Samples of discharge and vaginal fluid are placed under a microscope. An experienced health worker is almost always able to distinguish which type of infection you have just by looking at the sample under a microscope. A culture test is available should a further diagnosis be needed. In some cases a Pap smear will show an infection is present. A sample of fluid from the penis can be examined or cultured to see if a male is carrying an infection that may be passed to a female partner. Males are seldom checked for these diseases, since they are most likely to occur in the vagina.

Treatment. Antibiotics are usually prescribed for vaginitis. These drugs may create problems of their own and upset the balance of bacteria needed to maintain a healthy vagina. Some people are using alternative treatments. (See *The New Our Bodies, Ourselves* under "Vaginitis" for some of these treatments.)

➤ Yeast infections can be very annoying and hard to eliminate, especially during pregnancy. The health worker may suggest using antifungus creams in and around the infected area, and vaginal suppositories may also be used. If it is a severe case or one that keeps recurring, medication may be prescribed.

With your permission, the health worker can paint the inside of your vagina and your cervix with a substance called gentian violet. This procedure really helps a lot of girls and women, although a small number have a severe reaction to the procedure. Ask your health worker to check for a reaction before applying gentian violet. Because of its bright purple color, it can stain your clothes, so use a sanitary pad after the procedure.

If you find yourself getting recurring yeast infections, check *The New Our Bodies, Ourselves* for some very helpful remedies.

➤ Trichamoniasis, or trich, can be cured by taking a drug called Flagyl. Sexual partners must take the treatment together or they will continue to pass the trich bug back and forth. Do not drink any alcohol during this treatment, because it can cause severe nausea. Some people suggest avoiding vinegar and mayonnaise too.

Tests have shown that metronidazole, the drug used to make Flagyl, may have dangerous side effects. Pregnant girls should not take this drug, because its use during pregnancy may be harmful to the unborn baby. If you have trich and you are pregnant, you are in a no-win situation, since Flagyl is the most effective treatment for this disease. Talk this over with your health worker. There are some sulfa creams and self-help remedies that might help. Look up Flagyl in *The New Our Bodies, Ourselves*.

➤ BV: The treatment for this disease is similar to that for trich. Usually the male partner is not treated, but if the disease persists, your partner should be treated too.

> The best treatment for trich and BV is to prevent it in the first place by not having unprotected sex.
>
> Use latex condoms and other safer-sex methods!

Follow-up. In the case of yeast infections, if the symptoms don't go away within four weeks after you begin treatment, go back to the clinic. Also, try some of the techniques suggested under Prevention. Have no sexual contact with a partner until the disease is cured.

For the other infections, if symptoms persist, or if you and your partner continue to pass the infection back and forth, go to the clinic together to be checked and treated.

Prevention. These methods apply to all types of vaginitis:

➤ Keep the genital area clean. Wash with soap and water at least once a day.

➤ Don't use perfumed powders or deodorants or bath preparations in the genital area.

➤ Don't wear pants that are tight in the crotch.

➤ Use barrier protection during intercourse.

➤ Contraceptive jellies may slow down the growth of yeast infections.

➤ Cut down on sugar. High sugar intake can interfere with your body's normal chemical balance.

➤ Use plain white, unscented toilet paper.

➤ Wear clean, light-colored cotton underwear.

For females:

➤ Always wipe your vagina *before* wiping your anus (wipe front to back).

➤ Never put anything from your anus into your vagina without washing it first!

➤ Don't douche. Repeated douching is not good for your vagina.

➤ Wear cotton underwear, or at least panties with a cotton crotch.

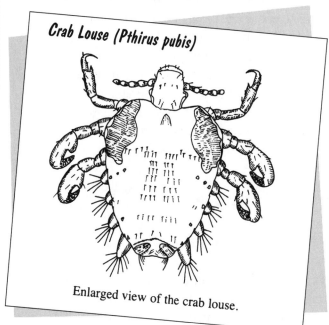

Crab Louse (Pthirus pubis)

Enlarged view of the crab louse.

Parasites

These final STDs are caused by parasitic organisms that jump from one body to another. They are more of a nuisance than a disease, but they can be a very uncomfortable nuisance.

PUBIC LICE (CRABS)

What Are They? Pubic lice are little animals the size of a pinhead, yellowish-gray in color. They feed on human blood and like to live in moist, hairy spots—for example, in pubic hair, eyelashes, underarm hair, and chest hair. They are commonly referred to as "crabs," because they look like tiny crabs.

How Are They Passed? Crabs are passed through close contact with a person who has them. The crabs from the infested person hop onto another person, pet, upholstered furniture, or bed to make themselves comfortable in the new host. Since they need blood to survive, they cannot live for more than twenty-four hours without a live host. Their eggs, however, can live without a host for almost a week.

The crabs move from one host to another, especially if you are touching each other's bodies. But even if you just borrow the clothing or sleep in the bed or sit on the couch of someone who has crabs, you can catch this STD. They are *highly* contagious.

What Are the Symptoms? The first symptom of crabs is usually an intense itching in the site where the crabs have established themselves. They are generally found in pubic hair, so your crotch may become unbearably itchy. Crabs can move to other body hair and eyelashes as you scratch them and then touch other places on your body.

You can see crabs without a microscope. Nineteen-year-old Angelica said,

Me and my boyfriend spent the night together at his place and a couple of days later I'm itching like crazy and I see these bugs crawling around in my eyelashes. It was the grossest thing.

If you look closely, you may even be able to see the eggs the crabs left to hatch on your body.

Some people may not feel any particular itching even though they have crabs. These people may not know they have them until they pass them on to a partner.

Tests and Diagnosis. If you don't find the crabs yourself, a health worker at the clinic can take a sample of hair or skin from an itchy area and see the crabs or their eggs under a microscope.

Treatment. Plain soap will not kill crabs, but special soaps and shampoos that will kill them are available both by prescription and over the counter. The most effective product needs a prescription, because it contains a powerful pesticide that can cause allergic reactions. It works very quickly and effectively if you follow the instructions exactly. Pregnant girls should not use it. Nor should it be used on babies or small children. Alternatives that are less

toxic may work almost as well. Check with your health practitioner or a pharmacist.

If you have crabs in your eyelashes or eyebrows, use ophthalmic petroleum jelly.

All your clothes, bedding, and blankets must be washed in very hot water with detergent and dried in a hot dryer, or you must have them dry-cleaned. Remember, the crab eggs can live for a week in clothing or bed linen or on stuffed animals or soft furniture; if you can't wash everything, make sure you store it for two weeks in a plastic bag. Tie the bag tightly shut.

Follow-up. You may have to repeat the treatment in two weeks. Keep checking yourself for crabs and eggs. Make sure all your partners are treated too. Otherwise you will keep passing the crabs back and forth.

Complications. The itching will make you want to scratch. The more you scratch, the greater the chance of moving the crabs from one site to another. Also, scratching can tear your skin and create an infection.

Crabs can carry diseases such as typhus, although this is very rare.

Prevention.

➤ Keep yourself clean. Shower at least once a day. Wash hair frequently.

➤ Keep your clothes and bed linen washed regularly.

➤ Don't have sex with someone who itches a lot, unless he or she has some other good reason for it. Check for crabs on his or her body.

➤ Try not to borrow other people's clothes.

SCABIES

What Are They? Scabies (*scay*-bees) are microscopic parasites that burrow under a person's skin and lay their eggs there.

How Are They Passed? They are passed when a person who has them touches another person.

That can be anything from shaking hands to making love. They are *highly* contagious.

What Are the Symptoms? The bug burrows under the skin and causes a red sore or series of sores, or raised reddish tracks along the skin. There is intense itching around the site.

Scabies can appear anywhere on the body. Sometimes it is confused with the beginning stages of poison ivy or poison oak.

Tests and Diagnosis. Go to the clinic or doctor's office. The health worker will prick out some particles from the infested area and examine them under a microscope. He or she will be able to see if scabies are present.

Treatment. Same as the treatment for crabs. Use a special soap prescribed by your health practitioner, or check with your pharmacist about an alternative. Use the soap exactly according to instructions. You may want to use two treatments to be sure to get the eggs that may have been left under your skin.

Follow-up. Make sure your sex partners are being treated too. Otherwise you'll pass the bugs back and forth.

Wash clothes and bed linen in very hot water and detergent; dry in a hot dryer.

Complications. Scabies usually itch terribly, so people scratch. Scratching can cause secondary infections and can spread the parasites to other parts of the body.

Prevention.

➤ Use proper hygiene.

➤ Wash regularly.

➤ Don't have sex with anyone who itches a lot, unless he or she has some other reason for it.

➤ Watch for sores, red spots, and patches on people's skin.

We hope you will always honor yourself enough to be careful. If that means getting yourself checked by a doctor every six months, do it. If it means using safer-sex methods every time you have sex with someone, do it. If it means postponing sexual activity altogether until you are older or in a committed relationship and willing to protect each other from disease and unplanned pregnancy, do it. Here's what Charmayne decided:

> If you don't have sex, you don't have to worry about "Oh, what if I get pregnant? What if I get an STD?" I know people who when they want to use protection they don't say anything, because they're afraid the person they're with won't like it. By not having sex, you don't have to deal with that. You don't have to worry about any of that. You know sex can be a big headache. For me, it's so much better to wait. I mean, I can have sex at any age. Right now I want to concentrate on getting my education.

RESOURCES

STD Hotline, Centers for Disease Control in Atlanta, GA (toll-free): 1-800-227-8922. This hotline is set up to answer questions and provide referrals regarding all sexually transmitted diseases.

HIV/AIDS Hotline (toll-free): 1-800-342-AIDS (2437).
HIV/AIDS Hotline in Spanish (toll-free): 1-800-344-SIDA (7432).
HIV/AIDS Hotline, Deaf Access (toll-free): 1-800-243-7889 (TTY).

Chicago Women's AIDS Project: 1-312-271-2242.
For recorded information about herpes and other STDs: 1-800-653-HEALTH (4325).

Reading Materials

The National Centers for Disease Control and Prevention (CDC) in Atlanta, Georgia, has excellent pamphlets available on HIV/AIDS and other STDs. Call the STD hotline: 1-800-227-8922 and ask the person who answers to send you the information you need. One booklet, called "Voluntary HIV Counseling and Testing: Facts, Issues, and Answers," is all about who should get tested and how to get tested for HIV.

Planned Parenthood puts out an easy-to-read, illustrated pamphlet called: "The Condom: What It Is, What It Is For, How To Use It." Call your local Planned Parenthood to find out how to get it or call the national Planned Parenthood office toll-free at 1-800-669-0156.

The New Our Bodies, Ourselves, by the Boston Women's Health Book Collective. New York: Touchstone, 1992.

Sacrificing Our Selves for Love, by Jane Wegscheider Hyman and Esther R. Rome. Freedom, California: The Crossing Press, 1996.

What You Can Do to Avoid AIDS, by Earvin "Magic" Johnson. New York: Times Books, 1996. An excellent discussion of HIV/AIDS in an easy-to-read question/answer format.

Protecting Yourself: Birth Control and Safer Sex

THE CHOICE IS YOURS

Consider this: Within the first year of having intercourse, four out of every five couples who don't use birth control will start a pregnancy. If you are a girl having sexual intercourse without using protection, it is not an accident if you get pregnant. *It is an accident if you don't get pregnant!*

Another fact: AIDS can kill you. Every year almost 20,000 teenagers catch HIV, the virus that causes AIDS. These teens now live with a disease that has no cure and that probably would have been prevented had they used protection.

These are scary statistics. You may decide to ignore them. We hope you don't. The information in this chapter will help you protect your health and your future. It may even save your life.

PROTECT YOURSELF

There are many good ways to protect yourself and your partner against both unwanted pregnancy and sexually transmitted disease (we discuss them beginning on page 286). So you might wonder why people would choose to endanger themselves by not using protection.

Here are a few reasons we heard from the teens we interviewed:

Sometimes people act without thinking through to the consequences of their actions. Maybe they say to themselves, "Why spoil the romance by planning too much?" They take chances with sex and assume they won't get hurt. When you're strong and healthy, it's hard to imagine that anything bad might happen that could change your life.

Another reason has to do with not being informed. Some teens aren't aware of how easy it is to get pregnant. Many don't know that having multiple sex partners or injecting IV drugs puts them at an especially high risk for acquiring HIV/AIDS and other sexually transmitted diseases (STDs). Some don't know where or how to get safer sex protection, or if they do know, they're embarrassed to get it and use it.

A third reason involves appearances. Some teens worry that it will be embarrassing if they come prepared with birth control/safer-sex protection. Instead of saying, "I want to be prepared just in case we do it," they say, "We probably won't have sex, so why look as if that's what's on my mind?"

Then there are a few teens who take risks with their sexual activity because they don't seem to care very much about themselves or other people. They may be thinking, What's the difference anyway? or It doesn't matter if I (or you) get pregnant or catch a disease. Sally, a high school senior from Boston, said she can't understand that attitude:

It seems really dumb to me nowadays to get pregnant if you don't want to. With all the precautions you could take, it just seems dumb. It's like you don't care about yourself a bit.

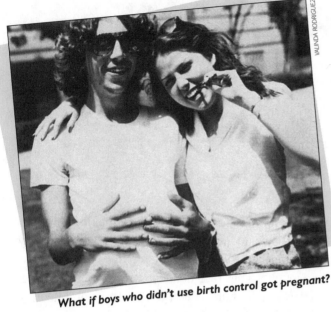

What if boys who didn't use birth control got pregnant?

Sixteen-year-old Wilson calls it the "smile today, die tomorrow" attitude. People who have goals for the future, who want more education or a good job, who plan to get married and raise a family, don't want to "die" tomorrow. They don't want an unplanned pregnancy or an incurable STD to jeopardize their plans. Many are choosing to wait until they're older, when they can better handle the responsibility of a sexual relationship, or if they do decide to have sex now, *they use protection every time*.

MYTHS ABOUT SAFER SEX

A lot of our ideas about safer sex come from what we hear:

➤ If you have intercourse right around a girl's period, she won't get pregnant. FALSE

➤ If your partner is clean-cut, nice-looking, smart, healthy-looking (fill in the blank with your own adjective), then you won't get an STD. FALSE

➤ You can't get pregnant or catch an STD the first time you have sex. FALSE

➤ If you have unprotected intercourse for a while and you don't get pregnant, you probably can't get pregnant. FALSE

➤ If you and your partner only have sex with each other, you don't have to worry about STDs. FALSE

➤ You're too young to get pregnant. FALSE

➤ Only gay people and IV drug users get AIDS. FALSE

Too many people continue to believe these myths about sex until they get pregnant or get sick with an STD. They may think, Oh, nothing's going to happen to me, instead of realizing they are pushing their luck. The truth is, *each* time you have unprotected sex, you are taking a big chance.

MEDIA INFLUENCES

How are any of us going to learn the truth about safer-sex methods when the media set us up for something very unreal? Movies show all sorts of torrid sex scenes, but they rarely show a boy putting on a condom. You never see a girl putting in her diaphragm. For that matter, you hardly ever see two people banging noses when they kiss or squirming around to find a comfortable position or getting up because they have to go to the bathroom. Fantasy love scenes always work out perfectly. Real life doesn't.

In reality, if you don't want to get pregnant or catch an STD, you must abstain from having sex or you *must* use protection every time you have sex.

PARENT-TEEN COMMUNICATION ABOUT PROTECTION

Studies show that teenagers who have received good sex education at home are less likely to get pregnant, less likely to catch an STD, and less likely to have casual sex than teens who haven't received good information. Brianna, a seventeen-year-old from California, said:

> I use my diaphragm every single time we have sex. If I didn't and I got pregnant, I couldn't ask my parents for help. They'd be so angry with me for being irresponsible. It would be really hard for me to admit to them that I was just being stupid and not taking care of myself, because they talked to me so much about protection and all that before I started having sex. They made me promise I would always be careful.

For teens who have *not* discussed sex with their parents, fear of discovery is one of the main reasons they don't get protection. They don't want to let their parents know they are having sex or thinking about having sex, because they're afraid their parents would stop them from going out with their boyfriends or girlfriends if they knew that. A seventeen-year-old Missouri girl told us:

> I was scared to go to my mom when I needed birth control. My boyfriend used a rubber sometimes, but not always. He kept telling me to get on the Pill, but I was scared my mother would find them if I got some. There isn't any place in my house to hide them, because my mom goes through our drawers and even under the mattress when she cleans up. I was stupid, though, because one of the times my boyfriend didn't use a rubber I came up pregnant. So my mom found out the hard way.

A sixteen-year-old mother from Chicago explained:

> The only kind of birth control my mother told me about was, "Keep your dress down and your pants up." I snuck out and got some birth control pills, but she went through my purse one day and found them. Maybe if my mother would have trusted me enough to tell me a little more about birth control and not get mad at me about it, I wouldn't have gotten pregnant. But it's too late now.

Boys have similar stories. One sophomore in California said:

> If I had rubbers in my drawer, my mom would find them for sure.

Many teenagers and their parents have trouble talking to each other about a lot of things. It seems that the times when you could use the most communication are often the times when you have the least. Of course, sex is probably the most difficult subject of all to discuss with your parents, but it's definitely worth the effort. Parents don't want their teens getting into a heavy sexual relationship before they're old enough to handle the emotional and physical consequences of sex. But almost all parents said they would rather help their teens find and use protection than have them take chances with pregnancy or STDs. A mother of three said:

> For me, it's AIDS and some of those other STDs that are so dangerous. I just want to make sure my kids know that they should never have sex without using protection. There's too much at stake.

You may not want to bring up the subject of sex with your parents because you feel embarrassed or ashamed of what you're doing or planning to do. Sometimes you may not be thinking about having intercourse right away, so you don't want to give your folks the idea that it's something you *are* considering. Parents are often a good source of information about sexuality and protection, however; they can offer advice and help you get the protection you need. Parents can also help support teens who want to wait before having intercourse. Either way, the rewards of talking usually outweigh the desire to remain silent.

A number of parents are very much opposed to premarital sex, or at least to teenage sex, and they *would* be upset to learn that their teenagers were considering it. You will make your own decision about whether to talk to your parents about sex. But even if you feel there's no way they would understand, or you're afraid to give them the opportunity to come through, don't let that keep you from being safe. *If you are sexually active, get protection and use it.*

CHOOSING TO WAIT: ABSTINENCE

There is only one 100 percent sure way to avoid pregnancy and sexually transmitted disease: complete sexual abstinence. Complete abstinence means not having *any* sexual activity—no making out or oral sex or penetration.

Many teens who practice abstinence have some sexual contact with each other, but they choose to avoid certain practices, like oral sex or sexual intercourse. It's important for you and your partner to discuss sex and decide together what you feel comfortable doing and what your limits are.

Except in a situation where one person is forcing sex on another (see page 227), you are *always* free to choose abstinence. Even if you've already had sexual intercourse, *from now on* you can decide not to. Abstinence is the cheapest and most effective method of birth control and protection against sexually transmitted disease. You don't have to buy anything or use anything. You just have to be prepared to say no and mean it.

Seventeen-year-old James said:

Why sweat it out every month when you can have a great time with each other and not have to worry?

Lili, his girlfriend, added:

I promised my mom I would wait till I was in college before I had sex—you know, intercourse—with James. And that feels okay to me. We have a great time together. From what I've seen, I think we have a better relationship than a lot of couples who are doing it.

Like Lili and James, most teens don't want to worry about the problems that go along with sexual intercourse; they just want to have fun and feel good about each other.

BEING RESPONSIBLE ABOUT SEX

There are teenagers who have decided that abstinence is not for them. It's a decision that can't be taken lightly, because it carries a lot of risks, but if you do choose to have sexual intercourse, you can make that choice responsibly and learn how to protect yourself. In the next sections, we'll discuss how to do that.

Step One: Making Sex a Conscious Decision

Many people grow up feeling shy or guilty or maybe even scared about sex, because they don't learn much from their families or at school except "don't do it." Then they see sex glamorized everywhere—on TV, in the movies, in newspapers and magazines, in music, in advertising—and the underlying message they get is "Go for it! Do it!"

When we hear "Don't do it!" and "Do it!" at the same time, it's no wonder we feel confused. And it's no wonder we don't always make responsible decisions about sex. Michele and Brian, two seventeen-year-olds who helped us with this book, explained:

Brian: When you're still in high school, you have to deal with the whole guilt thing about "Oh, you're too young to be having sex." If you're only in junior high, it's even harder to deal with. So if you're not supposed to be doing it anyway, you can't really let yourself plan for it by getting birth control, because that just adds to your guilt.

Michele: That's right. You're taught that you shouldn't be doing it, so when you do it, you have to tell yourself, Oh, well, I couldn't help myself. I was drunk. Or I was too stoned to know what I was doing. Or we just got carried away like in the movies. That's why it's so hard to use protection, because that would be admitting that you were thinking about what you were doing.

To use protection the very first time you have sex, you have to make a big mental leap from "I'm not a sexually active person" to "I'm going to be a sexually active person and I want to take care of myself." The more shame or guilt or uncertainty you feel about becoming sexually active, the harder it is to plan for it by getting protection.

TAKING YOUR TIME: Teens say it is a lot easier to talk about sex and use protection when you and your partner have been going out for a while. Lucy, an eighteen-year-old from San Francisco, helps out at a birth control clinic near her home. She told us she and her boyfriend spent over two years together as a couple before they decided to have intercourse:

> When you're our age you want everything to be so romantic. Free and spontaneous. That's why so many kids tell me they don't use birth control— because it isn't spontaneous. I remember the first few times Kevin and I had sex. We didn't know what we were doing at all. The whole thing was anything but romantic or spontaneous. I was trying to put in some foam and it got all over everything. I waited till the last minute to read the instructions, and there I was in the middle of everything trying to figure out how to use the stuff. It got all over my hand and everyplace else. It was embarrassing, sure, but it was also pretty funny. We spent a lot of time laughing about it.

Some teens don't use protection because they rush into having sex. Unfortunately, rushing into sex can make the experience less than what you hoped it might be. It can also make you very insecure while you wait to find out if you're pregnant or have an STD. Stuart, a senior from Detroit, said:

> Sometimes when you're getting ready to have sex, you feel like you don't have time to put on a rubber—even if you have one with you—because it happens so quickly sometimes. You get into it so fast. But if you talk first, or go a little slower, take some time with each other, then you have a chance to think about using protection.

Girls may have a harder time than boys admitting to themselves that they're becoming sexually active and preparing for sex, because of the double standard about sex (see page 105). Most boys feel pressured to have sex. Girls are usually warned not to. So if a girl comes prepared with protection, she may worry that her partner or other people will think she's "loose" or "an easy lay." Because many girls have been taught not to think about sex until

Mr. Right comes and sweeps them off their feet, they feel they have no power in sexual decision making. Patricia, a fourteen-year-old from a suburb near Cleveland, said:

> I think it's up to the boy to use birth control. I feel like my boyfriend is sort of slowly leading us up to intercourse, and I think I'll be able to say no. But if we do it, I think he ought to have birth control, especially at first. It's up to him, because it's his idea in the first place.

Patricia's passive attitude is dangerous, since *she's* the one who will have to deal most directly and personally with the pregnancy if it happens. That's why many sexually active young women are deciding that their health, their safety, and their future are more important than worrying about what people may think of them. They carry condoms to have them available when they need them. And those girls who have decided to wait before having sexual intercourse are feeling stronger about not letting themselves be talked into sex before they are ready.

Step Two: Deciding to Use Protection

Protection falls into two main categories: protection against pregnancy and protection against sexually transmitted disease. To be safe, we have to think about both categories. Methods that prevent pregnancy do so by blocking, killing, or immobilizing sperm, or they change the girl's hormonal balance so she doesn't release ripe eggs. These are called birth control, or contraceptive, methods. Methods that block or kill the germs or viruses of sexually transmitted diseases are called safer-sex methods. While safer-sex methods also may protect you from unwanted pregnancy, many birth control methods do *not* protect you against sexually transmitted diseases.

Teenagers tell us they know that they *should* protect themselves against both pregnancy and STD infection when they have sex, but they forget to use protection, or they forget to buy it, or they just think this one time nothing will happen. One teen described the scenario he imagines goes on inside the head of a person trying to decide about using protection:

I Need to Get Protection	***No, Don't Worry About It***
I'm too young to have a baby.	I'm sure my partner doesn't have any STD. He (or she) is clean.
I don't believe in abortion.	
I don't want to catch an STD.	I'm probably too young to get pregnant anyway.
I'm afraid of getting AIDS.	I don't have the money to buy protection.
I promised my parents I would be careful.	It's too much hassle.
I want to be safe.	Life is short—why worry?
I want my partner to be safe.	Having a baby will bring us closer.
I have plans and having a baby or catching an STD would wreck those plans.	Just this once, nothing will happen.
	I forgot to buy it.
	I'm too embarrassed to use it.
	My mother would find it.
	Rubbers don't feel good.

A girl from Ohio, who's a senior in high school, said:

One of my friends has been pregnant three times. Three times, can you believe it? Every time I talk to her, she's complaining that she just got pregnant. But when I ask her why she doesn't use protection, she says because she doesn't think she'll get pregnant!

This girl's friend may have reasons she's not even aware of that keep her from using birth control. Maybe she hasn't accepted the fact inside herself that she's sexually active, or maybe she doesn't know enough about protection or is afraid to get it. Maybe, too, she isn't comfortable enough with her partner to bring up the issue of protection. Fifteen-year-old Ginny said:

I think birth control is embarrassing. I wouldn't want to spoil the romance of being out with a really cool guy by talking about birth control.

And Estelle, a sixteen-year-old sophomore from Los Angeles, said:

There's this one dude I've had my eye on for a long time; if I could get me a piece of him, I wouldn't bother with no birth control.

Both Ginny and Estelle seem to be willing to take a big chance with their own lives just to please the boys they're with. Perhaps if they could imagine themselves waiting for their missed period to come or waiting for the results of their HIV test, they might realize that no romantic moment is worth the risk and worry of unprotected sex. Julie, an eighteen-year-old from New York, told us she used to be the same way:

I didn't use any birth control for a pretty long time, because I was afraid of saying anything to the guys I was with. I was afraid to tell them how scared I was of getting pregnant. I was too scared to even let myself think about it. I would let these guys tell me, "Oh, don't worry, I'll take care of you. I won't get you pregnant." As if they had some magic. I was putting them ahead of me and letting them do it their way. I had absolutely no respect for myself or what I needed, which was to really feel safe.

Actually, many young men *are* concerned about unplanned pregnancy too. Luis, a senior from Florida, said:

Before guys say no to rubbers, they ought to really think about what would happen if they don't use them. If we got pregnant instead of girls, I bet we'd be more interested in using them.

Seventeen-year-old Timothy had this warning:

I got my girl pregnant and now half my paycheck goes to her for child support. That's why I tell all my friends it ain't worth it. Use protection.

Abby was sixteen when she got pregnant. She and her boyfriend split up just before the baby was born:

> Tiffany is six months old now, and I have no time for myself anymore. I can't even go to the bathroom or brush my teeth without wondering what she's getting into. I never have energy to get any homework done with her always needing me, so I'm thinking that maybe I should drop out of school for a while. It's just too hard. Not that I'd give her up or anything, but I have to admit I didn't realize my whole life was going to be completely turned upside down just because we didn't use protection.

When you have unprotected sexual intercourse, there's also the baby to consider. You and your partner need to discuss what you'd do if you started a pregnancy, because it can be a real shock to discover that each of you has a different idea about how to handle it. Would you have an abortion? Who would pay for it? Would you put the baby up for adoption? Would you keep the baby? Who would care for it? Would you get married? Lots of teens say they wish they had remembered about the baby *before* they had unprotected sex. As fifteen-year-old Patrick told us:

> You've seen the bumper sticker that says "Shit happens," well that's my life for sure. When Sherrie came up pregnant, I thought she'd have an abortion, but she doesn't believe in it. So here I am, a father.

While many teen parents, like Patrick and Abby, struggle to be good parents and provide as much love and care for their children as possible, most wish they hadn't had a child so early in their lives. It's an overwhelming responsibility. (See Chapter 12 on page 369.)

These days both boys and girls realize that protection doesn't just mean protection from unwanted pregnancy. It also means protection from HIV/AIDS and other STDs. Some contraceptives, like the Pill or Norplant, are extremely effective against pregnancy, but they don't protect either females or males from disease. Tawnie said:

My cousin was only twenty-two when she died from AIDS. She and her boyfriend were only having sex with each other for the whole time they were together, so they didn't think they had to use condoms, but he had used IV drugs before they met, and he didn't even know it but he had HIV. He gave it to her, and now she's dead.

It is shockingly easy to catch HIV or some other STD if your sex partner has it. Latex condoms are the best protection. If you are going to have sex, we hope you will use them.

Step Three: Deciding on a Safer-Sex Method and Getting It

Now you are faced with the decision of which method of protection is best for you and your partner. There is no *perfect* form of protection except abstinence. Every method has advantages and disadvantages.

It's a personal decision. The best method for you may not be the best method for someone else. And the best method for you now may be different from the one you might choose at some point later in your life. The goal is to find a method of protection that *you feel comfortable using,* because if you don't feel comfortable with it, there's a good chance you won't use it, and *protection only works if you use it properly every time you have sex.*

Greg, a sixteen-year-old from Wisconsin, uses latex condoms, which some people call "rubbers":

> I can't imagine stopping in the middle of everything to get dressed again and go out to the store to buy a rubber. It would totally spoil the whole thing. So you have to keep some rubbers with you. They're so cheap you might as well buy a few extras to have them on hand. Then you're always prepared.

Cheryl and her boyfriend weren't as prepared as Greg:

> Me and Joey always talked about using birth control, and he kept saying he was going to get some rubbers just in case. But he never actually

got around to it. He kept putting it off, and then we'd be screwing anyway. We were lucky for a few months, but then I got pregnant. I was only fifteen when it happened, and I couldn't believe it. I thought I was going to die.

Clearly, talking about using protection is not the same as using it. Talking won't keep the sperm from traveling up the vagina to reach the egg. Talking won't keep the STD germs from infecting you either. So although it's important to talk to each other about using protection, it's even more important to use it when the time comes.

There are a number of different issues—like effectiveness, ease of use, protection from STD infection, and cost—to consider before deciding on a method. In the section entitled "Methods of Protection," we list each method and discuss these factors. You will probably want to read through that section carefully before making your choice.

GETTING PROTECTION: Of course, before you can use a method, you have to purchase it. Here's what a few teens said about that:

> *Allen (sixteen):* I'd start laughing, I'm sure. It would probably take me a half hour to build up the courage just to go into the store.

> Ginger (sixteen): I would feel really embarrassed if I bumped into somebody I knew when I was going in or coming out of one of these clinics. Everybody knows what you're there for.

> *Steve (seventeen):* Getting protection is harder than using it. I usually spend about ten minutes outside the store psyching myself up to go in. The first time was the worst. I was sure everybody was watching me, so when I went in I tried to act real casual. I acted as if I'd done it a million times, but when I paid the cashier, I just about tripped over myself getting out of there.

Many health clinics these days are making an effort to help teenagers protect themselves by offering condoms free or at very low cost. In most towns and cities, there are clinics that give low-cost family planning counseling to teenagers. Some high schools

have clinics right on campus. The U.S. Department of Health is also prepared to help you protect yourself from disease and unplanned pregnancy. Recent cutbacks in government spending may have limited the number of these clinics and the hours they are open. Look in the phone book under your county government's Health and Human Services Department for the telephone number of the clinic nearest you and call for an appointment (see "Visiting a Family-Planning Clinic" on page 310).

If you would prefer seeing a family doctor, you may want to test his or her attitude about sex and birth control by asking a general question, such as "Do you think teens should use birth control?" or "Do you think it's okay for teenagers to have sex?" You'll be able to tell by the answers whether your doctor will help you and keep your visit confidential, if that's important to you. Some parents have already discussed safer sex with their teenager's doctor and given permission for the doctor to provide information and protection to the teen.

METHODS OF PROTECTION

NOTE: There can be a big lag time between when a book is written and when a reader reads it, so you may want to check with your local family-planning clinic to find out whether any new types of protection have been developed since the printing of this book.

Use a Barrier Method

We want to let you know that we're very biased about methods of safer-sex protection. There are many ways to protect yourself from unplanned pregnancy, but there are only a few ways to protect yourself from catching sexually transmitted diseases. The methods that protect against STDs are called barrier methods, because they place a barrier between you or your partner and the germs or viruses. In the discussion below, we've placed a star next to the most effective barrier methods. They will protect you both from unplanned pregnancy *and* from catching an STD. Please consider using a starred method. We want you to be safe!

Abstinence Methods

ABSTINENCE: Complete abstinence (no sexual activity with another person) is a 100 percent sure way to avoid both unwanted pregnancy and sexually transmitted disease.

LOVEMAKING WITHOUT INTERCOURSE:

One excellent form of birth control is to make love without having sexual intercourse. Heterosexual couples throughout history have developed techniques for giving each other sexual pleasure without putting a penis anywhere near a vagina. In fact, by focusing on intercourse, couples sometimes overlook the intense pleasure other forms of sex can bring. Teenagers from all across the country told us they experience intimacy, passion, tenderness, and orgasm in many ways that they say offer equal or greater satisfaction than intercourse.

Lovemaking without intercourse does not protect against STDs. Oral sex and mutual masturbation can transmit STD germs, so if you are engaging in either of those two activities, read about barrier methods you must use to protect yourselves (page 288). HIV viruses and other STD germs and viruses can pass through cuts you may have on your hands or other parts of your body. Menstrual fluids can carry HIV and other STDs if the girl is infected. Semen carries the germs if the boy is infected. *Get tested for STDs before you begin a relationship and again after three to six months.* If you are both negative, have sex *only* with each other, and do not use IV drugs, you are probably safe from passing or catching STDs after one year together.

Protect Yourself
A Simple Guide to Birth Control and Safer Sex

Method	Pregnancy Protection	STD Protection	Health Choice
Abstinence	Best	Best	Best
Condoms with foam	Excellent	Excellent	Excellent
Condoms	Good	Excellent	Excellent
Foam	Good	Fair	Excellent
Diaphragm	Excellent	Poor	Excellent
Cervical cap	Good	Poor	Good
The Pill	Excellent	No protection	Some risk/some benefit (see page 301)
Depo-Provera (injectable)	Excellent	No protection	Some risk/some benefit (see page 305)
Norplant (implant)	Excellent	No protection	Some risk/some benefit (see page 307)
IUD	Excellent	No protection	Serious risk (see page 309)
Withdrawal	Poor	No protection	Serious risk (see page 309)

Condoms are the best protection against STDs, including HIV and HPV. Use condoms together with other methods for excellent protection from pregnancy *and* sexually transmitted disease.

Other issues to consider are cost, availability, storage, and your comfort level using the method with a partner.

Remember, protection only works if you use it properly *every* time!

Barrier Methods

*MALE CONDOMS: Also called rubbers, safes, Trojans, prophylactics, sheaths, bags, protection.

What Are They? Condoms, in one form or another, have been used by men for hundreds of years. Modern condoms are thin latex or polyurethane sheaths that fit over a boy's erect penis to catch the sperm and fluid that come out during ejaculation. Condoms are the *only* effective temporary form of birth control that males can use. *They are the best form of safer-sex protection available besides abstinence.*

Condoms have two jobs. The first is to keep semen out of the female vagina so that a pregnancy can't happen. The second is to protect both partners from STDs in heterosexual and homosexual relationships. The condom wearer is protected because the condom covers his penis and keeps germs out. The partner is protected because if the condom wearer has HIV or some other infection, his fluids won't be able to enter her or his body.

Effectiveness Against Pregnancy and STDs. If used perfectly, which means using a *new* condom correctly every time you engage in sexual intercourse, this method is 97 percent effective against pregnancy and STDs. In reality, heterosexual couples don't always use condoms every time, or they use them improperly— or, rarely, the condom has a tear in it— so the effectiveness rate is closer to 88 percent. *If a girl uses foam or a diaphragm with spermicide while her partner uses a condom, the effectiveness rate jumps to nearly 100 percent.* For excellent protection against passing STD germs in

male homosexual relationships, one partner can use a condom and the other a spermicide if they engage in anal intercourse.

The male must use condoms to protect himself against disease if a female partner uses a nonbarrier form of birth control (the Pill, Depo-Provera, Norplant, IUD).

Types Available. There are a variety of condoms to choose from. Consider cost, texture, lubrication, and fit. Try different brands to see which one works best for you.

Latex or *polyurethane* condoms offer the best protection against STD germs. Lambskin condoms are also available but *do not* protect against HIV because they are more porous; the germs can pass right through them. A few men are allergic to latex and polyurethane; they can use a lambskin condom against their skin with a latex or polyurethane condom over that for protection. This is nicknamed "double-bagging."

Care of Condoms. Sometimes people apply lubricant to help the condom-covered penis slide more easily into the vagina or anus. *Use only water-soluble lubricants with condoms,* because oil lubricants can damage the latex. Don't use Vaseline,

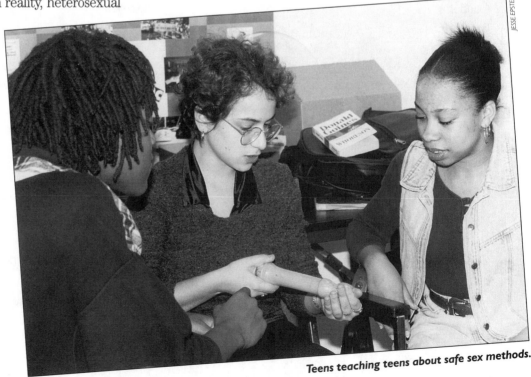

Teens teaching teens about safe sex methods.

JESSE EPSTEIN

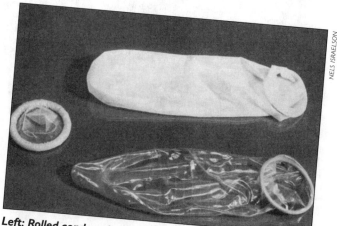

Left: Rolled condom, before use.
Upper right: Unlubricated, regular-end condom.
Lower right: Lubricated, receptacle-end condom.

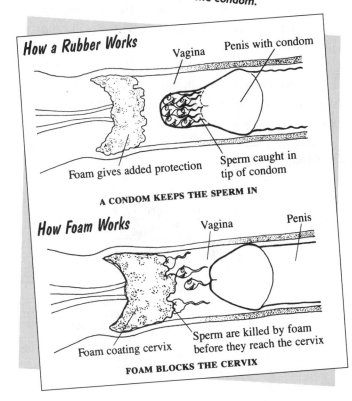

How a Rubber Works

Vagina
Penis with condom

Foam gives added protection
Sperm caught in tip of condom

A CONDOM KEEPS THE SPERM IN

How Foam Works

Vagina
Penis

Foam coating cervix
Sperm are killed by foam before they reach the cervix

FOAM BLOCKS THE CERVIX

mineral oil, baby oil, or hand cream with your condoms. You *can* apply K-Y jelly, Astroglide, Probe, or Ortho lubricant, or you can use saliva or water. If the partner is using foam or spermicidal jelly, that gives extra protection and also creates lubrication.

Condom packages have expiration dates on them, because old condoms can dry out and develop flaws. Don't use a condom past its expiration date, and don't keep condoms in your pocket, wallet, backpack, or car for too long. Too much exposure to sunlight, air, or extreme temperatures can ruin them.

Buy only as many as you think you can use in a month or two.

How to Get This Method. Condoms are sold in drugstores and markets usually on a shelf in the main part of the store. In some stores, they are kept behind the counter, and you must ask for them. They are also available from health clinics, including county or city health or hospital facilities.

Condoms can be bought from wall dispensers in the men's rooms of some public facilities, but if the dispenser hasn't been resupplied recently, you run the risk of buying old condoms. Make sure the expiration date is clearly printed on the package. Throw the condom away if it's past the expiration date. It's better to waste a little money than take a chance on catching an STD or starting a pregnancy.

Cost. Condoms range in price from around 30 cents each to a little more than one dollar each. Check with your clinic or at the Department of Health for free or low-priced condoms.

How to Use Condoms. The male must be sexually aroused before putting on a condom. It is made to fit over an erect penis and will not stay on a soft penis. The time to put the condom on is as soon as you're erect, and before the clear fluid called "pre-ejaculate" comes out of the tip of your penis. That fluid can contain sperm or STD germs, which you don't want to pass on to your partner.

Open the packet carefully. You'll see that the condom has been rolled into a little circle. Take it out, and holding the top half-inch between your fingers, unroll it over the penis. Leave some extra room at the tip to catch the semen and fluid during ejaculation. Many condoms have "reservoir" tips to catch the fluid. Look for that when you buy yours. The reservoir tip should be pointing outward, away from the boy's body.

To keep out air bubbles and help it stay on, squeeze the condom lightly as you unroll it in a downward motion toward your body. On occasion, a person might start the condom inside out. If this occurs, throw out the condom and use another. The same is true for an unrolled condom; it is very difficult to get an unrolled condom on a penis.

Take a few trial runs in private, opening the packet and unrolling the condom onto your penis. That way you'll feel comfortable doing it when you need to. If you like, during sex play your partner can put it on for you.

You can add water-based lubricant to the outside of the condom once it is on your penis, to help ease penetration.

Removing the Condom. After intercourse, use one hand to hold onto the condom near the base of your penis while you pull your still-hard penis gently out of the vagina or anus. If you wait till your penis softens, the condom may come off when you pull out. The idea is to keep the ejaculate inside the condom and not let it ooze out. Ejaculate is full of sperm, which can start a pregnancy. It may also be full of STD germs.

Once the boy's penis is completely out and away from his partner's body, he removes the condom and *throws it away.* Then, if possible, he should wash

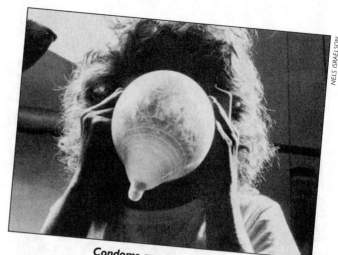

Condoms are strong; they don't burst easily.

and dry his penis. If that's not possible, let the penis air-dry or wipe it off with a tissue. Throw the tissue away. Don't let the uncovered penis touch your partner's body.

It rarely happens that condoms break or come off during intercourse, but if that should happen, you may get pregnant or catch an STD. Using foam or spermicidal jelly inside the vagina or anus along with

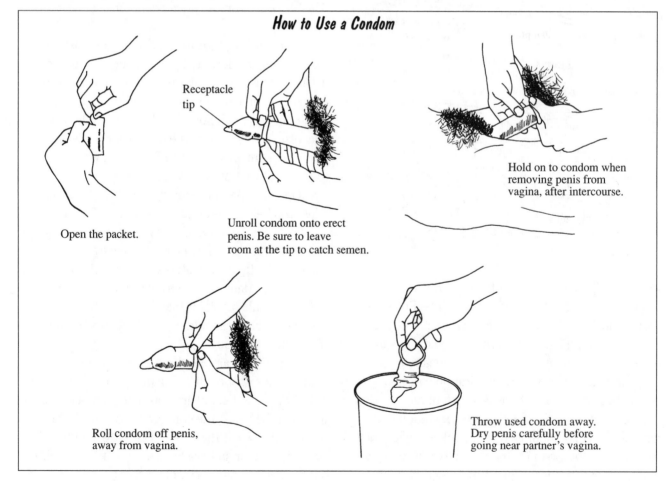

How to Use a Condom

Open the packet.

Receptacle tip

Unroll condom onto erect penis. Be sure to leave room at the tip to catch semen.

Hold on to condom when removing penis from vagina, after intercourse.

Roll condom off penis, away from vagina.

Throw used condom away. Dry penis carefully before going near partner's vagina.

a condom creates backup protection. We recommend it highly.

In the unlikely event of breakage, males should pull out, urinate, and apply spermicide to the tip of their penis to give themselves protection from STD infection.

Advantages. Condoms are cheap, convenient to obtain and carry around, easy to use, and the only method available to males (at the time this book was being written). They don't hurt your body or your partner's body in any way. You use them only when you need them. Aside from not having sexual activity at all, condoms are the best protection you can use to prevent STDs, especially HIV, from spreading. Eighteen-year-old Hillary said:

> Most people I know carry condoms these days. You just never know when you're going to be in a situation where you might need one, and it's too scary to not use one. I would say now that I would never have sex without using a condom. I mean at least till I'm married.

Taylor told us:

> I've been using condoms for a couple of years now, mainly for STD protection. When Becky and I first started going out, the one time I didn't use a condom happened to be the same time she forgot to take two birth control pills in a row, and she got pregnant and had to have an abortion. I won't make that mistake again!

Disadvantages. Probably the number-one complaint against condoms is that some people think they reduce sensation during intercourse. As Alvin told us:

> It's just not the same as being bare.

Putting yourself at risk for an unwanted pregnancy or a sexually transmitted disease, however, is far from pleasurable, and the reality is that unless you are abstinent, condoms are the only way to protect yourself from catching HIV/AIDS or other STDs. You have to decide what's more important to

you—the feeling of the moment or the length of your life—because not using condoms can be life-threatening.

Some boys talk about not liking condoms without ever having tried them. Try one of the new lubricated condoms. Also some condoms are thinner and fit a little more snugly than others, allowing for more sensation for you. Ribbed condoms may give your partner more pleasure.

To get used to how condoms feel, try masturbating with a condom on. Fantasize about sexy things while you put one on your penis. During sex, let your partner put one on for you if he or she is willing. Do whatever you need to do to make condoms okay for you. Remember, your health and your future depend on it.

*FEMALE CONDOM

What Is It? A female condom, also called a vaginal pouch, is now available. It is a double-ringed, cylindrical polyurethane pouch that a woman places inside her vagina to keep out semen and germs. The female condom can be a good choice for a couple who are having intercourse if for some reason the boy will not or cannot wear a male condom.

NOTE: The latex male condom and the female condom tend to stick together during intercourse, so they should not be used at the same time.

Effectiveness Against Pregnancy and STDs. Female condoms are new. There are fewer studies of their effectiveness than there are of male condoms. When the female condom is used by women who might not otherwise use a barrier method during sex, however, the transmission rate of STDs is significantly reduced. At this point, with "perfect use," meaning you use it correctly every time you have intercourse, the female condom has a 90 percent effectiveness rate against pregnancy. That is quite a bit lower than the perfect-use effectiveness rate of the male condom: 97 percent. So you might consider using a hormonal method, like the Pill or an implant or shot for birth control, together with the female condom for protection against STDs. Then you have increased protection against pregnancy without having to rely on your male partner to protect you.

Types Available. At the time this book was printed, there was only one type of female condom on the market, called Reality.

How to Get Them. They are available at family-planning clinics and many drugstores and markets.

Cost. They cost about $2.50 each. Check with your clinic for lower prices.

How to Use Them. The female condom is inserted into the vagina like a tampon or a diaphragm (see diagram). If you have never used a tampon, you may want to try putting one or two fingers into your vagina and moving them around a little to get used to the feel of it.

The female condom has two rings: an inner ring, which goes all the way into the vagina to fit around your cervix, and an outer ring, which stays outside the lips of the vagina. You lubricate the closed end with a water-based lubricant and push the inner ring into the vagina, just the way you would push in a tampon or diaphragm, with your finger. Take out your finger and leave the outer ring hanging about an inch outside the lips of your vagina. It looks a little different, but offering a girl the opportunity to protect herself against sexually transmitted diseases definitely makes it worthwhile. The boy's skin is bare, but the girl is protected from sperm and seminal fluid touching her vagina. During intercourse, make sure the penis enters the vagina through the opening in the outer ring. The penis should not go between the outer ring and the girl's vagina, which can happen if you are not careful.

If you are planning to use this method, we highly recommend that you buy one or two female condoms just for practice. Try to put them in while you're alone. See if you can insert them easily. If you are very close with your partner, practice together. Just don't have intercourse until one of you is protected.

To Remove. After intercourse is over, carefully pull it out and throw it away (see diagram).

Advantages. It's a great method for girls whose male partners have said they won't wear con-doms. Now you can say, "Okay, you don't have to wear one—I will." They are good protection against unwanted pregnancy and against STDs. They are easy to obtain and fairly inexpensive if you don't have intercourse too frequently. Girls who want to be prepared can carry the small packet in their purse or backpack.

Another advantage is that the female condom can be inserted up to eight hours before intercourse, so it won't interrupt you during lovemaking. Also, there are no side effects to worry about. You use the female condom when you need it and then throw it away.

Disadvantages. The main disadvantage is that female condoms are not as effective against pregnancy as some other methods. For girls who are already on the Pill or using Depo-Provera or implants, however, none of which offer *any* protection against STDs, the female condom is a good supplement to give you that STD protection.

Some girls worry that a parent might find the condom if they leave the packet in their drawer or in their purse. This problem exists with most forms of protection, and female condom packets may be small enough to go unnoticed.

Another disadvantage is that a girl has to feel comfortable touching her vagina to be able to insert the condom. And she has to feel good enough about protecting herself to explain the method to her partner, who is bound to notice the condom sticking out of her vagina!

Finally, for girls who have intercourse regularly, the cost is higher than some other methods. As more girls choose female condoms, more manufacturers may produce them. Then marketplace competition may bring the price down.

*SPERMICIDES

What Are They? Spermicides are chemical agents that keep sperm from traveling up into the cervix. Sperm that don't travel up the cervix into the fallopian tubes can't join the egg to start pregnancies (see page 38, about fertilization). A few studies indicate that spermicides may disable HIV and other sexually transmitted disease germs too, which means they may protect against STDs as well as against pregnancy.

When inserted into the vagina, spermicides coat the walls and block the entrance to the cervix so sperm and germs can't get in. When inserted into the anus, they coat the lining of the anus to help block STD germs.

Effectiveness Against Pregnancy and STDs.

Spermicides when used alone in the vagina during intercourse have a 94 percent perfect use effectiveness rate against starting a pregnancy. That means if 100 girls use spermicidal foam or creams or jellies or film or suppositories perfectly every single time they have intercourse, 94 will not get pregnant. The reality is that people don't use spermicides perfectly every time they have intercourse, so the effectiveness rate is really around 75 percent. Even a 75 percent prevention rate is a lot better than not using any form of birth control at all, but we don't think you should rely on spermicides *alone* to prevent pregnancy. We recommend that girls use a spermicide at the same time their male partners use a condom, for close to 100 percent protection against both pregnancy and STDs.

The combination of spermicide and condoms is the best form of birth control and STD protection for teenagers: easy to use, inexpensive, no side effects, and very effective.

Types of Spermicides.

There are many different types of spermicides to choose from: contraceptive foam; contraceptive creams or jellies; contraceptive film; and contraceptive suppository capsules. All effective spermicidal products available in the United States contain either nonoxynol-9 or octoxynol-9. The two are equally effective.

How to Get Them.

They are all available in family-planning clinics. They are also available at drugstores and some markets. You do not need a prescription.

Cost.

The cost varies from product to product. Individual foam applications come in separately wrapped packages that look like tampons. They cost about $15 for six to eight applications. A small can of foam with applicator is about the same price. A 3.8-ounce tube of cream or jelly costs about $11 to $12.

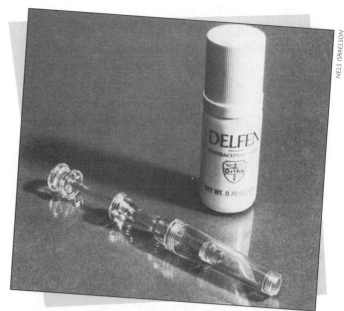

Foam with applicator.

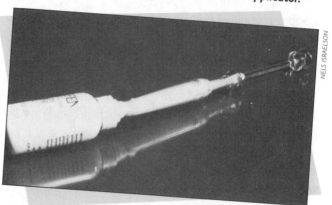

Filling the applicator.

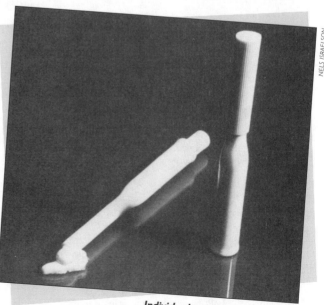

Individual applications of foam.

How to Use Them. All spermicidal methods come with straightforward instructions. If you get them at a family-planning clinic, the counselors there will teach you how to use them. If you buy yours at a store, take it home and practice inserting it. If you don't have the privacy needed to practice in your room, take it with you into the bathroom or shower and practice there. The idea is to insert the spermicide deep into the vagina so that it covers the cervix. If the male partner is not wearing a condom, we recommend using two applications of spermicide.

Foam, the most commonly used spermicide, comes in two types of containers: in a can with multiple applications, and in a package containing individually wrapped single applications. The first time you buy the can, be sure you purchase it with the "applicator kit," which gives you the special insertion applicator you need to put in the foam. Keep the applicator, and after that you can buy less-expensive refill cans, which come without the applicator. The individual foam tubes have their own applicator.

To use the canned foam, shake it, attach the applicator, and fill it with foam by slightly bending or pressing down on the top nozzle. There will be good instructions in the kit. Once the applicator is full of foam, remove it from the nozzle and insert it into your vagina (or anus), as far up as you can without

hurting yourself. Then push down on the applicator stick to shoot the foam into your vagina (or anus). Most people like to lie down while they are inserting foam. Many boys like to insert the foam for their partners while they are making love. Foam begins working immediately and lasts for about one hour.

Spermicidal jellies and creams can be used together with a diaphragm (see below). For girls who don't use diaphragms, spermicidal jellies and creams can be purchased with an applicator stick. Fill the applicator with the jelly or cream and insert it deep into the vagina without hurting yourself. Then push on the plunger to release the spermicide. You may want to lie down to insert this method.

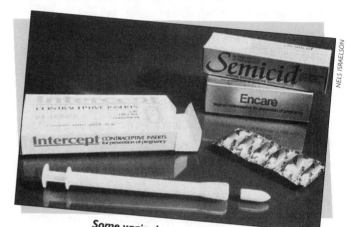

NELS ISRAELSON

Some vaginal suppositories and an applicator used for birth control.

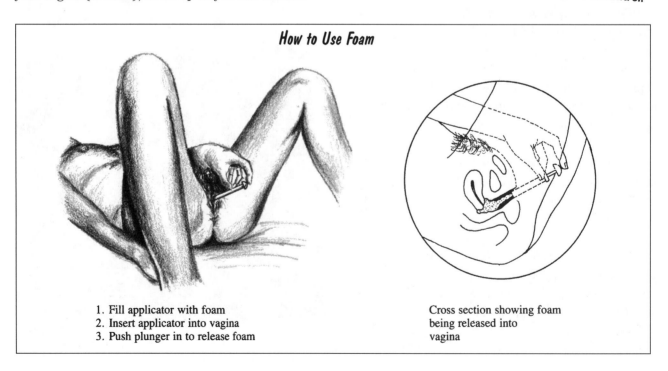

How to Use Foam

1. Fill applicator with foam
2. Insert applicator into vagina
3. Push plunger in to release foam

Cross section showing foam being released into vagina

Spermicidal cream and jelly begin working immediately and last for several hours. Don't stay in a vertical position for too long. Without the diaphragm holding them in place against the cervix, spermicides will ooze out the vagina when you go to the bathroom or walk around too much.

When you insert **contraceptive suppositories and film,** wait fifteen minutes for the agents to become active and coat your vagina (or anus). If you have intercourse before the suppository or film has time to become potent, you will not be protected. After the initial fifteen-minute waiting period, contraceptive suppositories and film are effective for one hour.

NOTE: Because spermicidal suppositories and film are potent for one hour, if intercourse lasts longer than that or if you decide to have intercourse a second time, you must reinsert the method and wait another fifteen minutes for it to take effect.

For pregnancy protection, don't swim, douche, or bathe for at least six hours after your last intercourse. Give the spermicide the time it needs to kill and immobilize all the sperm inside your vagina. If even one sperm makes it up into your cervix, you could get pregnant.

Care. Keep the spermicide away from extreme heat. Check the expiration date on the package, and do not use past that date.

Advantages. Foam, suppositories, film, and contraceptive jellies and creams are easy to use; they have few, if any, side effects; they are relatively inexpensive; and they are easy to get without having to go to a doctor. They are like condoms in that you only use them when you need them, so they don't affect your body all the time.

Some people like using spermicides because they add lubrication to the vagina or anus, making intercourse more comfortable.

Using foam and condoms together is the favorite form of birth control/safer sex among the teenagers we interviewed. This is what fifteen-year-old Chris, a sophomore from Chicago, said:

> I feel like I'm too young to take the Pill or get an IUD. I haven't even had a pelvic exam yet, so I don't want to be messing around with doctors' appointments.

My sister told me about foam, and I went to the drugstore and got some. I got the kind that looks like Tampax, and you put it in the same way.

Gloria, a senior from Los Angeles, said:

> Foam and rubbers are just about the only kind of protection you can use when you need it and forget when you don't need it. I carry around those little tubes of foam when I go out with my boyfriend, and it's just like carrying tampons, which everybody does.

Disadvantages. One main disadvantage is that a few people have allergic reactions to certain kinds of spermicidal products. If that happens to you or your partner, you may feel a burning sensation when you urinate or your vagina may feel swollen. You'll have to stop using that particular product and try another. But get yourself checked out at a clinic to be sure the burning isn't being caused by an STD. A male partner can protect himself by using a condom. Carol, a college freshman from Boston, had this experience:

> I went out with this guy and we used foam. Well, he didn't use a rubber, and after he pulled out he felt sore, and when he went to pee it burned him. He thought I had given him the clap [gonorrhea], but I knew I didn't. It turned out he was just allergic to the foam, so the next time we used a different type and he used a rubber.

Some couples don't like using spermicides, because they can be kind of messy. Keep some tissues nearby to wipe your hands and outside your vagina or anus. Other people don't like them because you have to insert them during lovemaking, just before intercourse. But many couples who use spermicides find ways to incorporate their use into foreplay and lovemaking, perhaps allowing the male partner to insert them.

If a girl doesn't feel comfortable touching her vagina, she may not want to use these products. If she wants to learn, she can practice by gently inserting one or two fingers partway into her vagina and get used to what that feels like.

Another disadvantage is that some teens are wary of keeping spermicidal products around for fear their parents might discover them. Pauline said:

> I was always afraid my mom would find my foam, so I stopped using it. But when I got pregnant, my mom was really mad. She said, "Why didn't you use birth control?"

Finally, as we mentioned before, spermicides have a relatively high pregnancy rate when used alone, as Shirley, a seventeen-year-old mother from Dayton, found out:

> See this baby? She's a foam baby. Loreen was born nine months after I used foam, so I guess I did something wrong or it just didn't work very well.

Because of experiences like Shirley's, remember to use foam, or one of the other spermicides, together with male condoms for almost 100 percent protection.

THE DIAPHRAGM AND THE CERVICAL CAP: Please note that we didn't star these methods, because while they offer good protection against pregnancy, they may not offer adequate protection from STDs unless they are used together with the male condom.

What Are They? The diaphragm (*dye*-uh-fram) is a shallow rubber cup that fits inside the vagina to cover the cervix. It is soft and flexible and comes in different sizes to fit different women. The cervical cap is similar to the diaphragm, except it is smaller and fits more tightly around the cervix. Girls choose to use one or the other, not both at the same time.

The cervical cap creates a suction around the cervix, keeping sperm out. You use a small amount of spermicidal cream or jelly inside the cap to kill any sperm that might break through. The diaphragm has a looser fit than the cap. Its purpose is to hold spermicidal cream or jelly around the cervix to block sperm from entering.

Effectiveness Against Pregnancy and STDs. When used properly, every time you have intercourse, the diaphragm provides a 94 percent effectiveness rate against pregnancy. The cervical cap has a lower rate, 91 percent. The real effectiveness for both is lower than that, about 82 percent, because people don't always use the diaphragm or cap perfectly every time. In rare cases, they may be dislodged by deep thrusting movements during intercourse.

These methods do not protect the vagina from STDs, so we recommend using them along with a male condom. **When a couple uses both a condom and a diaphragm or cap, their protection against pregnancy and STDs is nearly 100 percent.**

How to Get Them. Diaphragms and cervical caps come in different sizes, because women come in different sizes. To get the proper size for you, you must be fitted at a family-planning clinic or a doctor's office.

The procedure is very simple: At the clinic or doctor's office, someone will talk to you about the different methods of protection available. Before you decide on the diaphragm or cap, discuss the pros and cons with your health practitioner. Then you will lie on the examining table with your legs bent and your knees apart. The practitioner will place a gloved hand inside your vagina to feel around your cervix. Then she or he will take a sample diaphragm or cap and insert it to see if it fits. If it fits well and covers your cervix, it is the proper size. If it slips around or feels too tight, the health practitioner will take that one out and try another size.

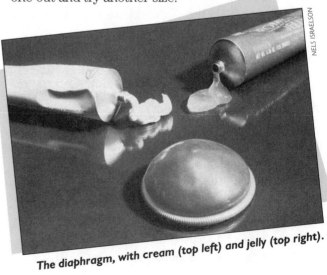

NELS ISRAELSON

The diaphragm, with cream (top left) and jelly (top right).

She or he will demonstrate how to apply the spermicidal cream or jelly and how to put the diaphragm or cap inside your vagina yourself. *Make sure you practice putting in and taking out the diaphragm or cap* before you leave the clinic. Insert and remove it enough times to give yourself confidence that you'll be able to do it on your own. Remember, when you need to use it, the health practitioner won't be there!

If for any reason the doctor or nurse forgets to give you time to try it yourself, don't be shy about telling her or him you would like to practice. That way, if you have trouble putting it in or taking it out, you can ask for help.

Cost. A diaphragm costs about $25 to $35; a cervical cap costs about $30. The exam will cost anywhere from $40 to $200, depending on whether you use a public health clinic or a private doctor. For teenagers there may be a sliding scale, and they may allow you to pay in monthly installments.

How to Use Them. You will have practiced inserting and removing the diaphragm or cap at the clinic, but you will probably want to practice a few more times at home. The diagrams on this page should help.

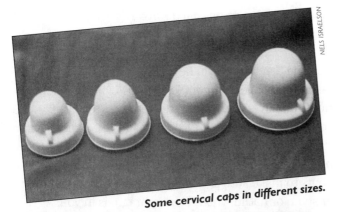

Some cervical caps in different sizes.

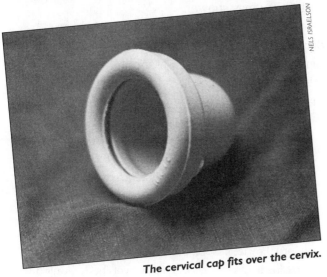

The cervical cap fits over the cervix.

You have an important role to play in this exam. Tell the doctor or nurse how the device feels to you. If it is very uncomfortable, make sure to say so. That probably means it doesn't fit well. Remember though, it may feel a little funny just because you aren't used to having something inside your vagina. Discuss this with the health practitioner.

USING A DIAPHRAGM: First, put about one tablespoon of spermicidal cream or jelly on the inside of the diaphragm. That's really all you need. Some people overdo it and put on so much that the diaphragm slips around inside. Spread the cream or jelly around with your finger to coat the inside and the rim. After the diaphragm is covered with jelly or cream, it is ready to be inserted into your vagina. Some women like to lie down; others stand with one leg up on a chair or the toilet seat; others insert it while seated. Experiment with different positions to see which is the easiest and most comfortable for you. Fold the diaphragm and slide it up into your vagina. You have to push it all the way in so the back rim goes past your cervix and the front rim stops at the pubic bone. You'll be able to feel your pubic bone at the top front of your vagina.

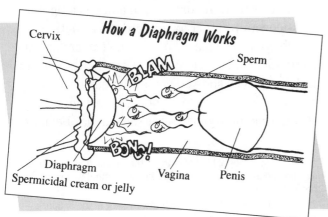

How a Diaphragm Works

Cervix

Sperm

BLAM

BONK!

Diaphragm

Spermicidal cream or jelly

Vagina

Penis

Since your vagina does not open into the rest of your body except through the tiny opening in the cervix, there's no way for the diaphragm to get lost inside. When you've placed it correctly, it will fit comfortably and stay in place. Sixteen-year-old Elizabeth told us that the first time she tried to put in her diaphragm, "It totally slipped out of my hand and flew across the room!" Larra had a similar experience:

The couple of times I tried to put it in, I spent about a half hour in the bathroom with that thing slipping and sliding all over the place. The jelly was all over my hands and my legs, and I couldn't get a grip on the diaphragm enough to push it up far enough so it would stay in there, so it kind of hung halfway out. What a mess! Finally a friend told me not to use so much jelly. I was using so much because I wanted to make sure I wouldn't get pregnant, but when I cut down on the jelly, it was much easier to put it in.

The diaphragm can be inserted up to six hours before you have intercourse, but the closer to the time you have intercourse the better, especially if you are physically active while it's in (like dancing or running or standing a lot). After intercourse you *must* leave the diaphragm in place for at least six hours to make sure it works properly. *Do not douche** or swim or bathe while the diaphragm is in your vagina. You may shower.

Some girls say they wouldn't want to use a diaphragm because they wouldn't want to have to touch themselves. Sixteen-year-old Rebecca, a high school junior from Los Angeles, said she used to feel that way too:

I used to think I'd never be able to use a diaphragm, because I couldn't even think about putting it in. I thought that whole area down there was gross. But one day, one of our counselors took the girls in our group to the women's clinic near our school and they did this demonstration for us where they let us look at their cervix, and some of the girls in class even did it too. Everybody wanted to look, because I mean really it's a part of your body that you don't even know anything about. Everybody's cervix looked a little different. Some were big, some were little, some holes were open pretty big and some were pretty tight. They showed us how the diaphragm goes in and covers up that hole in the cervix. It made it seem logical.**

USING THE CERVICAL CAP: The cervical cap is quite a bit smaller than the diaphragm and has a tighter fit. It covers your cervix and creates a suction which holds it in place. You fill the cap about one-third full of spermicidal jelly or cream, then insert it the way they showed you at the clinic. You can put the cap in up to *forty* hours before intercourse. If you have intercourse after the cap has been in

How to Apply Spermicidal Cream or Jelly to a Diaphragm

The diaphragm

Rim with spring inside to allow the diaphragm to fold so it can enter the vagina

Coat the diaphragm with about one tablespoon of spermicidal cream or jelly.

Spread the cream or jelly around the inside cup of the diaphragm and along the rim.

*A douche is a special kind of bath for the vagina. It is an unnecessary procedure since the vagina has its own natural cleansing process.
**Thanks to Carole Downer and Ginny Cassidy of the Feminist Women's Health Center in Los Angeles, 1978.

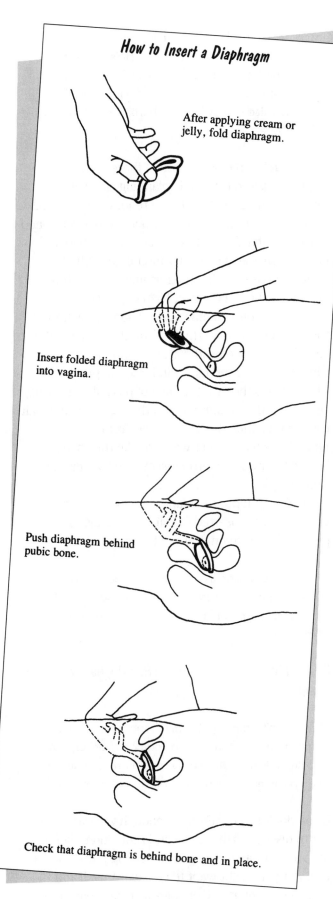

How to Insert a Diaphragm

After applying cream or jelly, fold diaphragm.

Insert folded diaphragm into vagina.

Push diaphragm behind pubic bone.

Check that diaphragm is behind bone and in place.

place for more than forty hours, you may want to use an applicator to apply a little more spermicide into your vagina. (Some health practitioners caution against applying more spermicide. They say it can cause the cap to slip. Check with your clinic.) After intercourse you must keep the cap in place for at least six to eight hours. *Never douche* while the cap is in place. Do not swim or take tub baths. Showering is just fine.

To avoid infection or irritation to the cervix, some practitioners think the cap should not be worn for more than forty-eight hours at a time. Others say you can keep it in place for up to seventy-two hours before removing it. That means that with the cap you can have continuous protection for a whole weekend. However, as we said earlier, neither the cap nor the diaphragm alone offers 100 percent protection against pregnancy or STDs. To increase your protection, have your partner use condoms too.

Care. The diaphragm and cap require little care. After use, just wash them with warm water and regular face soap, then dry them and put them away in their cases. Be careful not to put any oily substance (like Vaseline) on them; that can deteriorate the rubber. Also, do not boil them or use very hot water or keep them near high heat, all of which may weaken the rubber. You can sprinkle a little cornstarch on them to keep them fresh, but do not use any powder containing talc. Studies show that talc can cause cancer.

From time to time, hold the device up to the light to check for cracks, holes, or tears. If you discover a hole or tear, it's time to replace your diaphragm or cap. To be safe, replace your diaphragm about every two years.

Because proper fit is important for both devices, you may have to change sizes if you gain or lose more than ten pounds, if you've been pregnant, if you've had a baby or an abortion, or if you've grown a lot taller or broader since your original fitting. Whenever you have a gynecological exam, bring your diaphragm or cap along with you to have the fitting checked.

Advantages. Both the diaphragm and cervical cap have a lot of advantages. They are safe. They have very few negative effects and no permanent side effects. The diaphragm has been used by women in one form or another for hundreds of years. Both products are easy to obtain at any family-planning clinic. They offer good protection against pregnancy, and they offer some protection against the transmission of STDs, in particular chlamydia and gonorrhea. You use them only when you need them. Once you buy them, they should last for two years, so they are a good value for your money. Although you have to use them with spermicidal jelly or cream, one tube of spermicide gives you many applications.

Bonita had been on the Pill for a year but didn't like the side effects she was experiencing, so she switched to a diaphragm:

> I went back to the clinic and told them I wanted to stop using the Pill because it was making me have really strange periods and I was getting really bad headaches, and that made me scared of what it might be doing to me. So we talked about all the other methods, and it seemed like the diaphragm was my best choice, so I got one and I've been using it for about six months now. I haven't gotten pregnant yet, so I guess it works.

Although most girls who use the Pill or other hormonal methods experience few or no negative side effects, for girls who cannot or do not want to use hormonal methods, the diaphragm or cap is a good choice.

Another advantage to the diaphragm or cap is that it can be put in ahead of time, before lovemaking. Jennifer said:

> Since my boyfriend and I don't have sex that often, mostly because we don't have that many places we can go to be alone, we pretty much know when we're going to do it, and that gives me plenty of time to put in my diaphragm before we go out.

These methods can also be incorporated into your lovemaking, as Irena, a seventeen-year-old from Los Angeles, told us:

> My boyfriend and I are really close, and he helps me put in my diaphragm. Like, he'll put the jelly on

for me and he'll hold me while I put it in. That relaxes me and makes it easier. He's really into using birth control, because once he got a girl pregnant and he nearly freaked out over it. He had to raise money for her abortion, and it was a big scene.

Disadvantages. Both of these methods require a visit to the family-planning clinic or doctor's office for fitting, and both require that you feel comfortable enough with your body to put your hand in your vagina. For girls who have not yet had a pelvic exam (see page 250) and for girls who feel uneasy about touching their vagina, the diaphragm or cap may not be the best form of protection.

Another disadvantage is that some girls find they are allergic to particular brands of the spermicide that must be used with diaphragms and caps. Changing the brand may eliminate the problem. There is also the disadvantage of possible discovery, since both the diaphragm and the cap come in small cases which must be stored away from excessive heat. Some teens don't want to take the chance of having their birth control discovered by a parent or sibling.

Unless you put the diaphragm in beforehand, it will have to be inserted during lovemaking, before penetration. Sixteen-year-old Dolores said:

> Those diaphragms are messy. You have to go into the bathroom and say, "Oh, excuse me, I have to go to the bathroom now," and the guy knows all about it.

Susi, a high school junior from Seattle, had the same complaint:

> I wouldn't want to put in my diaphragm with the guy around. I mean, could you be in front of your date and say, "Oh, excuse me honey, I'm going to go put in my diaphragm now?" I couldn't do that.

If you don't feel comfortable enough with your partner to discuss birth control and protection, then perhaps a diaphragm or cap is not the right method for you. But you might want to consider this: If you don't feel comfortable enough with your partner to discuss birth control and protection, how are you going to keep yourself safe from pregnancy and STDs?

Hormonal Methods

The following methods introduce synthetic (artificially or chemically made) hormones into a girl's body to prevent pregnancy by interrupting her regular cycle of fertility. They are extremely effective against undesired pregnancy. Unfortunately, they offer absolutely *no* protection against sexually transmitted diseases. For full protection, we recommend that you use them together with the male or female condom.

MONOGAMY: It's important to say a word about monogamy here. Monogamy (mah-*nah*-gah-mee) means being involved in *one* relationship. Two people who are monogamous have sexual relations *only* with each other. As soon as one of them has sex with anyone else, they are no longer monogamous.

Monogamy will not protect you from pregnancy, because if you are having sexual intercourse without using birth control, you will probably get pregnant. Once the boy's sperm meets with the girl's egg, pregnancy begins.

But if neither you nor your partner has any sexually transmitted disease to begin with, monogamy *can* be a form of safer sex. **You must both test negative for HIV and other STDs in a clinic or doctor's test.** Since HIV does not show up immediately, you must have two successive tests, three to six months apart, and test negative on both to be certain you don't have HIV. That means a couple has to be monogamous for at least six months, preferably a year, and test negative on the STD tests to feel safe not using a barrier method during sexual relations.

Until your second test results come back, use a barrier form of protection. After that, if you have both tested negative, and you are not using IV drugs or having any form of sexual relations with anyone else, you probably do not have to worry about catching an STD. That means for as long as you are monogamous you can use a hormonal method of birth control alone, if that is what you would prefer.

Even ONE time with someone else or ONE time sharing IV needles or engaging in other risky practices puts you at risk again, however. A nurse practitioner said:

> The girls that come into our clinic aren't really all that comfortable asking their boyfriends about their sexual practices, and that's risky. I tell them, use condoms along with their Pill or Depo [a birth control method that is injected] or whatever. Then you *know* you'll be protected from STDs. I think teens are taking way too big a chance if they don't use condoms.

THE BIRTH CONTROL PILL

What Is It? The Pill is a small round tablet made of synthetic hormones. To understand how the Pill works, first read about the female menstrual cycle starting on page 36. The purpose of the Pill is to keep the girl's body from being able to maintain a pregnancy. One type, called the combination pill, works by stopping ovulation altogether. It contains both estrogen and progestin (synthetic progesterone). Girls on this Pill don't release ripe eggs, so pregnancies can't start. Another type, called the progestin-only pill, doesn't contain estrogen and does not stop ovulation. It increases the mucus around your cervix to block sperm from entering the cervix. It also inhibits the egg's journey through the fallopian tube.

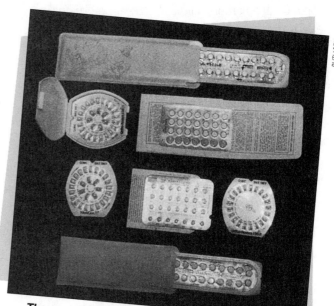

RUTH BELL

There are many different brands of the birth control pill.

While you are taking this type of pill the lining of your uterus may temporarily change to become less nurturing for a pregnancy, should one occur.

The Pill, in one form or another, has been available since the early 1960s, and it has been and is used by millions of women and girls throughout the world. As of now, there is no birth control pill for men.

Effectiveness Against Pregnancy and STDs. The Pill is extremely effective against pregnancy. Fewer than one girl in a hundred who takes it according to instructions will get pregnant. Some girls do not always remember to take their pills, however, so pregnancies do occur.

The combination pill is the most effective type of birth control pill, but it also has more potential side effects than the progestin-only pill. Discuss this with your health practitioner when you are deciding about which pill to take.

The Pill does *not* protect you in any way from catching sexually transmitted diseases, so please don't allow yourself to fall into a false sense of security if you take the Pill. If your partner doesn't use a condom when you have intercourse, you are at risk for HIV/AIDS and all the other STDs out there today. (Please read the STD chapter, beginning on page 253.)

How to Get It. The birth control pill must be prescribed by a doctor. You can go to a private doctor or to a family-planning clinic. At the appointment, a health practitioner will ask about your medical history. The Pill is not a good form of birth control for people with certain medical conditions. But neither is becoming pregnant or catching an STD.

After you and your health practitioner discuss your medical history, you should receive a thorough physical checkup, including an internal exam (see page 250). Eighteen-year-old Leah went to a local family-planning clinic to get the Pill. She said:

> Anytime I have to have an examination, I always freak out. But they were so nice to me it wasn't too bad. They were so neat about it—they tried to cool me out and make me relax. And then when it was over, they gave me the pills and told me how to use them. They were super nice people.

Who Should Not Take the Pill

The Pill—in particular, the combination pill—is especially dangerous to the health of women with the following conditions:

Blood-clotting disorders.

Breast cancer or a family history of breast cancer.

Cardiovascular disease.

High blood pressure.

Liver tumors or certain liver diseases.

Pregnancy.

Stroke or family history of stroke.

Women with the following conditions are *advised* not to use the Pill, or to use the Pill only under the supervision of a medical practitioner:

Diabetes.

Active gallbladder disease.

Active mononucleosis.

Family history of hyperlipidemia.

Gilbert's disease.

Heavy smokers.

Migraine headaches.

Nursing a baby.

Undiagnosed abnormal vaginal bleeding.

Sickle-cell anemia.

At the clinic, you'll talk to the health practitioner about whether the Pill is safe for you. Weigh the risks versus the benefits to help you decide. You want to find a method you are going to use properly and consistently. If you choose the Pill, the health practitioner should explain exactly how to use it. *This is the time to ask all the questions you may have.* Remember, don't leave the clinic until you understand exactly what to do. Learn what kind of pill you will be taking (combination, low-dose estrogen, or progestin-only) and what to do if you forget to take a pill.

Although most girls are very careful about taking their pills, it's not unusual to forget once in a while.

Evie, one of the girls we met in Boston, said she forgot more than just once:

> I wasn't taking my pills regularly. I couldn't stand to swallow them, so I'd sort of let myself forget to take them. That's how I got pregnant. I missed too many and they just didn't work for me.

As Evie found out, not taking the Pill every day can result in pregnancy. The Pill works by keeping a certain level of hormones in your body over a twenty-four-hour period. If you forget a pill, your body won't receive the required amount of hormones for that day, leaving you vulnerable to pregnancy.

It's a very good idea when you have intercourse to use condoms even though you're on the Pill to protect against sexually transmitted disease. It is especially important to use condoms as a backup during any month you forget to take one or two pills. Use condoms until you have completed that cycle and have your next menstrual period. If your period is very late, keep using condoms and call the clinic for advice.

Important: Don't ever start taking birth control pills without going through a complete physical exam at the clinic or doctor's office. Don't ever borrow pills from a friend or take pills prescribed for someone else. Each person is different, and the dosage of hormones in the different kinds of pills varies. The doctor will prescribe a dosage that is suitable for you, given your size, your weight, your medical history, and your menstrual history.

Cost. The Pill costs approximately $20 for a one-month supply. On top of that, before the Pill can be prescribed, you must have a complete gynecological exam, which may cost from $40 to $200, depending on the clinic you go to or the doctor you see. Call first to check prices. Your medical insurance may cover the cost, or there may be a sliding scale for teens. Check the public or nonprofit clinics in your area for lower prices.

How to Use It. Pills come in packets of 28 pills or 21 pills. If your packet has 28 pills, you take one pill every day. If your packet has 21 pills, you begin taking a pill on the fifth day after your period begins and continue taking them for twenty-one days. Bleeding should begin soon after that. Then you start the cycle over: On the fifth day after bleeding first begins, you start taking your pills again.

In the beginning, it takes about a month before the Pill becomes effective. You must use another form of birth control for a month or two while your body adjusts to it. Carolyn didn't understand how the Pill works. She said:

> I used to think that taking the Pill meant that you would just take one before you had sex each time. I thought it was like taking aspirin for a headache—you took a pill when you had sex.

You don't take one pill each time you have sex, as Carolyn mistakenly thought. Each pill contains about twenty-four hours' worth of chemical hormones, and you need a whole month's worth to make it work. You must take one pill every day, at about the same time every day, in order to achieve the maximum effectiveness. You take it whether or not you are having intercourse that day.

Advantages. There are many advantages to taking the birth control pill, which is why millions of women use it. Sarah is eighteen, and she has been using the Pill for one year. She said:

> You've got to use a spontaneous kind of birth control. I mean what if you're driving home from the movies and you go parking and it's twelve o'clock at night? What are you going to do then? Drive around all night looking for a place that sells rubbers?

Other girls told us:

> You don't have to plan on the Pill. It's real convenient. And I feel safer with it.

I was using foam before, and that was messy, so I wouldn't always use it. The Pill doesn't get in the way at all.

I got my pills at a family-planning clinic when I was only fourteen, and nobody gave me any hassle. I had been having sex with my boyfriend for a couple of months, and we weren't using anything, and I started getting really worried that we were taking too many chances. I feel so much safer now.

The best thing about the birth control pill is that it really works. If you take your pill every day according to instructions, you can be almost 100 percent sure you won't get pregnant.

Another advantage of the Pill for some girls is that it brings your period on at a predictable time each month. In some cases, doctors prescribe the Pill as a way to regulate menstruation for girls whose periods have never been on a regular schedule. Being on the Pill may also help reduce the cramps

and premenstrual tension that many girls experience. Fifteen-year-old Francie, a ninth-grader from California, said:

I used to get real bad cramps with my period, so bad that I couldn't do anything but stay in bed for the first day or two. Now that I'm taking the Pill, my cramps aren't as bad. That's an extra bonus I wasn't expecting.

Also, the Pill might help clear up your skin, as it did for Geri:

I never had any problems with the Pill. In fact, it cleared up my zits, and after a couple of months I even lost weight. I've never had any headaches or anything with it like other girls told me about.

Disadvantages. As we said earlier, the most serious disadvantge of the Pill is that it does nothing to protect you against sexually transmitted diseases. Unless you and your partner are in a long-term, monogamous relationship, and unless you have both tested negative for STDs, by using the Pill without condoms, you are leaving yourself vulnerable to infection. Boys who want to protect themselves against STDs will want to use condoms even if their partner is on the Pill. If the boy will not use condoms, girls on the Pill can protect themselves from STDs by using the female condom (page 291), a form of spermicide such as foam or contraceptive suppositories, or a diaphragm or cervical cap. This is important. Your life may depend on it.

There are side effects and health problems associated with the birth control pill, but the reality is that these problems happen to a relatively small percentage of women. We advise you to read through this section before you start taking the Pill and to discuss the complications and disadvantages thoroughly with your health practitioner and with your sex partner.

The Pill interrupts your body's normal menstrual/ovulation cycle. Therefore, we recommend not taking the Pill until you have had regular periods for at least one year. If you start taking the Pill before your menstrual cycle is functioning regularly and

---

Menstruation and the Pill

Although girls who are on the Pill bleed each month, they don't really menstruate. Menstruation is part of the full fertility cycle, which includes ovulation (see page 36 for a full discussion of menstruation). Since the Pill stops the release of ripe eggs (ovulation) and interferes with the buildup of the lining of the uterus, the bleeding you experience while on the Pill is not true menstrual bleeding. It is caused by a drop in the hormone level toward the end of the pill packet.

Missing a Period on the Pill: Some people do not get their periods during their first month or so on the Pill because their body needs time to adjust to the sudden change of hormones. If your period doesn't come when it's supposed to, call your clinic for advice. They may have special instructions for you.

With some of the newer pills, girls have more menstrual irregularity, which makes some girls worry more about pregnancy. Be sure to check with your clinic if your period is late or doesn't come at all.

rhythmically, you may experience problems later, when you choose to go off the Pill.

Cassie told us about a complication that made the Pill impossible for her to take:

> Ever since I started taking the Pill I had these terrible, really really terrible headaches. Like migraines. They came just before my period. I decided it wasn't worth it and I went off the Pill.

Bobbie had a different problem:

> There have been times during the last six months that I've been on the Pill that I've felt so depressed I couldn't even do anything. I just wanted to stay in bed with the covers over my head. I thought it was just me, but then my friend told me that maybe the Pill was causing it. If that's what it is, I'm going off the Pill right away.

Severe headaches and depression are not uncommon conditions associated with the Pill. Some girls say that their skin problems get worse while they are on the Pill, and some say they gain weight more easily and feel bloated more of the time. A weight gain of ten pounds or more is an indication that you should not take the combination pill. You may have better results with the progestin-only pill.

DEPO-PROVERA

What Is It? Depo-Provera is the brand name for a drug manufactured by the Upjohn Company, which contains synthetic progesterone. It is injected into a girl's body once every twelve weeks. The protection against pregnancy provided by one Depo-Provera injection lasts three months. It suppresses ovulation, thickens the consistency of cervical mucus, and weakens the uterine lining, making it unable to support a pregnancy. It is a popular form of birth control in the United States and also throughout the world.

The Pill and Good Nutrition

Studies show that synthetic estrogen interferes with your body's ability to absorb vitamins and minerals. The particular vitamins mentioned are the B complex (including B_6, B_{12}, riboflavin, thiamin), C, and folic acid. Zinc absorption may also be affected.

Without adequate supplies of B vitamins, your body may be more susceptible to anemia and depression. Vitamin C is important in fighting off infections, but do not take more than 1 gram per day if you are on the Pill. Vitamin C can increase your body's absorption of estrogen, which may have negative effects. Zinc deficiency can lead to skin and hair problems.

Food sources for these vitamins and minerals are:

Vitamin B_6: whole grains, liver, wheat germ, meats, fish, soybeans, nuts, corn, bananas, organ meats.

Vitamin B_{12}: milk, eggs, meat, cheese. Strict vegetarians and vegans are advised to take B_{12} supplements.

Riboflavin (B_2): brewer's yeast, milk, organ meats, whole grains, seeds, leafy green vegetables.

Thiamin (B_1): whole grains, bran, rice (especially brown rice), pork.

Vitamin C: citrus fruits, leafy green vegetables, fresh strawberries and other berries, tomatoes, potatoes, cabbage, bean sprouts, green pepper, squash.

Zinc: Oysters, yeast breads, wheat germ, dark muscle meats.

If you smoke and drink alcohol while you are on the Pill, you further deplete your body's nutritional resources. A good multivitamin/mineral supplement may help. Check with a nutritionist or health practitioner.

Smoking and the Pill: As Planned Parenthood says, smoking and the Pill are a deadly mix. There are many reasons not to smoke. Cigarettes alone are deadly! If you are on the Pill and smoking more than fifteen cigarettes a day, you put yourself at high risk for many serious medical conditions, such as heart disease, lung disease, and stroke. Try to cut back on cigarettes. Better still, try to quit smoking altogether.

***Effectiveness Against Pregnancy and
STDs.*** Depo-Provera is highly effective in preventing pregnancy. Only one woman out of every two
hundred and fifty who take this drug will get pregnant. That is a 99.6 percent effectiveness rate, as
high as that of the Pill.

Like other hormonal forms of birth control,
Depo-Provera is great protection against pregnancy
but no protection at all against sexually transmitted
disease. If you use this method for birth control, be
sure to have your partner use a condom to protect
both of you from STDs.

How to Get It. This method is available at
family-planning clinics and doctors' offices. Call to
make an appointment. When you go in, you will be
asked about your medical history—what illnesses
you've had, what illnesses run in your family, and so
on. You will be given a pregnancy test, to make sure
you aren't already pregnant. This birth control
method should not be used during pregnancy. You
will receive a thorough examination, including a
pelvic exam (see page 250). At the end of the exam,
the health practitioner will discuss with you whether
Depo-Provera will be a safe method for you. If it is,
he or she will administer the Depo shot, either in
your upper arm or in your buttock (backside). This
will protect you from pregnancy for three months.

*You must return to the clinic every twelve
weeks to receive another shot, if you do not want
to get pregnant.*

Cost. It generally costs between $30 to $40, or
sometimes more, for each three-month injection,
about $12 per month. You will need a full medical
exam the first time you go in for your injection, and
that will cost an additional $40–$200. Some clinics
have sliding scales and allow teenagers to pay in
installments. Medicare or other health insurance
may cover some or most of the cost. Discuss cost
when you call for your appointment and find out
what arrangements can be made.

How to Use It. This is the easiest of all methods to use: you don't have to do anything except
show up at the clinic for your next shot! Be aware of
any side effects you may be experiencing and report

them to the health practitioner during your next
appointment. If you have severe side effects (see
below under "Disadvantages"), call the clinic immediately and report what is happening.

One question a lot of girls ask is, "If I use this
drug for a long time, will I be able to get pregnant
after I stop using it?" The answer is that more than
three-quarters (75 percent) of the women using the
Depo-Provera method get pregnant within a year
after stopping it. More than 90 percent get pregnant
within two years of stopping the drug. Teenagers
who have never had a child or women who have
used Depo-Provera for many years may experience a
longer period of infertility after stopping the drug
than those who never used it or those who have
already had one child.

Advantages. The main advantage of this form
of protection is that you do not have to do anything
to make it work. Once you receive the injection, you
have as much protection from pregnancy as is currently possible, short of abstaining from intercourse
altogether. Your protection lasts twelve weeks. Then
you renew the protection by having another shot or
starting to use another method of birth control.

For some girls Depo-Provera creates scantier
menstrual periods or even no periods at all. If you
are used to heavy, painful menstrual periods, you
might enjoy decreased cramping and lighter flow.
Check with the clinic if you have no periods at all
just to be sure there is no problem. On the other
hand, in some girls, bleeding increases and comes
irregularly for the first six months.

Depo-Provera may help protect some women
from endometrial cancer (a kind of cancer that affects
the lining of the uterus) for at least eight years after it
is discontinued. It does not seem to increase the risk
of cancer of the cervix, ovary, or liver.

Disadvantages. The number-one disadvantage is that you have to go to the clinic every three
months for an injection. Some girls don't mind that
at all, but if you do not like shots, you may have trouble "remembering" to show up for your appointment.
Definitely weigh this factor into your decision about
which method to use. If you know you hate shots,
consider using another method.

Because Depo-Provera interferes with a girl's regular menstrual flow, some girls worry that they are pregnant when their periods don't come regularly. This can be checked with a pregnancy test until you get used to the way your body reacts to the drug.

A number of girls experience weight gain, a bloated feeling, breast tenderness, headaches, fatigue, and dizziness. Some girls do get heavier, irregular periods on this drug. And some girls have reported severe depression, acne, and hair loss due to taking Depo-Provera, although this is not common. Unfortunately, if you experience unpleasant side effects there is *no way* to stop the drug until it runs its three-month course. It cannot be neutralized or reversed. So once you receive the shot, you cannot change your mind during that three-month period.

There have been some studies linking DMPA, the hormonal substance in Depo-Provera, to a condition that may speed the growth of already existing tumors in women under thirty-five.

You must not use this drug (or any hormonal method of birth control) if you are pregnant, because it can lead to low-birth-weight babies.

Finally, a number of girls just don't feel comfortable using synthetic hormones. They don't like the idea of tampering with the natural functioning of their bodies. For these girls, barrier methods or abstinence are better alternatives.

NORPLANT

What Is It? Norplant is a contraceptive device that comes in the form of six small sticklike capsules, each containing a large supply of slow-release synthetic progesterone. The hormone capsules are implanted under a woman's skin (subdermal) in the upper, more fleshy part of her arm. They can protect her from pregnancy for up to five years.

Norplant works by continually releasing a low dose of progestin into a girl's body, interrupting her natural fertility cycle and causing her cervical mucus to thicken; it may also contribute to the temporary inability of her uterus to nourish a fertilized egg. When a girl has the Norplant capsules removed, her normal fertility cycle and functions resume.

Effectiveness Against Pregnancy and STDs. Of all the methods available, Norplant has the most effective record against pregnancy. For every one hundred women who use Norplant over a five-year period, between three and four will get pregnant. In other words, fewer than one person in a hundred get pregnant per year.

Norplant provides *no* protection against the transmission of STDs. We strongly recommend that the male partner use condoms together with this method. If he won't, the female partner can use a female condom or spermicide to protect herself against STDs.

Who Should Not Use Norplant?

Norplant has possible side effects that make it an unwise choice for some girls. Girls should not use Norplant if they themselves have now or have had in the past: heart disease, blood-clotting problems, stroke, breast cancer, or acute liver disease. Girls who have a family history of those diseases should also consider using other forms of contraception. In addition, girls who have had unexplained bleeding from the vagina or girls who are pregnant or breast-feeding a baby should not use Norplant.

Like other progestin-only contraceptives, Norplant may create cardiovascular problems for smokers. If you are a smoker, we advise you to stop smoking before using this method of birth control.

How to Get It. Norplant is available at family-planning clinics. Call for an appointment. At the clinic, the health practitioner will ask you questions about your medical history, illnesses you might have had, health conditions common to your family, etc. Some girls have health conditions that might get worse if they use this method, so the health practitioner will want to go over that with you. Your physical exam will also include a blood pressure check, a breast exam, a pelvic exam, and a Pap smear to test for cervical cancer.

You will be asked to return to the clinic during the first seven days after the start of your next period, when the implants will be inserted. This is to guarantee that you are not pregnant, although sometimes people have one period even if they are pregnant. Girls who have had unprotected intercourse since their last period should ask to have a pregnancy test done for added protection.

Use some other form of birth control/safer-sex protection like condoms until the Norplant is inserted.

Just before insertion, the health practitioner will numb the skin on the upper part of your arm with some anesthetic. When the area is numb, he or she will make a small cut in the skin and place the six capsules inside. It takes about ten to fifteen minutes to complete this procedure. Girls say that even though it sounds bad, it doesn't hurt except for the initial prick of the anesthetic needle.

After the device has been inserted, you will wear a bandage on your arm for a few days. You should not do any heavy lifting or stretch your arm in any extreme way during that time.

You must return for a checkup within three months of the insertion, and then every year after that. After five years, the old capsules will be removed and you can decide whether or not you want to have new ones inserted. If you do have a new batch put in, that will protect you for another five years. If you decide not to reinsert Norplant or if you have it removed before the five years are up, you will be without protection. Unless you want to get pregnant, use another form of contraception.

Cost. Norplant costs between $500 and $700 for insertion and about $100 to $200 for removal. That's a total cost of around $600 to $900. (Five years of birth control pills cost around $1,100.) Medicaid or your personal health insurance may cover the cost for you, and some clinics may have a sliding scale or be able to make special arrangements for payment. Check with your clinic or doctor.

How to Use It. Once Norplant is inserted, that's it. You don't have to do anything to protect yourself from pregnancy for five years, except go back to the clinic or doctor for a checkup each year.

Remember, however, that although you are protected from pregnancy, you are *not* protected against sexually transmitted diseases. To protect against STDs, you or your partner can wear a condom.

Removal. Although in the majority of patients it takes no more than fifteen to twenty minutes for the capsules to be removed, in some girls removal is more problematic because the capsules have become embedded in deeper tissue. In these cases, removal may be difficult and scarring may occur. Scarring may also occur after insertion.

Advantages. Norplant is very easy to use and very effective against pregnancy. It doesn't require any care other than yearly checkups. If you decide you want to become pregnant, the rods must be removed. Some girls experience lighter periods, or even no periods, when they are on Norplant, especially during the first year or two.

Disadvantages. The main complaint against Norplant is that it tends to cause irregular bleeding during the first year of use, so girls can't predict their periods. In some people the bleeding is light; in others the bleeding is excessive. Irregular bleeding becomes so much of a problem for some girls that they choose to have the rods removed during the first year. Since Norplant costs so much to insert and to have removed, some clinics suggest using a progestin-only pill for a few months as a test to see if irregular bleeding poses a major inconvenience for you. If it does, you may not want to use Norplant. Talk this over with your health practitioner when you go in for your first appointment.

Other possible side effects include headaches, acne, breast tenderness, hairiness, depression, nausea, and nervousness. Some women experience weight loss; more experience weight gain. These conditions are commonly associated with all contraceptive methods that contain hormones. Once your body adjusts to the hormones, the side effects usually lessen or disappear. In some cases, however, the side effects become so inconvenient and disruptive that girls decide to have Norplant removed.

Girls whose bodies tend to form excessive scarring may consider that a disadvantage, because the potential for scarring exists at the site of implantation and removal.

Some girls say they don't want to use Norplant because they want to be in charge of their own body. They don't like the idea of having some foreign substance implanted under their skin, and they don't like the idea of playing around with their natural menstrual cycle. These girls prefer using one of the other methods of safer sex.

Finally, from the perspective of protection, Norplant may offer a highly effective protection against pregnancy, but it does not protect you in any way from sexually transmitted diseases. Since there are so many dangerous STDs around these days, we hope you will keep yourself and your partner safer by using male or female condoms along with Norplant.

Other Methods

THE IUD: We don't recommend that teenagers use the IUD. Many women have had long-range fertility problems due to infections related to IUD use. In fact, the risk of developing pelvic inflammatory disease (see page 50), which can lead to permanent infertility, is double for women who use the IUD as their method of birth control. The IUD may also increase your chances of catching some STDs.

FERTILITY-AWARENESS METHODS: If you've read the section starting on page 36 about a girl's menstrual cycle, you know that there is a time during every month when a girl releases ripe eggs from her ovary. This time of ovulation is a girl's fertile time, the time when she can get pregnant. By using fertility-awareness methods, such as checking cervical mucus and keeping a menstrual/ovulation calendar, a girl can learn to predict her time of ovulation.

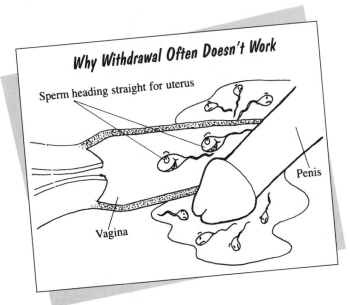

Why Withdrawal Often Doesn't Work

Sperm heading straight for uterus

Penis

Vagina

The fertile time can change from month to month and from cycle to cycle. That's why guessing about it doesn't work, and why this is a complicated method to use. To learn more about fertility awareness, we recommend taking classes that are offered at many family-planning clinics and local hospitals. Women who have learned this procedure say it is satisfying to understand how your body works well enough to be able to predict ovulation.

Fertility awareness does *not* protect you in any way from catching a sexually transmitted disease.

WITHDRAWAL: Withdrawal requires that a boy take his penis out of the girl's vagina *before* ejaculation (coming). Unfortunately, even if a boy is able to pull out before his final orgasm, drops of seminal fluid containing sperm escape from the penis into the vagina throughout intercourse, and those tiny drops are enough to start a pregnancy. They are also enough to pass a sexually transmitted disease.

When a boy tells a girl, "Don't worry, I'll pull out in time," he is talking about using withdrawal as his method of birth control. When a girl believes him, she usually ends up very sorry that she did.

Furthermore, withdrawal does not in any way protect the boy from catching a sexually transmitted disease from his partner. We recommend condoms for boys who want to be responsible about their own health and the health and safety of their partner.

EMERGENCY BIRTH CONTROL (AFTER-INTERCOURSE CONTRACEPTION): Although we hope you will use protection every single time you have intercourse, we know that sometimes people mess up. We also know that on rare occasions, safer-sex methods fail to work properly.

If you have unprotected intercourse or if your method fails in some way, there are some postcoital (after intercourse) measures you can take to help reduce your risk of pregnancy. The treatments are simple, effective, relatively safe, and legal. But *you must act within seventy-two hours—three days—or less* from the time of intercourse for these methods to work.

What Is It? Postcoital birth control prevents a fertilized egg from being implanted in the uterus. It is a combination of synthetic hormones designed to make your uterus a hostile environment for the fertilized egg. The egg will not be able to implant and develop.

How to Get It. A girl who thinks she may have gotten pregnant has to go to a family-planning clinic fast. Time is very important, because this treatment probably works best within the first two days after intercourse. It may not work at all if you wait longer than seventy-two hours.

It consists of a special combination of hormone pills, just like birth control pills but often in higher doses, designed to meet your particular body's needs. Health practitioners at your clinic will discuss options with you. Some girls receive a combination of estrogen and progestin. Some receive progestin

---

Visiting a Family-Planning Clinic

In every state in the United States, there are clinics that offer safer-sex and birth control methods free or at low cost. To find a clinic near you, look for an advertisement in your local newspaper's classified section or look in the business pages of your phone book under Clinics, Family Planning, Health Clinics, Medical Clinics. You can check the white pages if you know a clinic's name. Planned Parenthood is listed in the white pages. State or county clinics will be in the Government section under County Government: Health and Human Services. If all else fails, call your local hospital and ask for a referral to the nearest family-planning clinic. Sometimes the hospital itself will provide the services you need in an outpatient clinic.

There are also many women's health centers and clinics throughout the country that are excellent sources of information and service.

How to Use the Clinic: The procedures in each clinic vary. Usually you call to make an appointment and then go in at a scheduled time. When you call, ask about their fees. Ask if they have a sliding-fee scale for teens. Clinics usually have a way for teens to pay according to how much they can afford. If you have absolutely no money, see if some arrangements can be made for you. Remember, these people want you to use protection. In most instances they will do their best to accommodate you.

Some clinics have a special "drop-in day" so that people can come in without an appointment. Many clinics have a time each week set up specifically for teenagers. When you call the clinic, you can ask about drop-in days and teen days.

At the clinic, you may be asked to sit in a waiting room until a health practitioner is free to meet with you. You may meet with the health practitioner individually or as part of a group information session. In either case, someone will tell you about the different methods of protection that are available, and you will be given the opportunity to ask questions. *Don't be shy.* Ask your questions. That's why the staff is there and that's why you're there! If you have read this chapter and go to the clinic already knowing about some of the methods, you will be able to make an informed choice. Otherwise, you may find yourself being persuaded to use the kind of protection the clinic thinks is best for you.

The Pill, Norplant, Depo-Provera, and the diaphragm or cervical cap must be prescribed by a doctor. If a girl decides to use one of these methods of birth control, she will be examined by a doctor or health practitioner, who will explain how to use the method. Before you leave the clinic, you will be given either the method you have chosen or a prescription to get it, with instructions for how to use it properly. That's all there is to it.

Even though most protection is for girls to use, condoms are usually also available at family-planning clinics. In fact, clinics often give condoms away free of charge or at very low cost. Clinics are for both males and females, and couples are encouraged to come in together, because you both can benefit from the information about protection, pregnancy, and STDs. The more informed you are, the safer you can be.

It's nice to go together as a couple or to bring a friend along with you so you will have someone to talk to while you're sitting in the waiting room. If you're nervous, having a friend along may help.

Some teens prefer going alone, because they consider this a very private matter and they don't want anyone else to know about it. Do whatever makes you feel most comfortable. The people at the clinic will no doubt be friendly and helpful since they believe that sexually active teenagers should use protection. They are on your side.

If for some reason the people at the clinic are not friendly, and if they do not treat you with respect and answer your questions carefully, you have every right to leave and take your business elsewhere. If there is no other clinic in your area, you have a right to voice your complaint to the manager of the clinic. Remember, you deserve to be treated with dignity and respect. You are acting responsibly by getting protection.

only with some danazol (a synthetic androgen drug). Never try to treat yourself with birth control pills without calling your clinic for advice; misuse could have serious health consequences.

Postcoital treatment often causes severe nausea and vomiting. Also, it may affect the timing of your next few menstrual periods, so be careful to use protection if you have intercourse again. Until your cycle becomes regular, you will not be able to judge your fertility time accurately, and if you do not use a barrier method of contraception, you are likely to get pregnant again.

If for some reason this postcoital treatment doesn't work and you find that you are pregnant, you should be aware that there is potential danger to your baby. The high dose of hormones used to try to stop the pregnancy can have a negative effect on the developing fetus. You may want to consider abortion in that case. (See Chapter 11, on page 313.)

Safer-Sex Methods for Sex Acts Other Than Intercourse

Because sexually transmitted diseases are spreading at epidemic rates, and because many STDs can be caught from sexual contact other than penis-vagina intercourse, we want you to know what some people are doing to protect themselves from catching STDs.

Germs thrive in and are passed to and from warm, moist body areas—for example, the mouth, vagina, penis, and anus. Many germs live in blood and are passed through cuts in the skin. Any place that has an opening through which blood and/or other body fluids can escape is a potential carrier or receptor of germs. To be safer in all situations, the idea is to put a barrier between your body and the other person's germs, or if you are the infected person, to use a barrier to prevent your germs from infecting someone else.

To be effective, barriers must be used properly every time you engage in any sex act. You must use a new barrier with each new act, and you must throw away the old barrier after use. Be very careful when you remove and dispose of the used barrier. Use latex gloves or plastic wrap or tissues to touch the barrier once it has been used, because it could be

covered with germs, then wash your hands with soap and water afterward if possible.

Here are some ways people have devised to protect themselves during sex acts other than intercourse.

LATEX CONDOMS: An unprotected penis can potentially transmit or receive many STD germs, like HIV, human papilloma virus, syphilis, gonorrhea, herpes, chlamydia, and others. Boys who do not want to catch STDs must protect themselves during oral sex as well as during intercourse. Girls who do not want to catch STDs must protect themselves as well. Make sure the boy you are with uses a condom during penis-mouth sex. For vagina-mouth sex, partners may use an oral barrier.

ORAL BARRIERS: These are protective materials made of latex or impermeable, flexible plastic used to cover a potentially infected area, like the mouth, the penis, the anus, the vagina. Another term used is dental dam. To keep germs from spreading during mouth-contact with any of these areas, partners can cover the area with a layer of thin latex; some people use plastic wrap (like Saran wrap), although we don't know how effective that is. Sensations are still felt, but the area is protected. *Do not* use thin plastic bags, which do not provide protection and can cause suffocation.

LATEX GLOVES: Finally, for some sex acts involving hands—like mutual masturbation or finger-vagina or finger-anus manipulation—people are advised to wear thin latex gloves, like the gloves medical people use. These gloves help keep germs from passing from one person to another should you have a cut on your skin. You can buy them in the drugstore.

RESOURCES

Planned Parenthood health clinics are in every state of the United States. Usually located in urban areas, they are a good place to go for birth control and safer-sex protective methods.

Planned Parenthood Hotline. 1-800-230-PLAN (7526). You can call this toll-free hot line to be connected to the Planned Parenthood clinic nearest to you. They will answer your questions and help you.

Department of Health Clinics

These are government-run public clinics that provide birth control and safer-sex services. Look at the agencies listed under the name of your county. Check the headings for Birth Control or Family Planning in the business pages.

Books

The New Our Bodies, Ourselves. New York: Simon & Schuster, 1992. Written by the Boston Women's Health Book Collective, this book is a wealth of information on women's health and sexuality. There is an extensive section on birth control and safer-sex protection. Advanced reading level.

Sacrificing Ourselves for Love, by Jane Wegscheider Hyman and Esther R. Rome. Freedom, CA: The Crossing Press, 1996. Excellent discussion of the ways women can choose to take care of themselves in love relationships. Advanced reading level.

The Internet

If you have access to a computer with a modem, you can reach the World Wide Web and find the latest information about birth control and safer-sex protection. Go to a Net search machine and type in safe sex or contraception.

So You Think You Might Be Pregnant

Girls can get pregnant. Boys can't. That certainly doesn't come as a surprise to any of you, but we wanted to say it at the beginning, because it will help you understand why we've written this chapter the way we have. A lot of the chapter is directed to the girls who read it. Very often it is the teenage girl who has to figure out what to do about an unplanned pregnancy by herself—without the support of the boy or man who participated in the conception. In the end, the girl is the one who decides what she wants to do about the pregnancy, and we believe that is her right. Her body is involved, and too frequently, if she makes the choice to continue the pregnancy, she is left to raise the child alone.

We hope that if you are a boy involved in a pregnancy, you'll want to support your girlfriend as she decides what to do. If she chooses to have the baby and chooses not to put it up for adoption, we hope you will join with her in the parenthood. Children need and benefit from having loving, involved fathers as much as they need and benefit from having loving, involved mothers.

HOW CAN YOU TELL YOU MIGHT BE PREGNANT?

To get pregnant, a girl has to have had sexual intercourse or have been with a boy who ejaculated very near the opening of her vagina. *If you have been having intimate sexual activity with a boy, you could be pregnant,* even if you're very young, even if you've had intercourse only once, and even if you were using some method of birth control.

First Signs of Pregnancy

A missed menstrual period is usually the first sign of pregnancy. But even though they are pregnant, some women have a period that is shorter than usual, with less bleeding. It probably won't seem normal. So if you miss a period or have a period that doesn't seem quite right, *you may be pregnant.* If you miss a period and have even a few of the other signs of pregnancy, that's a pretty sure indication that you are pregnant—but it's still not 100 percent sure. The only way to tell for sure is to have a pregnancy test (see page 315).

A pregnancy won't go away just because you ignore it, and it won't go away because you wish for it to go away.

FEELINGS ABOUT A POSSIBLE PREGNANCY

You may have lots of feelings, thoughts, and fantasies about a possible pregnancy. Some people feel

Here are some signs of pregnancy:

➤ You miss your period or your period is lighter or for fewer days than usual.

➤ Your breasts are tender and seem to be bigger.

➤ You have to urinate a lot.

➤ You feel sick to your stomach in the morning or late afternoon or all the time.

➤ You feel bloated or crampy.

➤ You're more tired than usual, and you feel sleepy during the day, or you get dizzy.

➤ Your appetite has changed.

➤ You are moodier than usual.

➤ Your clothes feel tighter.

Not everyone who is pregnant has these symptoms, and not everyone who has these symptoms is pregnant. But if you had sexual intercourse with a boy and you have some of these symptoms, plan to have a pregnancy test done as soon as possible.

angry, upset, scared, shocked, and very sad when they find out they are pregnant. Others feel happy, glad, excited, and joyful. Most people feel very mixed—happy, sad, angry, and scared all at once. There are no right or wrong feelings. You don't have to be ashamed about having your feelings or about feeling confused. Lots of people do. Here's how fifteen-year-old Carol put it:

We were having sex on the safe days, and I wasn't very sure about it, but I wasn't getting pregnant, so after a while I started thinking, Well, maybe I can't get pregnant. Then one month I didn't get my period. I didn't want to face it—I kept putting off telling my boyfriend. It was funny because I was sort of glad to find out I could get pregnant, but I was miserable about being pregnant.

Sixteen-year-old Bev, a sophomore from San Francisco, told us:

Last semester I got pregnant, and I would sit in bed at night, every night, and say, "I don't believe this. This can't be happening to me. Go away. Leave me alone. I can't handle this." I mean, I know that sounds ridiculous, but I didn't know anything, and I was so frightened I just thought I'd force my body not to be pregnant.

You may feel very alone. Try to put your thoughts and emotions into words; it will help you get clear about the decision you face—whether to end your pregnancy or to continue your pregnancy and have the child. You can write in a private diary or journal. You can talk about your feelings with someone you trust, someone who can help you sort out your confusion. Don't let your confusion or fear or anger prevent you from acting, as Roberta, a fourteen-year-old from New Jersey, did:

I thought I was pregnant because I missed my period, but I tried not to think about it. I didn't want to talk to anybody because I was too scared. My mother would have never let me forget it, so I didn't want to tell her, and I didn't want to tell any of my friends because I was afraid word would get around school. But finally I told my boyfriend. He found out where I could get a test done, but I was scared. I'd make an appointment at the clinic and then I wouldn't go. Weeks were going by and finally I talked to my counselor at school, who I really like. She was great. She explained everything to me. I went and got the test, and it wasn't so bad. But what came out was that I was already five months pregnant, so now I have to have the baby. I can't have an abortion because I'm too far along.

Some people, like Roberta, think they might be pregnant but don't go for a pregnancy test right away because they think it will be a hassle or they worry it will hurt them or they think they'll feel embarrassed. Some people worry that an adult will give them a lecture or they won't have enough money or they won't be able to get to the doctor's office or clinic. Many people don't go for the test because they don't want to face knowing for sure that they are pregnant.

It's natural to feel worried. But if you want to have a *choice* about how to deal with the pregnancy, you have to have a pregnancy test done early—as soon as you suspect you might be pregnant.

Girls who already know they don't want to end the pregnancy still should be tested early, because they need good medical care right away. As a pregnant teen you must eat right, take special vitamins, and be checked by a doctor periodically. You must also *stop taking drugs, stop smoking, and stop drinking alcohol.* To be born strong and healthy, a fetus needs good care while it's still in your uterus (prenatal care), and it needs a drug-free, alcohol-free, and smoke-free environment in which to develop.

If you are pregnant and want to have the baby, we recommend reading the chapters about pregnancy, childbirth, and postpartum (after the baby is born) in the book *The New Our Bodies, Ourselves.* There are other good books about pregnancy and childbirth available in bookstores and libraries.

DETERMINING WHETHER YOU ARE PREGNANT

To find out if you are or are not pregnant you need two kinds of tests:

1. a urine or a blood test
2. a pelvic exam

See the following sections called "The Urine Test," "The Blood Test," and "The Pelvic Exam" for a detailed explanation of these three types of pregnancy tests.

Where to Get a Pregnancy Test

The urine test is available at doctors' offices, hospitals, clinics, or special pregnancy labs. (You can also use a home pregnancy test, which may be purchased at a drugstore.) Most places that do urine tests also offer the blood test and a pelvic exam. The fee for a pelvic exam and a urine test can range from no fee at all to more than $100, depending on whether you go to a public clinic or a private doctor.

The phone book lists places offering free pregnancy testing, counseling, and help with problem pregnancies. Be aware that some of these may be organizations that oppose abortions under any circumstances. While you are trying to decide whether to continue your pregnancy or not, you may prefer talking with someone at an organization committed to a woman's right to choose for herself whether to have an abortion or not.

When you find a place, call for information. You don't have to give your name if you don't want to. Ask if pregnancy tests for teens are available. Ask whether you can consent to your own health care, meaning you do not need the signature of your parent or guardian, and ask whether your confidentiality will be respected so that no one else will be contacted. Ask about cost. If money is a problem for you,

As soon as you find out for sure that you are pregnant, the decision is yours whether to continue the pregnancy and have a baby or end the pregnancy by having an abortion. If you don't get a pregnancy test right away, you won't have the same choice. Usually by the time your body starts looking pregnant it will be too late to have a simple abortion.

Those of us who wrote this book believe, along with the majority of people in the United States, that it is a woman's right to be able to decide whether to keep a pregnancy or have an abortion. Abortion is legal. If you find out you are pregnant and you decide early enough that you don't want to be pregnant, you can end the pregnancy legally and safely.

However, abortion is a last resort. Choosing whether to continue a pregnancy or end it can be a difficult and emotional decision. A better way to avoid an unwanted pregnancy is to keep it from happening in the first place if you can. Unless sex is being forced on you, you and your partner have the choice to use birth control and safer-sex methods every single time you have sexual intercourse.

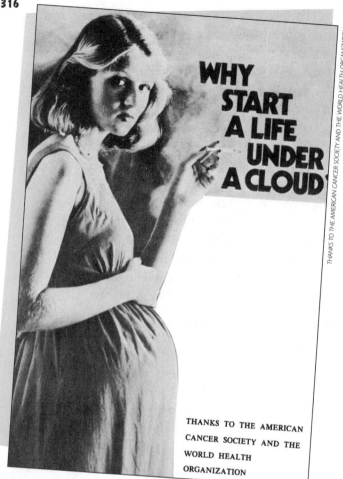

WHY
START
A LIFE
UNDER
A CLOUD

THANKS TO THE AMERICAN
CANCER SOCIETY AND THE
WORLD HEALTH
ORGANIZATION

THANKS TO THE AMERICAN CANCER SOCIETY AND THE WORLD HEALTH ORGANIZATION

Beware!

Studies by doctors and research institutions have proved that taking drugs, smoking, using caffeine, and drinking alcohol can each cause serious complications for the unborn fetus.

Drugs are especially dangerous. All drugs, even aspirin and cold remedies, cross from the mother's body to the developing fetus. Cocaine, amphetamines, LSD, heroin, and other illegal drugs can cause birth defects or addiction in the baby. They can lead to severe developmental problems in young children. Check with your doctor before taking *any* drugs, even a prescribed drug, while you are pregnant.

Heavy smokers tend to have low-birth-weight babies who are more susceptible to infant death and brain damage.

Caffeine—in cola drinks, coffee, tea, and "stay awake" drugs, such as No-Doz—can cause deformities in the fetus.

Alcohol can stunt fetal development both physically and mentally and can lead to fetal alcohol syndrome, a harmful developmental condition.

If you are having sexual intercourse without using effective birth control, *be aware that all the drugs, alcohol, and cigarettes you use are not only bad for you, they're also bad for your baby should you become pregnant.*

ask if you can pay in installments. Some places have reduced fees for people who can't afford to pay. There may even be clinics that offer free pregnancy testing for teens. If you make an appointment, get directions about how to get there.

Trying to find a good place to get an affordable pregnancy test done can seem overwhelming, but don't be put off by what might seem like a lot of red tape. Fifteen-year-old Donna from New York City had this experience:

I called a clinic. At first I got a recorded voice asking me to use my touch-tone phone to select who I wanted to speak to and push the right button. I was so nervous I almost hung up. Then when I finally got to talk to a person, she was pretty nice. When she said that it would cost $100 for a urine test and pelvic exam I almost started crying. The lady was understanding that I couldn't pay. She told me to call another number, where I could get a pregnancy test for free.

You may want to ask a parent or a friend to help you get the information you need. It can be comforting to have another person involved, especially if you feel worried or confused.

THE URINE TEST: If you are pregnant, a special hormone called HCG is released into your urine. A urine test can tell whether HCG is there. A chemical is mixed with your urine, and if the urine reacts one way, it means you are pregnant; if it reacts another way, it means you are not pregnant. The urine test may not be accurate before two weeks after conception or after four or five months after conception.

There are several kinds of urine tests available. Most family planning clinics now use a newer test that can be accurate from around ten days after conception, a little before your period is due. The price of this test fluctuates, but may be as low as $5 for teenagers, depending on the clinic. You may be asked to bring a sample of your first urine from the morning, although most clinics can run the test using a sample of urine produced at the time of your visit.

To collect urine in the morning, when you get up on the day of the test, instead of urinating in the toilet bowl, hold a clean, dry jar under you and urinate in that. Try to get at least a half cup of urine in the jar, then cover the jar. If you aren't going to bring the urine sample into the lab or do a home test right away, store it in the refrigerator, or if you can't do that, put it in some other cool place (away from the heat). If the urine is too warm, the test may not be accurate. The first urine of the morning is usually the most concentrated and will produce the most accurate result.

You can do a urine pregnancy test yourself at home. Kits are available for sale at drugstores and some markets. It is very important to follow the instructions *exactly* and to remember that these tests are sometimes not accurate. If the test shows you are pregnant, you should see a doctor for a pelvic exam to make absolutely sure. If the test shows you are not pregnant *but you still do not get your period,* have another test done at a lab.

Urine tests done at home or at a lab may not always be accurate because:

➤ You didn't use your first urine of the morning.

➤ The sample got too warm by the time it was tested.

➤ You are too early in your pregnancy for the HCG to show.

➤ You are too late in the pregnancy for the HCG to be recognized.

➤ The jar wasn't clean. (If it had chemicals or perfume or soap in it before, that might affect the test. Wash the jar thoroughly with hot water and make sure it is dry before using it.)

➤ You are taking drugs or medicine, such as aspirin in large doses, marijuana, Thorazine, Mellaril, heroin, methadone. Drugs and medications can affect the test.

If the urine test says you are pregnant, believe it. You are probably pregnant, especially if you have other symptoms. To be absolutely sure, have a pelvic exam.

THE BLOOD TEST: HCG is also released into your blood when you get pregnant. A sample of your blood is taken, and then a special lab test is run to see if HCG appears.

The blood test for pregnancy is like other blood tests. You go to the doctor's office or clinic and a nurse or a doctor takes a sample of blood from your body. Usually, they draw the sample from a vein in your arm. It may hurt for a second as the needle sticks you. Some nurses and doctors are so skilled at taking blood that they can do it almost without your noticing.

There are two kinds of blood tests. The RRA test is accurate fourteen to seventeen days after conception, or when your period is just several days late. The RIA test is more sensitive and can tell you whether you're pregnant within a week to ten days of conception. In general, the blood test is more expensive than the urine test. Usually, blood tests are done if there is some question about the accuracy of the urine test.

THE PELVIC EXAM: Read pages 250–252 for a description of a pelvic exam. Millions of women have pelvic exams every year. It's the way to check for infections inside your vagina or in your reproductive organs, and it's the way to get a Pap smear to check for abnormal cell growth. If you are having sex, it's important to have a pelvic exam done at least once a year to check for STDs and other general health concerns.

During this exam, the doctor can see by looking at your cervix and feeling your uterus whether you are pregnant and about how far along in your pregnancy you are. If you are pregnant, your cervix, which is usually pink or red, will look bluish (because of the enlarged veins filled with blood). Also, your uterus will feel bigger and softer than normal. If you ask, the doctor may let you hold a mirror to see for yourself how your cervix looks.

An ultrasound (sometimes called a sonogram) device may be used to get a more precise determination of the fetus's age. This painless procedure involves scanning your abdomen with an electronic wand to produce a sound wave picture of the inside of your uterus on a special TV screen. Ask the doctor if you can see it too.

Lots of women and girls feel uneasy about pelvic exams. That's natural. It takes practice to get used to a doctor examining your insides. But don't let your uneasiness keep you from getting this important exam, especially if you think you might be pregnant.

In Texas, seventeen-year-old Dorrie had this experience:

> When I missed my period, I told my sister and her girlfriend, and they were great. They took me to a birth control clinic to get the test done. The clinic was real busy, and I felt like they were rushing me. Everything seemed real impersonal, like they didn't care about you very much. I asked if my sister could come into the examining room with me when I went in, and at first they said no. But I just about cried, and I promised them I would do better with my sister in there with me. Finally, someone talked to the nurse and she said okay. This nurse was wonderful. Really. She told me all about what she was doing, and the exam was fine. Even my sister learned a lot of stuff she didn't know.

It can be very helpful and comforting to go with someone you trust when you have your tests done. Some places let you bring a friend (even your boyfriend) into the examining room. Some girls prefer to go alone. Decide what will make you most comfortable. Suzanne, a high school senior, said:

> I went alone for the test, because I didn't really have anyone to go with me. The guy I got pregnant by went back to his old girlfriend, and I was too embarrassed to tell anybody else about it. I felt pretty funny walking into the clinic, but the people there were so nice I relaxed right away.

Most places that do pregnancy tests for teenagers are set up to make you feel comfortable. Everyone understands that you may be nervous, worried, and upset. Lots of times there will be counselors there to talk with you and explain the proce-

dures. They may explain the choices you have if you are pregnant. Your visit and your conversations should be confidential. Check to be sure that is the policy of the testing place you visit.

If for some reason you're not happy with the way you were treated, you have the right to make your complaints known to the director of the clinic.

FEELINGS ABOUT FINDING OUT YOU ARE PREGNANT

The results of your test will come back almost immediately, so you will know whether or not you are pregnant right away. If you are pregnant, you may feel relieved to be sure at last. You may even feel glad or proud of the fact that your body can get pregnant. But at the same time you may feel depressed and panicky. It's important to try to sort through your feelings so you can think clearly about what you want to do now. Thirteen-year-old Patricia said:

> I knew I couldn't have the baby. I mean, I thought, I can't have a baby, I'm just a kid myself. But I had been so worried and so miserable and so sick that I was really glad to find out for sure that I was just pregnant and not dying of some disease or something. I mean, I hated that I was pregnant, but at least I knew I could do something about that.

When you find out for sure that you are pregnant, you may feel like crying. Lots of girls do. People will understand. You may feel angry and want to scream at the guy with whom you got pregnant. Luisa said that's how she felt:

> I'm so angry I can't stand it. I told Noah I wasn't using birth control, but he said, "Oh, don't worry, I know what to do." How could I have let him talk me into doing it? I was stupid, but he kept saying, "Don't you love me?"

Barbie, a sixteen-year-old from Denver, said she felt her pregnancy just wasn't fair:

> Why me? I know lots of girls who are doing it, and they aren't pregnant.

If you think you may be pregnant or if you think your girlfriend is pregnant, you have some hard decisions to make. If this is an unplanned pregnancy, there may be no perfect solution, and you will have to figure out the best possible choice for you. You will have lots of mixed feelings regardless of what you choose. There are problems connected with all your choices—abortion, parenthood, and adoption.

Help yourself by talking over your feelings, fears, doubts, and concerns with someone you trust. Try to talk to your parents if they are available. Meet with a pregnancy counselor at a birth control clinic like Planned Parenthood or talk to a counselor at school or your community center.

Most important, make the decision that you feel is right, given your situation and your beliefs.

IF YOU ARE PREGNANT, THESE ARE YOUR CHOICES

When you know for sure you are pregnant, you may continue the pregnancy and have a baby or you may choose to end the pregnancy by having an abortion. It will probably help you to make your choice if you answer the following basic questions for yourself honestly:

➤ Can I raise a child?

➤ Can I have a baby and allow the baby to be adopted?

➤ Can I have an abortion?

Throughout this chapter there are stories from pregnant girls who decided yes, they did want to become mothers and raise children. When you read the stories, you'll have a better sense of what being a teen mother is like.

If you don't think you are ready to be a mother, you have two choices: You can have an abortion, which will end your pregnancy. (Abortion is discussed in detail starting on page 324.) Or you can have a baby and give it up for adoption. (That choice is discussed on page 357.)

Some teenagers know what they want to do about pregnancy. For others, the decision is confusing, painful, and difficult. Your feelings about teen parenthood, marriage, babies, adoption, and abortion will influence your decision. Try to understand where your feelings are coming from before you decide what to do. Are you worried about what your parents and friends will think? Are you feeling pressure from your boyfriend? Do you have strong religious feelings about this? Can you sort through all those views to decide what *you* think and feel? Here are some of the reactions and experiences other teens have had when faced with the same decision:

Brenda (sixteen): I love little kids, so I was glad to have my own. My mother helped me and I got welfare.

Brenda went back to school to get her high school diploma and hopes to go to school to become a paralegal. Brenda's mother, who has young children of

It is common to feel alone and unlucky when something negative happens to you. Perhaps Barbie doesn't know that most girls who have unprotected sex *do* get pregnant. It could be that her friends practice safer sex and use birth control. Perhaps she didn't know about friends who had abortions.

Some girls who find out they're pregnant feel as if they're being punished for having had sex. Fifteen-year-old Monique said:

We got stoned, and he wanted to have sex, and I didn't, but after a while we did it anyway. And the next day I thought to myself, I'm going to be punished for that. And I was right, because I just found out I'm pregnant.

Pregnancy is the natural consequence of having sex without using birth control. Sometimes when we think we've done something irresponsible, however, we feel guilty and we feel that we are being punished or should be punished for what we've done.

her own, cares for her grandson while Brenda is in school.

Jo-Ellen (seventeen): My boyfriend wanted me to have the baby. We were going to get married anyway. I planned to go to college at night.

Jo-Ellen decided to have her baby, but when Jo-Ellen was nearly six months pregnant, her boyfriend, Bill, decided he wasn't ready to settle down. They didn't get married. Bill sees the baby once in a while and helps out a little with expenses. Jo-Ellen's living at home with her baby, but she's uncomfortable there. When the baby gets a little older, Jo-Ellen wants to put her in day care and try to get a job. Then she hopes to find a place of her own to live. Of course, all that takes money, which she doesn't have.

Denise (fifteen): Both my sisters got pregnant when they weren't married, and they had the babies, and I think they've had it really rough. I want to have a better life than that. It's tough raising a child on your own, especially when you're as young as I am. I'm having an abortion.

Denise had the abortion, and she said she felt bad for a while, but now she can't imagine what her life would have been like if she'd had the baby.

Lisa (sixteen): I didn't believe in abortion. I thought it was killing. I tried to raise my baby, but I couldn't manage. My son is in foster care, and that is not good for him or me.

WHAT'S THE MALE'S ROLE IN YOUR PREGNANCY?

If you are a male involved in a pregnancy with a teenage girl, you may have strong feelings at this time too. It's natural to want to be part of the decision; it's natural, also, to feel very confused and wish you weren't in this situation. All sorts of feelings are normal. The young men we spoke with were proud, happy, and concerned about their girlfriends. They also felt worried, anxious, guilty, and confused. Some felt disbelief—how could this happen? Others felt angry at themselves, their girlfriend, or at the situation. Some felt like running away. A few maintained

---

The decision about your pregnancy is one of the most serious you will ever have to make. Help yourself in these ways:

➤ Read through the rest of this section so you can be clear about your options, your rights, and your values. Even if you think you know what you want to do, read on to find out how other people handled the same problem.

➤ Talk with someone you trust, someone who is realistic and supportive. Weigh the advantages and disadvantages of each choice. Discuss your needs. Talk about your feelings. *Figure out how you are going to manage the choice you make.* If you don't have anyone to talk with, call your nearest Planned Parenthood or birth control/family-planning clinic. These places have understanding counselors on their staff who will be able to help you make a decision that's right for you.

➤ Share your feelings with the guy involved with the pregnancy. Many guys want to take their responsibility about pregnancy seriously. If he is willing, talk to him about his feelings. Find out what he has to say. Let him know what you're thinking. He may be able to help you sort through your choices and help you pay the costs of whichever choice you make.

The decision is yours and you will have to live with its consequences. There is no one right choice to make. But be sure to make your decision as soon as you can to keep your options open. If you choose to end the pregnancy, the *earlier* in the pregnancy you do it, the easier it is. If you choose to have the baby, the sooner you get pre-natal care, the better.

that they had no feelings at all about it, but most of the boys and young men we met with were ambivalent about the pregnancy—they had a lot of mixed feelings.

In our society, guys are often taught that it's not cool to be afraid or sad or to worry. Men are often taught that they're always supposed to be in control of the situation. But of course men worry and feel fear and sadness, and of course men are panicky and out of control sometimes. Everybody is.

If you're having strong feelings about this pregnancy, it helps to talk with a close friend, a parent or relative, a minister, or a teacher you like a lot. You can call a local Planned Parenthood to find out about talking to one of their counselors. You may be embarrassed or feel bad that you and your girl got into this mess, but with help and understanding, you'll be able to find the best way through it too.

Most of the attention will probably be on the girl. She's the one who gets pregnant, she's the one who has to go for the test, and she's the one who has to have the abortion or go through the childbirth. It may seem that there's no role for you in this process, but that's not true. Often how you feel about the pregnancy depends on how old you are, your financial situation, and your feelings about the girl involved. No matter whether you feel close to her or not, the truth is that you have a responsibility to help her in any way you can, since you were one-half of the process of creating the pregnancy. If you show her you care and that you want to be a part of it, and if she wants you to be there, you can participate at all stages. Sixteen-year-old Stanley told us:

> I really care about Brenda and I was so worried when she told me she was pregnant. She had to go through a lot, but I told her I would be there for her.

Like Stanley, a lot of boys are concerned about the girl's feelings and well-being. They wonder, Will she be okay? Have I hurt her? Your girlfriend may act very differently now that she's pregnant. She may be depressed and angry and feel panicky about what decision to make. You may have to be extra-patient with her at this time.

If the girl you have made pregnant is not your girlfriend, you may wonder what your role should be in the decision-making process. Some guys get scared and angry, because the reality of the pregnancy makes them realize that they are not really interested in such an intense relationship. They find themselves dealing with a heavier situation than they intended. Even if you are not in a relationship, or if you don't want to stay together anymore, it's important to help a girl who became pregnant after having sex with you. That's the right thing to do. It's your responsibility. The girl's difficult situation will be a little easier if you show concern and interest in her well-being. Talk to her and help her make plans. Eighteen-year-old Bob told us:

> She wasn't my girlfriend. We had sex a couple of times, then she tells me she's pregnant. I didn't want to have a baby, period! And definitely not with her. I could tell she was scared when she said she didn't tell anyone, and then she cried. I told her I wasn't ready to have a baby but I would help her get an abortion. That's what she wanted to do also. I talked to my older sister, who knew of a place. I went with her to have it done, and I called her a couple of times after that to see how she was doing.

As a male involved in a pregnancy, there's a lot to think about and a lot to decide. You may feel as though you don't know what to do. Your decision about how much to be involved will have an effect on at least two people's lives—three if the girl decides not to have an abortion.

It's not uncommon for boys to feel proud and excited that they helped start a pregnancy. When you first find out about the pregnancy, it's easy enough to forget that being a father is a serious, time-consuming, and important responsibility that will totally change your life. Do you want that responsibility? Are you ready to handle it? Talk to other young fathers about what life is like for them. An eighteen-year-old guy from Wyoming told us:

> My brother and his girl had to get married because she was pregnant, but they separated a year after the baby came. It was just too hard a life. They kept fighting with each other, and pretty soon Dave moved out and left Paula with the baby.

I didn't think that was fair. Now that my girl's pregnant, I really think she should have an abortion.

Steve, a seventeen-year-old from San Antonio, had a different feeling:

I think it will be nice to have a baby. Everybody in our family loves babies, and they'll all help us out. They're real understanding and are behind us. We're much closer now that we're having a baby.

You and your girlfriend may discuss getting married and keeping the baby. For some people that will seem like the only decision to make. For others of you, that will definitely not be the right decision.

Before you and your girlfriend choose to have a baby, find out who's going to be there to help you out. How do your families feel about it? Will you be able to finish school if you want to? Where will you live and how will you support yourselves? Who's going to take care of the baby while you and your girlfriend work or go to school?

Many teenage marriages don't last because marriage isn't easy for anybody. Getting married and having a baby right away is even more difficult. It takes a real commitment to each other and a willingness to work together and adjust to hard times.

Some of you may feel that you are more ready to have a baby then you are to get married. Carl, a sixteen-year-old from Detroit, put it this way:

In my family, my mother raised six of us and she never got married, so I mean, not being married and having a kid is no big deal. That's how I see it. I'll take my responsibility like a man, but there's no way I'm ready to get married, not at sixteen.

Carl may think being single and having a child is no big deal, but for most people it is a very big deal. Childrearing is hard work. Taking care of an infant and being there to provide love, food, shelter, and care twenty-four hours a day is a tremendous responsibility for one person. That's why we recommend using birth control if you are sexually active and not ready for the responsibility of raising a child together (see page 279).

Once a girl gets pregnant, many relationships break up before there's even any discussion about marriage. In New Jersey, fifteen-year-old Dominic said:

Her parents never liked me. When she got pregnant, they just shut me out, and after a while I said to hell with them and I stopped seeing her. I never even knew if she had the baby or not.

And in Florida, seventeen-year-old Jerry said:

I am embarrassed about the way I treated Linda when she got pregnant. I was afraid she'd start pressuring me into marrying her, so I told her I didn't even think it was my kid. I mean, underneath I knew it had to be, but I said that, and it made her feel really bad. I told her she better get an abortion, and I gave her the money for it. She wanted to have an abortion anyway, but I didn't know that until after I bad-mouthed her. She broke up with me right away after that.

Some guys act the way Jerry did and pretend the baby isn't theirs, even though they're pretty sure it is. It's natural to feel like running away from the problem, because you're facing a big responsibility when you accept your part in the pregnancy. But if you were there for the conception, it's up to you to be there for the pregnancy too. It's also up to you to find out about safer-sex/birth control methods to avoid another pregnancy until you're ready for one.

Sometimes the girl doesn't know exactly who made her pregnant. Sometimes she'll say she thinks it's you, but you don't think so. There is a blood test that can verify whether you are the man involved in the pregnancy. This is a genetic test that compares many different factors in your blood with similar parts of her blood and that of the baby. If she continues the pregnancy, and takes the matter to court, and proves that you fathered her child, you will be held legally responsible and you will be required to pay child support.

Guys who know they don't want the responsibility of parenthood may try to persuade their girlfriend to have an abortion. Bruce tried to talk Kathy into having an abortion, but she didn't want one:

Kathy wanted to have the baby, and there wasn't anything I could say. My parents even offered to pay for the abortion, but she didn't want to, so now she's married to some other guy and they have my *baby. That feels pretty weird.*

You can't force a woman to have an abortion. You also can't force her to have the baby. In the long run it's her decision. But if you talk about it together, then you have a better chance of finding a solution that will be best for both of you. Later in this chapter, on page 349, we will discuss your rights and responsibilities if you do become a father.

TALKING WITH YOUR FAMILY

Many teenagers feel very anxious about telling their parents that they are pregnant or have gotten a girl pregnant. We've heard teens say:

My parents would kill me if I ever got pregnant before I was married.

They'll be so disappointed.

I promised them I'd used condoms because of AIDS. They'll be so mad at me.

Now they'll know I've been having sex. They'll kill me. They'll feel so ashamed in front of their friends.

They'll make me break up with Jimmy.

They'll force me to have an abortion.

My mom will never let me forget it.

My dad will kick me out of the house.

Parents have feelings too. Most parents will be upset that their teenage daughter is pregnant or that their teenage son got a girl pregnant. They are likely to feel that you are too young for this to happen. They may be very distressed about the pregnancy because you are not married, and their first reactions will probably express their surprise, confusion, fear,

and disappointment. Then they may get very angry. They may cry, they may make you feel terrible, but after they get over the first shock, their reactions may change. Parents are usually more understanding than you give them credit for, and generally they are very concerned about your health and happiness. Most parents can be helpful to you if you let them.

Before you talk to your parents about the pregnancy, try to clear up some of your own confusion. Try to figure out what you think *you* want to do about the pregnancy. Mentally go through the choices and understand what's involved in each of them. That way you will feel better inside yourself when you talk to them. You'll know what your options are, and you can help your parents see the different options too.

One of the pregnancy counselors who worked on this section said:

Whenever I'm talking to teenagers who are worried about telling their parents, I always advise them to practice what they're going to say. I tell them to go over everything with a friend or with someone they trust. That way it's easier when they finally meet with their parents.

A few parents will just not be able to handle the fact that their teenage child is involved in a pregnancy. Their own upbringing and their own ideas of what is right and wrong will not allow them to be understanding. You have to decide whether your parents will be able to handle the news or not. Of course, if you choose to go through with the pregnancy, the girl's parents, at least, are *bound* to find out. If you are a minor (under eighteen), some states require that to have an abortion you must notify your parents and/or get their consent. It is important to find out about the laws in your state. (You can call the National Abortion Federation at 1-800-424-2280 for this information.) If your state requires parental notification and/or parental consent, and you believe you cannot involve your parents, you may be able to make your own decisions without your family. There are usually legal ways around this requirement. Clinics such as Planned Parenthood may have a counseling staff to help you.

Only the pregnant girl can sign the consent form legally allowing the abortion to be performed, so no one can force you to have an abortion if you don't want one. If you feel you are being coerced into either having an abortion or having the baby, speak to a counselor or close friend immediately. Get help figuring out what to do.

THE CHOICES EXPLAINED

The Abortion Choice: Deciding to End the Pregnancy

Abortion is *legal*.

The earlier you are in your pregnancy, the easier, safer, and cheaper it is to have an abortion.

For a teenager, having an abortion is safer than having a baby, because of the possible complications of pregnancy and childbirth.

Having an abortion does not, except in rare instances with serious complications, affect your ability to get pregnant again.

You *must* use birth control after an abortion if you don't want to get pregnant again.

Each year about one and a half million women have abortions. Of those, over three hundred thousand are girls between the ages of eleven and nineteen. If you decide to have an abortion, you are not alone.

An abortion is a medical procedure that removes the fetus from the uterus *before* it develops into a baby that can live outside the mother.

Normally, when a girl gets pregnant, an egg from her body and a sperm from a male's body unite in the fallopian tube, and the resulting fertilized egg moves down into the uterus and attaches itself to the lining of the uterus, where it continues to grow. (For more on this, see page 38.)

The fertilized egg is called an embryo, and at one month the embryo is the size of a pea. At the end of two months, the embryo, which is now called a fetus, is about one inch long and is beginning to take human shape. At three months the fetus is about

three inches long and is beginning to develop recognizable body parts. When the fetus is about eighteen to twenty weeks (four and a half to five months), the woman can begin to feel it move. Between twenty-four and twenty-eight weeks, the fetus may be able to live outside of the mother under intensive hospital care. Some babies can survive at this stage.

DETERMINING HOW FAR ALONG IN YOUR PREGNANCY YOU ARE: Most doctors can figure out how pregnant a woman is by counting the weeks from her last menstrual period (LMP). For example, if you started your last period on January 1 and it is now February 12, you are about six weeks pregnant LMP. That means it's been six weeks since your last period.

Actually, you are probably only four weeks pregnant, since conception (when the egg is fertilized by the sperm) usually takes place about two weeks after a woman gets her period. But to make calculations easier, doctors often go by the date of your last period, and in this section we will use the same method. Some abortion facilities use ultrasound to determine the true length of pregnancy. (This is an X-ray-type picture of your uterus made using sound waves.)

The method of abortion used will depend on how long you have been pregnant. Abortion is easiest, safest, and least expensive in the first three months (twelve weeks) from your last menstrual period. Although abortions can be performed safely and legally up to twenty-four weeks LMP, more complicated procedures are necessary, involving more risk. These late abortions can also be more costly, and it may be more difficult to find a facility that will agree to do them. (See page 333 to learn about the different types of abortions.)

We urge you to come to terms with being pregnant as early as possible. If you choose to continue the pregnancy and have a baby, you will need to get good prenatal care. If you choose to have an abortion, the earlier you do it, the better, so don't put off having your pregnancy test. As soon as you suspect you might be pregnant, have the test and make your decision early about what to do.

Some girls are too afraid and unhappy to decide about abortion right away. We advise you to talk over your feelings about abortion with a close friend, a parent, a favorite relative, or a counselor. Find someone whom you trust and feel comfortable with. Try to find someone who will listen carefully to what you have to say, someone who will help you make up *your* own mind, not tell you what *they* think you should do.

If your parents are understanding, they are the best people to talk to. They may also be able to help you find a place and help you pay for the procedure if you choose to have the abortion. Many teenagers we talked with said they were glad they had confided in their parents about this decision. And most parents we met want to help their children, especially when their children are in trouble.

IS ABORTION RIGHT FOR YOU? Abortion is legal, and as a teenager you have the right to have an abortion if you want one. Abortion is also controversial, and you will have to decide what you believe is "right" for you. Young people say:

> Abortions are okay for other people, but not for me. I don't believe in it for myself.

> I'm worried that I would regret it years later.

> I feel so lucky to be able to have the choice. If I got pregnant now, I would never be able to have the baby. I don't think abortion is killing. After all, the fetus couldn't possibly live on its own when it's only two and a half or three months.

> My mother got pregnant for the fourth time when she was over forty and she had an abortion. She said it was a blessing.

> Abortion is my right as a woman.

> I think abortion is a sin. If people don't want to have babies, they shouldn't have intercourse.

> My religion tells me that abortion is murder. If you get pregnant then the only right thing to do is have the baby.

There is a lot to think about when you are trying to decide whether or not to have an abortion. But it's a good idea to consider what will happen if you don't

have an abortion. Are you ready to be a mother? How will having a baby now affect your life? How would you feel about giving your baby up for adoption? These are important questions because if you don't have an abortion, you *will* have a baby.

If you decide to have an abortion, do it as soon as possible. Mary Elizabeth is seventeen. She comes from Rhode Island and got pregnant last year. She decided to have an abortion. Here's her story:

> I was raised to think that abortion is killing. I saw some of those films that they show you about babies being left to die in garbage pails after an abortion, and I thought it was like murder. I couldn't imagine how anybody could have an abortion. But then, when I got pregnant, I had to think about it a different way. I had to think, What can I do for a child? What kind of life would a child have with me? I knew if I had a baby I wouldn't be able to give it up. I just knew that. I knew I couldn't go through nine months of being pregnant and then go through childbirth only to sit up and give my baby away to somebody else. So I decided to go to an abortion clinic to find out what I could do. They explained all about the simple kind of abortion I could have if I did it early. They showed me what it would be like. They told me what to expect. I got to thinking, This sounds okay. I got to thinking, This is better than having a baby who might have a miserable life because I can't provide it with anything. And I also got to thinking that I didn't want to have a baby yet. It would wreck *my life*. I have so many things I want to do before I become a mother.

Lurene, a sixteen-year-old from Washington, D.C., made a different decision. She told us:

> At first when I found out I was pregnant I thought I would have an abortion, but when it came down to it, I couldn't do it. I was brought up very religiously, and I had a real fear of abortion. So I've decided to keep my baby. I feel like this, I chose my own way to go, so I have to take the responsibility that comes with it. And I know I'm making the right decision for me, because I'm in love with my baby and it's not even born yet.

Other teenagers explained their opinions this way:

Joan (fourteen): I know what it's like to grow up without a father. My father left when I was three, and my mother had to raise us alone. She had to go to work, and my brothers and I ran wild. I always felt bad about not having a father, so I don't want to do that to my kid.

Penny (sixteen): My boyfriend wants me to have the baby. He says he'll support it. But I want someone to give me more than money. I want someone to help me take care of it—be a real father. I just can't see us being together for the next eighteen years!

Mike (fifteen): I feel bad about Suzi having an abortion, but I know I'm not ready to be a father. I'm still a kid myself.

Georgia (sixteen): If I had this baby, I'd have to live at home for the next three or four years. My mother said she'd take care of the baby while I went to school, but then I'd be so dependent on my mother. I think she'd always throw it up in my face that she was taking care of my kid.

Choosing to have an abortion is never an easy decision. Yet the alternatives can be more devastating. Here is sixteen-year-old Tina's story:

Wanting to have an abortion does not mean that:

➤ You hate children.

➤ You never want to have children.

➤ You are a bad person.

➤ You do not love your boyfriend or girlfriend.

➤ You like the idea of having an abortion.

It means that you have decided not to have a child now. Most teenagers who choose to have an abortion do not like the idea of having one, but they feel that it is the best choice for the situation they are in.

When I got my period my mom warned me about having sex and getting pregnant. She had a real thing about it. At the time, I thought, "What is she talking about? I'm not into having sex. I'm only thirteen." Then I started to date this older guy, and after having sex just a couple of times, I got pregnant. Well, I didn't tell anyone, and when I was seven months pregnant my mom found out. She was upset at first but then said that she would help me out. So now I'm living at home with Becky, who is now two. My mom acted as if she understood that I made a mistake and that I had "learned my lesson." I never got birth control because I promised myself that I wouldn't be having sex.

I had this old friend from school who wasn't my boyfriend or anything. He was nice to me and Becky. One night I went out with him, and it wasn't meant to happen but we had sex this one time in the back of his car. Of course, with my luck I came out pregnant. I freaked out! I just couldn't let my mom find out. I couldn't deal with the whole thing. So I think I denied it for a while. After having Becky, I felt that abortion was wrong. I didn't think I could do it. Then I thought how I couldn't have another baby for Becky's sake. I finally talked to a counselor at my school, and she helped me find a place to go for the abortion. But when I went they told me I was already eighteen weeks pregnant, so they wouldn't do it. I called three other places, and finally I found a clinic that would do it, but it cost more money than I had. I was so scared and depressed. I mean I was really freaked out. I was hoping that I would never have to tell this guy about being pregnant. It was all such a big mistake. I didn't want him to be my boyfriend. I wanted to make believe that this whole thing never happened. I finally had to tell him. He didn't try to talk me out of the abortion. He was actually helpful and gave me some money so when I put it together with the money I had, there was enough to pay for the abortion.

Although Tina feels certain she made the right decision, she has a very clear message for all the girls she knows: if you're having sex, use birth control.

She says:

> I went through hell just because I just couldn't deal
> with preparing for having sex or with my mother
> finding out that I hadn't "learned my lesson." I was
> just ignorant about birth control. But I've grown a
> lot because of this. I will never, *never* put myself in
> that position again.

When Rebecca found out she was pregnant, she
knew she wanted to have an abortion. She called
Planned Parenthood right away to make an appointment. We met her there when she went back for a
checkup, and this is what she said:

> I had a girlfriend who had her first baby when she
> was sixteen, and she told me she had really
> wanted to have that baby. She said she wouldn't
> think about having an abortion. But after she had
> the baby, she realized what a big responsibility it
> was. She was up half the night, and she never got
> to go out. So when I got pregnant, I knew there
> was only one choice for me: to have an abortion. I
> wouldn't want to have a baby until I could take
> care of that baby myself. I want to have my own
> job and make my own money before I have a
> baby. I want to be able to afford babysitters and a
> good place to live, and I don't want to have to
> depend on my parents. I wouldn't even want to
> depend on my boyfriend, because he could leave,
> and then where would I be?

THE YOUNG MAN'S ROLE IN ABORTION: The boy
with whom you became pregnant can have as much
of a role as he chooses and you allow him to have. If
you have been in a loving relationship together, you
may feel that the pregnancy you created belongs to
both of you. You may both have come to the conclusion that abortion is the best decision to make. Guys
can be supportive during this time by showing concern, helping you plan for the abortion, giving financial support toward it, and accompanying you to the
procedure.

If you are a young man involved in a pregnancy,
you probably have lots of mixed emotions about both
pregnancy and abortion. Sometimes it's hard to
express your feelings or even know what they are.

Give yourself an opportunity to sit quietly and think
this through, to figure out what *you* feel about pregnancy and abortion, so you'll be able to communicate your feelings to your girlfriend. Without
communication, misunderstandings between partners are very common. Ron, age fifteen, told us:

> I was very upset, because I was worried about
> Lori and how all this would affect her. I was
> worried about whether she would be okay after
> the abortion. I thought I had to be strong for her,
> so I acted "cooler" than I was really feeling. What
> came out after we had this big fight was that she
> thought I didn't care.

We spoke to a male counselor who works with
young men whose girlfriends are pregnant and having abortions. He told us that most boys are concerned about the safety and well-being of their
partners. He said that many of the young men he
works with have feelings of sadness, anxiety, guilt,
anger, and relief all at the same time.

> I advise the guys I counsel that whether their
> relationship with their partners is good, bad, or
> broken up, they must take responsibility for
> supporting their partners at this time. It is
> important to reassure her that you care about her
> and what is going on.

For the pregnant girl, how a boy reacts is very
important. Some boys are very supportive. Some
may prefer you have an abortion because they aren't
ready to become fathers, but they will understand
and participate if you choose to have the baby.

Other boys panic when they find out you are
pregnant. They may accuse you of sleeping with
other guys. They deny being involved in the pregnancy, or they insist you "get rid of the baby." Many
girls are left alone to make this emotional decision,
because the boy who took part in the conception
can't face his responsibility. Molly told us about her
boyfriend, "He was there when it was fun. As soon as
it got complicated, he disappeared."

Some boys put heavy pressure on their girlfriends *not* to have an abortion. Kevin told us:

My girlfriend wants to have an abortion, but it's my baby she's killing, and I want that baby. I told her we'll get married. My mom will help us take care of the baby; we'll make it. But she says no way; she says she wants to go to college and can't be having a baby now.

YOUR LEGAL RIGHTS: No one—whether it's your boyfriend, husband, or parents—can legally force you to have an abortion, nor can they legally force you to have the baby. No doctor, clinic, or hospital can legally do an abortion unless they have *your* written consent. Don't sign anything until you read it first, and if you don't understand the language, ask to have it explained to you.

> If you have any questions about your rights, or if you believe a doctor or clinic has violated them, call the National Abortion Hotline at 1-800-424-2280, or call your local chapter of the American Civil Liberties Union (ACLU), a local chapter of the National Organization for Women (NOW), or Planned Parenthood.

The United States Supreme Court legalized abortion in 1973 in a case called *Roe v. Wade.* Since then a number of political and legal changes have limited a woman's access to abortion. These changes affect teenagers as well as older women. Particular laws that make it easier or harder to obtain an abortion vary from state to state. Some state laws make it more difficult for a woman who is eighteen or younger—legally, a minor—to obtain an abortion without parental consent or notice.

Find out what the particular laws are in your state by calling the toll-free Abortion Hotline (1-800-424-2280). If you are under eighteen, ask the Abortion Hotline counselor if your state requires parental consent for minors to have an abortion. If you feel you cannot inform your parents about your pregnancy, discuss your dilemma with the counselor. Ask where you can go for help. Some clinics, like Planned Parenthood, have lawyers and a counseling staff to support you. The Hotline counselor will have the names and addresses of these places.

Regardless of the law, some doctors and clinics require parental consent, because they are afraid of lawsuits brought by angry parents. Make sure you are clear about your doctor's or your clinic's consent rules.

FINDING AN ABORTION PROVIDER: In your community, there may be many places, few places, or no places at all that provide abortions. If you live in or near a big city, there is probably at least one abortion clinic there, and there are probably several doctors who do abortions privately. Some clinics do not offer as good a service as you will want. Some charge more than you should pay. That's why you should check around and choose your doctor or clinic carefully.

> To find out about abortion services in your area:
>
> ➤ Call the **National Abortion Federation** at 1-800-424-2280 (a toll-free number). This organization has information about clinics all over the United States.
>
> ➤ Call the **Planned Parenthood** clinic nearest you. This national family-planning organization has offices in almost every state. Look in the phone book for their number or call 1-800-230-7526 to be automatically transferred to the closest Planned Parenthood office.
>
> ➤ Check the business pages under Abortion, Family Planning, Health Agencies, or Birth Control.
>
> ➤ Call a women's group or women's health clinic in your area.

Assessing Abortion Services After you have the names of some clinics, doctors, or hospitals that perform abortions, take a little time to check them out. Phone or drop in for a visit. You'll be able to tell a lot by how you are treated (is the staff friendly and willing to answer your questions?) and how the health facility looks (does it appear to be well run and clean?).

In our experience, it's a good idea to have someone you trust help you with this assessment, so if you can, include your boyfriend or your parent or a friend with whom you can share ideas and impressions. Sixteen-year-old Karen from Connecticut told us about her experience.

> I was pretty sure about my decision to get an abortion, but I got real upset when I had to call the different places. I mean, it was bad enough I had to go through having it, but making the arrangements was something else. My best friend Julie helped me so much. If I had to give girls in my situation advice, I would tell them that if you have someone you can trust, let them help you out. It really makes a difference.

Use this checklist to help you make your choice. Consider:

➤ The kind of attention you get over the phone—are all your questions answered with respect?

➤ If you need your parents' consent and if the doctor or person in charge will notify your parents even if you don't want them involved.

➤ The kind of abortion that will be done.

➤ How long you can expect to be at the facility. Will everything be done in one visit?

➤ The kinds of anesthesia offered. After you read about anesthesia on page 332, you may know whether you want local anesthesia, general anesthesia, or augment anesthesia. Some clinics offer only local anesthesia, because it has fewer risks. Not offering a choice of anesthesia isn't necessarily an indication of poor service. You may need parental consent for general anesthesia if you are under eighteen years of age.

➤ Emergency backup procedures. What hospital is used if hospital services become necessary? Is the health facility equipped to provide blood transfusions or oxygen?

➤ Whether anything in your medical history would interfere with your getting an abortion at that particular medical facility.

➤ The fee. How much will the entire abortion and postabortion checkup cost? If you have Rh-negative blood, you will need a special shot of Rhogam (see footnote, page 333). Ask if that is included in the price or if it is extra. How much extra? Do they provide birth control services? Also, find out in what form they accept payment. Many clinics will not take a personal check but require insurance, cash, Medicaid, or a certified check or money order; some take credit cards.

➤ Whether you can talk with a counselor by yourself, if you would like that. Some clinics offer only group counseling sessions. That can be wonderful, but some people prefer a private session to feel comfortable.

➤ Whether you can bring someone who is close to you (your boyfriend, your mother, a friend, your sister, anyone you choose), and ask whether that person can be allowed into the abortion room with you—if you'd like that. Some people feel much better with a friend holding their hand during the procedure.

➤ Whether the person doing the abortion will be a licensed physician. It is illegal for anyone but a licensed physician to do an abortion.

➤ If there will be a staff member in the abortion room just for your comfort and support.

Use this list while you're on the phone and go through all the points. You'll be able to tell a lot about the kind of service they give by the way they listen to and answer your questions. If you have a choice, select the health facility that sounds as if it will offer you the best care. Should you have some concerns about your choice, call the number we listed above for advice. Remember, don't be afraid to ask questions. You have a right to receive the best care possible.

Finally, try to find out if there's a chance that you will encounter people opposed to abortion on your way into the health facility, what these abortion opponents are likely to do, and what help you can expect. People who are very strongly against abortion sometimes demonstrate outside of clinics to try to prevent patients from entering. They feel that abortion is murder. This can be very upsetting. Many clinics have escorts who will meet you outside and accompany you to your appointment. There are often alternative entrances to avoid protesters.

Remember, abortion is legal. The majority of people in this country do not believe abortion is murder. They believe it is a woman's right to decide about abortion and that no one should be able to interfere with your choice.

PAYING FOR THE ABORTION: The fee for abortion varies according to the type of procedure used and the duration of the pregnancy. Different facilities may charge different amounts. Here is an example of a fee schedule for a New York City clinic.

6 to 12 weeks—$350	19 to 20 weeks—$750
13 to 14 weeks—$450	21 to 22 weeks—$975
15 to 16 weeks—$550	23 to 24 weeks—$1200
17 to 18 weeks—$650	24 weeks—$2,000

Most health facilities will not do the abortion unless you have proof that you are able to pay for the procedure with insurance, cash, a certified check, or Medicaid. Some facilities accept credit cards. Most places will not take a personal check. Ask about payment when you call to make your appointment.

Abortions are expensive. And late abortions are much more expensive than abortions done within ten to twelve weeks. (See pages 333–337 for information about types of abortions.) You will have to be resourceful in getting the money together if you don't have it. Here are some suggestions:

➤ You may be eligible for Medicaid coverage in some states. To find out if yours is a state where Medicaid pays for abortion and under what circumstances, call the National Abortion Federation at 1-800-424-2280 or the National Abortion Rights Action League (look in the telephone directory for the office nearest you, or call their national office at 1-202-973-3000).

➤ In some states, if you are under twenty-one years old, pregnant, and wish to have an abortion, you may be able to receive "expedited Medicaid" to cover the cost of the abortion. You do not need parental consent and you may not have to prove financial need. You must go to your local Medicaid office with proof that you are pregnant, your birth certificate, your social security card, and proof of your address. You will receive a Medicaid authorization letter that you can take to a clinic. This notifies the clinic that Medicaid will pay for the abortion.

➤ Talk with your parents if you can, or talk to some other adults you trust. See if they will lend you the money.

➤ Ask the boy who was part of the conception. It's only fair that he pay at least half, since he had half the responsibility for the pregnancy and you're the one who has to go through the procedure.

➤ Ask some of your friends for small loans. Tell them it's for a personal emergency if you'd rather not tell them it's for an abortion. Remember, while you may feel afraid to let people know you need an abortion, they'll find out you were pregnant for sure if you stay pregnant.

➤ Call the clinic or doctor and ask about a reduced fee or a partial-payment plan (where you pay some money at the time of the abortion and then pay the rest in installments). Many clinics have been cheated by women who asked for a payment plan and then never paid their debts. That's why not many places offer such a plan anymore. For the sake of other teens, if you are allowed to pay in installments, be sure to continue paying until your debt is cleared.

➤ See if your private health insurance will pay for the abortion, although this choice will probably have to involve your parents.

If you cannot raise the money for your abortion, call the National Abortion Federation at 1-800-424-2280. They may be able to help you find a place that has a fee that you can afford. They will give you information about Medicaid funding for abortion in your state, tell you about clinics that offer reduced fees, and provide information about groups that help women get abortions if they are having difficulty raising the money.

Remember, late abortions cost more than early abortions, so the longer you wait to get the money, the more expensive the abortion will be.

RISKS AND COMPLICATIONS ASSOCIATED WITH ABORTIONS: For teenagers, abortion is safer than childbirth. But as in any medical procedure, sometimes there are complications. For an early abortion (up to twelve weeks), the risk of complication is about one percent. The later the abortion, the higher the risk. Usually, signs of complication will show up within the first few days after the abortion. The most frequent problems are infection, tearing of the lining of the uterus, blood loss (losing more than a pint is serious), and incomplete abortion, which means the doctor missed some of the tissue that was part of the pregnancy.

Fortunately, abortions performed under safe and medically sterile conditions considerably reduce the chances of complication. If your abortion is to be performed with general anesthesia, this adds some risk. The staff at the clinic will give you instructions to follow—for example, not to eat or drink anything for twelve hours before the abortion if you are having general anesthesia. The instructions are designed to keep you safe.

After the procedure, watch your recovery carefully. Follow *exactly* the aftercare instructions given to you by the clinic. (See page 338 for an example of aftercare procedures.) If you experience excessive bleeding (ask the staff before you leave how much normal bleeding to expect), fever, or extreme pain, call your doctor or clinic immediately.

Having an uncomplicated abortion *does not* decrease your chances of having a healthy baby in the future. But every time you have an abortion, you run the risk of having complications, which could interfere with future pregnancies. That's why it's so important to use birth control until you decide you *want* to get pregnant.

There may be some emotional complications to deal with also. While most girls feel okay about their decision, they may also feel upset before the procedure and sad afterward. Many girls feel blue at times about having to face such a choice. But the overwhelming majority of young women feel relief about not being pregnant any more.

Occasionally, a young woman has second thoughts after the fact about her choice. Some girls feel guilty, sorry, and victimized for having had an abortion. One teenage mother we met in Michigan had had an abortion two years before her first baby was born. She told us that she is sorry she had the abortion:

I wish I had thought more about my decision to have that abortion. At the time I was so desperate, I didn't know what else to do. After all, I was only fifteen. But I don't think it's right to say that abortion isn't killing just because the fetus is too small to live outside the mother. That's not the point. If you don't have the abortion, the fetus will grow to be big enough to live. That's the point.

Sometimes young women who have ambivalent feelings about their abortion avoid using birth control and end up getting pregnant again. It's almost as if they're replaying the situation in the hopes of feeling differently the next time. We met eighteen-year-old Carrie, from Philadelphia, at an abortion clinic where she was waiting to have her second abortion. She spoke to us quite openly.

I can't believe I'm back here, since I had an abortion this time last year. I said, "I'm never doing this again." I felt so guilty last time. I wasn't going to have an abortion this time, but when it came right down to it, I just couldn't go through it all and have a baby. Yeah, I didn't use birth control. Maybe I felt that if I had to do it again, I would make a different choice. This time I'm not having sex till I'm really ready to have a baby, or I'll use birth control. This time I'm gonna deal with it and take care of business, if you know what I mean.

Sometimes women have negative feelings about the abortion experience itself. Carmen, a nineteen-year-old college student, reported:

It was degrading. The place I went treated us like we were on an assembly line. You got shuffled around from room to room. I woke up crying.

Abortions don't have to be performed under "assembly line" conditions. They don't have to be scary and degrading. Many women's clinics are set up to make the experience a dignified and respectful one. If you bring a friend or loved one with you, that will give you extra support. Evaluate the services well before you go for your abortion. You may have more choices than you think.

Some girls feel guilty after an abortion. Their sense of guilt about the abortion may really come from feeling mad at themselves for having gotten pregnant in the first place. Instead of feeling guilty, they can learn from this experience to use birth control from now on *every time* they have sexual intercourse.

It's helpful to try to think through your ambivalent feelings about abortion before you go in for the procedure. Consider carefully whether you'd be more grieved by having an abortion or by having a baby you aren't ready to care for. Afterward, if you find yourself having recurring negative feelings about the abortion, consult a counselor. There may be other problems causing you to dwell on your abortion experience. **Remember, the best solution to the abortion dilemma is to abstain from sexual intercourse or use effective birth control whenever you do have sex, so you won't have to make this hard decision again.**

ANESTHESIA: While childbirth can be very painful, abortions are usually less so. Early abortions tend to be much easier, with far less cramping than late abortions or childbirth. Of course, each person is different, and how you experience your abortion will be individual to you.

To help you cope with possible discomfort or pain, doctors and clinics provide a variety of painkilling substances called anesthesia. There are two basic types of anesthesia: *local,* which just affects the cervix (the opening to the uterus), and *general,* which affects your whole body and puts you to sleep. Another method, called *augment,* combines a local anesthetic with a drug that causes you to be partially asleep.

Local anesthesia, like the shot you get in your mouth for dental work, is injected into the cervix. This numbs the area around the cervix. It can be very helpful. Since there are few nerve endings in the cervix, the shot is generally not very painful. It does not numb the entire uterus, however, so you may still experience some cramping.

A number of clinics and hospitals offer general anesthesia to put the patient to sleep during the procedure. This is usually given by injection before the abortion. If you are having this type of anesthesia, you will probably be asked to bring someone with you to help you get home, because you may feel groggy afterward. General anesthesia will make the abortion painless, since you'll be asleep, but when you wake up you may feel cramping, and some people also feel dizzy, disoriented, or nauseated. For the most part, it takes longer to recover from general anesthesia than from local anesthesia. Furthermore, since it affects your entire body, it is potentially riskier. *You must not eat or drink or swallow anything*—not even water—for twelve hours before having general anesthesia.

In a first-trimester abortion (under twelve weeks), general or augment anesthesia is not medically necessary. Some teens choose to have general anesthesia anyway, however, because they are worried about possible discomfort, and some health care providers suggest it, because they are afraid teens will become upset during the abortion. General anesthesia is more commonly used for abortions performed after twelve weeks, which take longer and may be more uncomfortable.

Some doctors and clinics give you a choice of anesthesia; others provide only one type of anesthesia. If you wish to have a choice, ask about that when you are checking for a place to have the abortion.

Remember, no matter what kind of painkiller you use, after the abortion you will still probably feel cramping as the medication wears off and your uterus returns to its pre-pregnant size. This is normal.

HAVING THE ABORTION: In an abortion, the contents of the uterus are removed, including the embryo or fetus and the lining of the uterus, which normally gets expelled every month with your period. There are several methods of abortion. The method you have will depend on how far along in your pregnancy you are and on the preferences of doctors in your area. In this section we will describe in detail the most common types of abortion.

Please note: How abortions are performed varies to some degree from place to place. Therefore, the information in this book may be slightly different from the way it is where you live.

TYPES OF ABORTION

Vacuum Suction (Vacuum Aspiration) Abortion.
This is the most common method of abortion. It is a first-trimester abortion method used *only* if you are less than twelve to fourteen weeks pregnant counting from your last menstrual period. During this type of abortion, the contents of the uterus are removed through a tube that is inserted into the cervix (the opening to the uterus). The tube is attached to a source of suction, which gently removes the contents. This method of abortion has the least chance of complications and is considerably less risky than pregnancy, labor, and delivery. It takes about five to fifteen minutes and can be performed in a doctor's office, a clinic, or a hospital. You do not have to stay overnight, but you should plan to stay at the clinic for about four to six hours. Time is needed before the abortion for explanations, pregnancy tests, and counseling, and time is needed after the procedure for recovery. The anesthesia most often used for this type of abortion is local anesthesia. Some women choose to have general anesthesia.

If you're receiving a vacuum suction abortion, plan to arrive at the facility on time. Bring a book or a friend to talk with. It's a good idea to bring a friend for support and encouragement.

First, you will have lab work done: A urine test to make sure you're pregnant, a blood pressure check, and a test to see what type of blood you have. If you have something called Rh-negative blood— about one in ten patients do—you will probably need to have an injection of a medicine called Rhogam within seventy-two hours after the abortion. This will keep you from having certain complications with your next pregnancy.* Some places also do a sonogram, sometimes called ultrasound, which uses sound waves to take a picture of your uterus to determine more accurately the size of your pregnancy.

After the lab work, many clinics and doctors offer patient-education sessions to a group of patients or to an individual patient. In this session, a nurse or counselor will talk to you about what to expect in the abortion, answer any questions you have, and discuss with you your decision to have an abortion. She wants to determine that *you're sure* you want an abortion. These sessions can be very helpful and reassuring. They are likely to include information about methods of birth control and how to use them, so that after the abortion you won't get pregnant again until you choose to. (See page 279 for a complete discussion of birth control.) Here's what Debby, a sixteen-year-old girl from Los Angeles, told us about her pre-abortion counseling session:

> I went to a women's clinic for my abortion, and everyone was really great. About five of us were there at the same time for abortions, and first we all had urine tests and blood tests and stuff like that. I really liked doing the urine test because they let us do our own. First we took turns going into the bathroom to pee in this little cup. Then we came out and mixed a drop of pee with something they gave us and we watched what happened. One girl found out she wasn't really pregnant after all, and we all cheered for her. Then, after that, we all went into this dressing room where we sat around talking about what the abortion would be like. The head of the group was a counselor who had had an abortion herself, so she told us about what it was like for her. That really made me feel better. I figured if she could do it, so could I. We talked about whether it might hurt. One person said that she'd had an abortion that didn't hurt at all, but someone else said she heard that it did hurt. We also talked about our feelings about abortions and pregnancy. One person started crying a little, and everyone was real supportive and told her it would be okay.

Debby was part of a group counseling session. If you prefer private counseling, ask if they offer that option when you call the abortion provider.

After the counseling session, you will be called

---

* Most people have Rh-positive blood. Some people have Rh-negative blood, which means their blood has a slightly different composition. It is perfectly normal, but if an Rh-negative woman is carrying an Rh-positive baby, birth or abortion can cause her body to build up antibodies against the Rh-positive blood from the fetus. These antibodies may affect a future pregnancy and harm the next Rh-positive fetus. If Rhogam is given within seventy-two hours after an abortion or childbirth, it will prevent antibodies from forming in the woman's blood. Rhogam can be expensive. If you can't afford it, ask for financial assistance. If you have Rh-negative blood, **it is very important to have Rhogam after every abortion or delivery.**

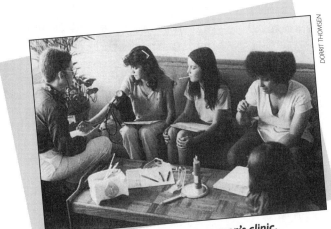

A group counseling session at a women's clinic.

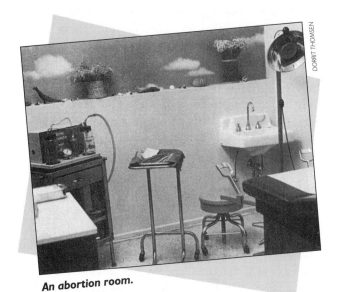

An abortion room.

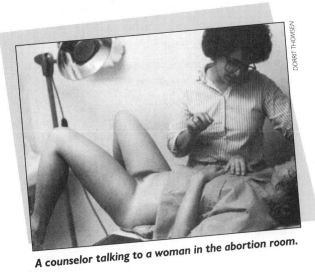

A counselor talking to a woman in the abortion room.

when it's your turn for the abortion. You can ask if your friend is allowed in the abortion room with you. Some places let you do that. Usually there will be a counselor with you to hold your hand and reassure you. Ask about that when you call for an appointment.

The room where the abortion is performed usually looks like any doctor's examining room. You'll be asked to undress from the waist down and cover up with a surgical cloth; some places ask you to undress all the way and put on a hospital gown. The doctor will first give you a pelvic exam, to check that you really are pregnant and that you are less than twelve weeks pregnant. If there is a question about how far along you are, some places require an ultrasound, or sonogram, to confirm the size of the fetus.

If you're having general anesthesia, you will probably get an injection in your arm, fall asleep, and wake up after the abortion is over. Often, with general anesthesia, an IV (intravenous line) is placed in your arm.

If you are having local or no anesthesia, about a half hour before the abortion, the doctor or nurse may offer you some medication to relax you. It will probably be a tranquilizer. If you are allergic to some drugs, let the nurses know that. Also, be sure not to use any drugs or alcohol at home before you come; mixing drugs could be dangerous to your health. If you have taken something, be sure to tell the doctor or nurse. (For a complete discussion of the different types of anesthesia, see page 332.)

After the pelvic exam, the doctor will insert a speculum into your vagina to hold the walls open (see page 251). If you are having local anesthesia, the doctor will inject it into your cervix to numb the area. The injection takes a few seconds and may feel a little uncomfortable. Since the cervix is not very sensitive, you should not feel the shot very much. Try to relax during the shot. Breathe deeply and hold someone's hand.

For the abortion, your cervix has to be opened wide enough to allow the suction tube to enter the uterus. The suction tube is about as wide as a piece of chalk. Usually the cervix has only the tiniest opening, and forcing it to open wider for the abortion often causes cramping and pain. Local anesthesia should considerably reduce that discomfort.

To open your cervix, the doctor will use a dilator. Dilators come in different sizes, from the size of a matchstick to the width of a thumb. The doctor will start stretching open the cervix using the smallest dilator and then gradually bigger ones until the opening is wide enough for the abortion. The further along you are in the pregnancy, the wider the opening has to be.

Dilating takes about two minutes. You may feel sharp cramps at this time or strong pressure. Use your breathing to help you relax. Relaxing will help ease whatever pain you may experience.

After the cervix is open, the abortion can begin. A clear plastic, hollow tube with a suction tip is

---

Here's how to use your breathing to help you get through the abortion:

➢ Relax as much as you can. Let your legs flop apart and your arms hang loose. Let your mouth drop open.

➢ Try not to let your toes and fingers curl up tight. Hold someone's hand if you want, and try to keep your toes relaxed.

➢ Blow out all the air in your lungs and take a deep breath. Watch your stomach rise as you breathe in. Then breathe the air out and watch your stomach fall. This deep breathing will help you relax.

➢ Try not to breathe too quickly or you may become faint.

➢ Make noise if you have to. Keep breathing deeply for as long as you want to. The dilation lasts for only a few minutes.

---

inserted into the cervix. It is attached to a suction machine. When the machine is turned on, gentle suction is produced in the tube. The doctor moves the tube around in your uterus for a few minutes to clean out the embryo or fetus, the tissues surrounding it, and the excess lining of the uterus. If this hurts, try to relax and use your breathing techniques. The more you relax, the less it will hurt.

Once the fetus and tissue have been removed from your uterus, you are no longer pregnant.

The doctor will then check for any remaining tissue inside the uterus. With a special utensil, he or she will gently scrape along the inside of the uterus to be sure the fetus and loose tissue have been completely removed. This may take an extra minute. The whole abortion itself takes no more than fifteen minutes.

If you have not had general anesthesia, you will be awake, and you may feel mild to heavy cramping. That's because your uterus, which is a muscle, is contracting back to its pre-pregnancy size.

As soon as you feel ready to get up, usually only several minutes after the abortion, you will put on a sanitary napkin, to catch any bleeding, and dress. You will then go into the recovery area, where you can relax and have something to eat or drink. Your companion may be allowed to come with you into the recovery area.

This is how one fifteen-year-old girl described her feelings right after her abortion:

What a relief! I mean, *what a relief!* All I can say is thank God abortion was a choice for me, because I just could never have made it with a baby.

Besides relief, your feelings may include sadness, fear, regret, worry. We'll talk more about those feelings a little later (see page 338). After an abortion, you are likely to continue bleeding and cramping for a while; most women do. If the cramps stay strong for more than twenty or thirty minutes, ask the nurse for some pain medication. The bleeding may last just a few hours or it may last several days. Some women stop and then start again. **If you have very heavy bleeding—heavier than your normal menstrual flow—be sure to call the doctor or clinic right away.** That may be a sign of infection, an incomplete abortion, or some other complication.

You will be given instructions on how to care for yourself after the abortion. Follow them carefully, because your body needs a chance to get back to normal. We also discuss aftercare instructions on page 338. Many facilities routinely give medication to help the uterus contract, which limits the bleeding, and antibiotics to prevent infection.

D-and-C Abortion (Dilation and Curettage).

This type of abortion can be done between twelve and sixteen weeks of pregnancy and takes about seven to fifteen minutes to perform. It can be done in a doctor's office, a clinic, or a hospital. General anesthesia is usually used, which means you are put to sleep during the procedure.

It is similar to the suction abortion. Your cervix will be dilated (opened) as in the suction abortion, but since the fetus is larger, the doctor will use a curette—a scraping instrument—to remove the fetal tissue and excess lining from your uterus.

There is slightly more risk with this kind of abortion, because your pregnancy is further along and the fetus is larger. Also, scraping is a bit more complicated than the suction technique.

The aftercare process is similar to that with a vacuum suction abortion.

D-and-E Abortion (Dilation and Evacuation).

This type of abortion combines both the vacuum aspiration and dilation-and-curettage methods of abortion. It is usually done after twelve weeks of pregnancy. Depending on the state and the facility where the abortion is performed, the upper limit for performing the D-and-E abortion is between sixteen and twenty-four weeks. It takes between fifteen and thirty minutes. The procedure can be performed in a clinic, a properly equipped doctor's office, or a hospital. Usually the patient is under general anesthesia (put to sleep), but it can also be performed with local anesthetic and a tranquilizer.

A later abortion is more complicated than an earlier abortion, because the fetal tissue is larger and the uterus is softer and easier to injure. Since later abortions require a higher level of skill, many practitioners or health facilities will not do them. An ultrasound examination, or sonogram, which uses sound waves, is usually required to verify the actual size of the fetus.

With the D-and-E method of abortion, the cervix needs to be opened wider than with a first-trimester abortion, since larger instruments must be inserted into the uterus to remove the pregnancy. Some health facilities use a piece of sterile seaweed, called laminaria, to dilate the cervix. The laminaria is the size and shape of a wooden matchstick and is inserted into the cervix at least six hours prior to the abortion. You may be asked to come in two days before the abortion to have the laminaria inserted, which may be less stressful to your cervix. As the laminaria absorbs fluid, it expands and causes the cervix to open over a two-day period, easing the discomfort of speedier dilations. The abortion is performed on the third day. At the time of the abortion, the laminaria is removed. Dilators will open the cervix even wider, so the doctor can insert forceps, a curette, and a vacuum suction tube to loosen and remove the fetal tissue and the uterine lining. You may be given a drug called oxytocin to help your uterus contract. This slows down the bleeding that usually occurs after the procedure. Some facilities also routinely give antibiotics to prevent infection.

The aftercare is the same as for the vacuum aspiration abortion.

Induced Abortion.

This type of abortion is used between sixteen and twenty-four weeks. It is a medically induced miscarriage, and it is the most stressful type of abortion. This method is not used frequently, since a D-and-E is safer, has fewer complications, and is less traumatic. During an induced abortion, a liquid—usually saline (salt) or prostaglandin (a hormone)—is injected through your abdomen and into your uterus. After several hours, it causes contractions to occur and the fetus to be expelled. In rare situations, if prostaglandin is used and you are more than twenty weeks pregnant, the fetus may be expelled alive and able to live outside your body for a number of hours. This may create an extremely upsetting experience for you if you are awake and see the baby. After the fetus is expelled the doctor may scrape out any remaining tissue with a sharp instrument called a curette.

An induced abortion is always done in a hospital and involves a stay of twelve to forty-eight hours. The complication rate for an induced abortion is higher than for earlier abortions, but no higher than for a full-term pregnancy and delivery.

If you are having an induced abortion, here is what the experience may be like: In the hospital you will undress and put on a hospital gown. You will lie on a hospital bed. The nurse will numb a patch of skin on your belly with local anesthetic and then the solution will be injected. The doctor puts a needle through the abdomen, about three to six inches below the belly button. This feels like pressure to many women. Some fluid from inside the uterus is withdrawn, and it is replaced by a hormone called prostaglandin or by saline, a salt solution. If saline is used, you may feel bloated and thirsty. It's good to drink a lot.

About five to fifty hours later, the uterus will begin to contract and push out the fetus and other tissue inside your uterus. This can be painful. There's no way to know in advance how long it will take or how painful it will feel to you. After the fetus is expelled, the uterus shrinks back to its pre-pregnancy size. That causes cramping.

This type of abortion can be very hard on you physically, because it takes a long time and can be painful. It is also difficult emotionally, because when the fetus comes out, if you are awake you will see that it looks like a baby. Between sixteen and twenty-four weeks, the fetus goes through a lot of growth and development, it becomes larger, and by twenty-six weeks, develops the potential capacity for life outside the mother's womb. For these reasons, if it is possible for you to have the abortion during the first three months of pregnancy, that is by far the better choice.

Some hospitals offer counseling and some don't. It will be very helpful to have someone to talk with before and after the experience. If the hospital allows it, try to bring your boyfriend or an older woman you like and trust (your mother, your sister, your aunt, a counselor) to stay with you during the abortion. An adult woman who has been through childbirth may be able to reassure you and support you.

Aftercare is the same as for a suction abortion (see page 338).

Abortion-Inducing Medication.

Certain medications have been found to cause abortion. For example, low doses of the common cancer-fighting drug methotrexate, combined with a drug called misoprostol, which causes uterine contractions, proved 96 percent successful as an abortion agent for women who wanted to end their pregnancies within the first two months. These two medications are already legal and widely available in the United States. Having this type of abortion involves using a combination of injections and pills or suppositories (medicated preparations inserted into the vagina that melt at body temperature), all of which are administered by a doctor. It is a two-step procedure. First an injection of methotrexate is given, and a week later the second drug, misoprostol, is given in a pill or suppository form. This combination of drugs causes the uterus to contract and expel the pregnancy. Most patients experience cramping, sometimes severe, and bleeding after receiving misoprostol, but there are no major side effects or complications that we know of at this time. Not all doctors are willing to prescribe such drugs, because they may be worried about potential lawsuits. This is a new and somewhat controversial procedure. If a woman takes the injection and then does not return for the pill or suppository, a damaged fetus may develop. So if you choose this method of abortion, you *must* follow through with the second visit.

The drug called mifepristone in the United States and RU-486 in France* has been shown to end a pregnancy up to seven weeks after the last menstrual period. Using this method involves three visits to a health facility; one visit to take mifepristone, a second visit to take another drug, misoprostol, which makes the uterus contract, and a third visit to verify that you are no longer pregnant.

The Morning-After Pill.

See page 309 for more information on this alternative, called "emergency birth control."

PHYSICAL AFTERCARE: Most girls have few physical aftereffects from the early, suction-type abortion. They feel fine right away and can leave the clinic within an hour. It is normal to feel tired and have cramps for several days after the abortion while the uterus shrinks back to its normal size. Bleeding is also normal, and it varies from none at all to a light-to-moderate flow for two to three weeks. Bleeding can start and stop and start again, but it should never be heavier than your heaviest periods. If it is, call the clinic or doctor to tell them what you are experiencing. If you are bleeding extremely heavily

---

* This drug has been used in Europe and will soon be available in the United States. As of the printing of this edition, it was not yet available.

and your clinic isn't open, go to the emergency room of your local hospital. Pregnancy symptoms sometimes last up to a week after an abortion. Recovery from later abortions may require a little more time.

No matter what type of abortion you have had, you must take care of yourself afterward by following the instructions your clinic or doctor gives you. The following is an example of postabortion instructions:

- ➤ Watch for fever. Take your temperature in the morning and at night for about five days after the abortion. If it goes over 100.5 degrees, call the doctor or clinic.

- ➤ Watch your bleeding. It may stop and then start again. It may last a few hours or a few days or over a week. It shouldn't be heavier than your normal period. If it is heavy and lasts a long time, call the doctor or clinic.

- ➤ Expect your next normal period to come in about four to six weeks. It's important to know that **you can get pregnant before your next period if you have unprotected intercourse. Get and use birth control! Don't risk another unplanned pregnancy.** If you do not get your period within four to six weeks, call the doctor or clinic.

- ➤ Call the doctor if you have severe pain or cramping or an unusual vaginal discharge.

- ➤ For two weeks, to prevent irritation and infection, don't take a bath, swim, use tampons, have intercourse, or douche. In other words, don't put water or anything else into your vagina. You can shower and wash with a washcloth.

- ➤ Take it easy for a day or two and don't do anything strenuous. Pay attention to what your body needs, and rest if you are tired. After that you can resume normal activity as soon as you feel like it.

- ➤ **Have a checkup two weeks after your abortion** to be sure everything is going well and your body is back to normal.

After the abortion, if you continue to have pregnancy symptoms—swollen and tender breasts, increased urination, tiredness, weight gain—you may still be pregnant. In very rare cases, the abortion does not remove the fetus. Sometimes an embryo is developing in some place other than in the uterus. This is called an ectopic pregnancy. Report your symptoms to the doctor or clinic immediately and go in for a checkup.

If you live at home and you haven't told your parents about your abortion, it may be hard to take care of yourself the way you should, especially if you have a lot of bleeding and cramping. You may try to pretend that everything's fine, when really you're not feeling well at all. Sally told us that happened to her:

After my abortion I didn't feel like doing anything for a couple of days. Nothing serious, I just felt crampy, lonely, and sad. But I didn't tell my parents, so I had to pretend I was okay. We had to go on this hike—it was planned and everybody was going, and I was feeling so bad. But I figured, If I don't go, everyone will be asking me what's wrong. I might have been able to tell my mother, but I just couldn't tell my father. He'd be so disappointed if he knew.

EMOTIONAL AFTERCARE: You may have a lot of strong feelings for a while after the abortion. Many people experience a deep sense of relief, but lots of girls also feel sad. It's very natural to feel both.

Other emotions are common too. For some girls it is confusing to feel so ambivalent—positive and negative at the same time—about something they have done. Nineteen-year-old Alisha told us that it took her a long time to accept that she felt sad about making what was, for her, the right choice. She said, "I never imagined that I might not welcome my first pregnancy. For me, it was a loss—not having that pregnancy happen at the right time."

Here are some of the feelings other young women have experienced after an abortion:

Anger. You may be angry with the reaction you got from your boyfriend, parents, or friends, or you may be angry with the poor care you got from the doctor or people at the clinic. You may be angry with yourself for getting pregnant in the first place—that your birth control didn't work, that you were careless, that you got "caught" when you know other people who have intercourse and haven't gotten "caught" yet.

Anger is natural after an abortion. You aren't bad or sick or mixed-up to have such feelings. But if you keep your anger inside, it will make you confused and depressed. Talk with someone you can trust. Fourteen-year-old Susie went to a counseling center in Los Angeles. She said:

> After the abortion, I was so angry at my boyfriend Billy I couldn't stand him. Everything he did got me mad. The counselor helped me to see that my feelings were pretty normal. After all, *I* had to have the abortion, not Billy. I talked to him about how I was feeling, and in fact we had a big fight about it, because he said he couldn't help it if boys don't get pregnant. When we made up, I was really glad I told him what was on my mind. And now we're both totally committed to using rubbers.

Guilt. Guilt is what we feel when we do something that we don't feel right about, when we go against what we believe in. You may feel guilty for having an abortion, for not telling your parents, for not telling your boyfriend, for not using birth control, or for having sex in the first place. Some girls feel guilty for being relieved that they're not pregnant anymore. They feel they should have been punished, and guilt is a way of punishing themselves. Some girls grow up being told that abortion is wrong, so they feel very guilty for having one. Many girls are disappointed that they had to have an abortion, even if rationally they think it was the best decision for them.

If you chose an abortion, you probably did so because you weren't prepared to be a parent. You were taking care of yourself. Faced with a very hard decision, you made a choice. You may feel that being pregnant and having an abortion was a mistake, but remember, everyone makes mistakes. Perhaps continuing the pregnancy and having a baby would have been a bigger and more long-lasting mistake for you and for a baby. If you feel uneasy about abortion,

make sure you do not put yourself in that situation again: *Use birth control every time you have intercourse.*

Depression. Some depression after an abortion may be caused by the drop in your body's hormones when the pregnancy is ended. But most postabortion depression is caused by conflicting emotions. You may feel angry, guilty, sad, disappointed, and vulnerable all at once. You may not feel good about your relationship with the guy involved, or you may not be feeling good about where your life is at the moment. You may feel isolated and alone with your feelings. Try to figure out what you are feeling (see Chapter 5, Emotional Health Care, beginning on page 153). Don't be too hard on yourself. You did what you thought was best. It's important to know that even if you are feeling depressed now, you probably won't always feel this way. It takes time to get over a loss, and having an abortion is a kind of loss.

It's helpful to talk to someone about what's going on with you, someone who is understanding, nonjudgmental, and a good listener. This may be a friend, a counselor, or an understanding adult in your life. Niki, who is sixteen, felt depressed after her abortion.

> Actually, when I look back on it, I think I was feeling, you know, a little shaky before this pregnancy thing happened. I really liked this guy, but it wasn't like he was my boyfriend or anything. Anyway, we were together, smoking and all that, and we had sex. Then he avoided me like nothing ever happened. I felt awful, because all along I knew I would become pregnant. Well, I'm like that. I always worry about getting pregnant, but this time it really happened. I didn't want to face him and tell him, 'cause I couldn't take him being mean to me, like, "get away from me." So I had the abortion. Thank goodness my girlfriend was real supportive. Afterwards, when I was real down, she took me back to the counselor at the clinic. She was understanding, and I went back to speak to her a couple of times. She helped me through it. That was about a year ago. God, I never thought I would feel good again.

If your feelings about your abortion bother you intensely, seek professional help. (See page 179 for information on how to find help.)

Fear. Sometimes you may feel scared because you think you ought to be punished for having an abortion. You may worry about not being able to have a baby when you are ready to have one. Seventeen-year-old Lynn said:

> I've had two abortions, and I'm worried because I've heard that too many abortions can keep you from being able to have a baby. I really want to have children when I get older, so hearing those warnings scare me.

Having an abortion will not keep you from getting pregnant again, unless you had very serious complications. But remember, each time you have an abortion you run the risk of having complications, so *avoid problems by using birth control.*

Strength. Many girls feel more self-confident after coping with an unplanned pregnancy. You may feel more competent, since you were able to handle things and make the best of a difficult situation. That was LaTisha's experience:

> I felt very grown-up after the abortion. I didn't fall apart. I knew that if I could pull something like this off, I could take care of myself when I had to. It's a good feeling.

Several girls we met said that after their abortions they were much clearer in themselves about who they would have sex with and who they wouldn't have sex with. Also, they found it a lot easier to take a stand about using birth control and safer-sex precautions. As Suella said:

> Once you've gone through an abortion you know you don't want to do that again. It makes you stronger to say, *No sex without condoms.*

Feelings About Sex. After an abortion, many young people get reliable birth control for the first time, so they feel less anxious about having sex. For others, after an experience with abortion, having sex can seem risky. It hits home: sex has consequences. Some young people feel turned off by sex for some time. If this is how you feel, respect it. Don't push yourself. Abstain from sex for as long as you want to, because your sexuality will always be there when you're ready for it. If you had mixed feelings about having sex in the first place, now is the time to reassess whether you are ready for the responsibilities and emotional demands having sex imposes on you. Many girls told us that after the abortion they decided not to have sex until their partners agreed to use condoms each time. *Condoms are effective at preventing pregnancy and AIDS.* They are cheap and easy to use (see page 288). Seventeen-year-old Laura reported:

> I was glad when my counselor told me I couldn't have intercourse for two weeks after the abortion. She also coached me on talking to my boyfriend about using condoms. Still, I didn't want to have sex for a long while after the abortion. I kept thinking that I was going to get pregnant again.

Barbara, a family planning counselor who specializes in working with teens, urged us to note that after an abortion, many young people say, "I don't need birth control. I'm never having sex again!" She stresses the importance of being realistic. She tells all the young people she counsels:

> *Be sure you have a plan for what method of contraception you will use when you do have sex again.* Because even if you feel like you'll never have sex again, it's pretty likely that you will have sex again someday, and you will want to protect yourself so this doesn't happen again.

Deciding to Continue the Pregnancy: Having a Baby

If you are pregnant and choose to continue the pregnancy, you are deciding to have a baby. Deciding not to have an abortion is a decision to have a child.

Whether you keep the baby or give him or her up for adoption, the fact that you had a baby will change your life and your child's life forever. It's not just a question of whether you think you can handle the pregnancy, the childbirth, and the raising of a child for eighteen or more years. It's whether you think your child will get the kind of love, attention, caring, and commitment he or she deserves. This is not a decision to be made by default. Give it thought and careful planning. Make sure you really *want* to have a baby and can care for one.

LET'S LOOK AT WHAT'S INVOLVED: Having a baby is a lifetime commitment. Your baby will only be a baby for a very short time. He or she will become a toddler, a preschooler, a school-age child, and after only twelve years a teenager like yourself. He or she will have a personality and will of his or her own. Your child will sometimes seem cuddly and lovable and at other times act in a way that you will find hard to handle. That's not because your child is "bad," but because that's what children are like. Remember back to when you were a baby and a small child. No one is always sweet and pleasant and adorable, and you probably weren't either. As a parent you will have to sacrifice a lot of your time, energy, and attention to your child, because healthy, normal children need their parents' love and help. If your child should be sick or have chronic problems, he or she will require even more help and attention. Understand the commitment to another human being you are making when you decide to give birth.

In this section we will try to help you sort through the options open to you if you decide to continue your pregnancy. We will ask you to consider whether you really want to be a parent now, if you are ready to give a child what every child needs, or whether you are willing to give birth to a baby for someone else to adopt.

ADVICE FROM TEEN PARENTS: We asked teen parents what advice they had for other teens who were considering parenthood. Here's what they said:

➤ "Babies are a constant thing. They take *all* your time. You should know that. Even if you think you had experience, let's say with your younger brothers and sisters. If it's *your* baby, it's different."

➤ "You have to know that your life changes totally. It's not like your life is ruined now that you have a child. It's not like that. It doesn't have to be a completely negative thing. But you're not going to be able to go out or run around or party the way you used to. If you want to hang out or be with your friends all the time, then don't have a child and don't get pregnant."

➤ "Even though your life changes, you can do it if you're willing to put your child first. *You* have to come second now."

➤ "Don't get pregnant to keep your boyfriend. It will push him further away. If he's going to go, being pregnant won't stop him."

➤ "Some girls see other girls who are pregnant and they think they're getting all this attention. When they see a baby they say, 'Oh, he's so cute! I want someone to love me too,' but that's not right. You have to give them love before they'll love you. If you just want someone to love you, but you can't make all the sacrifices, and you aren't able to provide for a child—get a puppy."

Tiffany, age seventeen, with a three-year-old son, gave this advice:

If I could have changed anything, I would have waited. That's what I want to say to everybody who reads this book. Just wait, even if your hormones are running wild, protect yourself. Don't think, Oh he's protected—I don't need anything. *Protect yourself and wait* to have a child. It's not the worst experience in the world, but it's hard, very hard, and I think a child could benefit if you have your life together. Not to say that we are not good parents, because we are, and I love my son to death, but I mean, wait to have a child.

DECIDING TO BECOME A PARENT: We asked teens why they had chosen to become parents. Sixteen-year-old Marla was attending a meeting at a center for pregnant and parenting teens when we met her. She said:

When I was first pregnant with Evie, I was only fourteen. I could have had an abortion, but there was just this feeling that I wanted to have somebody to depend on me. I wanted to have this little baby who would just love me. Something of my own. I wanted to give my baby everything I never had.

Like Marla, many girls have a romantic view of what motherhood will be like:

I like having someone who needs me.

A baby's skin is so soft. They're so sweet and cuddly.

I'm going to be a great mom. I'll always be there for my baby. I want to give my baby all the love I never had.

Some boys feel that way too. Eighteen-year-old Brendan told us:

Angie and I didn't choose to get pregnant, but we were planning to get married anyway. I remember being in the doctor's office with her, waiting for the results of her pregnancy test. When they told her she was pregnant, I felt okay, because I've always looked forward to having kids.

It's pretty easy to visualize parenthood as a way to have someone to love you, as a way to offer love yourself, as a way to be needed and wanted. The creation of a human life—a baby—seems like a miracle. Many of us have very positive, even romantic feelings when we think about having a baby of our very own. We imagine how good it will feel holding a soft little snugly baby. We picture dressing our baby up and taking him or her out for a walk and having everybody say, "Oh, what a beautiful baby."

In reality, a baby can be wonderful *and* a baby can be very, very demanding. A baby is work. Hard work. A baby needs you twenty-four hours a day— you have to feed the baby, change his or her diapers, play with the baby, and attend to the baby when he or she is sick or upset. That means you as the parent must be there *all the time*. The baby doesn't stop needing you because it's time for you to go to bed or because you want to see a movie or be with your friends or because you want some time to be alone. The baby doesn't understand your needs. That's not because the baby is "bad" or "spoiled." That's what being a baby is all about. And if you want to give your baby what he or she needs to grow up feeling good about himself or herself, then you or some

other loving, caring person has to be there *all the time. Be sure you have the energy, the strength, the unselfishness, the resources, and the help you need to raise a baby before you decide to have one.*

Some teens said that they welcomed parenthood because they felt that it would make them more independent. Carmen told us she found out it was the opposite. A baby made her more dependent:

When I was pregnant, at fifteen, I knew for sure that I wanted to have a baby. I thought that it would do a lot for me. If I had a baby, it would be like I would have my own family, I would be the mother, and no one could tell me what to do. It was a chance to be grown up. I'd have freedom.

Well let me tell you how it really went down. Everyone was so nice to me when she was born. They always asked me how I felt, and they all wanted to see her and hold her. I liked having a newborn. That part was pretty easy for me. But now she's two. She's still cute, but she's going through a thing now and she's hard to be around. I've been on my own for a year now. At first it felt like a lot of freedom, but now I see that it's such a heavy responsibility. Sometimes it gets to me, because I see my friends who don't have kids and their lives seem so much easier. I would have to say that if you're pregnant, I wouldn't recommend motherhood as the best way to be independent, because you really don't have any freedom at all. Of course, you couldn't have told me that when I was fifteen.

Marina also found that it was much harder than she imagined to raise her child:

After I had Kira, I couldn't believe how my life changed. I couldn't stand just sitting home all the time watching her, so I started going out and leaving Kira with my mother, and if my mother wouldn't watch her, I'd drag her along with me. When she was real little, she used to get up a lot during the night, and I hated getting woken up. So sometimes I would just let her cry and cry and it would wake everybody in the house up and we'd all be miserable in the morning. Then when she was about nine months old, Kira got so sick I had to take her to the hospital. She was in there for almost two weeks. I was so scared that she was going to die because I didn't take care of her the way I should have. That's when I decided I had to grow up and take some responsibility. I decided I'd have to change and not go out partying or running around. I wanted to be a good mother.

Like Marina, you may be ready to have that beautiful baby who will gurgle and coo and love you. But you may not be ready to deal with a sick baby or a screaming, demanding, fussing baby who wakes you in the middle of the night and who makes you stay home when you'd rather be out with your friends. Both parts of the picture are real, as all parents find out.

It doesn't matter at what age you become a parent, if you're not prepared for the hard part you'll be shocked. Many older parents, in their twenties and thirties, say that they weren't at all ready for the way a baby changed their lives. They weren't prepared for how much work it is to have a baby.

Probably no one is ever completely ready for parenthood, and everybody has some mixed feelings about taking on such a responsibility. But it's easier to be a parent if:

➤ You are grown-up yourself.

➤ You like children and enjoy being with them for hours at a time.

➤ The mother and father are both ready and willing to participate in bringing up their child.

➤ You have support from other adults who are willing to help you and listen to you.

➤ You have enough money for a suitable place to live, food, clothing, toys, doctor's bills, babysitters.

➤ You are ready to change your lifestyle to make time for a baby.

➤ You feel worthwhile as a person and have your own interests.

When you find out about your pregnancy, talk to other teenage parents to see what life is like for them. Some people are finding ways to make their lives work. Other people are having a very hard time. Of course it would be easier to make the decision if you could look into the future and see how being a parent will work out for you. But since that's not possible, the next best thing is to listen to other teenage parents. In this chapter you will meet some.

MAKING REALISTIC PLANS: We spoke with a counselor in a special program for pregnant and parenting teens. She told us that once a teenager decides to continue her pregnancy, together they discuss the importance of making realistic plans *before* the baby is born. She emphasizes that pregnancy takes nine months both because it takes nine months for a fetus to develop into a baby and because it takes nine months to prepare for becoming a parent. (We suggest you read the section "Consider the Support That May Be Available to You," starting on page 350. This will give you information about services available to you, and may help you in your decision about your pregnancy.)

Questions to Ask Yourself If You Are Considering Having a Baby.

WHO CAN I COUNT ON TO HELP ME OUT? Being a parent is so demanding, it's hard to do unless you have lots of support emotionally and financially. You will need someone to share in the everyday care of your child. All parents need this regardless of whether they are fourteen or thirty years old. Many pregnant teens we spoke to felt that "it would just work out," but being a parent will not just work out. You will need help, people you can count on. This can be a husband, boyfriend, mother, father, grandparents, other relatives, or a combination of people.

WHAT RELATIONSHIP WILL I HAVE WITH MY BABY'S FATHER? Think about your relationship with the baby's father. Talk to the father and decide how much help and support you can count on realistically. Lots of boys say, "Oh, yeah I'll be there for you. I'll support you," and then they disappear from your life or find another girlfriend. Of course, some young fathers are very involved with their children even if they are not married to the mother. Richard said,

> We were definitely too young to get married. Legally, I know that I'm supposed to support Terrance until he's eighteen, but that's not real. The best I can do for him is stay in school and get myself together so one day I can do that. There's lots I can do besides give him money. I spend a lot of time with him. Some guys say, "You babysit that kid a lot" because he's always with me. But I tell them, "He's my son. I'm not babysitting him, I'm taking care of him."

Although you may hope that your pregnancy will keep you and your boyfriend together, it often works the other way, and you end up raising the child without his support. That is what happened to eighteen-year-old Sylvia:

> I wanted to marry my daughter's father, and after I was pregnant he moved in with me and he helped me some. But during the first several months after she was born, he moved out because he wanted his freedom. After a while he just said, "Never mind."

Fifteen-year-old Rita said:

> We broke up when the baby was six months. It was hard, 'cause he got this new girlfriend and someone just told me she's pregnant too. When I had the baby, he said he would stick by me. He even lived here with me and my mother. He didn't like it, though. He never got along with my mother. I never thought of not having my baby, and I knew that I was too young to get married. My mother helps out a lot, so it's not too bad.

Today, a lot of teenage mothers have babies without getting married or having partners. But babies need males in their lives too, so if the father is not going to be involved, think about finding a positive male role model to help you raise your baby—your own father, an uncle, an older brother, a friend from school—some male who is willing to make a long-term commitment to your child, who can help you. Jennifer, age seventeen, has a two-and-a-half-year-old son.

> I knew right away that I didn't want anything to do with his father, because he just hangs out and I don't want him to have influence on my son. My boyfriend has been with us for about a year now, and he treats him like his own son.

Some teens do get married. Susan, seventeen and Neil, eighteen, have a one-year-old daughter, Molly. Neil said,

> It's not easy, but we're doing it. We are both really into Molly. My parents help us out a lot, even made this apartment for us in the basement of their house. We're both in school, so we're juggling a lot right now. Yeah, it would have been easier if we waited, but that's not how it worked out.

The vast majority of teenage marriages end in separation or divorce. It's very difficult to take care of your baby and your relationship if you do not have a diploma, job skills that can enable you to get a decent-paying job, or support from your family. Tom and Becky married when they were eighteen and Becky was three months pregnant. Their son, Luke, is five now. Tom told us:

> When I look back, I regret the marriage most of all. It's hard to think about abortion now, because I can't wish Luke wasn't here, but Becky and I really weren't ready for marriage. We loved each other, sure, but we've had so many problems over these last years—money problems especially. I was struggling with a job and night school and Becky was trying to find a job. After a while, we would spend all our time together—which wasn't very much anyway—fighting. We hurt each other a lot. We're separated now, and that's hard on Luke, because he lives with Becky but he misses being with me. I see him as much as I can, but the tension between me and Becky is hard for him.

AM I WILLING TO PREPARE SERIOUSLY FOR HAVING A BABY? Teenage mothers and their babies face a higher risk of pregnancy and childbirth complications than older mothers do, because teenage bodies are still developing, and often teenagers do not take proper care of themselves. To help avoid complications, get prenatal medical care as soon as you decide to continue the pregnancy. Good care means regular monthly visits to the doctor, or sometimes twice monthly. It means eating a healthy diet, exercising daily, taking special vitamins, not smoking or drinking, and staying away from drugs.

If you want to have a healthy baby, take a look at your eating habits and other activities. The fetus is completely dependent on you; he or she is fed through what you put into your body. If you are taking drugs, they go to the fetus. If you smoke, that goes to the fetus. If you drink alcohol, that affects the fetus too. If you eat healthy foods, like vegetables and protein, your fetus has a better chance of developing into a healthy newborn. If you drink lots of coffee and soft drinks and fill up on fatty junk food, your fetus suffers. *For this reason, eat well and do not smoke or use drugs or alcohol while you are pregnant.*

DO I KNOW ENOUGH ABOUT PREGNANCY AND CHILD-BIRTH? We spoke to many teenage parents about their experiences and what they thought teens should know if they are faced with a pregnancy decision. Kendra, a sixteen-year-old mother of a six-month-old girl, thought that it was very important to tell teens what pregnancy and childbirth are really like. She went to a prenatal clinic as soon as she admitted to herself she was pregnant. She also attended childbirth preparation classes to give her the information she desired about pregnancy and childbirth. Here is what Kendra told us about her prenatal care experience:

When I first realized I was pregnant, I was scared because I knew I wouldn't have an abortion. After a while, I kind of got used to the idea that I would have a baby, and I wanted my baby to be healthy. I was lucky, because my counselor at school told me about a clinic that specialized in teens, and they were nice and told me what was happening; like how the baby was developing and what was going on in my body. The nurse explained the tests and exams I had to get. I didn't realize that

she would be examining me down there so much and that I'd have so many blood tests. It turned out that I had so many blood tests because it came out that I was anemic. I didn't have enough iron in my blood, so they kept having to check my blood. I had special iron pills to take.

When I first went to the clinic, the nurse told me that everything I ate, drank, or smoked also went to my baby. To tell you the truth, that made me scared, because before I realized I was pregnant I drank and I smoked pot. I worried about that the whole time I was pregnant. During the first appointment they checked my blood and my urine to see if I had diabetes, anemia, the Rh-negative blood factor, or a kidney or bladder infection. They also gave me some special vitamins for pregnancy and told me about the foods I should be eating. The doctor examined me inside. I won't tell you that I wasn't embarrassed because I was. When she explained why they were examining me like that, I did feel a little better. She said that they wanted to see how far along I was and if I had any infections. Not only did the doctor use her fingers to feel inside my vagina, but she felt inside my rectum too. Of course she wore rubber gloves.

Kendra's pregnancy was pretty normal. She describes it here:

I remember that in my second month I was tired all the time and I had to pee a lot. Then my clothes started to feel tight, but nobody really noticed I was pregnant. I think that in the fifth month I began to look pregnant and I felt the baby move. Then I started to gain more weight (I gained 35 pounds). In about the fifth month, my boobs got tremendous and the area around my nipples got darker and wider. I hated getting so big. I felt fat and old. I started getting some backaches, and in about my seventh month my ankles started to swell. It was hard, because I was still going to school. The baby seemed to be squashing my insides. I could only eat little meals because I had terrible heartburn. On top of that, I was constipated, which made matters worse. Finally, in my ninth month, the baby dropped, moved lower down, so I felt better, but I felt like I had to go to the bathroom all the time. By that time I couldn't wait to deliver. It was hard for me to find a comfortable position sleeping. Maybe it sounds as if I'm complaining, and I know that some of the girls in my pregnancy group had it worse. One girl got hemorrhoids, another got stretch marks, and another girl was nauseous all the time. I didn't have any of that. Emotionally, during my pregnancy, I was very sensitive, I cried a lot, got into arguments with my boyfriend and sister. My doctor said the change in my hormones was affecting me. I found out later they affect nearly everybody who's pregnant.

Kendra and her boyfriend and her sister went together to childbirth preparation classes to find out about the pregnancy and what to expect from childbirth. Darlene, a sixteen-year-old mother of a one-year-old, said that she wished that she had taken a childbirth class, because during the birth she felt totally unprepared. She didn't know what to expect, and although the nurse was nice to her, she felt panicky and screamed much of the time. After she was in labor for twenty-four hours, the doctors had to do an emergency cesarean section, because her son was showing signs of distress. (A cesarean section is an operation where the doctor makes an incision in the abdomen and uterus wide enough to remove the baby. One in four or five deliveries is done this way.) Although her son turned out to be fine, Darlene had to stay in the hospital for an extra week while she healed from complications. She felt alone and scared. Her boyfriend was no longer in the picture, and her mother worked days, so she could only visit at night.

Every birth is an individual story. Some are wonderful; some are scary. The sooner you begin to prepare yourself for childbirth, the less scary the experience will be. So if you make the decision to have a baby, contact your hospital, clinic, or doctor's office to arrange prenatal care and childbirth education classes right away. Take the time you need to

prepare yourself for the major life change that is about to occur.

TEEN PARENTS TALK ABOUT THEIR PARENTING EXPERIENCES: Basically, when you decide to have a child, you give up your own childhood. Your baby needs you to be a grown-up. Your baby needs you to put his or her life before your life. We sat in on a young parents' group at a youth center in New York City. It was clear that having a baby had completely changed the life of every teenager in that room. Because these young parents found they couldn't be the good parents they wanted to be without help, they came to the youth center for support. All of

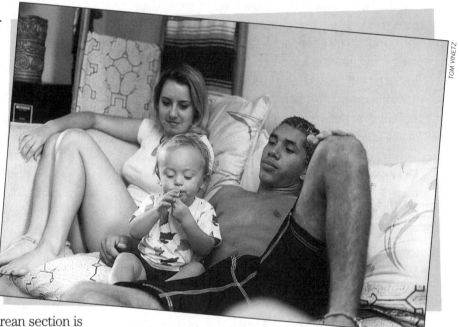

them agreed that being a parent is extremely difficult. Here's what they told us about their everyday experiences as parents:

Kerry and Tim are both nineteen, and their son Kevin is two and a half. Kerry told us:

I take him to the day care because Tim leaves very early in the morning to get to his job. Most of the time Kevin's a sweet kid who listens up pretty good. Lately he's going through this thing where he just sits on the floor, screams, and kicks me. He doesn't want to go to the day care. He cries when I leave him, but I have to finish high school, so I go. Yesterday I just went into the bathroom and cried.

The teacher, she said he's okay in about five minutes, but I'm upset all morning.

Carmen, sixteen, has a one-year-old daughter, Lourdes:

She's still not sleeping through the night, so I get up with her at least once. My mom says I should just let her cry, but she's in the room with me, and when she sees me she won't let up till I get up and walk around with her. Then when she finally goes back to sleep, I'm wide awake. Some mornings I'm so tired I can't get out of the bed, so I just roll over and go back to sleep. I'm not doing well in school.

Seventeen-year-old Carla's son is three and a half.

I worry because his day care teachers tell me he doesn't get along with the other kids. Sometimes he'll come up to a kid who's playing and just bites the kid and takes the toy away. She said that kids his age do this and that I shouldn't worry. Where we live, Willie is always with grown-ups, it's me and my mom and grandma. I wish he would play with the other kids better. I worry that he won't have friends.

Lottie, who is fourteen, told us:

I think the hardest thing for me is people's attitudes. I mean, I go in the street with my baby, she's dressed nice, and I have her in this nice carriage. People stare at me because I look so young. They see it's my baby because how I treat her. They look at us and they shake their heads. They are so rude!

Shareen, age sixteen, said:

Yeah, I was in the supermarket yesterday and Tanya decides to have a tantrum 'cause she sees candy and I won't give it to her. People started to stare at us because she was screaming, and I know they thought I was abusing her because I'm a teenager. I just bought her the candy to shut her up. Then I was mad at her for making me look bad.

Vanessa brought up another issue that seemed to be of concern to several of the girls in the room.

Tasha can be so sweet, but when my boyfriend comes around she acts all bratty, like she doesn't want him to be with me. It's hard, 'cause I have to deal with her and then he gets an attitude about her.

Being a parent is trying. Many of these teens admitted that they often wish they hadn't gotten pregnant in the first place. But they were all grateful for the advantage they had by being in a support group where they could share their feelings with other parents. They weren't isolated. They could get advice and comfort from one another. For young parents who are alone or without proper resources, raising a child is extremely difficult, physically and emotionally. Angela, for example, does not have any child care. She, herself, was sexually abused as a child and she said:

When you have a daughter, it's very hard. Like for me, it's very hard to leave my daughter with anybody, because I worry so much about if somebody might hurt her. I'd rather drag her everywhere with me, because at least I know where she is. I just don't trust leaving her with anybody else.

Teen parents have a special set of challenges, since they are young and not prepared to be economically self-supporting. Often they must live with relatives, complete their education, juggle jobs and schooling, and put their children in day care, when they can find adequate day care. This responsibility at such an early age tends to be extremely stressful. And when parents are stressed out, regardless of their age, children are shortchanged. Seventeen-year-old Maria told us:

My mother had me when she was sixteen, and we kept having to move because nobody wanted us. My mom married my stepfather basically to have a place to live. He kept losing his job, so my mom always had to work, and she had different people watching me. My stepfather's way of disciplining me was hitting, and he was always calling me "stupid." I don't think it's good to have kids when you're still a teenager unless you have good people to help you.

Carol, who's now twenty-three, didn't have anyone to help her. She had to make it on her own:

I left home at seventeen because my father kicked me out. He called me a slut for having sex with my boyfriend, so I moved in with some friends and then drifted from place to place. It was pretty nice being on my own, but it was also very lonely. I hardly had any friends, and I didn't know what I was doing with myself. Now when I look back on it, I think I must have been very immature.

My boyfriend and I got along pretty well. We used birth control some of the time but not always. At seventeen I just didn't think I would get pregnant. Jimmy and I talked about what would happen if I got pregnant and he said, "I'll take care of it." You know how that goes. Anyway, in the beginning of my pregnancy everything was cool. Jimmy said we'd get our own apartment and that would be great. Then when I was four months gone, he tells me he can't handle it, so I should get an abortion. To make a long story short, we split. I just couldn't get myself to have an abortion. I even made four different appointments, but I never showed up.

I was so scared, I tried to forget I was pregnant. I didn't take care of myself. I'll tell you right now I was dumb, because Ray was extra small when he was born, and he has a hearing problem, and I'm sure that was because of all the drugs I did. Finally, when I was six months pregnant, I called a hot line for help and got information about a maternity residence. They put me up and gave me food and clothes and a place to stay, but for a while they kept pressuring me to give the baby up for adoption. That was hard for me, because no way did I want to give the baby up.

Well, my delivery was pretty easy, but I didn't like being in the hospital at all. I felt sorry for myself, because I was in this room with married women who were going home to their husbands and people who cared about them, and I didn't have anyone who cared about me.

When I left the hospital, Ray and I lived with another friend of mine until I could get on welfare and get my own place. I thought it would be okay then, but the first few months were like a nightmare. I could only afford this dumpy place. The heat would go off all the time, and Ray was sick a lot. I had bad dreams, and Ray and I were sleeping in the same bed, and so I kept being afraid I'd roll over and crush him. I really thought I was going to go crazy.

Let me tell you, it wasn't easy. I don't think it's ever easy for a single parent without money.

Carol stayed on welfare for a couple of years, but when we interviewed her she was working and going to college at night. At five, Ray goes to school during the day and to a babysitter's while Carol goes to school. Carol is worried that she doesn't see Ray enough.

Even when you do have help, and when money isn't a problem, life for a teen parent is still difficult. We heard from Susan and Neil before. They live with their daughter in an apartment Neil's parents made for them in their house, and both Susan's parents and Neil's parents help them out financially. Susan said:

Neil's in his last year of high school and I'm a junior. He goes to school during the day and I go at night, so you can see we don't get much time to be together. Here's what a typical day is like for us: We get up about seven and Neil gets ready for school and I feed and change Molly. Then I have breakfast and clean the house and take Molly to the supermarket. When we get back, Molly has a nap and I try to fix things up or catch up on chores. Then Neil comes home for lunch and that's when I get a chance to go out by myself. I need that hour because being cooped up with Molly all day isn't easy. I love her very much of course, but I do need a break. When I get back, Neil goes back to school and I finish feeding Molly. Then sometimes she'll take a short nap in the afternoon and that's when I try to study. Neil has a job until six, and when he comes home I rush out the door to get to my class on time. Neil takes over with Molly. He plays with her and gives her a bath and puts her to sleep.

When I get back from school about nine, we hang out together for a while. That's really the only time we get to talk to each other. And then sometimes we have to use that time to study. We're usually in bed before eleven, and we take turns getting up with Molly in the middle of the night.

YOUNG FATHERS: We wanted to include a special section for young fathers, because many people assume that teen fathers are not involved with their children and don't care about them. We have found that many young dads *are* interested in their children but find it hard to meet their financial responsibilities. As Jerry said, "When you are young and don't have an education and don't have a well-paying job, doing the right thing seems overwhelming."

Remember, there are many ways, besides financial support, to be involved as a father. The most important by far is to spend time and have a relationship with your child. This lets the child know you care. It helps your child feel worthwhile as a person and builds self-esteem. Eventually, all children ask, "Who is my daddy?" And when you have been there throughout his or her life, your child will know you and know you tried. Daryl, age nineteen, has a four-year-old son.

I take William to the park and play ball with him a couple of days a week. He's just a little guy, but when I come by to pick him up, he's ready. He looks up to me. He needs me.

Regardless of whether or not you are married, you can be emotionally supportive to your child's mother both before and after the baby is born. Spending time with her, listening to her worries and concerns helps her know that she is not alone. You can encourage her to eat right, exercise, rest, and not smoke, drink or take drugs. Many prospective fathers go to the doctor with their partners and attend prenatal childbirth preparation classes with them. You can practice childbirth exercises together and coach her during the delivery. Once the baby is born, you can help her take care of the baby. We spoke to Kendra's boyfriend, Matt. He said,

I spent a lot of time with Kendra while she was pregnant. She was moody a lot, but I tried to make her feel like she looked good to me even when she was really upset about gaining weight. I went with her to some of her doctor's visits. And I tried to make sure she ate right. We both gave up smoking. That was hard for me. I used to still drink and smoke pot sometimes, but I never did it around Kendra.

Steven, age sixteen, who is a new father, told us:

I told Lori, "I'll watch the baby. You go out. You need a break."

Giving the child's mother a break is important, because parenthood is very stressful and all parents need a break. But remember, babies need love and attention every day, all day long. They need to be cared for and cherished every single day of their lives. If you are able to give emotional support to the mother and love and time to your child, you will help that child grow into a self-confident, loving human being.

If you are not married to your child's mother, it is important to establish legal paternity, even if your name is on the birth certificate. The actual procedure varies from state to state. Usually both mother and father sign an affidavit (a legal paper) that states that you are the child's father. This is necessary for your child to receive benefits through you—such as social security, insurance, and veterans' benefits. Establishing paternity is the only legal way for an unmarried father to establish his rights to visitation and custody. If there is disagreement about whether or not you are the father, you can take a blood test. The test compares many different factors in your blood with similar parts of the mother's blood and the child's blood.

Only about one in three teen mothers is married when her child is born, and by the time the child is three, a high percentage of these marriages have ended. Often parenting teens spend most of their child's life with different partners. But remember, even if you are not with your child's mother, you can still be an involved parent, and it's always better for your child if you are. Then your child grows up knowing that he or she is loved.

Consider the Support That May Be Available to You

When you are pregnant, we encourage you to take a realistic look at the services that are available to you. Our society does not give parents much assistance, yet all parents, no matter what their age, need a lot of help. You may have to be very assertive about getting the support you need. Look for the following services in your area. Many are not available everywhere:

➤ Prenatal care—from clinics, hospitals, private doctors—which includes checkups and health care while you are pregnant.

➤ A maternity residence, where you can stay during pregnancy and for a while after giving birth, or a residence where you can live with your child.

➤ Childbirth classes to prepare you for pregnancy and delivery. A delivery without preparation can be frightening and lonely. Check at your local hospital, the Department of Health, or your prenatal clinic.

➤ Parenting classes to help you learn how to care for your baby and child.

➤ A pregnant and parenting program or group for teenagers.

➤ Support for staying in school—help from your parents and or the school district.

➤ Day care—someone to take care of your child while you are working or in school. Good day care is hard to find. Make this a top priority while you are still pregnant.

➤ A job-training and placement program.

➤ Subsidized housing—sign up as soon as you are pregnant. Subsidized housing, like good day care, is extremely hard to find. Check with your social worker.

➤ Income assistance (welfare).

➤ Food stamps or other government programs to help provide nutritious food.

➤ Clothing and other items for infants—sometimes available from churches, temples, service clubs, community centers.

➤ Child-support payments from the father of the child. If the father is not paying child support, contact your social worker or legal aid.

➤ Foster-care placement for your child or for you with your child.

➤ Adoption assistance.

To Find Out About These Services:

➤ Call your local city or county Department of Health and ask if they offer services for pregnant and parenting teens. You can either call directory assistance or look up the number in the phone book. (For example, in New York City, we called the New York Women's Healthline, at 1-212-230-1111, which is part of the New York City Department of Health. They offer referrals to needed services.)

➤ Ask your doctor.

➤ Call Planned Parenthood. (To find the Planned Parenthood office nearest you, look it up in the phone book or call the toll-free number 1-800-230-7526. You will automatically be transferred to the Planned Parenthood nearest you. Ask to speak to a counselor or a social worker.

➤ Call a social service agency in your area.

➤ Speak to your school counselor.

➤ Talk to someone at your community center.

The cost of services and the amount of time they will be available to you differs from place to place. Some services may be free or low-cost. Some services may be covered by Medicaid, which is government health insurance. (You may be able to use Medicaid through your family or on your own.) Try to figure out with a counselor how long you can count on these services being available to you at reduced cost.

(continued)

At the time this book was published, states were starting their own welfare and workfare laws in response to the federal Personal Responsibility and Work Opportunity Act of 1996. These laws may affect how much financial support you can count on from the government. Since benefits are determined on a state-by-state basis, we encourage you to find out the situation in your state.

Even if many of the services you need are no-cost or low-cost, having a child is still *very* expensive. Consider whether you will have enough money to care adequately for your child. If you are not married, you are entitled to child support from the baby's father. Many fathers do not pay on time or at all, however, and the government has a great deal of difficulty making them do so.

It is very important for you to stay in school during your pregnancy and to return to school after you give birth. You must have at least a high school education if you are going to be able to hold any decent job that will enable you to support, or contribute to the support of, a child. It is illegal for a school to make you leave because you are pregnant or parenting. Many schools have special programs or services for pregnant or parenting teens. Some schools offer on-site child care or help with securing a family day care arrangement. Call your local school district office to find out its policy. Also, consider going on for a degree beyond high school. Since most well-paying jobs require certain skills, such as computer literacy, acquiring these skills at your local community college may be essential to obtaining a well-paying job.

You may find a great deal of help by joining a young parents' support program if one exists in your city or town. If none is available, you can set up a support group of your own by seeking out other young parents in your area and meeting with them on a regular basis to share information and stories. Those of you in the group may choose to organize a play group for your children or a babysitting co-op in which you help each other with babysitting. Being a parent home with a young child all day can isolate you from adult companionship, so it is important to find ways to be together with other parents and develop ways to assist one another.

If you need a place to live during pregnancy or after you give birth, you may be able to use a residential (live-in) program. If such a program exists in your area, usually it is time-limited—you can use it for only a year or two—and you must agree to follow through with certain goals. For instance, Inwood House, in New York City, offers young mothers-to-be a place to live and child care after giving birth, but they must agree to attend school, learn about child care, prepare for becoming self-supporting, and leave when they are twenty-one.

If you cannot manage caring for your child when you first give birth, but believe that you will be able to manage in the near future, you may be able to use foster-care placement. This option is discussed in greater detail starting on page 352.

It is also possible to carry your pregnancy to term and give birth, but decide to place your child for adoption. This option is discussed in greater detail in the section beginning on page 357.

ARRANGEMENTS FOR YOUR CHILD IF YOU CAN'T TAKE RESPONSIBILITY

If you have decided to carry your pregnancy to term, and everything proceeds normally, you will give birth. Then you will be faced with the decision of becoming that child's parent or finding someone else to care for the baby. There are a variety of ways to proceed, but it is not easy to find a good home for a baby on a temporary basis. *The conditions that are best for your baby allow him or her to remain in one place for a long time.* Babies and small children need stability for their own sense of security. They crave and need a home base and one or two caring adults who will always be there for them. Babies and children who are shifted from one child care arrangement to another suffer from lack of a permanent family and a permanent place to call their own. Perhaps you know about that from your own experience.

Making Informal Arrangements. Sometimes you can arrange to have your child cared for by someone you know. These arrangements are not made through the courts, and there is no formal, written agreement. If your parent, relative, or friend agrees to care for your child until you are able to take care of him or her, you can make a private agreement with that person. You should consider the protection offered by a legal contract, however, even if someone in your family provides the care. Legal contracts can help prevent misunderstandings.

An unmarried mother has the legal right to her child even though the child is living temporarily with someone else. If the mother and father are married, they both have legal rights to their child. If they are not married, the baby's father has the *same rights* as the baby's mother, but he must legally establish paternity through the courts. The actual procedure for doing this varies from state to state. Call a lawyer or legal aid to find out the procedure in your state.

Here is an example of an informal arrangement: Karen got pregnant when she was fifteen. She was living at home with her mother, brother, and sister. Karen's mother told her there would be no room for the baby, and Karen felt she was too young to live on her own. The baby's father had moved out of state and wasn't interested in taking care of the baby. When Derrick was born, Karen looked for someone to care for him temporarily. Her mother's close friend Mrs. Rowan said she would be able to care for Derrick. Karen brought Derrick to Mrs. Rowan's to live and she visited him three times a week at least. Sometimes she took Derrick home for the weekend. When the child was two years old, Karen got married and took Derrick to live with her and her new husband. Karen's arrangement with Mrs. Rowan worked out very well for everyone. Karen kept in close contact with her baby and he felt attached to her.

Karen was lucky, because many of these informal arrangements do not work out so well. Your legal rights to your child can be taken from you if it can be proved in court that you have abandoned, neglected, or seriously mistreated your child. That is what happened to Joyce, who was sixteen when Matthew was born. Joyce's boyfriend, Joe, was seventeen. Neither of them was able to take care of Matthew, so a friend of Joyce's aunt, Mrs. Quentin, agreed to take him. Mrs. Quentin had always wanted a son after raising three daughters of her own. Joyce and Joe said that they hoped to take Matthew back in eighteen months, after Joe graduated from high school and got a decent job. They said they would visit Matthew at least once a week. Mrs. Quentin agreed. Within six months, Joe and Joyce broke up. Joe moved out of the state to live with his new girlfriend, and Joyce became very depressed. Matthew looked a lot like Joe, so Joyce found it harder and harder to visit him and take care of him. Pretty soon she stopped visiting altogether. Matthew became very attached to Mrs. Quentin and her daughters. He was part of the family and thought of Mrs. Quentin as his mother. After Joyce failed to visit or call for six months, Mrs. Quentin hired a lawyer to try to adopt Matthew legally. Joyce was notified of this action, and she was told that she could have free legal services if she needed them. Joyce decided not to fight the adoption because she knew she couldn't be a good mother to Matthew. She felt that he was better off living with Mrs. Quentin.

If you make a private arrangement for your child, it's up to you to visit the child and help out as much as you can. If you neglect your duties as a parent, the person who cares for your child may try to have your legal rights taken away from you. *A child's emotional well-being and sense of security depend on knowing that he or she is loved and appreciated.* If you cannot or do not give that care and affection to your child, he or she might be better off with someone who can.

Temporary Foster Care.

Girls who decide to continue their pregnancy but cannot take on the responsibility of caring for the baby can decide to give the baby to another family *temporarily*. This arrangement is called foster care.

Several different types of foster care are available. To learn about your options, call a lawyer, the department of child welfare in your state, or one of the agencies listed on page 366. In this section, we will describe some of the arrangements you can make.

Rules about foster care differ from state to state. To find out about the rules in your state, contact your local department of child welfare or a local service agency.

KINSHIP FOSTER CARE. Since a teenager's parents aren't legally or financially responsible for the care of their grandchildren, they may be able to receive foster-care funding if the grandchild lives with them. This is called kinship foster care. In some states, grandparents are not eligible for this type of funding if the parent of the baby also lives with them. In that case, they may be eligible to receive regular public assistance or add the baby to an existing budget if they are already receiving public assistance.

Other relatives, such as aunts and uncles and older siblings, can have their homes approved as kinship foster homes too. Kinship foster parents are

Foster care is help for parents who can't take care of their child *now* but think they will be able to take care of their child in the *near* future. A licensed agency will place your child in an approved foster home for a certain amount of time. *You are still the child's mother or father,* so you must be actively involved in your child's life by visiting regularly and helping out financially if you can.

It is not good for a child to live separately from his or her parents for a long time, so most states do not arrange long-term foster-care placements. If you don't think you can manage being a parent for your child, it is probably better to allow your child to be adopted by a family that is able and eager to take care of him or her.

treated by the state much as other foster parents are. They go through the same kind of investigation. They are monitored once kinship foster care begins, and they receive foster-care money and medical coverage from the state. The foster-care agency sends caseworkers on a regular basis to check on the well-being of the child. It is important to understand that with all foster care, the agency has the right to remove the child at any time.

VOLUNTARY (NON-KINSHIP) FOSTER CARE. You can also place your child temporarily in an approved foster home. The government pays a foster-care family to care for your child. This is not an around-the-clock babysitting service for your child; it is a place where he or she can be cared for until you can provide adequate care yourself. That means you must have some plans to care for your child in the near future—after you graduate from high school, as soon as you find an apartment, or when you get a job. Many agencies can help parents make foster-care arrangements:

➤ State Department of Child Welfare operates its own foster care homes and cooperates with other voluntary agencies.

➤ Private foster-care agencies in your area (call the state department of child welfare for information about these agencies).

➤ Religious organizations: Catholic Charities, United Federation of Jewish Philanthropies, Federation of Protestant Welfare Agencies, placements made through local churches or temples.

➤ Groups that oppose abortion, such as Birthright or Right-to-Life.

➤ Charitable organizations like United Community Services.

➤ Maternity homes or shelters will sometimes help you arrange foster care.

To contact these agencies, look in the white pages of the phone book for a listing under their name. If you live in a very small town, try the phone book of the biggest city near your home. The library should have

---

Legal Rights

The decision to use foster care is yours unless the government can prove that you are unable to care for your child, in which case a judge may place him or her in foster care without your consent.

Even if you are a minor and your parents have legal responsibility for *you,* they *don't have legal responsibility for your child.* Your parents or relatives may be able to receive public assistance for caring for your child or act as kinship foster parents (see page 352 for more details).

Both parents of the child, whether they are married or not, must consent to foster-care placement. When a mother places her child in foster care, she must name the father unless he is unknown or it can be shown that naming him would be harmful to the child. If the father refuses to admit that he is the father, he can be taken to court in a paternity suit.

If one of the parents does not consent to the foster-care arrangement, a judge will decide whether to place the child in foster care even without that parent's consent. The judge can also decide that some other arrangement would be better for the child.

phone books from neighboring cities. Or call directory assistance. Talk with a school counselor, hospital social worker, or staff member at a local youth center.

If you know before your baby is born that you will want to make use of foster care, get in touch with the agency while you are still pregnant. The arrangement will be easier, and you will feel better knowing that you have someone to look after your baby right away.

The agency you contact will assign a social worker or counselor to help you make the arrangements and write up a legal agreement concerning the care of your child. The worker will answer your questions and assist you in making your plans.

Some children in foster care are placed in a private foster home, licensed and paid by the state and approved by the agency, where the children live as part of the foster parents' family. Some children in foster care are placed in a child care institution run by the agency. These children live in a group setting and are cared for by hired child care workers.

The final decision about where your child is placed is up to the social service agency, but you can request that your child be placed in a family, and you can ask that the family be of a particular race or religion. Usually, the agency will try to honor your request if the staff thinks it's reasonable and if the agency has the facilities. Marilyn tells how she secured the placement she wanted:

When Frankie lost his job, he couldn't get another one, because he got sick, so I had to go to work. We couldn't afford babysitting for our baby, and there wasn't any day care near us that would take a one-year-old. So we talked to our baby's doctor, who put us in touch with an agency that arranges foster care. We told them that we had a friend of Frankie's family who was a foster mother to another kid, and they got in touch with Mrs. Polk and said the baby could live with her until we got on our feet again. Mrs. Polk loved kids. She kept our baby for a year, but we visited him every weekend, and he always knew that we loved him and would take him back as soon as we could. It took us a year to get it together, but then we got Mark back, and now we're all together again.

This poem was written by a fifteen-year-old girl who spent her childhood in six different foster homes.

REALITY

*Her eyes were of wonder
As she saw her new home.
She quietly began to ponder
All the places she had been sent to roam.*

*Alone at night she would cry
(Her mother's death came as a shock),
Hoping and praying the days would
   pass by,
Having something to say but not wanting
   to talk.*

*Now on the verge of insanity.
No one will listen.
Is this the fault of fate or society?
For now her eyes no longer glisten.*

Foster care is recommended as a last resort, because temporary placement is usually not as good for a child as permanent placement. To feel secure, children need to know that they are loved and will be cared for on a permanent basis. Children in foster care sometimes don't have the opportunity to experience that sense of being wanted, because they may be shifted from one home to another. Anna, twelve, told us she spent her life in ten different foster homes. Now she's in a group home and has no contact with her birth mother.

You and the agency staff members working with you should explore all other possibilities for helping you care for your child—welfare, family day care, help from parents and relatives, and adoption—before you decide to use foster care.

If you and the agency agree that foster care is the best thing for your child, they will ask you to sign an agreement that legally transfers the care and custody of your child to an authorized agency. When you sign that agreement, the agency becomes the legal guardian of your child.

Be sure to get a copy of the agreement and

keep it in a safe place. If any legal problems come up, you will need it. If you have to contact a lawyer, he or she will want to see the agreement.

The agreement will probably be written in confusing legal terms, so be sure to have the agency explain everything to you in language you understand. Remember, your rights and your baby's rights are at stake. You may even wish to speak to a lawyer before signing the agreement. If you don't have much money, you are probably eligible for *free* legal assistance. Ask about it.

The agreement will state your *obligations* as well as your *rights.* Since foster-care laws vary from state to state, you will need to find out what is true in your state. You are usually *obligated* to:

➤ Visit your child.

➤ Plan for the future of your child.

➤ Meet with and consult with the agency about this plan.

➤ Contribute to the support of your child if you are able.

➤ Inform the agency of any change in name or address.

Failure to meet your obligations could lead the agency to file a petition to terminate your rights as a parent. In some states you can lose your parental rights if you fail to visit your child regularly over a six-month period, or if a year goes by without your planning for your child's discharge.

Be sure that you understand the foster-care agreement you sign. The agreement will say how often you are supposed to visit your child, how long your child will be kept in foster placement, and whether you have to give any money toward the cost. The agreement will also say that you have to keep in contact with the agency's social worker and work toward being able to care for your child.

Follow the rules of the agreement completely. If you do not, you risk losing your rights to your child.

REALITIES OF FOSTER CARE. Once you sign the foster-care agreement, your child is the legal responsibility of the foster-care agency. The agency can make decisions about your child that you may not agree with. For example, the agency can transfer your child to another home without your consent; they can refuse you the right to take your child for an overnight visit; they can decide that you are not able to care for your child, and they can bring your case to court. You have the right to appeal in court any decision made by the agency.

If you do not follow the instructions in the foster-care agreement, the agency may decide you are an unfit parent and set up court proceedings to release your child for permanent adoption. This is how Janis lost her daughter, Suzi:

Janis was seventeen when she gave birth to Suzi, and she agreed to place her daughter in foster care until she was able to find a suitable place to live, get a job, and arrange child care. Janis visited Suzi twice a month for the first three months, but after that she didn't see Suzi for almost a year. She told her social worker that she was busy looking for a job and just could never make the visits. She missed appointments with the social worker too. When the social worker called, Janis said she was living with a new boyfriend who didn't like children, but she didn't want to give up her rights to Suzi because she was sure she could persuade her boyfriend to accept Suzi. Janis didn't call her social worker or make any attempt to visit Suzi for six months more, and the agency took the case to juvenile court.

Though Janis knew about the hearing, she didn't show up in court. The judge decided to order the court to begin proceedings that would make Suzi eligible for permanent adoption. At that point, Janis tried to fight the ruling, but the court ultimately decided that she had not been a fit mother and would not be a fit mother in the future. Suzi was adopted within a year, and Janis lost all rights to her.

Your child will be released to you at the time and under the conditions stated in your foster-care agreement. Voluntary placement may expire on a specific date or at the occurrence of a specified event, such as when you get your own apartment. At that time, the agency must return your child to you or go to court to extend placement. If the agency feels you have not met the terms of the agreement and that you can't take good care of your child, it can refuse to return the child to you. If you don't agree with this decision, you will have to appeal it in court.

FEELINGS ABOUT FOSTER-CARE PLACEMENT: A lot of teenagers who put their children into foster care do so because they feel they have no other options. They want the best for their child, and they know *they* can't provide such care. Here is how three teenagers described their situations:

Mary (fifteen): I could never give my baby up for adoption, but I really couldn't take care of her myself either. My mother and I never got along, and after I got pregnant she made me move out. I've been living here and there since then, and that's really not the best situation for a baby. Welfare won't pay for me to have my own place, because they say I'm too young. They said I

Voluntary Foster Care Is Voluntary

This means that no one can force you to put your child in foster care—the decision must be yours. However, your child can be placed in foster care without your consent in the case of neglect or abuse that is proved in court. If an investigator from the state child welfare agency feels that your child is in danger, the child may be removed from your care prior to a court ruling.

➤ You have the right to legal representation. If needed, free legal services must be provided.

➤ You have the right to have your child returned to you under the conditions of the agreement you signed, unless otherwise ordered by the courts.

➤ You have the right to supportive services to enable you to meet the agreed conditions.

➤ You have the right to visit your child.

➤ You have the right to a fair hearing if the agency prevents visits or fails to provide services to you.

---

should go into a foster home with my baby, but no thanks! Then you got a curfew and rules and stuff like that, and I've been on my own too much already for that. So foster care for Tammy seemed like the only way. I get to visit Tammy at least once a week, and I'm going to start a waitressing job and save enough to get my own place together. By that time I'll be old enough for welfare to help me out, and then I'll get Tammy back. I feel like it's the right way for us.

Gregory (sixteen): My girlfriend and I are still living at home. We want to live together as soon as I can get a job that pays enough, but right now I'm finishing school. Melinda's mom is very sick, and it would just be too much for her to have the baby around, and her dad travels a lot, so he can't be counted on to help. And my mom, well, she was really mad when she found out about the pregnancy. She never liked Melinda. She thought Melinda was a bad influence on me, and she told me she doesn't ever want to see Melinda or the baby around here. I keep hoping she'll change her mind someday, but right now Mel and I figure the baby will be better off in a foster home.

Trina (sixteen): When I was pregnant, I lived in this home for pregnant girls. I thought of adoption, but I kept changing my mind. When I had the baby, I needed more time to figure things out, so I put Maria in foster care. Now I'm living with my older sister. It's crowded there 'cause she's got four of her own kids and it's only a two-bedroom apartment. She said she understands how hard it is to give up my baby. She plans to move into this big house next month, and she said me and Maria can live down in the basement.

Many of the teenagers we spoke to said they have very mixed feelings about having put their children in foster care. Jody, a sixteen-year-old mother from Texas, said:

I felt so empty after I left the hospital without the baby. There just wasn't anything else I could do, but it's very hard for me to visit her. When I'm with her, I don't want to leave. I can see that she thinks the foster-care mother is her mother. The foster family treats her so well. She's always clean and dressed in pretty things, and she has so many toys. God, I never had so many toys. But it really hurts me when I hear her call her foster mother "Mommy," and I feel like maybe I don't have a right to her anymore.

Brian is a seventeen-year-old father. He and his girlfriend Sarah visit their son every week, but Brian said that's just not like living with him:

When Sean took his first step, he was with his foster mother, and somehow it's beginning to feel like he's going to grow up without me. I'm really trying to get something going for us—to find a job that can support us all—but until then I guess me and Sarah are just going to miss out on some of those important moments.

Beverly, a seventeen-year-old from Washington, told us:

I used to wake up in the middle of the night with the same dream. I'm walking on the beach, and I see my daughter with her foster family. I try to catch up with them but I can't. I run as fast as I can, but even when they see me, they ignore me, like I'm not really there.

Seeing your child in a foster-care situation is bound to bring up lots of feelings like these, and you may also worry that your child isn't getting good care, because of course not all foster care is of the quality you would want for your child. In fact, some foster-care homes are abusive and dangerous. You have a right to report any sign of mistreatment to your social worker.

Talk all your feelings about the placement over with the social worker from the agency, or with some other person you trust. It will make you feel better to share your worries and your sadness and to get out your anger. Your mixed emotions are natural.

It's also natural to have an emotional reaction to getting your child back when the placement is over. It will almost certainly take time for you and the child to feel comfortable living together after having

been separated. Give yourself the time it takes to get adjusted. Talk about your feelings, the negative ones and the positive ones, with someone who will understand. You're not bad or mean or wicked to have mixed feelings about being a parent. Most parents have mixed feelings about being parents.

Your child may have a difficult time accepting you back too. He or she will probably suffer from a natural sense of loss after leaving the foster-care home. The agency social worker or some other caring adult in your life may be able to help you learn how to handle your child's reaction to the separations he or she has had to endure, first from you and now from the foster family he or she may have learned to love.

Adoption Is an Option.

Another option is to choose to allow your baby to be permanently adopted. In adoption, you give over your rights as a parent to another person or family. Legally, you will no longer be considered the child's parent.

Many years ago people thought it unacceptable for an unmarried woman to keep her baby. There were few services and little support available to help her cope with her situation, so a large number of unmarried women put their babies up for adoption. Patricia remembers her experience:

Standing at the nursery window and staring at my one-day-old daughter, I had no idea what I was in for. I was just doing what everyone told me was the right thing to do—giving her up for adoption. Being only sixteen years old myself, the possibility that I could raise her was never even discussed. That wasn't the way it was done then.

Today, the majority of single mothers keep their babies. It is estimated that only 2 to 4 percent of teen mothers choose adoption. But given all the options, if you find yourself with an unwanted pregnancy, adoption is definitely a wise and caring option to consider:

➤ A teen mother who places her baby with adoptive parents has a better chance of completing her education and is less likely to live in poverty.

➤ The baby is more likely to live in a home with two parents and have social, economic, and educational advantages.

➤ The adoptive parents are likely to be older and more established in their careers and have more education. They're ready to take on the full-time responsibilities of raising a child and have gone to great lengths emotionally, financially, and legally to become adoptive parents.

Most mothers choose adoption because they love their baby and believe that their child should grow up in a family that very much wants to raise a child and is prepared to do so. Fourteen-year-old Luanne told us:

> I don't believe in abortion, but I know I can't raise a baby—not now anyway. I know I could do it if I really struggled but that's not the life I want for me or my child. I want my baby to grow up in a family that could give her all the things I never had. They told me that I could go into a foster home, but my baby would be my responsibility. I couldn't do that. Like, there's no good decision here, but I could live with adoption easier than I could with trying to raise a baby now. One day I want to have children, but not now.

Emily, a seventeen-year-old, said:

> At first I planned to keep my baby, but I chose adoption to give my kid all he deserves. I knew I couldn't handle the responsibilities of having a baby. I heard of a good adoption agency. They helped me choose the best parents for my kid, and I think they did a very good job. Although I miss my baby I'm glad I made the decision of putting him up for adoption. I feel it was best.

Mary and her boyfriend are both sixteen. Mary explained:

> I didn't know I was pregnant till it was too late to have an abortion. I was one of those people who got their period until I was four months pregnant. Anyway, I felt strange but I didn't think I was pregnant. I know some places would have done the abortion, but for us, it wasn't right. Jon thought I might really want to keep it, but he admitted that he thought we were too young. I was actually relieved, because I felt that way too, but I wanted Jon to say that. I read something about adoption, and I said, "Let's just check it out." I think that when they said we could choose who would have our baby, it seemed like we could do it.

Knowing in your head that adoption may be a better option for your baby doesn't always mean you can accept it in your heart, or that it's the right option for *you*. Don't let anyone pressure you one way or the other. There are some choices available to you about whether to place your child with an agency, whether to arrange an open adoption, in which you can have contact with the adopting family, whether to answer an ad and arrange the adoption yourself with the help of a lawyer. Think through your choices and talk them over with people you trust. At the back of this chapter we list some toll-free telephone numbers to call for more information. We encourage you to speak to an authorized not-for-profit adoption agency in your state, or to your state department of child welfare, to find out the particular laws and types of adoption choices in your state. You can also contact legal aid.

Placing a baby for adoption can be very difficult emotionally, and you should not go through it alone. Janine said she felt overwhelmed by her experience:

> The way I came to terms with her adoption was to stop feeling. I didn't do it on purpose, and I didn't even realize I was doing it. It just happened. Whenever I thought of her, I felt like I was thinking about a neighbor child, no real connection. Sometimes I felt scared, but I wasn't sure why. Maybe because I was afraid of being ostracized by "society."

If you are considering adoption, it is very important that you get good counseling before and after the adoption takes place. A good counselor will listen to you and let you come to your own conclusions. If you make the decision carefully, after exploring all your other options and alternatives, adoption can be a loving decision for your child.

No one can make you give up your child for adoption. Even if you are underage, no one can force you to sign an adoption surrender, and the baby or child cannot be put up for adoption without your consent. The only way your child can be taken from you legally is through a court decision that you are an unfit parent.

In this section, we will help you look at adoption, and will give you the information you need to decide if this is the option for you.

Adoption laws are different in every state. A few states allow open adoptions, in which the birth parents and the adoptive parents get to know each other (see page 359). Some states have laws against open adoptions. All adoptions are finalized by a judge after the baby has been with the adoptive family for a specific period of time. Adoption is legal and binding. In some states there is a "grace" period, during which you can change your mind about the adoption after the surrender is signed, but that involves getting a lawyer and going back to court. There is no guarantee that the judge will determine that it is in the best interest of the child to return him or her to you.

Both biological parents must consent to the adoption, even if they are not married. Only when the father or mother is legally declared unfit or cannot be located does he or she lose the right to consent.

If the biological parents disagree about whether to put the baby up for adoption, the court decides what to do. Patrick and Leeann were in that situation. Sixteen-year-old Leeann told us:

> I figured that if he wasn't going to marry me, I wasn't going to be able to raise the baby myself. I didn't even want to raise *his* baby, so I decided to give the baby up for adoption. That way he'd never see it and he'd always know that he made me give his baby away because he wasn't man enough to take care of his responsibility.
>
> But when it came time to sign the adoption papers, Patrick wouldn't sign. He said he wanted the baby and that he would keep the baby with him and his mother. We went to court, and the judge gave custody of the baby to Patrick and his mother. I was so mad I felt like killing Patrick.

Leeann said in her opinion the decision wasn't fair. She felt the judge didn't have the right to give her baby to Patrick. But the judge saw that Patrick was the father and that Patrick's mother had agreed to care for the baby, so he decided it would be a better solution than putting the baby in an adoptive home. If it is possible and in the best interest of the child, the court will usually place the child with one of the biological parents.

TYPES OF ADOPTION. There are two main categories of adoption: closed and open.

CLOSED ADOPTION. The names of the birth mother and the adoptive parents are kept secret in a closed adoption. Fourteen-year-old Tawana's adoption plan was a closed adoption:

> I went to an adoption agency and told them I couldn't possibly take care of my baby, because I don't have anyone to help me out. After my son was born, I signed surrender papers, and the agency put him with a family. I'm a Baptist, and I wanted my son to be raised that way. I also wanted him to go to a family that had other kids, because I'm an only child and I always wished that I had a brother or a sister. They told me they found a home that met my issues but that they legally couldn't tell me who the adoptive parents were. It's like I had no rights to speak with him or write to him, and I couldn't even get any information about how he was doing. They said I could register with an adoption information registry, and when he's eighteen, if my son wants to find me, maybe he'll get in touch with me.

OPEN ADOPTION. The birth mother (or parents) and adoptive parents are known to each other. In this type of adoption, the birth mother (or parents) may choose who adopts her child. A wide variety of adoption situations may be considered "open," ranging from having birth parent(s) and adoptive parents send letters and photos to each other (through the agency) as the child grows up, to the birth parent(s) and the adoptive parents carrying on an ongoing relationship with each other. In either case, the adoptive parents have all parental rights to the child. Carolyn and Ramon were both seventeen when their daughter was adopted in an open adoption:

> I don't think I could have gone through with it if I didn't know who was going to get my daughter. I would always be worried that she wasn't being taken care of. My counselor at the adoption agency was wonderful. We talked a lot about all the options. Not that it was easy to decide on adoption—I wouldn't say that. The counselor asked us to make a list of things that we thought were important for our baby to have. I wanted it to be a couple who had a good marriage, since my parents got divorced when I was three. And I wanted my baby to grow up with grass and trees and a yard to play in. It was important to me that she have a big family, brothers and sisters and aunts and uncles, like that, and that the parents be in their thirties. Ramon agreed with my list and added that he wanted the mother to stay home with the baby when she was young. My counselor picked out three families that met the requirements. They showed me pictures and a letter that they had written to the birth parents. I picked out the first family of the three. When Ramon saw the album, he agreed that the first family was his choice too. Then they showed us more pictures. We arranged to meet the family in a local park with my counselor there. I think we were all very nervous, but after we calmed down we really hit it off. The thing that impressed me was that they seemed kind. He was a teacher and she was a social worker who planned to stay home with the baby until she went to nursery school. They agreed to send us pictures every year so we would know how she was doing. I felt so relieved!

There is a trend toward more open types of adoption. To work successfully, counseling is essential. Agencies that arrange open adoptions will provide counseling or be involved with services that do provide counseling (see the Resource section at the end of this chapter, page 366, for the names of some open-adoption agencies). Open adoptions can be set up through an agency or through an attorney in an independent (sometimes called private) adoption. Sheryl, an adoptive mom who worked through a private agency in the Northwest, said:

> My little boy's adopted, and his birth mom sees him pretty regularly. She's married now and they come over on holidays and share birthdays with us. I think because she's such a part of his life, my son doesn't have any of those weird feelings like "Who is my real mom?" I don't think he spends much time thinking about it at all. He just knows he has a loving family *and* a birth mom who loves him.

TWO WAYS OF ARRANGING EITHER OPEN OR CLOSED ADOPTION

AGENCY ADOPTION: The birth parents give up their child to the agency, and the agency places the child in an adoptive home. The agency usually offers counseling services to the birth mother both before and after placement. The agency also conducts a home study to approve of an adoptive home and provides follow-up contacts and counseling with adoptive families. The birth mother receives free prenatal medical care, paid for by the agency; she also gets a place to live while pregnant if needed, and free legal services. Many authorized adoption agencies offer open-adoption arrangements. This may be a family chosen from the list of families selected and approved of by the agency, or a friend or relative of the birth mother who the agency has studied and approved.

The agency may be a public adoption agency, run by the state, or a private adoption agency authorized by the state. Lillian, age sixteen, contacted a private, state-authorized, nonprofit adoption agency when she was five months pregnant.

> My counselor at school told me about this agency, and since I was so nervous she actually called them when I was in her office. The social worker there seemed nice, and she set up an appointment for me. When I got there, Susan (the social worker) told me that the agency would pay for all my pregnancy expenses if I decided to give my baby up for adoption, but she didn't try to pressure me, which was good, because I wouldn't have liked that. She asked me about my situation and how I had come to think about adoption. She

really listened to me. I told her that the baby's father was not really my boyfriend. He knew about the pregnancy and said that he wasn't ready to be a father and that I should "get rid of it." I'm Catholic, and I could never have an abortion. Another reason I wouldn't consider abortion is that I'm adopted myself and that if my birth mother had had an abortion I wouldn't be here.

I get along well with my mother and father, but I hadn't told them about the baby, because they would be so disappointed with me. They wanted me to go to college, and I did too. My mom especially had really high hopes for me, and I knew that she would be so embarrassed in front of her friends. Maybe that's not supposed to be important, but to me it was. Anyway, my biggest worry was that I didn't want people to know about my pregnancy.

To make a long story short, Susan helped me find a way to tell my parents. That was a big relief! They were upset at first but actually were pretty supportive after they got over the shock. The agency gave them their own counselor, which helped. At first they said that *they* would raise the baby, but that's not what I wanted. I decided to go to a maternity residence when I began to show, because I didn't want my friends to know I was pregnant.

Susan had me list all the characteristics I wanted the adoptive parents to have, and she showed me an album of adoptive families that the agency had, with pictures and letters to the birth mother. I chose the ones that seemed the best to me, and I actually met them. In person I didn't feel so comfortable with them, so I ended up choosing another family who I liked right away.

After I had the baby, the nurse put him in my arms, and he looked right at me. I couldn't stop crying, because I wanted to keep him. I was so confused. I didn't expect to feel that way. Susan had told me that I might, but I really didn't think I would. We decided it would be best for me not to sign the surrender papers until I was sure of my decision. She explained that women get very depressed after they have a baby, which when I look back on it was exactly how I was feeling. I signed a consent form which allowed the agency

to place the baby in short-term boarding care for thirty days, while I tried to figure out what I wanted to do. I could visit my son whenever I wanted and I could change my mind at any time. After three weeks I decided that my original plan was right. No one tried to convince me to go through with the adoption, and that helped. But once I decided, I just wanted to get it over with as soon as possible, but we had to go over all the legal documents, because they wanted me to understand what I was signing. I signed the surrender papers, and the agency contacted my baby's father, and he signed too. Susan said I could come and talk to her whenever I wanted, which was good because even though I know I made the right decision, I have a lot of feelings about the whole thing. Anyway, I gave the adoptive parents a letter to give to my son when they thought the time was right.

I am writing to you to tell you that I love you very much and I hope that you do not hate me for giving you up for adoption. I spent a lot of time making this decision. I wanted you to have more than I could give you. I am doing this for you. I chose your family. I met your parents and know that they will love you very much. I want you to know that I am also adopted and that I love my parents like real parents. I am enclosing a picture of myself.

> *Love,*
> *your birth mother*

INDEPENDENT OR PRIVATE ADOPTIONS. These are arranged by a lawyer without the backing of an agency. The adoptive family goes through a home study and is certified by a social worker before the adoption. The birth parents give their child directly to the adoptive family at a pre-arranged time, often right in the hospital after birth. You can arrange this kind of adoption with someone you choose, such as a friend or relative or a couple you pick from an ad.

A number of birth parents meet possible adoptive parents by answering an ad in the newspaper, since many people who want to adopt advertise in local newspapers. Birth parents may also arrange an independent adoption through a doctor or lawyer or someone else who might know a couple wanting to adopt.

Sometimes pregnant teens are offered money by

a doctor or lawyer or someone else to give their baby up. *This is illegal!* Usually the person who arranges it makes a lot of money for doing it, and the couple who wants to adopt the baby pays a very high price. Their only qualification for adopting your baby is that they are willing and able to buy a baby. Having a lot of money has *nothing* to do with being good parents, so this is a very risky way to deal with your life and your baby's happiness.

The counseling offered to birth parents and adoptive parents in independent adoptions may not be as thorough as it is in agency adoptions. You can ask for counseling services to be part of the agreement. Since there is no agency, medical care and living expenses may be paid for by the adoptive parents. Lorna, age sixteen, went through an independent adoption for her second child:

I had Jared when I was only fourteen. I'm still living at home with my mom, my three brothers, and Jared, who's a handful, but there's a lot of us to give him attention. When I came out pregnant again, I think I didn't want to believe it, because I felt that I was just getting on my feet after having Jared. And as soon as I started looking pregnant, my mom and I had a lot of words. I don't believe in abortion, but I knew I couldn't raise another one. I started reading the papers and there were these ads from couples who couldn't have kids and were really interested in adopting. My mom helped me call a couple of the ads. When we finally talked to a couple who sounded good, we asked them to send us a picture. My aunt, who's a social worker, told us about a lawyer who specializes in adoptions, so we met with him and then we arranged to meet the couple together. We liked this couple because they seemed caring. She was a kindergarten teacher. They showed us pictures of their house and of a barbecue they had on the Fourth of July. It seemed like they had a big, close family. Our lawyer and their lawyer talked. The adoptive parents had to have a social worker approve of their home and everything. They agreed to pay all of my medical expenses and my pregnancy expenses, like when I went upstate to live with my mother's friends at the end of my pregnancy.

We agreed that they would come to the hospital when I had the baby. I live in a state where you have to wait forty-eight hours after the birth before signing surrender papers. That was hard, but I did it, but when they took my baby home from the hospital, I felt very sad. While I was still in the hospital, I got to talk to the hospital social worker about how I was feeling, but it wasn't like I had anyone to talk to when I came home.

Many adoption professionals agree that private, state-authorized, not-for-profit agencies offer the most complete adoption services, with counselors available throughout the process. Independent adoptions can be more risky. Of course it is up to each girl or each birth couple to decide how to proceed.

YOUR RIGHTS. It is important to know that if you are considering placing your baby in an adoptive home, you are entitled to certain rights, some of which are guaranteed to you by law. The following "Birth Parent Bill of Rights" is based on one prepared as a public service by Spence-Chapin Agency, a New York–area non-profit adoption resource.

While not all of the rights mentioned are available everywhere, this list should be used as a guideline when exploring adoption resources in your own area.*

THE IMPACT OF ADOPTION ON YOU: Choosing adoption is a process, not just a one-time act that you forget about after it is over. That's why counseling is so important. A good counselor will help you examine all your choices and feelings carefully. If you choose adoption, the counselor will help you recognize it as a choice made out of love for your child. Being able to choose who will adopt your baby may be an important and reassuring factor in your decision.

The following is a document created by a committee of birth parents dedicated to issues important to birth parents and adoption,** to be used by birth parents when giving their child to an adoptive family. We decided to reprint it here to show the love, hope, and caring of the birth mother:

* If any of the rights are not granted by the adoption resource with whom you are working, or if you have any questions or concerns, you can call Spence-Chapin, at 1-800-321-LOVE (5683), for advice on how to access these rights.

** The Spence-Chapin's Birth Parent Advisory Board, New York.

A Birth Parent's Bill of Rights

1. You have the right to be free from pressure. This is an important decision, and you need time to make it. Your adoption resource should assist you to plan for your child's future, not insist that you make up your mind before the baby's birth, or even immediately afterward.

2. You have the right to total confidentiality. Even if you are a minor, placing a child for adoption is your decision alone and you should be treated with respect.

3. You have the right to get help with medical and other birth-related expenses. If you don't have health insurance or aren't eligible for Medicaid, your medical fees, including those of private doctors, should be paid for by either your adoption resource or by the adoptive family. Adoption agencies should also help you find temporary housing during your pregnancy if you need it.

4. You have the right to be put in touch with other women who have placed their babies in adoptive homes. Before making a decision, or afterward, you may wish to speak with someone else who has had the same experience and understands your feelings.

5. You have the right to counseling. A trained and impartial social worker familiar with adoption should be available to help you review all the options and make the best plan for you and your baby. This social worker should not be the same one who counsels the adoptive parents. You should be able to come back for counseling or to supply updated information at any time. An established agency understands adoption is a lifelong process, not a moment in time.

6. You have a right to choose your baby's adoptive parents. If you are working with an adoption resource, you should be presented with family profiles so that you can choose the religion, lifestyle, and education you would want for your child. If you are responding to an advertisement, you should talk with the family and ask for this information. It's a good idea to meet the family, so this should be an option for you.

7. You have rights related to the legal aspect of adoption. You should be able to review and familiarize yourself with all related documents and papers ahead of time, and you have the right to keep copies of anything you sign.

8. You have the right to peace of mind. Every prospective adoptive family should be screened to ensure they will provide your baby with an excellent and loving home. A home-study report should include the family's work history, physical and emotional health, financial situation, and personal history.

9. You have the right to request pictures and periodic progress reports of your baby.

10. You have the right to pass along pictures, mementos, and letters for your baby. Explain in your own words your love and hopes for your baby. You may arrange to have a letter given to your child.

11. You have the right to change your mind. Verbal promises or written agreements signed before the birth of the baby are *not* binding in any way. Surrender documents, signed after the birth of the baby, vary from state to state as to when your decision is irrevocable.

12. You have the right to an adoption resource that will stand by a child with health problems. You should not have to assume care for the child if he or she is born with medical problems.

13. You have the right to send the agency updated medical information. An established adoption resource will still be there for you if any medical conditions develop that should be known to your child and the adoptive family. Your adoption resource should be able to maintain medical records and provide this necessary service.

14. You have the right to be told about adoption "Reunion and Information Registries" that exist in many states. If the laws in your state make such provisions in the years ahead, you or your child can contact the registries in an effort to learn more about each other and possibly meet if that is agreeable to both of you.

I am entrusting this most precious gift to you knowing that we all share a solemn promise and lifelong commitment to this child, who is now "our" child. This is your child to fully embrace in your family; to protect, to enjoy, and to love forever. This is my child to love always, to care about, and to remember. I enter into this agreement with sadness, hope, and sincere thanks.

I feel that security and stability for my child can best be provided through adoption. Know that I thought long and hard about this and finally concluded that adoption was the most unselfish and caring decision I could make. Please impart my boundless love to our child, and again, accept my thanks and honor my trust in you.

***Meet some teens who have chosen adop-
tion:*** Elizabeth, a fourteen-year-old from Los Angeles, made the adoption arrangements while she was
still pregnant. She told us:

> I don't believe in abortion, but I knew I couldn't
> take care of a baby. I'm too young to be a mother.
> So when I got pregnant I knew I'd give the baby
> up. I got in touch with Catholic Charities, and they
> arranged it for me. I think about him sometimes,
> but I know I did the right thing by him. I know
> he'll have a better home than he would have had
> with me.

Rosa also decided to give her baby up for adoption.
We met her at a maternity residence in Detroit. She
was nearly nine months pregnant when she said:

> By the time I found out I was really pregnant, I was
> already six months gone, so abortion was out. I'm
> just in junior high school, and I know right now I
> couldn't be a good mother. I'm just a kid myself. I
> came here since I knew I couldn't stay at home.
> My counselor here went over all my choices.
> When they told me about adoption, that sounded
> like the best thing for my baby. I think that to give
> the baby to a family that really wants to have a
> baby is the right thing to do. My best friend was
> adopted and she has really great parents.
> Sometimes I wish that they were my parents.

FEELINGS ABOUT ADOPTION. It's natural to have
many powerful feelings about giving your child up
for adoption. You may know that adoption is the
best choice for you and your baby but still have
mixed emotions about it. Fifteen-year-old Carly
told us:

> I wasn't ready to be a mother, not at fourteen, so I
> really had no choice. I'm relieved the whole thing
> is over now. But whenever I see a baby about my
> baby's age, I feel sad. I wonder how she is and
> what she looks like. I hope she's happy. I know
> some people think that I must not care because I
> gave her up. That's just not true.
> 　I try not to dwell on it, but it's hard. I tell myself
> that I have to get on with my life. I want to do a lot

of things for myself before I can be a good mother
to anyone. If I had kept the baby it would have
ruined both of our lives. At least now my baby has
a chance.

Seventeen-year-old Myra gave up her baby for adoption last year:

> I know I did the right thing. The hardest part was
> dealing with everyone about what I did. My friends
> said, "How could you give up your own flesh and
> blood like that?" They told me that I was cold. My
> mom said she would keep it and raise my baby
> like it was her own. No, thanks, that wouldn't have
> been doing my baby a favor. In the hospital I could
> hear the nurses talking about me. That really hurt!
> Nobody can really make a judgment about me
> 'cause they don't know my situation like I know it.

Because pregnancy and giving up a baby for
adoption involve so many feelings, it will help to talk
with someone you trust both before and after the
adoption. Keeping your feelings bottled up inside can
make you depressed and lonely. Telling someone else
about what's troubling you almost always relieves
some of the pressure. Julie was sixteen when she
gave her baby up:

> After I had the baby and gave her up for adoption,
> I felt very empty inside. I had trouble sleeping,
> because I would keep dreaming about the baby. I
> had the same nightmare over and over again. I
> was holding a baby and singing to it. I felt all
> peaceful inside, because the baby was cooing
> and smiling. But when I went to give it a bottle, I
> realized I was just holding a blanket. The baby
> had disappeared.
> 　That dream kept haunting me. I'd remember it
> even while I was awake. Finally I called the
> adoption agency, and they gave me the name of a
> social worker to call. She was very nice, really,
> very nice, and she didn't mind when I kept crying
> about the baby. I always felt before that no one
> wanted to hear me talk about the baby. My mother
> kept telling me to try to forget it, and my best
> friend kept saying I should just not think about it
> anymore. But of course you can't just stop thinking

about something. I'm sure that I won't always be feeling this way, but for now it's comforting to be able to talk to my social worker. She's very understanding.

Fathers, of course, may also have strong feelings about giving their babies up. Seventeen-year-old Ruben is from Iowa:

It was heavy. I don't talk about it too much. I mean it wasn't like Sharleen was my girlfriend. We just had a good time together. I didn't see her for a while, and then the next thing she tells me is that she's pregnant and she's giving the baby up for adoption. I couldn't believe it! First I thought she was kidding. Then I swore up and down that I couldn't be the father, but deep down I think that I probably am. I haven't seen her for a long time now, but I heard she did put the baby up for adoption. Sometimes I think about that a lot. It was a boy, I heard. I keep wondering who adopted him. I wonder if he is mine. I wonder if he looks like me. I wonder how he's doing. I'm sure now that I want to have a kid of my own someday.

Ruben and other fathers we interviewed have been deeply affected by the experience of adoption. They think about their babies and wonder about them a lot. It's natural for that to happen, but feelings can be very strong, and fathers, too, can benefit from good counseling. Find someone to talk with who will listen and help you through this difficult time.

Most parents who give their babies or children up for adoption do it because they feel it is the right thing, the best thing to do under the circumstances. Sad, disappointed, and angry feelings are part of the experience for almost everyone, but there might also be a sense of your own strength for having been able to do what you felt was best for yourself and your baby. An eighteen-year-old boy from New York told us:

My girlfriend and I talk about the baby a lot. He would have been a year old this month. Father's Day just passed and I got very depressed, but I know we did the right thing. Jeannie and I both know we weren't ready to be parents. We couldn't have given our baby anything, and now he's

probably with parents who really wanted to have a baby badly. I think the whole experience made me and Jean grow up a lot. We're real careful now—like, we never take chances anymore by not using birth control or anything like that. We want to plan our lives and enjoy our lives. I think we're a lot closer now.

MAKING AN ADOPTION PLAN. It's best for your child if he or she is put up for adoption as soon after birth as possible. One important thing to consider is that most people want to adopt a newborn baby. It is sometimes harder to find homes for older children. Also, for your sake, it may be wiser to give up the baby before you live with him or her and grow attached as a parent. It is never easy to relinquish a child for adoption, since parents usually feel connected to their babies even before they are born. But the earlier the adoption takes place, the easier it is on both you and the baby. Make sure long-term counseling is part of your adoption plan, because counseling will help you deal with your feelings.

Most important, it is best for a baby not to be separated from the people who care for him or her. Even very young babies grow attached to the adults who take care of them, and the sooner your baby goes to his or her family, the better adjustment he or she will be likely to make.

If you can and are ready to make adoption arrangements while you are still pregnant, do so, but regardless of when you make the arrangements, you can't sign legal papers surrendering your baby for adoption until after he or she is born.

After the baby is placed with an adoptive family, the family is monitored and supervised for one to six months to make sure that the adoption plan is working out before the adoption is finalized. The amount of time the adoptive family is monitored varies from state to state.

At age sixteen, Patricia, who spoke before, gave up her daughter for adoption. She wanted us to let you know how her story turned out:

I married and had two more children, two sons, and life was good. Then when she was sixteen years old, my daughter found me. I felt as if I had been dropped into a pool of ice water that woke me; then a hot volcano of long denied feelings erupted. I had hoped she would find me, but I had no idea it would be like this. I was so grief-stricken, as if she had been born and given up just the day before. But it was safe to feel the sadness now that she was back in my life, because I could also feel the joy of our reunion. When we met in the airport six weeks later, we held onto each other and cried for several minutes. Our deep connection had been full, strong, and unbreakable.

It has been over eight years since she found me. She has since married and lives across the country from me, but we talk by phone and e-mail often. She has met most of her birth relatives on my side of the family, as well as her birth father. I'm ecstatic that she's back in my life. Yet sometimes I still feel deep pain for having been separated from her and for the loss of what might have been.

How to Make Adoption Arrangements

If you want your child to be legally adopted, you have to work through a licensed adoption agency or arrange an independent adoption through a lawyer. In either case, a state judge will give final permission for an adoption. To find an agency that can help you:

➤ Look in the business pages of your phone book under Adoption. You should find a listing for the Boys and Girls Aid Society. They are an agency that can help you with a variety of adoption choices. Call them to find out their policies.

➤ In the business pages under Adoption, you may also find a listing for Open Adoption agencies. Call for information about open adoptions. One such agency, Open Adoption and Family Services, has offices in Oregon and Washington State: 1-800-772-1115. Another open adoption agency, Spence-Chapin, at 1-800-321-LOVE, offers services in the East.

➤ National Council For Adoption (NCFA) 1-202-328-1200. This agency deals with closed adoption services in which the birth parent is not given the opportunity to know where her baby is being placed.

➤ The Department (or Bureau) of Child Welfare in your state. It is sometimes called Children's Services Division. Call them for information about adoption agencies.

➤ Catholic Charities; the Federation of Protestant Welfare Agencies; the United Federation of Jewish Philanthropies— these agencies can refer you to adoption resources

RESOURCES

Where to Get a Pregnancy Test

Department of Health Clinics. Check the phone book under the name of your state or county Department of Health.

Planned Parenthood. Call this toll free number: 1-800-230-7526.

Local Community Health Clinic. Look in the business pages.

Pregnancy Services or Family Planning listed in the business pages.

Abortion Services

National Abortion Federation, toll free, at 1-800-424-2280.

Planned Parenthood: 1-800-230-7526.

Health and Counseling Services for Pregnant or Parenting Teens

Department of Health: check your local phone book under the state or county agencies.

Planned Parenthood: 1-800-230-7526.

Your school health clinic or the school nurse.

Your local hospital.

Foster Care

Department of Child Welfare: each state has its own service.

United Community Services.

Maternity Homes or Maternity Shelters.

A social worker at your local hospital or health clinic.

Adoption

Adoption services are available in every state of the United States. Most arrange traditional closed adoptions. Open adoptions are legal in only a few states, but other states have made adjustments to their laws to allow more flexibility with adoption rules. To find out what options are available in your state, you can call one of the numbers listed here:

Department of Child Welfare: each state has its own service.

Spence-Chapin Agency: 1-800-321-LOVE (5683) (New York area)

Open Adoption and Family Services: 1-800-772-1115 (Northwest)

Helpful Organizations

In every state there are excellent resources for pregnant and parenting teenagers. We cannot list them here for want of space. We have chosen to list one, as an example. You can call for a referral to resources closer to where you live.

The Door—A Center of Alternatives. 121 Avenue of the Americas, New York, NY 10013. 1-212-941-9090. This center is in New York City, but counselors there have information about teen health centers in other areas. The Door provides support groups, prenatal and postnatal health care, counseling, adolescent parenting services, and many other health and education services not related to pregnancy. It has an alternative high school, HIV services, drug awareness and treatment programs, crisis intervention services, and legal aid.

Books and Publications

Foster Care Youth United. A magazine published every other month by Youth Communication, 144 West 27th St., Suite 8R, New York, NY 10001. Phone: 1-212-242-3270. This magazine is written by teens in the foster-care system. It will give you some insight into what it's like living in a foster-care household.

Open Adoption: A Caring Option, by Jeanne Warren Lindsay. Morning Glory Press, 1987 (6595 San Haroldo Way, Buena Park, CA 90620-3748. Phone: 1-714-828-1998).

The New Our Bodies, Ourselves, by the Boston Women's Health Book Collective. New York: Simon & Schuster. Latest edition. An excellent resource on all aspects of pregnancy and childbirth.

Teen Dads: Rights, Responsibilities, and Joys, by Jeanne Warren Lindsay. Morning Glory Press, 1993 (6595 San Haroldo Way, Buena Park, CA 90620-3748. Phone: 1-714-828-1998).

Teens Parenting, a series of books by Jeanne Warren Lindsay. Morning Glory Press, 1991 (6595 San Haroldo Way, Buena Park, CA 90620-3748. Phone: 1-714-828-1998). Easy-to-read, informative books on many aspects of life for pregnant and parenting teenagers.

What Do I Do Now?—Talking About Teenage Pregnancy, by S. Kuklin. New York: G. P. Putnam's Sons, 1991.

Changing Things 12

Sometimes it seems as if nobody cares. You would think all the focus on AIDS, gangs, child abuse, substance abuse, and teen pregnancy would bring sympathy and help for young people, but instead an atmosphere of blame seems to prevail. Lots of teens agreed with seventeen-year-old Bryon, who said:

> All the time people say we're dumber, greedier, lazier, more violent than any generation before us. We're the slackers. It's like they think we're the symbol for everything that's wrong with America.

Uma added this story about an encounter between her and her mother:

> One day, I was lying around the house, and I mentioned I was bored. My mom, usually a very nice lady, went ballistic on me. She said no wonder I was bored, that my friends and I never did anything for anybody, never thought of anybody but ourselves. I was blown away. At first I was just angry, like, What gave her the right to say those things? But I'm really surprised she saw us like that. My friends and I are good people. We care a lot about the world.

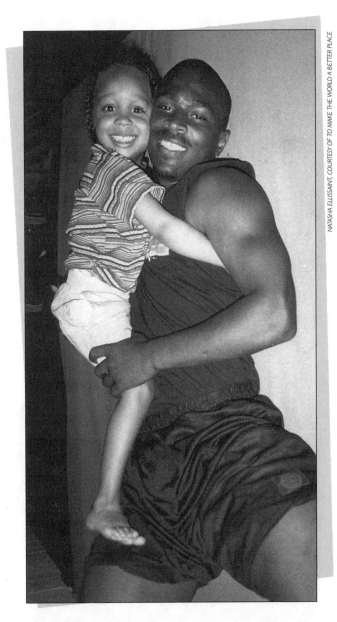

Teenagers all over the world are taking things into their own hands, lending their muscle and time to fixing up their communities and helping out people who are in need. They are solving problems with an energy and a spirit that often amaze adults and even surprise the teens themselves. As more and more teens discover they have a voice that deserves to be heard, they are finding creative ways to advocate for their ideas. Aaron, seventeen, told us:

> I think there's a big problem in this town with the police, who're always looking at kids to do something wrong. So I asked this cop if she'd be interested or if she knew any police that'd be interested in getting together with a group of kids. And the police just coming in regular clothes and just talking about why they have those feelings toward us and why they harass us so much and why they're so afraid of us. She liked the idea and said she'd try to get as many cops as I wanted,

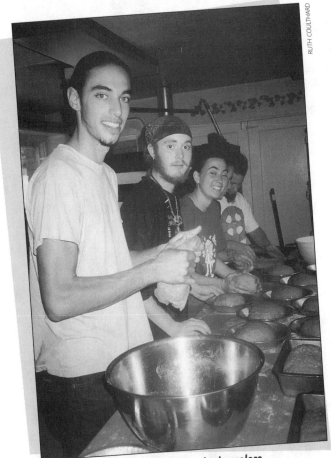

RUTH COULTHARD

Pax Panis teens bake bread for the homeless.

and she'd find a place to have it. Then I brought it up in my English class, and people just started flipping out on it, saying, "Man, I would love to talk to the cops." And not like they wanted to say "F——k you." But they actually want to let the cops know what they're feeling and how the relationship between kids and cops could be better. I was really surprised that so many people would be interested in doing it.

This chapter describes some examples of how one individual, or one small group of friends, or the teens in a community recognized a problem and decided it was up to them to fix it. They came up with their own solutions to problems—usually not fancy or complicated ideas but simple things that worked. Instead of being overwhelmed and disheartened by the world, they found out that what each one of us chooses to do can and does make a difference.

PAX PANIS

Once a week, a collective of young people in Southern Oregon gets together to bake bread and then give it away—fresh and hot—to homeless people, single mothers, seniors, runaways, anyone who's hungry. They call themselves Pax Panis, which means Peace Bread. Some of the teens in Pax Panis have been homeless or in need themselves. Some are high school dropouts. Many were already politically active before they started baking bread, but they all agree: baking bread and giving it away is a different kind of activism. Lily and Ati said:

> This is another aspect of our politics. It's more peaceful than our political struggles. It feels really good because here we can *create* something instead of our usual stance of fighting *against* something. It's so nice to give away warm bread to people who are hungry.

Braxton, one of the collective's founding members, said:

> I like the way the work is done on a community basis. Anyone can come and bake with us and anyone can have the bread we bake. I like that it's open for all people to help with and free for all

people to benefit from. When you create something this way, it's a lot more rewarding than just buying and selling. It's a way for us to reach out and act on our ideals.

And Tyler said:

When you're baking bread, you have a lot of time to talk while the bread is rising. It's nice to be part of a group. Doing work like this makes you a member of your community rather than just a resident of a place.

When the group began to expand, with new teens joining nearly every week, their vision began to expand too. They decided a community-wide garden would be their next project. Brian told us:

We started by asking around town to see if people would let us work their gardens for them, share the harvest with them, and then donate the rest of the food to soup kitchens, or set up free meals in the park. We got a lot of support right away, because of our bread-baking work. When I went to companies to ask for donations of seeds and tools, all I had to say was "I'm with Pax Panis" and they would say, "Oh, I've heard about the bread thing. I guess you're actually going to follow through with this new thing too." People knew who we were because of the work we'd done. Doors started opening for us.

In another action, Pax Panis raised money to travel to Guatemala with an adult adviser, where they delivered a donated ambulance to a very poor rural community. While there, they designed and planted the first fully organic garden in the area, and they helped a local man turn a garbage dump into a functioning recycling center. Tyler said:

Before we arrived, Felipe had already been working for months to transform the dump. He had this plan to eventually make it a financially self-sufficient recycling center by selling scavenged items, returning containers to major companies, and selling compost. We spent days helping separate nondegradables from partially decomposed compost. We also built a roof to provide shade for the workers at the site, and we laid a cement slab so trucks could drive in. When we left we knew that we had helped Felipe get further along the path to realizing his vision. It was a good feeling.

*   *   *

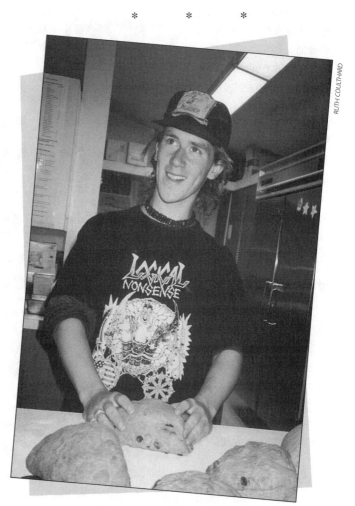

RUTH COULTHARD

Wherever you are, all you have to do is look around to see what needs to be done. Whatever you feel like doing, that's the place to begin. Ellen had spent time as a homeless teen on the streets of Seattle. After she got her life together, she returned to the same area to help out at the local teen shelter. She offered this advice:

You don't have to take on the whole world. I've lost my interest in big ideas and big corporations and the big plans of big government. I like to do the small, one-on-one things, like asking someone a question about their life and then really listening to what they have to say, finding out what someone needs right now and then trying to help them get it. Maybe it turns out that being listened to was all they really needed. Or maybe it turns out that hearing their story was what I really needed that night.

As you read this chapter, think about what in the world motivates you—something that makes you so excited or so outraged that you want to get up out of that chair and do something. What you actually do will be a combination of what you perceive needs doing, what you like to do best, and what you discover other people are already doing.

WHY BOTHER?

Why help? Because it can make a real difference. In fact, you don't have to do much; sometimes just your presence can be enough. Justine, who was seriously injured in an accident, said:

My friends came every day and just sat with me in my room. I would never have made it without them. But you know, the funny thing was, they kept worrying that they weren't doing enough, or weren't saying the right things. I wanted to shake them and say, "Don't you know how beautiful and wonderful you are?" They were keeping me alive day by day, but they couldn't see it—they were blind to their own magic.

Sometimes what you do seems like the only logical thing *to* do in a particular situation. But if you didn't do it, maybe it wouldn't get done at all. Cyndi, who lives in Oklahoma, told us,

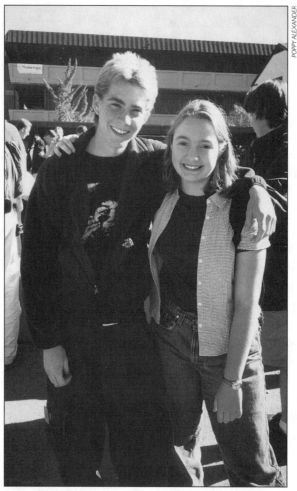

Good friends help each other.

My friend's mother was really sick, and they had no money for an operation. Social Services said she would have to be off work for 90 days to quality for a health card from the state. But she couldn't just quit her job and wait 90 days. I thought this was so dumb. I called our state representative up on the phone. They tried to get rid of me, but I wouldn't hang up. After I said I was twelve years old and I would call the newspaper and tell everyone about it, they put me right through. I told our state representative about the situation, and my friend's mom had her health card the next day. Even I couldn't believe it.

When you're feeling down, maybe a friend who's really depressed will call, and after you talk to her you realize that in helping her feel better, you feel better too. Miles, a high school student, told us about how helping a friend changed him:

My friend Cherie got pregnant. Another friend of mine was the father, but now Cherie hated him, and he wasn't handling the whole thing very well anyway. Then Cherie asked me to be her birth coach. I did it. It was incredible, going to the doctor, the classes, being at the birth. I don't think my friends or my teachers or my family really thought I could pull it off. I was a very withdrawn kid, and it was a big commitment. But this was the greatest thing that ever happened to me. It turned my life around. First off, I learned a lot about women. Also, when that little boy came out, and I held him, it was like I knew some big secret about life that most people didn't know yet.

Often helping is not even something you think about. A little kid falls off his bike, you stop and help him up. A friend is crying, you spontaneously say, "What's wrong?" and you drop everything you are doing at that moment to listen. Mica, sixteen, told us about the time she helped someone she didn't know very well:

I was at this party, and everyone there except me was drinking and smoking. I stayed all night, and at one point there was this boy lying on the porch who had thrown up and was really cold and blue-looking. He was lying in vomit and he was passed out. I tried to get other people to help me, but everyone was too drunk or stoned to really help much. They kind of put me down for even making a big deal about it. But I found a blanket and wrapped him up and I kept taking his pulse. Every once in a while I kind of woke him up by shaking him, and finally I got him to drink some water and walk into the bathroom and clean up. I think maybe I saved his life. And that night made it clear to me that drugs and alcohol are definitely not the way I want to go.

Louis, from San Diego, shared this story with us:

My friends and I were the only people who saw this train hit a pickup truck. So we stopped our car and ran down this hill to help. We worked together like we were all part of one machine; it was amazing. We got blankets from the car, we stopped people from bleeding, we removed glass, we held the kids. When the ambulances finally came, they asked where we came from. We pointed back and looked up at our car. It was way up there, on a huge cliff, nothing we would ever think of climbing down. But none of us could remember getting down as being difficult at all. I still wonder how we did it. But, mostly, I think it was just that we could have done anything because we *had* to do something.

Louis's story points out something that came up a lot: how good it feels to be a part of a group. It's not just what you and your group *accomplish* that's important; what also feels good is how you did it, the *process*. You feel part of something bigger than yourself.

THE TEEN THEATER MOVEMENT

Teens are coming together across the United States to create theater companies that write and perform original plays about important issues in teenagers'

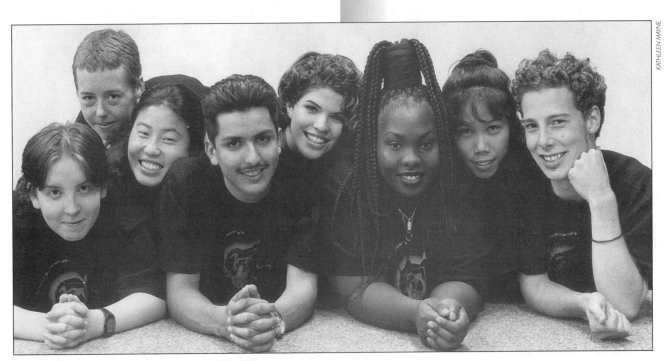

KATHLEEN MAYNE

1995–1996, the fifteenth season cast of IMAGES.

own lives. Teen theater troupes believe that when peers educate one another about things like sexually transmitted disease, rape, child abuse, violence, relationships, safer sex, racism, prejudice, emotional health care, and family matters, the learning that takes place is always more powerful than when it comes from school or books.

Teen theaters are usually sponsored by Planned Parenthood or the Red Cross or a local church or school or hospital. Often there's an adult director/coordinator, and sometimes more than one adult on staff, but teenagers themselves are always the core of the troupe. They choose the material, write the skits, design the props and costumes, and act the parts. They perform their shows for other teens in schools, religious groups, and residential centers, and sometimes they perform for adult audiences too.

The actors learn about sexuality, emotional and physical health, and substance abuse as part of their training. Keith, a teen theater member from the Midwest, said he's really glad about that:

My friends come to me and ask questions about sexuality, about addiction, about AIDS. They know we're highly educated in the facts, and I feel good about sharing the information. And even sometimes when they don't ask, I'm not afraid to bring up the subject or even confront them, because I've learned how dangerous some of that stuff is.

The plays these teenagers create come from their own life experiences, so a lot of their work as a group centers around sharing personal stories with one another and then developing those stories into performance material. A member of the Planned Parenthood Teen Theatre of Detroit, said:

We talk about sex in the company rehearsals. We talk about everything. There is nothing I can't tell these people. And sometimes when you can't answer your own questions, it feels really good to get feedback from everyone else. I've learned so much.

The performance skits range in length from short scenes to one-act plays, but they all have one thing in common: the message. Each play is about something teens need to know. One group had a skit about Prince Prophylactic (a prophylactic is a condom) fighting off an array of evil diseases. Another skit was about date rape, but they did it as a parody by turning the tables and accusing one of the male characters of making his car so tantalizing and irresistible that his date couldn't help stealing it. The whole point is to get the audience thinking and talking. Nakia said:

We end each performance with a little jingle. Then quick bow, grab a chair, and talk with the audience. Usually the audience is shy about asking us questions, so we start firing questions at them to see if they got the facts: "What's the most common STD?" "How long can HIV symptoms take to show up?" That gets things rolling, and then the talk just starts.

I'm really happy about the way we will just go in and tackle any issue.

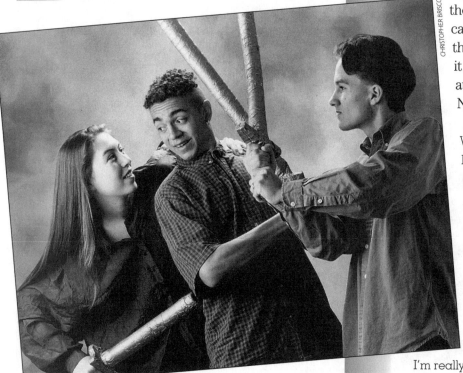

CHRISTOPHER BRISCOE

Three members of a teen theater group.

Clarinda, from the Crater Cabaret, remembered,

> One time, after seeing us do a scene about sexual abuse, a girl from the audience came up and told us the performance gave her courage. She said she'd been abused for years, and now she knew she had to tell someone and get help. Another time, some boy who hadn't spoken a word since his brother had died a couple of weeks before, came up to talk about it to two of the actors who'd done a piece about a kid dying of a drug overdose.

Ray, from Images, a teen theater company in San Diego, said:

> I guess my favorite moment of all time was during a scene called "Mythbusters." First of all we're talking about masturbation, and the audience is giggling, because it is very funny all the myths and taboos there are about masturbation. But then we get to birth control and the lies and myths there. And this silence descends. At one point I am going on about these fake "folk methods" of birth control, like the myth that you can't get pregnant if you do it standing up, and this kid in the front row turns to another kid, punches him in the arm, and whispers really loud, "See, I told you so!"

Though teen theater performances have a powerful effect on their audiences, the actors say they themselves probably benefit even more. They're picked, through interviews and auditions, for their interest in drama and their acting ability, but also for their individual life experiences. The goal is to put together a troupe of people who have different perspectives on social issues but who are all open to learning from one another. Guthrie said:

> Okay, so I'm deaf and I'm gay. Not a combination you'd expect to be picked in a very conservative town. But the Cabaret accepted me. They were some of the first people I came out to, and we created two scenes this year on gay issues because of me. At the same time, I worked hard on my speaking voice to get it to where other people could understand me. I guess you could

say the Cabaret helped me find my voice, in more ways than one.

Katherine, from the Detroit troupe, told us:

> I go to a school in the suburbs where there's a big emphasis on what's "perfect"—the perfect cheerleaders, perfect clothes, perfect hair; and it's a relief to get away to rehearsals with actors from the city; it helps me to know that the whole world does not have to be like my high school. Maybe by being in an interracial company, I'm more aware when someone at my school makes racist comments. I can say, "I work with people from that school, and what you are saying is wrong, it's just a dumb stereotype."

The actors in these theater companies all agree that when you get a bunch of teenagers together and encourage them to talk about personal things, share parts of their lives, and learn information that enables them to grow, the result is awesome. Angel put it this way:

> I watched drugs destroy and kill people I love. I watched them destroy me. I've got to say it again: the real high, the best high, the safest high, and the only good high is a natural high. So stay high on life. I tell my own story in every show. It's good for me to say it. And it's a lot easier to hear another teenager tell you it's okay to say no.

*   *   *

The teens highlighted in this chapter stress that they are just ordinary people, not saints or heroes or geniuses, and that they often started what became big or famous projects just by trying to help themselves. Enrico, who is disabled, is part of the independent-living movement that has helped many disabled young people get out of institutions and start living on their own. He said:

> Disabled people are always seen as invalids and I used to read that as in-valid. After my accident, I knew I could do a lot of things myself that people didn't think I should be doing. I was always

struggling to be recognized as "able." I moved out on my own over my parents' and my doctor's protests. I wanted to be independent, and I knew if I could do it, other people could too. So I went to a couple of the people I knew from the rehabilitation center and convinced them to join me. Then, eventually, I started going around to hospitals and institutions, talking to the disabled young people who were there to tell them they had the right to try to live on their own. They didn't have to be institutionalized just because they were in wheelchairs. Fighting for the rights of the disabled has grown into a life's work for me. And the independent-living movement has grown too. In fact, it's still growing.

THE POWER TO DO SOMETHING POSITIVE

You may wonder about what to do to make things better, or worry about whether what you do is exactly right or whether you yourself are even capable of being a help since your own life is not together in the way you'd like it to be.

That's all okay. Many teens told us that their decision to help others grew out of a personal crisis. For example, Melissa didn't set out to help anyone; she was the needy one:

When my boyfriend left me, I thought I would go crazy. I cried all night and tore up my room. Before the sun came up, I decided to go walk on the beach. I was really thinking about killing myself. But when I came out of the apartment, my neighbor's two dogs were sitting there, like they were waiting for me. I liked these dogs okay, but I didn't know them all that well. They walked to the beach with me. We watched the sunrise. I threw sticks for them. For the next few days, the dogs were waiting for me every time I left the apartment. One morning, I woke up and I felt better. I decided to go to school. I got ready to leave the apartment, feeling a little guilty that I couldn't walk the dogs. But they weren't there. They were lying down the sidewalk a ways, in front of their house. They lifted their heads a little and sort of hit their tails on the ground a couple of times, but they didn't want to walk with me

either—it was like we all knew the crisis was over. How did they know that? I mean, these were just plain old dogs.

Those dogs helped me so much, I decided I wanted to have dogs in my life. When I heard about the Dogs for the Deaf program, where you train dogs to help deaf people, I decided to volunteer there after school. And now I go almost every day.

Rachel, whose younger brother was riding his bike when he was killed by a drunk driver, told us:

This was the most awful thing that ever happened in my life. But my family decided we had to do something. So we raised money to have a sign put up on the road where Adam was killed— "Your actions affect others. Drive sober. Remember Adam." We've spoken out for stricter drunk-driving regulations. For my senior project, I put together a performance of dance and poetry, based on my own feelings and also on the letters people wrote us. I wanted to share my feelings so other people who lose a brother or sister won't feel so all alone, and so that other people who want to fight against drunk drivers will have some ideas of where to start.

Experience is a powerful teacher. Sometimes looking back at periods when we were hurting the most, the end of a relationship, the death of a loved one, a serious injury, we can see that growth comes out of that suffering, and power too—the power to try to make things better.

THE R.E.A.L. SCHOOL HIV PROJECTS

The Windham R.E.A.L. School (Regional Educational Alternative Learning), in Maine, is a high school for kids who have all been through hard times and suffering. Some have been in trouble with the law. Lots say they didn't think anybody cared about what they thought or did as long as they didn't create a problem. They are "at risk" for dropping out of school, failing subjects, homelessness, drug and/or alcohol abuse, teen pregnancy, and HIV.

The teens decided to tackle the issue of HIV. With the help of their teacher, a group of students developed three award-winning projects to educate the public about HIV. The first was an hour-long video called *R.E.A.L. Kids Talk About Real Sex*, which they showed to adults and students all over Maine. Marissa, one of the student directors, said:

> Too many people are ending up with HIV or some other STD. In fact, by the time I started my HIV education at the R.E.A.L. School, I felt it might be too late for me, because I'd already gotten an STD six months before our project started. That was a definite eye opener to the lifestyle I had been living. I'd always thought "it won't happen to me," but it did. Talking to people my age about HIV helped me to understand it all better.

Carla, their teacher, explained:

> We tried to figure out how to make talking about HIV interesting, and the kids decided the best way was to make a movie about it. Somewhere along the line the idea came up to present the information like a news report, with commercials and all. Each student picked a topic about HIV education and directed his or her segment. The student was responsible for gathering all the facts and deciding how to present them in a five-minute video with a commercial as part of it. We edited all the segments together into an hour-long film. It was a lot of work, but some very exciting things began to happen when people started hearing about what we were doing. We received a $300 grant from the State of Maine, Office of HIV Education, and we got invited to a Student Leadership Conference. Nothing like this had ever happened before for these kids! We also got invited to show the movie at the state teachers' HIV Education Conference.

The students decided to do a second HIV education project, and this time they wanted to use photography. To begin, they built their own darkroom and learned what they needed to learn about the technical aspects of photography. Then they contacted some of the HIV-positive people they had become friends with while working on their video and began taking black-and-white portraits of them. One of their HIV-positive friends helped them out in

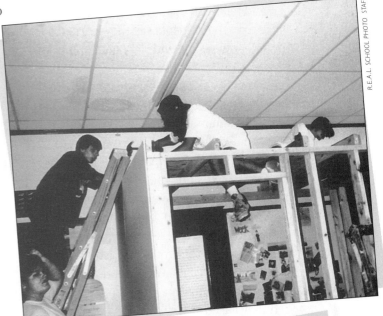

R.E.A.L. SCHOOL PHOTO STAFF

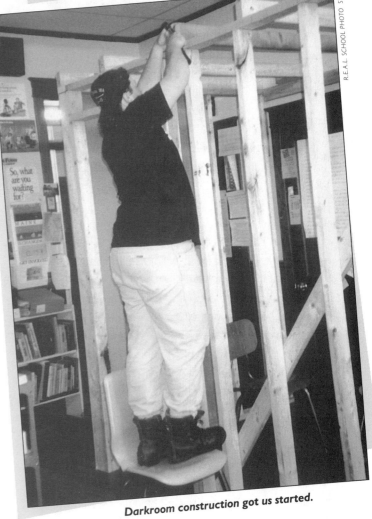

R.E.A.L. SCHOOL PHOTO STAFF

Darkroom construction got us started.

the darkroom on a regular basis. Others would come in and visit and talk with the students. As a result of these friendships, the students say they learned a lot about HIV and how people with HIV are coping with their lives.

The students chose twenty of the portraits to show in a photo exhibit, which they named the Vincent Boulanger Memorial Exhibit, after a young man they knew who had died of AIDS. The exhibit toured schools throughout Maine, helping to educate 2,500 students about HIV. In addition, their exhibit was shown at the largest art museum in the state.

To complete their project, the students collected the portraits into a poster.

By their third year, the group was getting a reputation for being very well informed about HIV, and they were invited to present a workshop on the subject, which they called *Getting Kids Involved in HIV Education*. About this time, they decided to make a public service announcement with the exhibit photos. It was thirty seconds long, showing each photo up close with the first name of the person in the photo, and reminding everyone that ordinary people get HIV.

Their next idea was to make another movie, *R.E.A.L.ities of HIV,* about the social impact of the disease—what it's really like to have HIV. This film won first prize at the Maine Student Film and Video Festival. Jason was the student director. He told us:

> For once in my life, I felt like I was having a positive effect on someone else's life, not the usual negative vibes I throw out. For the first time in my life I felt like king sh–t. People were coming up to me and saying, "Hey, I saw you on TV," and it wasn't because I was in trouble.
>
> I made people pissed at me by preaching so much about HIV. Lots of people I know don't have a clue about how someone gets HIV. Half the people don't even care, because they do so many drugs. I feel like an old fart sometimes trying to educate people.
>
> My personal life is a little weird. I'm actually abstinent presently, but I have used condoms when I was not. I'm afraid, because it seems like everybody is blind. They might just as well not have eyes. Working on the Peer HIV Projects

turned my thinking around and made me realize that HIV is a reality of everyday life.

> Before I was involved in the HIV Project, all the things I was popular for (flophouse, drugs, girls) I have a hard time admitting to now. Today I'm proud of what I know and what I did, winning prizes and awards and being encouraged in my work. If it wasn't for the people I met while doing these projects and my friends with HIV, I'd still be a go-nowhere and do-nothing instead of graduating from high school and into a photography program.

*   *   *

Young people talked about "hitting bottom" and feeling hopeless, but then pulling themselves back up by learning new skills, or speaking out, or connecting with others and insisting on change. Melanie, who lives in Montana, told us about the day she just couldn't stand the way things were anymore:

> My father was sexually abusing me and my sister. One morning I woke up and decided to tell. I planned the whole thing, I went to my aunt's house. It was a long walk, and when I got there I called the police and then I told my aunt. I didn't know who would support me, and I thought having police and family both there was the safest thing to do. Telling was the first step, but then I took my dad to court. And that was something I didn't do so much for myself but for my sister and for other girls too. It was like putting the other foot down, not just saying, "I am a victim," but saying, "I demand justice. For all of us."

Chantelle, who helped organize a referral agency for sexually abused teens, was also molested as a child:

> Even when sexual abuse has happened to you, you don't want to believe that it's true. And every time you hear a story about it happening to somebody else, you don't want to believe that it's true. And then you start adding up how many stories there are, just the ones that you have heard . . . and then you *really* don't want to believe

that it's true. You get to the point where you just know you *have* to do something to stop it.

WHAT IS "HELPING" ANYWAY?

It's important not to fall into the role of "I Am the Kind Helper and You Are the One Who Needs Help." Tina told us about going to Tijuana with her church youth group, to help out after a flood:

Inside this house where we were helping, I was digging two feet of mud out of a little girl's room, and I dug out her whole Barbie doll collection. It shocked me, because it was just like my Barbie doll collection. I guess I was thinking of them being so different from me. I was the great American, and they were the poor needy Mexicans. But when I saw her Barbies, I could feel her as a person in a way I hadn't before.

Bill, who has cerebral palsy and has been in a wheelchair since he was a child, said:

When I was growing up, I hated that word "help." Adults were always saying to other kids, "Be good and help Billy out." These little helpers were always being assigned to help me, but I could tell they didn't want to. They were just following orders. And of course, my part of the whole deal was that I had to be happy to be helped. When I turned sixteen, I became active in the disabled-rights movement. And one day someone said to me, "Why can't you accept help? If you can't accept it, you can't really give it out, either." And that made me realize that I had this really bad attitude about helping and helpers. It's great to be able to give help, but it's okay to accept help too.

Youth as Resources, an organization that works with youth offenders and the criminal justice system, uses the phrase "the dignity of the exchange," meaning that when you make a contribution and help others, it also helps you. In the program, everyone learns that society needs them as much as they need society. One student, Jamie, is a teen mother:

For my project, I visited elementary schools and talked to fourth- and fifth-graders about what it's like to be a teen mother, what it's like to try to go to high school with a baby, and work and deal with welfare. It's hard, and I think when the kids heard me talk about it, they got a sense of just how hard it is, and maybe they'll think twice before getting pregnant. I felt really good about it, like I was providing a service for the same community that was helping me out and my baby.

John and Lewis are also part of this program:

John: They always ask kids to "be good," you know. But it was too late for us. We were already in jail, too late to *be* good. But what I learned is that it is never too late to *do* good.

Lewis: I knew I was guilty, but I didn't care anything about my victims. Then they told me I was going to meet those folks I had hurt. I really was worried about it. But I got the message, "You are responsible as a human being for what you did to this other human being. And now you need to give something back." So part of what we do is work and send money to our victims.

John: And another part is to find something you can do to help the whole community. So Lewis and me coach a little kids' basketball team every Saturday morning.

Lewis: And our team is completely awesome.

For many teens helping means giving back to others some of the good things that were given to them when they needed help. Willie, who lives in a juvenile treatment center in the Midwest, told us:

I never had a father figure in my life, so this older guy helped me out. These five men in prison "adopted" ten of us in our cabin, and they sent us a video where they talked about stuff from their lives. It was real. Like about what had happened to them in high school, and what things were like with their own fathers, who were mostly mean or not there for them. They also talked about what being in prison was like. I got paired off with one of the men, and he had been where I am now, and he had thought very long and deep about what went wrong and what he had lost. He worried about me. He wanted me to get my feelings out, and he heard me when I started talking. He listened and he gave me good advice about what he knew.

So now my friend and I are "adopting" some younger kids who are getting into the same kind of trouble we did. We want to make the same kind of video, so that they won't find themselves doing all types of wrong things. We want to help them start caring about others.

TEENLINE, TEEN CRISIS HOTLINE, HELPLINE FOR TEENS

In most areas in the United States, there are toll-free phone numbers that teens can call to get help from other teens. Sometimes they're called hot lines, sometimes they're called help lines or teen lines or crisis lines; sometimes they're under individual area names, like Contact Chicago or Talkline for Teens, in Miami. Teens call in about relationship and family problems, drug- and alcohol-abuse issues, homeless/runaway situations, and suicide. The teen lines give them a place to vent their feelings and find a caring listener. Sometimes they offer the only hope for a teen in trouble.

Any teenager who's interested in volunteering at the teen hot lines can apply. LaVelle, who now works at Helpline in San Francisco, first found out about it when she called in for help herself:

I called because I had too much responsibility. My mother worked nights, and I was always taking care of my little brothers. One night I really thought I was going to kill one of them, I was so mad at him. I remembered hearing this number on the radio, so I called. The girl who answered said she could tell it was a really hard situation. She didn't know what I should do, but I could tell she wanted to comfort me. Just that someone wanted to comfort me was a big comfort.

Because of that night, I decided I wanted to work at the hot line too. Now on one of the nights that I don't have to babysit, I volunteer there. It

means I have even more responsibility now, but it feels good to know I might be there some night for someone who needed to call just like I did.

Before teens begin answering phone calls, they go through intensive training sessions, during which they learn how and where to refer people to get the kind of help they need, when to intervene with the authorities if the callers are in immediate danger to themselves or someone else, and mostly, how to be an effective listener.

Listening is what it's really all about, as two teens who staff phones in Missouri and Alaska told us:

Marla: Sometimes teens just want to talk without having to deal with critical looks or with their friends getting all sad and worried about them. When you call in here, you know that we want you to talk, that's why we're here, and we're not going to judge anyone or want them to shut up. I would never tell someone to stop crying or stop being mad.

Brandon: Before I started working at the Teen Hotline, I thought I would have to learn all the right answers to every problem. But no, what is important here is to help the caller come up with their own questions and then come up with their own answers. I mean, we are not dealing with math problems here. We are dealing with real live members of the human race.

Volunteers stressed that even after they complete all their training, they never feel alone when they're dealing with crisis calls that come in. First, you're an apprentice for a few months, with someone else right next to you to help you take calls. Then, when you start answering the calls on your own, there is always an adult mentor or facilitator in the room, and usually other teens are there as well.

Teens who staff the lines say you can choose how often you want to volunteer. Most of them work either one night a week or two nights a month. Noah works twice a month at a Teenline in the Northwest:

We don't get too many calls, just a couple most nights I'm here. Mostly we are like a big referral service. If a girl calls in and think she's pregnant, we can tell her where to get a free pregnancy test and counseling, or AIDS testing if that is what you need, or mental health counseling. In the Teenline manual, I have every number anyone could need. And after a while, you even get to know the people at most of the other crisis centers in the area, so you know who you're referring the callers to.

Charmaine works every other weekend at a Teenline in the Southwest:

We are not perfect experts here. We are just teens like the callers are, and we can feel really confused sometimes just like they do. You look at life, and sometimes you don't know what you are looking at. Sometimes people call in who are too young to even know yet that they are in real trouble. In the Teenline training, which is very intense and focused on the very serious situations, like a potential suicide, we learned how to offer emotional support, and what kinds of questions will help people keep talking until they can figure out for themselves what is wrong and what they want to do.

Sometimes teenagers call in with major crises— their life may be in danger through an attempted suicide, a beating, a fight with weapons, a drug overdose. Hot line volunteers learn how to recognize the difference between a caller who needs to talk and a caller who needs other kinds of intervention. Rasheed works for a crisis hot line in Los Angeles. He told us about the time someone called and said he'd just run away from home because his dad was drunk and beating him:

He called me from a pay phone, and it was one of those pay phones where you can't return the call. I needed to be able to call him back when I had information for him. So I had him promise he would call me back from another phone booth, and I was really relieved when he did. It was hard not to offer to get together with him myself or connect him with one of my own friends. But we're not allowed to do that, because you can see how it could turn into a real mess, and besides, what

they need to learn is that it's their life, it's their judgment what to do, and they have the ability to solve their own problems. What we can do is let them know what options are there for them, and what choices they have. In this guy's case we found him a safe house where there were adult counselors to help him.

Teens who work the phones say that although they know they are helping other teens who have problems, they are helping themselves too. C.J., from Atlanta, says:

Working here for two years has made such a big difference in my life. I was already turned on to the idea that I wanted to do something important in the world, but I didn't know where to start. I was shy and I was angry and I thought the world owed me something. Through the help line training I

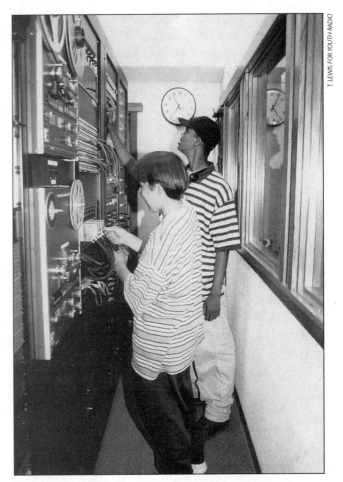

T. LEWIS FOR YOUTH RADIO

Youth Radio students in action. Checking the equipment before a broadcast.

realized that any changes that were going to happen in my life had to come from inside me. I learned to get in touch with my own power and how to let the teens who call us know that they have the power inside themselves too. Just the idea that they might have some power inside themselves to get in touch with is a big surprise to most teens. Just that idea is something. It is really quite a lot.

*　　　*　　　*

Lots of teenagers say they like to volunteer at service agencies or community centers in their neighborhoods. They give a few hours a week of their time. Djuna volunteers at a women's shelter in her city. She said,

I really like volunteering here because I've always felt strongly about wanting to help people who are in abusive situations and I really like working with kids. The work I do is to play with the kids and that's really important because a lot of these kids don't really know how to play. They come from situations where they don't really know how to have fun or be free because they've had to learn to tiptoe around and be quiet all the time. What's so great is that after a few weeks you can really see a difference. You can see them loosen up and relax.

For me it's been great because it's so easy to just get caught up in your life and feel like nothing you do really matters, but when you do something like this, you can actually see the difference you are making.

For some, volunteering turns into paid work when they have more time to give. Angie works at District 202, a center in Minneapolis for gay and lesbian youth. She told us about her job there:

I went from being a user of the center to a volunteer here to now a worker at the center. It doesn't seem like that big of a change to me. The change is mostly inside. I remember how much I needed this place when I first started coming here, and now I see how much other kids need it.

Gary, who learned masonry and carpentry in the Job Corps, told us:

I dropped out of high school; I was on the streets. There was a church basement where they used to let us hang out, and I liked it there. After the Job Corps, I came back and decided I would fix this closet in the basement so that kids could lock their stuff up. I was blown away when the church paid me for doing the work. This was my first paycheck outside of the Job Corps.

By volunteering at a place you may realize how much you enjoy doing a particular kind of work, which eventually directs you to a career in that field. But whether or not it leads you to your life's work, the moment you offer your services to help someone else or take a public stand for the values you believe in is often the beginning of a big change in your life. Travis said:

I started protesting timber sales. I thought I would change everything—or at least everyone's minds. But what really changed was me!

Aaron worked in a homeless shelter for a year:

What did it end up meaning for these people? I don't know. How much did I actually help? I don't know. I tried to do what was right. I cared a lot about them. We all did the best we could. And it's still alive for me. It still makes me choke up when I think about some of them. I haven't seen anyone from the shelter for almost a year now, but it's still going on for me. It's changed how I think about myself.

Listen to these testimonials from teens who feel they've changed because of the work they're doing:

I was really scattered. I didn't have a focus in my life. And then I started taking pictures of environmental protests, and all of a sudden I found I had a focus. All my energies got pointed in one direction.

Speaking out for animals helped me realize that I could be a force for good. I have a voice. I'm not just this polite little girl that does what she's supposed to do. I have something important to say.

The mural project gave me a forum for doing my art, a place to vent my emotions, a social life, and on top of all that a way for me to get connected with changing the city.

I was in a gang, so I know what it's like to be out there all the time running with the fast life. Now that I'm out and working in gang neighborhoods with little kids, I know that it's not just doing good for those kids. It's healing a place inside me too.

Through all of high school, I was afraid to raise my hand in class. Now I have spoken at rallies about the rights of children. I guess you could say I have gotten a lot better at speaking in front of people without feeling like I was about to pass out.

Teens from all over the country said not to worry about finding what seems like the biggest, most important project in the world. The important thing is that you are doing something positive for other people, and through that you're helping yourself too.

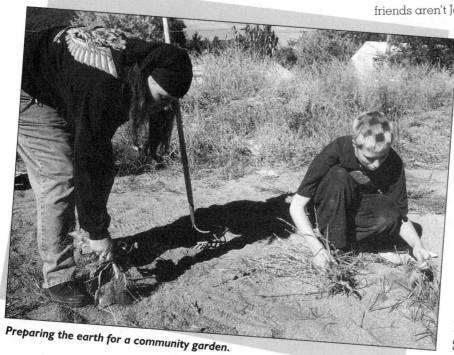

Preparing the earth for a community garden.

BEING TRUE TO YOURSELF

Especially as teenagers, lots of us feel the push to be like the people around us, to give up the ways we look and act and feel different and try to meld into the whole. But many teens discover that what is really important to them is just the opposite— exploring the ways they are unique and in that exploration finding out more about their own background, their own values, and their own experiences.

As Jacob discovered, by opening yourself up to the experiences of your own past, you may help others too:

None of my friends knew I was Jewish. I didn't know much about it either, because I wasn't raised with any religion. But I believe that it's important to know your roots, to know how you're the same as everybody else and also how you're different. So I shocked my parents and my friends by deciding to have a bar mitzvah—the Jewish rite of passage that you go through to be considered an adult. It was a lot of work, because basically I crammed three or four years of studying Hebrew and the Torah into one and a half years, but I did it, and now I feel like I am at least knowledgeable about what it means to come from a Jewish family. My friends aren't Jewish, but it was really good for them to learn about it too. So many people have prejudices against Jews, and by going through this with me, I think it made them more understanding of the whole culture that's behind Judaism.

Coya, at seventeen, set up campus-wide powwows at her college to celebrate her own Lakota identity and at the same time to give other Native Americans the opportunity to show pride in their heritage. The next year, she helped organize the first lesbian and gay high school prom in the Midwest. She said:

MICHAEL FOLEY

I don't feel like I'm consciously being an activist. I'm just doing stuff that interests me and that I care about.

Sokly, who also calls himself Don Bonus, is a Cambodian refugee who came to the United States with his family. He was having difficulties staying in high school and graduating. His life as a refugee was complicated by the violence in his inner-city neighborhood as well as by his desire to fit into American society while still staying connected to his Cambodian family and culture. During his senior year, he shot a film about his life. He called it *AKA Don Bonus*, which means "Also known as Don Bonus." He said:

The film started out to be about my struggles to graduate and just to survive my life during my senior year in high school. But it really is more than a self-portrait; it's about my Cambodian refugee family and neighbors and the ordeals we all face in the city. The film got lots of praise and won an award, and it's still being shown.

Making the film helped Sokly realize how much he wanted to remain part of the Cambodian community. After it was released, he encouraged his family to celebrate their culture by opening a restaurant:

I don't know a better way to start helping your people and your community than by providing good food, hospitality, and a warm environment where you can enjoy a traditional meal with family and friends. Having a restaurant is a lot of work, but it's worth it. We have lots of neighborhood people come in; and local workers on their lunch break. Lots of the Cambodians who come in are family friends. It's a place where we can feel comfortable and proud.

Sokly has plans to finish college and become a youth counselor for other Cambodian refugees. Sometime in the future, he also wants to make more films, but no matter what he does, he's committed to staying and working within his community.

Priya, a young woman in her twenties who helped start a substance-abuse recovery center in her community, also talks about how important it is to remember your roots, especially when your community is in crisis. She said:

People from low-income neighborhoods who become successful usually move out of the neighborhood, and that's sad for the young people in the community, because they don't get to see enough examples of successful adults. The more you have to look outside your community for examples, the less connected you feel.

NATIVE AMERICAN YOUTH ADVISORY COUNCIL

The Native American Young People's Wellness Program was established on the Yankton Sioux Indian Reservation in Lake Andes, South Dakota, to promote leadership and good health in the Native American teen community. About eighteen Native American teens make up the Wellness Program's Youth Advisory Council (YAC). Chaske Rockboy, fourteen, is the vice president of YAC. He said:

Through the council, we're learning how to become more Indian and do our traditional ways. We're learning how things were done in the old days, because our community needs leaders who will teach the next generation. This is the way our community will survive.

The students on the council participate in powwows, sweat lodges, sundances, and Native American Church rituals. Chaske explains:

I am a traditional dancer and go to powwows to dance and to visit with friends I haven't seen for a long time. I also sing traditional songs. I follow the drum. Ceremonies and the drum have kept our people together. When you hear the drum, you know people are in a good way. That's what's important to me.

When I'm having problems and need help, I go to a sweat and ask for help from the Great Spirit. It helps me to remember who I am and how I am supposed to be—a better person, a stronger person. The sweat lodge is for purification.

In YAC we learn how to prepare for the sweat by loading up the rocks and transporting them back to the sweat lodge. The wood has to be gathered for the fire. Then the rocks have to be heated and kept hot. Every time we have a sweat, we invite new people to come. That's how we recruit new members for YAC.

Along with training in traditional Native American activities, the members of the advisory council are also learning about health issues like domestic violence, substance abuse, sexually transmitted disease, teen pregnancy, alcoholism, and fetal alcohol syndrome. They pass the information they learn on to the other teens in their community. Frances, thirteen, said:

The workshops on date rape taught me that girls have the right to say no. I talked to my girlfriends about that, but they didn't understand the problem. It's not easy for girls here to feel strong about themselves. I'm going to keep talking to them until they get it. We also learned about what alcohol and cigarettes can do to your body. I told my friends about that too, and some of them stopped smoking because of it.

Brandon, age twelve, is also on the council:

We're opening a hot line. If you have problems, the hot line can help you. I'm kind of excited about the hot line opening up, because it'll give people a place to call when they're in trouble. We're going to help answer calls when it opens, and we've already helped put together the hot line manual and collect information about what kind of problems and questions teens have.

Council members know there are a lot of problems to deal with in their community stemming from extreme poverty, racism, and U.S. government policy, which for over two hundred years tried to wipe out traditional Native American culture and teachings. Many teens on the reservation are apathetic.

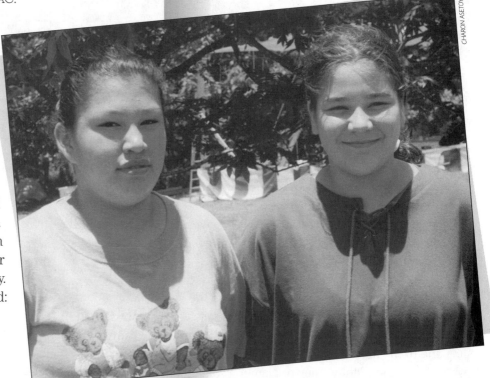

CHARON ASETOYER

They get involved with drugs and alcohol. They don't feel the future holds too much hope for them. The high school dropout rate is over 60 percent. The suicide rate is high too, and so is the rate of teenage pregnancy. Council members want to change that. They hope their hot line and their outreach will give Native American teens the feeling that there is a safety net for them, that the community cares about them.

The teens in YAC agreed that one big problem is the lack of activities available for teenagers on the reservation. Brandon said:

It's really boring here. There's nothing for teenagers to do. That's why everybody just hangs out on the street or stays home arguing with the people in their family. There's nothing to do.

The closest movie theater is 75 miles from their reservation. A water slide is 150 miles away. So YAC members decided they wanted to raise enough money to pay for field trips to those places.

The Resource Center gave them $100 as "seed" money, and with that, the council members started a food business to raise the necessary funds for their activities. Chaske describes it:

> The first thing we did, we had a bake sale. Then we had a taco sale, then a cinnamon roll sale, and we sold food at the VFW twice. We buy all the stuff we need out of the money we made the time before. The whole council decides what we're going to sell. We all have an equal voice. Each time we make money, the Resource Center matches what we make. It's a business. We've made over $1,000.

With their money the council has gone to the Northern Plains Tribal Art Show, about 150 miles from the reservation. They've also gone to the water slide and to the movies, and they put on a Halloween party for the community. They're planning some teen dances on the reservation. Chaske summed up his feelings about being on the council:

> I like the way in YAC that we help each other and help ourselves learn how to be together and work together and do the traditional things on our own. It makes me feel like I can put something back into the community. Knowing that I can do things for other people makes me high-spirited. It makes me feel like I'm out of the dark and walking in the sunshine.

*   *   *

WHAT TO DO?

When we talked to teens about what they'd like to change, they spoke about the environment, about homelessness, poverty, violence, and human rights.

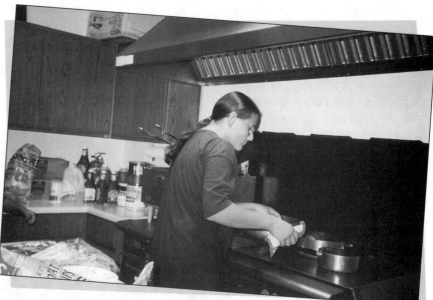

CHARON ASETOYER

Getting ready for a food sale.

They said they think everyone needs a decent education, a decent place to live, and the prospect of a decent way to earn a living.

YOUTHBUILD

YouthBuild began in 1978 when a group of thirteen-, fourteen-, and fifteen-year-olds from East Harlem in New York City decided they wanted to fix up an abandoned building in their neighborhood. Chantay, one of the original group, said:

> I remember we wanted to clean out a building to make us a home away from home or something. We weren't really sure how we could do it—we just knew we wanted to try.

They approached two of their favorite teachers and asked for help. David remembers:

> When they came to me and Dorothy, I said to them, "I don't think we can do it. It takes too much work. It takes skills. It takes money." But they said, "Come on, David. Let's go do it! We want to fix up that building." Well it took five years! But by the time we got through with that building, there were places for six young mothers to live with their children as well as two other single apartments, and three commercial units on the ground floor.

And we knew we had done something that was worth doing again.

The success of that building project spawned others in New York City, and eventually similar programs in over a hundred cities throughout the country. Now YouthBuild is a national organization in which teenagers and young adults fix up and rebuild old, abandoned buildings to create permanent housing for the homeless and for young people living in poverty.

The program is also about building confidence and self-respect for the young people who participate. One teen standing in a newly renovated building said as she pointed to a run-down place across the street:

It's a very good feeling when you see a building like that and then you see it finished like this. You see what our work can do.

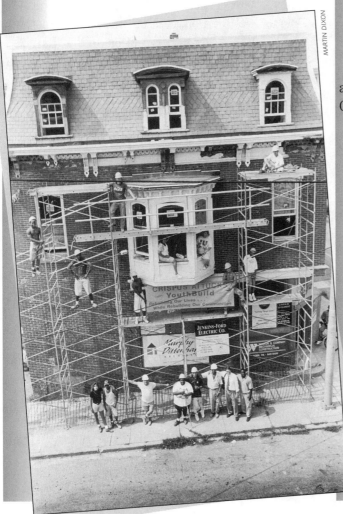

MARTIN DIXON

Young people want to take charge of their lives and make changes in the world around them. To do that they need education and marketable skills that can bring them economic independence. Through YouthBuild, teens and young adults who are without work or adequate education are offered the opportunity to learn a wide variety of construction skills, to earn their driver's license, to complete their high school diploma or GED, and to participate in leadership training. They receive a stipend for the work they do, but even more important, they receive good on-the-job instruction and academic tutoring so that when they graduate from the program they have skills and credentials. Connie said:

I'm studying to be an electrician now. That's what I want to become. It's hard because of the environment I live in. You can't be out with all the teenagers just hanging around if you want to get somewhere. You've just got to keep a strong head and go for what you want to go for.

Teens who want to join YouthBuild go through an application process and a rigorous orientation. One of the administrators said,

It's not a question of just wanting to work, it's a question of showing that you're ready to work. It doesn't matter to us if you're homeless or if you never finished high school or have been in a gang. We can help teens with their skills, but they need to come with an attitude that says, I want to do this and I'm prepared to do what I need to do to get something out of it. Young adults who express their initiative by showing up on time, by completing the application process, by being able to work with others in a group, by demonstrating commitment in the orientation, they're the ones who find success in this program.

YouthBuild participants learn that doing the best job they can really does matter, because people are going to live in the houses they build. As Connie said:

When I finish this place it's going to be terrific. They're going to *want* to live in here when I finish with it!

YouthBuild is a democratically run organization that believes adults and teens can work together, sharing responsibilities and successes. Young people who may have spent a lot of their lives feeling like failures end up feeling empowered by a system that respects their hard work and commitment. Eighteen-year-old Mike said:

It means a lot to me. It's really hard work, and you think you're never going to finish, but when you do it's a great feeling. I'm a father. I left school in the tenth grade, and I had no job or anything. It was really sad for me. Now I know I have leadership qualities. I have skills. I know I can get a good job.

*　　*　　*

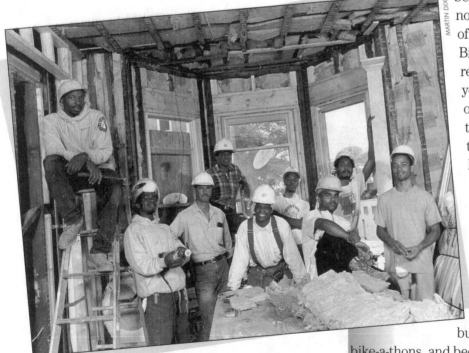

Teenagers realize that the world is complex and that to make things better, new questions need to be asked and new ways found to meet life's challenges. Many expressed disgust with a government that doesn't seem to be doing enough to help people. They complained about politicians who have no orig-

inal ideas or effective ways of dealing with the problems everyone knows exist. YouthBuild started from nothing and found a way to make more homes for the homeless *and* create jobs for young people. Bikes Not Bombs is another organization that took an old problem and found a new solution.

BIKES NOT BOMBS

When Bikes Not Bombs started in the 1980s, our country was sending weapons to Nicaragua during their civil war. The people in Bikes Not Bombs decided to send bicycles instead, both to give the local people transportation and to make a statement about how we can help one another peacefully. To date, the teens in Bikes Not Bombs have rebuilt and sent over 14,000 recycled bikes to Nicaragua. They now supply bikes to a program in Haiti too.

Since 1984, Bikes Not Bombs has run a Bicycle Repair and Recycling Center in inner-city Boston. The teens who spend time there believe in bicycles as a natural, nonpolluting, inexpensive method of transportation. In the "Earn-A-Bike" program, by volunteering to repair old bikes, any interested young person can earn a bicycle of his or her own. Hundreds of teenagers have earned bikes through this program, and they have learned how to build and repair bikes for themselves and others.

Teens and preteens learn from other teenagers who have already completed the classes in mechanics and bicycle repair. The teens who stay on to become instructors study business management, organize bike-a-thons, and become active in local clean-air initiatives. Antonio, now nineteen, has worked with Bikes Not Bombs in Boston for seven years:

I first came to Bikes Not Bombs when I was twelve years old. I had just moved to Boston from Puerto Rico and a friend told me about the Earn-A-Bike program. In those days we didn't even have a

MARTIN DIXON

center. We ran the Earn-A-Bike program in a park. A local bike shop and a hairdresser let us store our bikes in their basements, and on Wednesday evenings we used the bike shop for bike repair classes. I earned a ten-speed Raleigh, which is still in my basement, and now I have a mountain bike and a racing bike too, both of which I custom-built from the frame up.

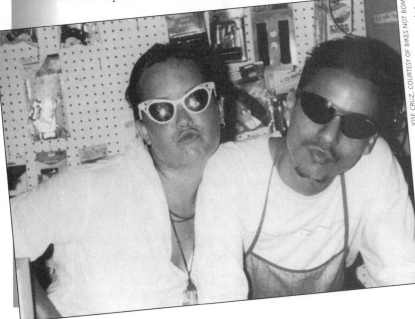

ANTONIO GONZALES, COURTESY OF BIKES NOT BOMBS

I took all the bike repair classes the group offered, plus the instructor training and the vocational training classes, and then I went on salary four and a half years ago when I was fifteen. Now I'm a shop manager and head mechanic. I also teach kids how to repair bikes, and I lead bike trips.

JOSE CRUZ, COURTESY OF BIKES NOT BOMBS

Bikes Not Bombs has helped set up bike shops in Nicaragua and Haiti that employ and train young people. In Nicaragua, one of the training centers is run by disabled teens and young adults, many of whom were injured in their country's civil war.

The teenagers in Bikes Not Bombs spend many weekends, holidays, and school vacations on the road, sponsoring community bike trips that may last anywhere from a couple of hours to a few days. In addition, these teens get involved in community health issues, teach bike safety to younger kids, gain environmental awareness, and advocate for the use of bicycles instead of cars.

*   *   *

Many of the teenagers we met believe the world can be a better place. They are motivated to use their energy and commitment to further that goal. They think in global terms, realizing that what each one of us does ultimately affects all of us on this planet.

Young people from twenty-eight nations around the world came together to talk about their concerns and their visions under the auspices of the United Nations. They drafted a proposal called "The State of the World Forum 1995 Youth Agenda for the 21st Century," in which they wrote:

Envision a world in harmony. Imagine a world without war, without violence and without poverty. Picture a world where every human being is able and encouraged to express their thoughts and desires without fear.

Teenagers all over are refusing just to sit back and wait for change to occur. They're putting their energy into making it happen. For example, Elias, a high school senior who lives in Oregon, believes that it's up to all of us to protect the environment. He himself is actively involved in actions having to do with saving the old-growth forests. He thinks that it's time for us to find new ways of doing things:

> We organized a roadblock at a timber cut. The blockade worked as a rallying point, and as a delaying tactic to keep the logging company from cutting the biggest, oldest trees. But it was just another roadblock where the environmentalists and the loggers were yelling at each other. It was very confrontational, touchy, polarized, angry. No one on either side was budging, nobody changed their mind about anything. I do feel we have to keep drawing the lines to save the forests, but I also know that the *real* solution is in all of us working together in cooperation, environmentalists and loggers, finding ways to help the timber communities and timber workers at the same time we help the environment. No real change is going to happen until we open up new ways of approaching old problems.

Jace is working for better housing conditions. He is part of an organization called Habitat for Humanity, which builds homes for low-income families:

> For my senior project in high school, I took part in building this house, and I felt so good about it. But then I looked around the neighborhood. And I'm thinking, Who is going to build all the houses for poor people? Why should anyone be homeless in this rich country of ours? I went into this with the idea of building one house at a time, but now I'm involved in the more political parts of the organization, advocating for lots more low-income housing.

Tovah, fourteen, started a website for vegetarian teenagers on the Internet:

> With the Vegetarian Youth Network, I'm trying to bring together young people so that we can empower ourselves and strengthen the vegetarian community so we can become stronger members of the global community. I believe that teenagers have to take responsibility for what we eat because what we eat has an impact on the world. We have to take responsibility for what we do too,

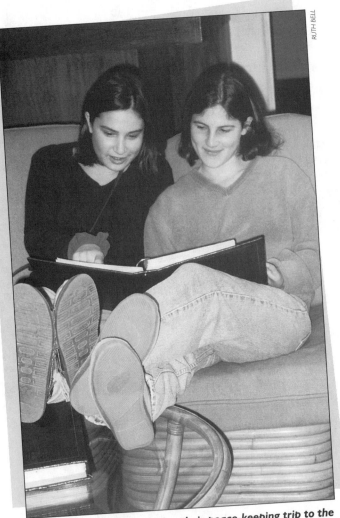

Two young women plan their peace-keeping trip to the Middle East with Earth Stewards.

because everybody's actions count. It's up to us to empower each other to heal the planet.

Four sixth-grade girls from Gloucester, Massachusetts, were concerned about how easy it was for kids to get cigarettes from the cigarette vending machines in their town. One of the girls said:

> The machines were unsupervised, so anyone could just walk up to a machine and buy cigarettes. So we came up with the idea of banning the machines.

The girls knew they needed the city council to pass an ordinance to ban the machines, but in order to get the city council to do that, they had to present an official petition to the council with enough voter signatures to warrant a public hearing. They spent the summer after sixth grade educating people, gathering signatures, meeting with city officials, and writing their proposal. By the time of the public hearing, they had collected 570 signatures.

Their proposal was controversial. Adult restaurant owners and business people talked against the ban, saying it would affect their profits. One of the four girls said:

> We couldn't understand how some people could think about making a few extra bucks when thousands of people are dying every day from tobacco-related illnesses.

At the end of the meeting, after hearing from both sides of the issue, the city council voted unanimously to ban the cigarette machines.

In northern California, the year Priya turned twenty, there were forty-two murders in her inner-city community alone. Eighty-five percent of all the violent crimes were either directly or indirectly connected to alcohol and drug abuse. The city responded to this by increasing arrests and incarceration by 250 percent. Priya joined with a group of friends and acquaintances, some young and some older, who had a different idea. They believed that to be really effective, the response had to be more long-term than just locking the offenders up. She said:

> We wanted to go for a solution that would involve education, health care, economic development, and drug treatment, so that people could overcome their addictions and the community could get healthy again.

After a year of meeting together, the group decided to put their efforts into starting a broad-based substance abuse treatment center. Called "Free At Last," their program helps people get off and stay off drugs. They provide health and education services that aren't readily available in many low-income communities.

Free At Last has outreach programs and a drop-in center staffed by over thirty community people, all of whom have been addicts themselves or have come from families involved with substance abuse. Many have been incarcerated. Many have been physically, emotionally, and sexually abused. So when a new person walks into the center, he or she sees familiar faces of people who have succeeded in changing their own lives. As Priya told us:

> It's important to remember where you come from. The people who work here and use the center are part of the community; they are known to each other. Through their own personal recovery, they become agents for change for everyone else in the community and they draw others into the center. Their own transformation is the attraction.

HOW TO BEGIN

Where do you start? How do you get something new going? Sometimes, like Tovah and the four girls from Gloucester, you have to point out that something that may not seem important to other people *is* important. Sometimes, like the Free At Last group and the teens in Bikes Not Bombs, you have to open your mind to new possibilities and figure out a whole new way of doing things, because the old way won't take you to the future you want. Mostly, you just have to have faith in yourself and know that what you have to say and what you want to do can make a positive difference.

Your activism may or may not be part of an existing program or national organization. It can grow simply from your own awareness of a problem in your community that you want to try to make better. We heard about several of these local actions through the Activism 2000 Project, which keeps track of teen action projects throughout the country (see Resource Guide, page 394). For example, some teenage girls got together in California because they didn't like the unfriendly atmosphere at a community health clinic in their neighborhood. The girls decided to set up some meetings with the director of the clinic to explain the ways they felt the clinic could improve. They convinced the director to hire teens as receptionists in the front office, in order to give the clinic a friendlier atmosphere. And it worked. Many more teens use the clinic for medical information and care now. The clinic director is happy, and the teenagers in the community are being better served.

Another local action happened in Louisiana, where some high school students were brainstorming ways to reduce the high rate of teen pregnancy in their community. They had the idea of starting a hot line for *adults*, staffed by teens. The hot line provides advice for parents on how to discuss issues like teen sexuality, abstinence, safer-sex methods, and STDs with their sons and daughters.

There is no magic formula for succeeding when you start out to do something that will make a difference. Remember, the very fact that you are both young and concerned enough to act can generate a lot of interest in the community. Here are a few guidelines for how to proceed:

SOME STRATEGIES FOR SOCIAL ACTION

Choose something that moves you. Act from your heart. In many cases, young people told us they had to find something they deeply cared about or they just got bored and quit.

Keep your inspiration alive. When you have your early vision, write it down somewhere. Keep a scrapbook of the photos or articles that got you excited about your project in the first place, so that if your vision changes or things get complicated, you'll be able to refer back to them.

Talk to everyone. Listen with particular care to those who have tried things like your idea before as well as to those who disagree with you. They'll challenge you to refine what you want to do. Try not to get weighed down by negativity or inertia.

Get a group together. Find others with similar interests. You probably aren't in this alone. It's usually more fun and more effective to work with other people.

Find out who has the power. Do your detective work. Research and interview. Use the phone, the library, the Internet, and people you meet. Write down the name, phone number, and e-mail address of anyone you may want to call on for financial or other support later on. While you research, start a list of the most influential people who might be able to help you. Don't be afraid to call community groups or government offices or the local media. Often it's to their advantage to speak with you.

Tell the World. Get the news out every way you can. If you are planning an event, telephone and send press releases.* Put up posters, write letters, fax information, use the World Wide Web, and follow everything up with more phone calls. The more interest you generate, the more likely you are to see some action. Make extra copies of articles and speeches, to hand out to reporters or whoever might want one. Give out business cards or flyers with your group's name and information about how someone can get hold of you. Start your own mailing list so you can get in touch with interested people.

Do It with Style. Proceed with confidence. Maximize the impact of your work. Appeal to people's senses. Use photographs, videotapes, charts, and graphs for visual impact; use music and recorded speech. Consider a skit or mural for a backdrop to focus attention. Your creativity in presenting your material will intensify your audience's involvement.

Shoot It. Have someone on your team videotape, tape-record, or photograph your event for future use. You may want to write an article for your school newspaper or a magazine. Someone else may want to write about you. It's useful to have a record.

Get Ready for Response. You may hear from a lot of people. You may get backlash; things will never go 100 percent the way you planned. You chose this project originally because it was

---

* A press release is usually a one-page—typed, double-spaced—statement about your event or organization that you send to newspapers and radio and TV stations.

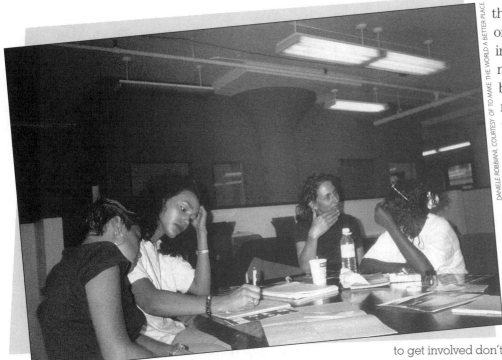

that's happening to you or someone you know or to deliver an important speech at a town meeting or to join with others to build housing for people in need. It might motivate you to volunteer at a homeless shelter, or visit a lonely neighbor, or offer your services as a tutor at a local after-school program, or address envelopes for a service organization you believe in. One of the teens who helped us with this chapter said:

The moments or turning points when people choose to get involved don't necessarily seem like any big deal to them at the time. It's not like there's a big fork in the road down there and you have to make this major decision which way to go. Almost every day there's the chance to do some good or make someone feel better, and it's those little acts of kindness or caring that all of us do that add up to making the world a better place.

important to you. Don't let setbacks discourage you—just keep yourself focused on the goal. Don't be afraid to compromise if necessary.

Look Back. Evaluate your work. Take a breather to reflect on what you've done. Meet with your group to evaluate how things went. Talk with the other teens who were at your event. Ask for a critique from a teacher or an expert in the field in which you are working. The purpose of evaluation is to look at the work you've already done to see what worked and what could be improved the next time.

Celebrate! Give a party! Celebrate your hard work and all the things you've learned.

YOU CAN MAKE IT HAPPEN!

Moving from not acting to acting is the first step. Nothing happens until you take that step. It might lead you to speak up against an injustice

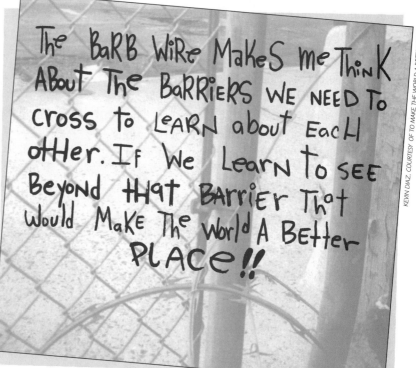

The BaRB WiRe MakeS me ThinK ABout The BARRiERS WE NEED To cross to LEARN about EacH otHer. If We Learn To SEE Beyond tHat Barrier That Would Make The world A Better PLAce!!

People who decide to participate aren't any particular kind of person. It's not a matter of being especially smart or kind or articulate or organized. It's just a matter of deciding that *you* want to do something to make things better. No matter what you decide to do, your participation will make a difference. And that's the truth.

Anne Frank was a thirteen-year-old Jewish girl. During World War II, she and her family hid from the Nazis in an attic above a factory for two years, aided by some Dutch friends. Shortly before the liberation of Holland, Anne and her family were betrayed and sent to Nazi concentration camps, where Anne died. The diary she had kept during her years in the attic was found and published after the war.* In it she made this statement of hope:

How wonderful it is that nobody need wait a single moment before starting to improve the world.

RESOURCES

There are literally thousands of organizations and activities to join and thousands more that need starting. Many of the best projects are happening at a neighborhood level. Check at your own school or community center or place of worship to see what service clubs and activities already exist in your area. Remember the slogan "Think globally, act locally."

The following resource guide is to help you connect on a national level with other young people who are working to make the world a better place. These are some examples of organizations and publications that can inspire you, provide you with information, and maybe become part of your life.

Organizations

Activism 2000 Project. P.O. Box E, Kensington, MD 20895. 1-800-543-7693. e-mail: ACTIVISM@aol.com. The Activism 2000 Project is a national network dedicated to keeping kids

* Anne Frank's book is called *The Diary of Anne Frank* or *The Diary of a Young Girl,* depending on the edition. There are many editions available. Check at your bookstore or library.

involved in political activism. The people there are friendly, informative, and easy to reach and have hundreds of ideas and contacts for political actions. If you call and report on your own activities, they may list you in their upcoming publications.

American Red Cross. 430 17th St., NW, Washington, DC 20006. 1-703-206-6000. www.crossnet.org/youth. (To reach them: call your local chapter. Their phone number is in your phone book.) By working with the Red Cross, you can educate others about HIV/AIDS, teach children how to swim, learn first aid and CPR, or work in the heart of the action as part of a disaster services team. There are so many different volunteer opportunities with the Red Cross that you may want to try out several of them. The national center estimates that around 100,000 teens are currently involved in local chapters around the country. It has been estimated that between 15 and 20 percent of the volunteers are under eighteen.

AmeriCorps. Corporation for National Service. 1100 Vermont Ave., NW, Washington, DC 20520. 1-800-942-2677. www.cns.gov. AmeriCorps is a national service program for Americans of all ages and experiences. AmeriCorps members earn educational benefits in exchange for one or two years of service. Opportunities are available to perform a wide range of services in the areas of education, human needs, public safety, and the environment. Once they have completed their term of service, members receive educational awards to help them pay back student loans, or finance college or vocational training.

Amigos de las Americas (AMIGOS). 5618 Star Lane, Houston, TX 77057. 1-713-782-5290, Fax: 1-713-782-9267. www.amigoslink.org. AMIGOS is an international, private, voluntary organization dedicated to youth leadership development, cross-cultural understanding, and providing public health services in Latin America. Teen volunteers go to Latin America on service projects that range from four to six weeks and work as health care workers alongside local people. Some of the services offered by teen volunteers have included community sanitation, dental hygiene, immunizations, and eyeglass distribution.

Amnesty International. Urgent Action Network. P.O. Box 1270, Nederland, CO 80466-1270. 1-303-440-0913. www.amnesty.org. Amnesty International is a Nobel Peace Prize–winning, worldwide human rights organization whose most important mission is to bring about the release of prisoners of conscience—individuals who have been imprisoned for their beliefs, color, sex, ethnic origin, language, or religion, provided they have not used or advocated violence. Urgent Action is a network of volunteers who agree to be "on call" to write letters in cases of emergency. Amnesty has a Student Action Network that you can contact at www.oneworld.org/amnesty/stan.html.

ASPIRA Association, Inc. National Office. 1112 16th St. NW, Suite 340, Washington, DC 20036. 1-202-835-3600. The mission of the ASPIRA Association is to increase the well-being of the Hispanic community in the United States by working with Puerto Rican and Latino youth. There are already clubs for Aspirantes ("those who aspire to something greater") at over 100 high schools, with more than 17,000 teens involved. The clubs work on drop-out prevention, leadership development, community service, and career exploration.

Bikes Not Bombs. 59 Amory St., #103A, Roxbury, MA 02119. 1-617-442-0004. Bikes Not Bombs promotes bicycles as a powerful tool for community empowerment and environmentally sustainable economic development. They send tools, trainers, and recycled bicycles to Nicaragua and Haiti and have established a bicycle recycling and youth-training center in inner-city Boston. They also organize bike-a-thons and bike advocacy events and publish a newsletter called *Spoke & Word.*

Center for Third World Organizing. Minority Activist Apprenticeship Program. 1218 E. 23rd St., Oakland, CA 94609. 1-510-533-7583. www.ctwo.org. This is an internship program for students of color who want to become community organizers. The program lasts eight weeks, six of them spent in the field. CTWO has been on the cutting edge of social change, recognized nationally for its innovative training and leadership-development programs for communities of color. They have the motto "We will either find a way or we will make one."

Free At Last. 1946 University Ave., East Palo Alto, CA 94303. 1-415-462-6999. e-mail: freelast@aol.com. Established to provide community recovery and rehabilitation services, Free At Last offers a drop-in center, a community meeting space, an outpatient program, an adolescent/young adult support program, residential shelters, and street outreach programs. They are a new model of recovery: in the community, by the community, and for the community.

Greenpeace. 1436 U St. NW, Washington, DC 20009. 1-800-326-0959 for general information about Greenpeace. http://www.greenpeace.org. The philosophy of Greenpeace is that governments and corporations will not take the necessary steps to plan for the future of the planet without pressure from the public. Volunteers are invited to contact them for information about joining Greenpeace environmental actions.

Guiding Eyes for the Blind, Inc. Office of Volunteer Services, 611 Granite Springs Rd., Yorktown Heights, NY 10598. 1-800-942-0149 / 1-914-243-2215. www.guiding eyes.org. Guiding Eyes for the Blind needs at least 400 puppy raisers a year, an individual or family willing to spend about two hours each day for about fourteen months taking their puppy for walks and teaching it good manners so that it will be ready to be trained to be a guide dog. GEB has training centers in seven states on the East Coast. There are other guide dog training programs throughout the country: for example, Dogs for the Deaf (10175 Wheeler Road, Central Point, OR 97502; phone: 1-541-826-9220) and K-9 Companions for Independents (P.O. Box 446, Santa Rosa, CA 95402-0446; phone: 1-800-572-2275).

Habitat for Humanity. Volunteer Support Services. 121 Habitat St., Americus, GA 31709-3498. 1-800-422-4828, ext. 214. www.habitat.org/CCYP. Habitat is a grassroots Christian ministry whose goal is to eliminate poverty housing from the world by building decent shelter for all people. They bring together volunteers of all ages and backgrounds to do the actual building and to organize communities around housing issues.

The Lela Breitbart Memorial Fund. 484 First St., Brooklyn, NY 11215. This small, nonprofit organization supports projects and individuals in the field of women's health and reproductive rights. It is named for Lela Breitbart, a patient counselor at Planned Parenthood and the Eastern Women's Center in New York City, who died at the age of twenty-four in a tragic accident. The fund honors her commitment to women's rights and women's health issues.

National Association for the Advancement of Colored People (NAACP). NAACP Youth and College Division, "Back-to-School/Stay-in-School" Program. 4805 Mt. Hope Dr., Baltimore, MD 21215-3297. 1-410-358-8900. www.naacp.org/pro-grams/school. The NAACP is acting to combat rising school dropout rates and truancy among black and other minority youth. Teen volunteers are recruited to serve as tutors and role models for younger kids. Local branches of the NAACP exist in most urban areas.

National Indian Youth Leadership Council. 325 Marguerite St., P.O. Box 2140, Gallup, NM 87305. 1-505-722-9176. This private, nonprofit foundation is dedicated to developing the leadership potential of young Native Americans. It has a strong focus on community building and service projects.

National Student Campaign Against Hunger and Homelessness. 11965 Venice Blvd., #408, Los Angeles, CA 90066-3954. 1-800-NOHUNGR, ext. 324. e-mail: nscah@aol.com. This is a student volunteer organization working to end hunger and homelessness. There are chapters in many cities throughout the United States.

National Youth Leadership Council. 1910 West County Rd. B, Rosesville, MN 55113. 1-612-631-3672. The NYLC is funded to help young people become better leaders in their communities. They provide resources (information and sometimes funding) for youth workers, teachers, educators, and youth organizations to develop service-oriented youth leadership programs. The council runs conferences, publishes a newsletter and brochures with start-up ideas, and serves as a network link for projects around the country.

Partners of the Americas (POTA). 1424 K St. NW, Suite 700, Washington, DC 20005. 1-202-628-3300. www.partners.net. POTA uses volunteers, including high school students, who are interested in furthering friendship throughout the Americas. They set up arts events and sponsor cultural action programs and community-based nonpolitical activities throughout Latin America, the Caribbean, and the United States.

PETA (People for the Ethical Treatment of Animals). P.O. Box 42516, Washington, DC 20015-0516. 1-757-622-7382. www.envirolink.org/arrs/peta. PETA is the largest animal rights organization in the world. Using many different approaches, PETA volunteers have successfully forced the cessation of cruel treatment of animals in laboratories, on factory farms, in the fur trade, and in the entertainment industry. They will send you a starter kit with information on how to create an animal rights activist group in your own community, and they have great brochures, books, leaflets and videos—all for free.

Special Olympics, International, Inc. 1350 New York Ave. NW, Suite 500, Washington, DC 20005. 1-202-628-3630. www.specialolympics.org. Special Olympics is an international movement that provides sports training and competition in a variety of Olympic-type sports for all individuals with mental retardation. There are opportunities for teen volunteers at all levels of the organization from local to international.

Student Conservation Association. P.O. Box 550, Charlestown, NH 03603. 1-603-543-1700. The conservation youth crew program places teen volunteers in wilderness management crews. Typically, the work involves trail maintenance and building and stream cleanup. Volunteers receive free room and board and spend the last few days on a wilderness outdoor adventure.

Students Against Drunk Driving (SADD). P.O. Box 800, Marlboro, MA 01752. 1-508-481-3568, Fax: 1-508-481-5759. SADD has programs for middle schools and high schools. Its goals are to prevent underage drinking and drunk driving, save lives, and eliminate the illegal use of drugs. SADD organizes peer counseling programs and community awareness projects. They have a manual for how to start a chapter at your school.

TreePeople. 12601 Mulholland Dr., Beverly Hills, CA 90210. 1-818-753-4600. TreePeople believes that trees should be planted in both urban and mountain settings to conserve and improve the environment. The founder of TreePeople started this work when he was still in high school. The organization publishes *The Simple Act of Planting a Tree,* a manual for people who want to organize tree planting in their own communities.

Vegetarian Youth Network. P.O. Box 1141, New Paltz, NY 12561. www.geocities.com/Rodeo Drive. e-mail: VYNet@mhv.net. An Internet youth network to teach and learn about vegetarianism and animal rights, share recipes, and meet pen pals.

Volunteers in Parks (VIP). U.S. Department of the Interior, National Parks Service Volunteers in Parks. 1849 C St. NW, Washington, DC 20240. 1-202-208-3100. Over 22,000 volunteers work in our country's national parks and historic sites. There are many kinds of jobs, from trail builders to guides to office staff and general maintenance. Volunteers under eighteen may become VIPs in the community where they live, so contact your local parks first.

Youth Advisory Council of the Native American Young Person's Wellness Program. P.O. Box 572, Lake Andes, SD 57356. 1-605-487-7072. This program promotes leadership, wellness, and the reduction of teen pregnancy and violence in the Native American community. It is located in South Dakota, but all Native American youth are invited to call or write or stop by and help out, or share their stories, or participate in traditional ceremonies.

YouthBuild USA. P.O. Box 440322, Somerville, MA 02144. 1-617-623-9900. At twenty sites around the country, YouthBuild trains young adults to build affordable housing in their communities and refurbish run-down properties. YouthBuild also sponsors Youth on Board, a program committed to ensuring that young people have their voices heard in all programs that concern them, by getting youth placed on boards of directors.

Youth Communication: Teens Writing for Teens. 144 W. 27th St., Suite 8R, New York, NY 10001. 1-212-242-3270 Fax: 1-212-242-7057. e-mail: Hefner@aol.com. This organization helps teens acquire the skills they need to become active in journalism and book/magazine publishing projects. Each year over 100 teens work on a maga-

zine called *New Youth Connections* as writers, artists, and photographers. Teens who write for another magazine, *Foster Care Youth United,* address foster-care issues and how to make the system more responsive to children's needs.

YMCA Earth Service Corps, at Metrocenter YMCA. 909 4th Ave., Seattle, WA. 1-206-382-5013, Fax: 1-206-382-7894. The YMCA Earth Service Corps empowers young people to be effective, responsible global citizens by providing opportunities for environmental education, action, and leadership development and by sponsoring international cross-cultural exchange programs. There is a network of clubs based in high schools and community centers, so check with your local YMCA first.

Children's Service Clubs

They're fun, they're learning experiences, they challenge the mind and the body and build character, they inspire community service and bring kids into the country and the wilderness. Many teens get their first service experience as club members, and they often continue as volunteer leaders with younger kids in the organizations. Another great thing about these clubs is that they make a huge effort to cut across race, religious, and economic barriers. You know their names, and you can always start as a volunteer by contacting your local chapters: Boy Scouts of America, Boys Clubs of America, Camp Fire Girls and Boys, Girl Scouts of America, Girls Inc., National 4-H Council, YMCA, and YWCA.

Publications

Children's Express. 1440 New York Ave. NW, Suite 510, Washington, DC 20005. 1-202-737-7377. www.ce.org. The mission of Children's Express is to give children and teens a significant voice in the world. CE is a news service produced by kids reporting on the issues that affect their lives. They have a great interactive website, and many of their publications have won national awards.

How to Make the World a Better Place, by Jeffrey Hollender, New York: William Morrow and Company, 1990. This book is subtitled: A Guide to

Doing Good—How You Can Effect Positive Social Change. It includes information about social problems and concerns and ways to get in touch with existing organizations. It also gives ideas for starting actions of your own.

The Kids Guide to Social Action, by Barbara Lewis. Free Spirit Publishing, Inc., 400 1st Ave. N., Suite 616, Minneapolis, MN 55401. Step-by-step advice on how to select a social problem, find a creative solution, and put it into action. Includes examples of young people who have made a difference.

New Youth Connections and **Foster Care Youth United Youth Communication.** 144 West 27th St., Suite 8R, New York, NY 10001. 1-212-242-3270, Fax: 1-212-242-7057. These two magazines are written by teens for teens about issues that are important to teens. Teenagers from the New York City area can submit articles to New Youth Connections. Teenagers from all over the country who are in or have been in the foster care system can submit articles to the bimonthly magazine *Foster Care Youth United.* Write or call them for more information. You can order their magazines and books by writing to the above address.

No Kidding Around!, by Wendy Schaetzel Lesko. Information USA, P.O. Box E, Kensington, MA 20895. The subtitle says it all: "America's Young Activists Are Changing the World and You Can Too." This inspiring book contains true stories of young citizen activists all over the country, and gives step-by-step pointers for every aspect of organizing. It is supplemented by an extensive resource guide.

Service Learning from A to Z, by Cynthia Parsons. SerVermont, P.O. Box 516, Chester, VT 05143. This is a stimulating book of ideas about service and citizenship written for children and adolescents, with practical recommendations for projects.

WorldLink. 3629 Sacramento St., San Francisco, CA 94118. 1-415-931-6952, Fax: 1-415-931-6038. WorldLink publishes and distributes *State of the World Forum Youth Agenda for the 21st Century,* a concise, moving, and well-written action plan for changing the world authored by young people from twenty-eight nations around the world. They also produce and distribute documentary videos about young people all over the planet.

YO! (Youth Outlook). Pacific News Service, 450 Mission St., Room 204, San Francisco, CA 94105. 1-415-243-4364. www.pacificnews.org. e-mail: yo@pacificnews.org. By and for teens, it is "dedicated to asking the unsafe questions, and raising unheard voices." $12 per year (6 issues). Also, Youth Outlook is well established on-line, with a great home page, past issues, and a constantly updated "Best of YO!" section.

Youth in Action Network. www.mightymedia.com. The network is an interactive on-line service for youth, educators, organization members, and school classes who want to learn about, and participate in, positive social action and service projects.

Index

(continued)